GYNECOLOGY

INTEGRATING CONVENTIONAL, COMPLEMENTARY, AND NATURAL ALTERNATIVE THERAPY

GYNECOLOGY

INTEGRATING CONVENTIONAL, COMPLEMENTARY, AND NATURAL ALTERNATIVE THERAPY

ADAM OSTRZENSKI, M.D., Ph.D.

Professor of Clinical Gynecology and Obstetrics
University of South Florida
Tampa, Florida
Visiting Professor
La Sapienza University
Rome, Italy
FIGO Expert Advisory Panel
on Surgical Techniques and Minimal Access Surgery
Former Professor and Director of Operative Gynecology
Howard University
Washington, D.C.

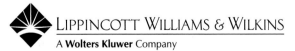

LIPPINCOTT WILLIAMS & WILKINS
A **Wolters Kluwer** Company
Philadelphia · Baltimore · New York · London
Buenos Aires · Hong Kong · Sydney · Tokyo

Acquisitions Editor: Lisa McAllister
Developmental Editor: Denise Martin
Production Editor: Thomas Foley
Manufacturing Manager: Colin J. Warnock
Cover Designer: Joan Greenfield
Compositor: Lippincott Williams & Wilkins Desktop Division
Printer: Courier Westford

Library of Congress Cataloging-in-Publication Data

Ostrzenski, Adam.
    Gynecology : integrating conventional, complemtary, and natural alternative therapy / Adam Ostrzenski.
      p. ; cm.
    Includes bibliographical references and index.
    ISBN 0-7817-2761-8
      1. Gynecology. 2. Generative organs, Female—Diseases—Alternative Medicine.
  3. Naturopathy. I. Title.
    [DNLM: 1. Genital Diseases, Female—therapy. 2. Alternative Medicine. 3. Naturopathy. WP 650 085g 2001]
RG121 .085 2001
618.1'06—dc21

                                             2001038036

10 9 8 7 6 5 4 3 2 1

To my mother for giving me life, love, and the guidance to become who I am today.

To my wife and best friend, Maria Molenda, Esq., for her unconditional love, her endless inspiration, and for all of the advice, support, help, patience, and understanding she has given me.

To my children Katarzyna M. Ostrzenska-Begahri, M.D.; Bartosz A. Ostrzenski, a law student; and my son-in-law, Farshad Baghari, for their continuous love and dedication.

To my granddaughter, Dahlia Beghari, for her constant love invigorates my life and revitalizes my sense of joy.

To my sisters Danuta and Judy, and their families, for all of their love and patience.

To my teachers, faculty friends, residents, students, and all those physicians who participate in my lectures around the globe, I have nothing but the deepest professional admiration for your brilliant minds and for the friendships we have shared.

CONTENTS

PREFACE

This book is designed as a gynecology reference textbook, integrating conventional, complementary, and alternative gynecology for students of allopathic and osteopathic medicine; residents in obstetrics, gynecology, and family medicine; and specialists in the field. By providing both basic and advanced gynecologic information, this book can serve a variety of healthcare providers for women. The range of conventional gynecologic information applicable to these different groups is delineated at the beginning of each chapter. The chapter structure is based on educational objectives recommended by the Association of Professors of Gynecology and Obstetrics (APGO) for medical students. The scope of fundamental knowledge of gynecology and obstetrics presented is in accordance with the requirements of the Council on Resident Educational in Obstetrics and Gynecology (CREOG) for residents. The information for practitioners in the field of gynecology is organized as recommended by the American College of Obstetricians and Gynecologists (ACOG) Educational Bulletins. The format of the textbook is, for the most part, customary, but subjects that have not appeared in other texts, particularly complementary and alternative gynecological therapies, have been included.

The newest approved modes of diagnosis and therapy in conventional, complementary, and alternative gynecology are incorporated and supported by specific references. Current information, from basic science to advanced clinical studies, is supported by evidence-based references. This provides an opportunity for the practitioner to easily refresh and advance his or her knowledge in the field and assists the student in learning not only conventional therapy, but also the complementary and alternative therapies.

This book is unique in integrating complementary and alternative medical therapy options into conventional clinical gynecological practice. The increased use of alternative medicine over the past decade is well documented and women tend to exploit alternative therapies more often than men do. This wide acceptance of alternative remedies creates a potential health risk, since approximately half of the alternative therapies are carried out by patients who have not consulted a professional health care provider.

Therefore, it is imperative for the allopathic practitioner to become familiar with the complementary and alternative gynecological therapies, as well as potential drug interactions, in order to share responsibility with a woman for her own health. On the other hand, the non-allopathic practitioner will also benefit from acquiring basic information in the area of conventional gynecology.

The physician, having respect for patient autonomy and personal values, should make complementary and alternative therapies accessible and an integral part of conventional health care. This is consistent with the patient's desire to select from a full range of therapy options. Since the clinical research in this field is still scant, this textbook introduces both the scientifically proven and the proposed indications for complementary and alternative therapies. These therapies have shown much promise. However, the lack of standards, as well as the inconsistencies in the fields' clinical medical training, will need to be addressed before practitioners can easily integrate complementary and alternative therapies into mainstream Western medicine.

One chapter, for instance, is devoted to the serious and actual potential for drug interaction between natural remedies and conventional prescription drugs. The chapter is designed in the form of a table for easy reference. The table includes: the name of the specific therapeutic remedy, its indication and dose, type of evidence for use, contraindication, potential or actual side effect, and drug interaction.

In order to avoid confusion, it is worthwhile here to provide the prospective user of this textbook with definitions of conventional, complementary, and alternative gynecology. *Conventional* medicine encompasses the practice of modern, scientific Western allopathic and osteopathic medicine. *Alternative* medicine encompasses traditional practice based on non-Western oriented biomedical methods and therapies. The role of *complementary* medicine is to enhance either conventional and/or alternative therapies. Integrative medicine combines conventional Western-oriented medicine with complementary and alternative medicine for optimal patient care.

Prof. Adam Ostrzenski, M.D., Ph.D.

ACKNOWLEDGMENTS

I am indebted to Lisa McAllister, Executive Editor, and Denise Martin, Developmental Editor, for their perceptive editorial advice, encouragement, and guidance, and to the staff of Lippincott Williams & Wilkins for the final preparation of this book. In addition, I am grateful to Jennifer Smith for her excellent illustrations; to Pamela Sherwill-Navarro, medical librarian at the University of Florida (Gainesville, FL), for helping me gather published scientific clinical material; to Farshad Bagheri, computer specialist, for his tireless efforts in keeping my computer system in order; to Bartholomew Radolinski, Georgetown University medical student, for assisting me with the preparation of this manuscript; to Patrick O. Fasusi, M.D., Chief of Anesthesiology and Medical Director of Premier Ambulatory Surgery of Washington, D.C., for his practical suggestions regarding pain management; and finally to Adam Radolinski, M.D., colorectal specialist, for his practical evocation in the field of colorectal disease.

MENSTRUAL CYCLE PHYSIOLOGY

EDUCATIONAL OBJECTIVES

Medical Students (1)	*Residents in Obstetrics/Gynecology (2)*	*Practitioners (3)*
APGO Objective No. 49	*CREOG Objective*	*ACOG Recommendation*
Physiology of menstrual cycle	No specific recommendation	No specific recommendation
Endocrinology of menstrual cycle		

DEFINITION

A menstrual cycle is a rhythmic, predictable, coordinated, and complex preparatory event of a woman's body for pregnancy, with particular changes occurring within the reproductive system (hypothalamic–pituitary–ovarian axis).

PHYSIOLOGIC MECHANISMS

The complexity and detail of menstrual cycle events are beyond the scope of this book; however, the presentation in general, and a schematic view will assist in clinical applications. For learning purposes, the menstrual cycle can be divided into four functional phases: the follicular phase, ovulation, the luteal phase, and menses. Occurring during the menstrual cycle in a sequential and harmonized, cyclic manner, neurohormones, ovarian hormones, intracellular autocrine communication (intracellular secreted regulating substances acting centrally or locally on receptors, or within the same cell), intracellular paracrine communication (intracellular regulating substances communicating from cell to cell by diffusion), intracellular intracrine communication (binding unsecreted regulating substances to intracellular receptors), and endometrial morphologic changes must all be carefully synchronized.

Role of the Hypothalamus

The preoptic and arcuate nuclei (a group of neurons), the pulsatile generators of reproduction located within the hypothalamus, produce and secrete gonadotropin-releasing hormone (GnRH), which travels through the hypothalamic–hypophyseal portal vascular system (the hypo-thalamic–pituitary portal capillary plexus) in the pituitary stalk to the pituitary gland, where it binds to specific receptor sites on target cell membranes (the gonadotropes) (2,3). Therefore, the adenohypophysis (the anterior pituitary gland) has no direct neuronal link with the hypothalamus. The hypothalamic neurohormone GnRH triggers a mechanism within the anterior pituitary, which leads to receptors triggering, evoking the release of follicular stimulating hormone (FSH) and luteinizing hormone (LH).

It has been demonstrated that, in the absence of a cluster of these neurons, gonadotropin-releasing hormone secretion from the hypothalamus ceases, and the pituitary gland can secrete neither FSH nor LH (Fig 1.1). Furthermore, it is a well documented fact that GnRH has dual functions in reference to pituitary gonadotropin hormones: to control and to regulate secretion of both FSH and LH from the anterior pituitary gland (4). Ovarian steroidogenesis comes to an end and the endometrial morphological cyclic conversion from the proliferative to the secretory phase stops, and endometrial atrophy appears when hypophyseal gonadotropin secretion is lost (5).

Gonadotropin-releasing hormone is a decapeptide, elicited in a pulsatile pattern, with 60- to 90-minute intervals during the follicular phase and 4-hour intervals during the mid-luteal phase, and a half-life of 2-4 minutes.

Neurotransmitters affect GnRH secretion as follows:

- Norepinephrine 1 stimulates GnRH secretion from the hypothalamus (6)
- Serotonin inhibits GnRH secretion from the hypothalamus (6)
- Dopamine inhibits GnRH secretion from the hypothalamus (6)

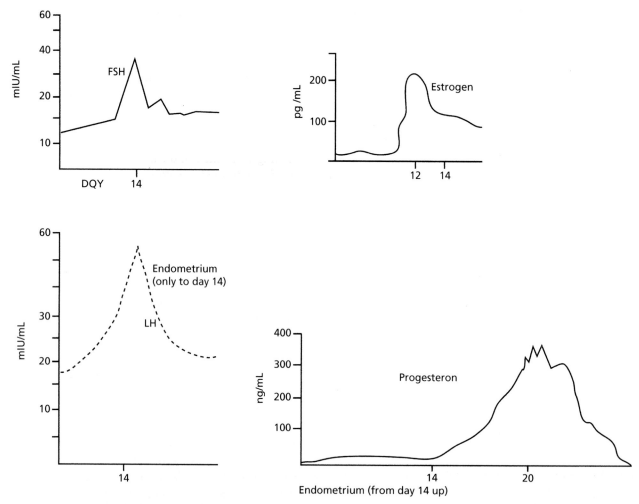

FIGURE 1.1. Gonadotropins, follicle-stimulating hormone, and luteinizing hormone. (Redrawn from Couchman GM, Hammond CB. In: *Physiology of reproduction. Danforth's obstetrics and gynecology*, 8th ed. Philadelphia: Lippincott Williams & Wilkins, 1999.)

Endogenous opiates and prostaglandins have been included as substances that may influence GnRH secretion (7). Endogenous opioids, such as β-endorphin, inhibit GnRH secretion from the hypothalamus (8,9). In addition, GnRH release is modulated by estrogens, androgens, and progesterone.

Role of the Anterior Pituitary

The anterior pituitary (anterior hypophysis or adenohypophysis) secretes a number of hormones such as corticotropin (ACTH), follicle-stimulating hormone (FSH), growth hormone (GH), LH, prolactin (PRL), and thyroid-stimulating hormone (TSH). Each has a specific role. The abnormal secretion of just one of these hormones may influence the function of all of them.

In the menstrual cycle, a prime role of the adenohypophysis is to allocate gonadotropins: LH and FSH. Hypothalamic GnRH controls and regulates the synthesis, stor-

age, and secretion of these hormones. Because GnRH is secreted in a pulsatile manner, FSH and LH respond accordingly, with a pulsatile mechanism. In addition to GnRH being in command, the FSH and LH secretory mechanism is adjusted by the feedback mechanism of ovarian hormones and regulatory peptides. This interrelationship between ovarian steroid hormones, regulatory peptides, and gonadotropins produces a homeostasis of FSH and LH in the range of 10 mIU/mL to 20 mIU/mL during the menstrual cycle, exception during the periovulatory/ovulatory phase. Lack of an adequate level of estradiol causes gonadotropin elevation above 40 mIU/mL, due either to a natural event, such as menopause, or due to prematurely diminished levels of estradiol secondary to ovarian disease (hypergonadotropic hypogonadism) or surgical castration (bilateral oophorectomy).

Follicle-stimulating hormone and LH are glycoprotein hormones with two chain structures: alpha and beta subunits. Both of them have identical alpha subunits, but different, specific beta subunits, which are responsible for precise biologic responses (10). Structurally, TSH and placental human chorionic gonadotropin (hCG) have identical alpha subunits, compared with gonadotropins, but different beta chains.

Role of the Ovary

In response to gonadotropin stimulation, the ovary initiates a dynamic process of steroidogenesis and undergoes morphologic transformation. The following divisions of the menstrual cycle are proposed for the purpose of interpretation of structural and functional changes within the ovary:

1. The follicular phase (from recruiting primordial follicles through preantral, antral, and preovulatory follicles)
2. Ovulation (releasing the ovum from the ovary)
3. Luteal phase (conversion of the dominant follicle to the corpus luteum)
4. Menses phase (comparatively, a functionally quiescent period, while the endometrium is sloughed)

Follicular Stage

In the follicular preantral stage, the primary oocyte becomes functionally active. The primary oocyte is transitionally suspended in the prophase stage of meiosis and is housed in the follicle. Between weeks 6 and 8 of fetal gestation, the mitotic division of germs cells is initiated, and 3.5 million oocytes are formed in one ovary (6–7 million in both ovaries combined) at the fetal age of 16 to 20 weeks, and decline to 2 million by the time of birth. Levels decrease to about 300,000 at puberty, and only 500 follicles from both ovaries will reach full maturity and produce an ovum (11–13).

In the early follicular phase, due to a reduction of ovarian steroidogenesis and to inhibin synthesis (inhibin is produced by the granulosa cells of the corpus luteum), FSH secretion is reactivated (14). While the menstrual cycle progresses, FSH pulsatile secretion intensifies and influences ovarian function. The growth of follicles in the preliminary stage does not require hormonal stimulation; however, FSH is essential to advance the follicles to the preantral stage, during which the increased, pulsatile pattern of FSH influences conversion of androgen to estrogen in the granulosa cells. Increased levels of estradiol and FSH increase the number of FSH receptors within follicles, and advance the follicle to the antral stage (13).

Antral Follicular Stage

In the antral follicular stage, the following events take place:

1. Two-cell and two-gonadotropin systems are created, in which thecal cells contain LH receptors with the ability to produce androstenedione and testosterone, and gran-

ulosa cells have FSH receptors with the capacity to convert androgens to estrogens (15,16).
2. Selection of the dominant follicle is usually completed by the 7th day of the menstrual cycle (selection ranged from day 5 to day 7). Upon selection of the dominant follicle, estradiol secretion steadily increases, causing progressive suppression of FSH secretion (13).
3. Increasing estradiol levels augment the bioactivity and quantity of LH at mid-cycle; in return, LH enhances androgen synthesis in the theca cells. At the same time, FSH activates LH receptors on the granulosa (13).
4. Modulating follicles respond to gonadotropins via ovarian regulatory proteins. Taking into account several aspects of the menstrual cycle—such as the meiotic arrest of oocytes and the resurrection of this process, angiogenesis and then cyclic vascular regression, and the generous blood distribution to the dominant follicle—it is clear that gonadotropins themselves cannot initiate these mechanisms. Therefore, additional mechanisms must contribute to complete this course of action. Several ovarian regulatory proteins play a role in this complex mechanism.

The following ovarian regulatory proteins are necessary to complete these processes:

- Inhibins (inhibin-A, inhibin-B) act via a negative feedback mechanism to regulate FSH secretion from the pituitary. FSH influences the manufacture of inhibins in the granulosa cells. Increasing levels of inhibin change control of the cycle from FSH to LH, together with estradiol, before the mid-cycle LH peak. Inhibin decreases in the late luteal phase, allowing FSH to resume its activity (13).
- Follistatin exhibits suppression activity on FSH (13).
- Activins (activin-A, -AB, -B) stimulate FSH secretion and enhance FSH influence on the follicles (13).
- Somatomedins (insulin-like growth factors, IGFs) express a functional and structural resemblance to insulin, and they participate in growth hormone activity. Circumstantial data suggest an effect on granulosa cell activity (13).
- The role of IGF binding proteins (IGFBPs) is to carry IGF in serum, to extend its half-life, and to adjust the effects of IGF on tissue. Six peptides have been identified that express the ability to bind IGF (17). The results from animal studies support the hypothesis that IGFBP-3 may act as an FSH antagonist; in this way, they compromise FSH simulation activity on the granulosa and theca cells (18).
- Müllerian-inhibiting substance (anti-müllerian hormone) is produced in the granulosa cells and may inhibit oocyte meiosis and follicular development (19).
- Fibroblast growth factor is a mitogen, and it exhibits the ability to stimulate angiogenesis and plasminogen activation. It also inhibits estrogen synthesis and FSH/LH receptor expression (13).

- Epidermal growth factor is a mitogen that promotes gonadotropin stimulation and suppresses the upregulation of FSH on its own receptors (13).
- Transforming growth factor opposes the epidermal growth factor; therefore, it increases LH receptors formed by FSH, and at the same time inhibits androgen synthesis in the ovary (13,20).
- Platelet-derived growth factor, together with growth factor and epidermal growth factor, participate in follicle prostaglandin synthesis (13).

The Preovulatory Follicle

The preovulatory follicle can be characterized by continuing oocyte meiosis, by an increase in size, by the production/accumulation of follicular fluid, and by the vascularization of the theca cells.

Approaching the finishing point of the oocyte's transformation, chromosomal reduction via the meiotic process is intensified (the meiosis is not completed until after spermatozoa penetration and the second polar body is released). When the dominant follicle achieves maturity, it is manifested by a peak of estrogens, about 24 to 36 hours before the LH surge, and sustained for at least 48 hours in the peripheral circulation (with an estradiol range of 300 pg/mL). This event triggers hypothalamic GnRH secretion, and the pituitary gland responds with an LH surge in a pulsatile pattern. LH is secreted with increasing intervals and amplitude. The LH surge usually occurs between days 11 and 13 of the menstrual ovulatory cycle. Simultaneously, under LH influence, luteinization of the granulosa cells takes place with progesterone production in the ovary (before granulosa luteinization, the adrenal gland produces progesterone; preceding the corpus luteum, developing follicles are not important contributors to progesterone levels in the follicular phase). However, the adrenal gland's secretion of progesterone is much smaller in quantity than that of the luteinized granulosa and theca cells (21). Estrogen priming is necessary for the impingement of preovulatory progesterone on pituitary positive feedback, and, eventually, for induction of the LH surge. One of the roles of progesterone is to make the follicle unresponsive to FSH stimulation.

In the preovulatory follicles, the FSH to LH ratio changes from greater than 1 to less than 1; at the same time, the pituitary gland exhibits positive and negative feedback responses to estradiol. With the changing FSH:LH ratio, the estradiol:androgen ratio within the follicular fluid is changing as well. When the estradiol:androgen ratio is greater than 1, the follicle becomes dominant, but if this ratio is less than 1, the follicle becomes atretic.

Ovulation

Ovulation occurs about 8 to 40 hours after the LH peak or 24 to 56 hours after the first significant increase in LH,

which is a measurable and reliable method of predicting ovulation (22). The LH surge commences 34 to 36 hours before ovulation (23).

The LH surge promotes the following follicular events:

- Resumption of the oocyte meiotic process.
- Intensification of intrafollicular plasmin (proteolitic enzyme) activity, which, in synergy with prostaglandins, dissolves the follicular membrane during the mid-cycle increase of FSH, allowing for the expulsion of the ovum. At the time of ovulation in the preovulatory follicle, the prostaglandin component within the follicular fluid is responsible for the *mittelschmerz* type of twinge pain reported by some women.
- Enhancement of angiogenesis within the follicle eventually prepares for corpus luteum formation.
- Triggering of ovulation.
- Increase of progesterone synthesis and secretion by the luteinization of the granulosa and theca cells.
- Regulation of receptor-binding low-density lipoprotein (LDL) transport of cholesterol to the cellular mitochondria (necessary for progesterone synthesis).

Luteal Phase of the Menstrual Cycle

The luteal phase of the menstrual cycle lasts 11 to 17 days (24). The hormonal milieu changes from estradiol being the dominant hormone in the preovulatory period to progesterone assuming the role as the dominant hormone. FSH sets up the most favorable preovulatory environment for follicle growth and menstruation, and it primes the granulosa and theca cells for the development of LH receptors, which facilitate progesterone synthesis. Peripherally, progesterone levels increase about 24 hours prior to ovulation, reaching their peak 3 to 4 days after ovulation, then sustaining that level for approximately 11 consecutive days. This process requires continued, tonic LH secretion. After the rupture of the follicle, the ovum is released, the follicle collapses, vascularization increases (vessels migrate into the granulosa cells, reaching maximum penetration by the 8th to 9th postovulatory days; this process is essential for the transport of cholesterol into luteal cells, which is necessary for progesterone synthesis. The granulosa cell layer is avascular before this event. The theca cells, derived from the theca and stroma, grow. The granulosa cells are luteinized (a process of the accumulation of lutein, a yellow pigment). The follicle undergoes its characteristic morphologic changes. Through this process, the follicle became the corpus luteum.

The corpus luteum is composed of not only small and large luteal cells, but also endothelial cells, fibroblasts, macrophages, and pericytes (25). It reaches maximum diameter of up to 2.5 cm, and its life span has been determined to be 13 to 14 days, unless conception occurs. When pregnancy occurs, hCG secretion from the product of conception stimulates the corpus luteum to synthesize progesterone. Gradually and progressively, the placenta takes over progesterone production at about 7 to 8 weeks of gestation.

Progesterone synthesis is directly related to the adequate, initial, and pulsatile FSH stimulation, and the LH surge and postsurge secretion.

The role of progesterone is to (a) suppress new follicular growth both centrally and locally, (b) convert the proliferative endometrium into the secretory endometrium, (c) create changes in the cervix and vagina, (d) facilitate endometrial implantation of the fertilized ovum, (e) support pregnancy during the early part of the first trimester, and (f) suppress pituitary secretions of FSH and LH through a negative feedback mechanism.

Coinciding with maximum vascular penetration into the granulosa cells, progesterone levels are at their peak by postovulatory days 8 and 9. On postovulatory days 9 to 11 the function of the corpus luteum becomes substantially less efficient. The secretion of progesterone demonstrates pulsatile characteristics in harmony with pulsatile LH secretions (26). There is no definitive answer as to why the corpus luteum regresses, and with it, progesterone synthesis and secretion. The most common theory offered to explain this process involves luteolysis promoted by estrogens and prostaglandins.

Role of Menses (Bleeding Phase of the Menstrual Cycle)

Menses is a cyclic endometrial shedding, manifested by vaginal bleeding. Women generally not only consider such regular, predictable events as a healthy occurrence, but menses also emotionally emphasizes their femininity.

Functionally, this phase of menstrual cycle is the most quiescent ovarian period; however, the continuation of the recruitment of follicles is taking place (the recruitment process is initiated during the late luteal phase, and it extends into the first few days of menses) (27). At the beginning of menses, reduced steroidogenesis continues at this low level for the first 5 days of the cycle.

The first menses (menarche) is expected, on average, at the age of 12.8 years (28) (between 11.5 and 13 years of age) in the United States, and if menarche does not occur by the age of 16, it calls for clinical investigation. The last menses is expected at the median age of 51.5 (between 48 and 55 years of age), and this is considered the beginning of menopause.

The gross appearance of menstrual effluent is dark, non-clotting blood. Occasionally, exfoliated endometrial tissue is noticeable, with a characteristic light fishy smell. Menses is expected at an interval ranging from 21 to 35 days (28 ± 7 days), with a duration of 2 to 8 days (averaging 3–5 days), and an anticipated blood loss of 30 to 50 mL (blood loss of ≥80 mL per cycle warrants clinical evaluation).

REFERENCES

1. Association of Professors of Gynecology and Obstetrics. *Medical student educational objectives,* 7th ed. Washington, DC: Association of Professors of Gynecology and Obstetrics, 1997.
2. MacCann SM, ed. The menstrual cycle. In: *Endocrinology, people and ideas.* Bethesda, MD: American Physiological Society, 1988.
3. Ryan KJ. The endocrine pattern and control of the ovulatory cycle. In: Insler V, Lunenfeld B, eds. *Infertility: male and female.* New York: Churchill Livingstone, 1986.
4. Schally AV, Arimura A, Baba Y, et al. Isolation and properties of the FSH and LH-releasing hormone. *Biochem Biophys Res Commun* 1971;43:393–399.
5. Knobil E. The neuroendocrine control of the menstrual cycle. *Rec Prog Horm Res* 1980;36:53–59.
6. Moore RY. Neuroendocrine mechanisms: cells and system. In: Yen SSC, Jaffe RB, eds. *Reproductive endocrinology.* Philadelphia: WB Saunders, 1986.
7. Brownstein MJ. Neurotransmission and endocrinology. In: Becker KL, ed. *Principles and practice of endocrinology and metabolism.* Philadelphia: JB Lippincott, 1990:52–56.
8. American College of Obstetricians and Gynecologists. *Precis V. An update in obstetrics and gynecology.* Washington, DC: American College of Obstetricians and Gynecologists, 1994:362.
9. Yen SSC. Neuroendocrine control of hypophyseal function. In: Yen SSC, Jaffe RB, eds. *Reproductive endocrinology.* Philadelphia: WB Saunders, 1986.
10. Catt KJ, Pierce JG. Gonadotropic hormones of the adenohypophysis. In: Yen SSC, Jaffe RB, eds. *Reproductive endocrinology.* Philadelphia: WB Saunders, 1986.
11. Baker TG. A quantitative and cytological study of germ cells in the human ovaries. *Proc R Soc Lond* 1963;158:417–423.
12. Peters H, Byskov AG, Himelstein-Graw R, et al. Follicular growth: the basic event in the mouse and human ovary. *J Reprod Fertil* 1975;45:559–563.
13. Speroff L, Galss RH, Kase NG. *Clinical gynecologic endocrinology and infertility,* 5th ed. Baltimore: Williams & Wilkins, 1994:183–230.
14. Roseff SJ, Bangah ML, Kettel LM, et al. Dynamic changes in circulating inhibin levels during the luteal-follicular transition of the human menstrual cycle. *J Clin Endocrinol Metab* 1989;69:1033–1037.
15. Dorrington JH, Armstrong DT. Effects of FSH on gonadal functions. *Rec Prog Horm Res* 1979;35:301–305.
16. Yamoto M. Shima K, Nakano R. Gonadotropins receptors in human ovarian follicles and corpora lutea throughout the menstrual cycle. *Horm Res* 1992;37(suppl 1):5–8.
17. Shimasaki S, Ling N. Identification and molecular characterization of insulin-like growth hormone factor binding proteins (IGFBP-1, -2, -3, -4, -5, and -6). *Prog Growth Factor Res* 1992;3:243–247.
18. Shimasaki S, Shimonaka M, Ui M, et al. Structural characterization of a follicle-stimulating hormone action inhibitor in porcine ovarian follicular fluid. *J Biol Chem* 1990;265:2198–2202.
19. Kim JH, Seible MM, MacLaughlin DT, et al. The inhibitory effects of müllerian-inhibiting substance on epidermal growth factor induced proliferation and progesterone production of human granulosa-luteal cells. *J Clin Endocrinol Metab* 1992;75:911–916.
20. Dodson WC, Schomberg DW. The effect of transforming growth factor-beta on follicle-stimulating hormone–induced differentiation of cultured rat granulosa cells. *Endocrinology* 1987;77:1411–1415.
21. Judd S, Terry A, Petrucco M, et al. The source of pulsatile secretion of progesterone during the human follicular phase. *J Clin Endocrinol Metab* 1992;74:299–305.

22. World Health Organization Task Force Investigators. Temporal relationship between ovulation and defined changes in the concentration of plasma estradiol-17 beta, luteinizing hormone, follicle stimulating hormone, and progesterone. *Am J Obstet Gynecol* 1980;138:383–390.
23. Hoff JD, Quigley ME, Yen SSC. Hormonal dynamics at midcycle: a reevaluation. *J Clin Endocrinol Metab* 1983;57: 792–796.
24. Lenton EA, Landgren B, Sexton L. Normal variation in the length of the luteal phase of the menstrual cycle: identification of the short luteal phase. *Br J Obstet Gynaecol* 1984;91:685–689.
25. Maas S, Jarry H, Teichmann A, et al. Paracrine actions of oxytocin, prostaglandin F2 alpha, and estradiol within the human corpus luteum. *J Clin Endocrinol Metab* 1992;74:306–312.
26. Fillicori M, Butler JP, Crowley WF. Neuroendocrine regulation of the corpus luteum in human: evidence for pulsatile progesterone secretion. *J Clin Invest* 1984;73:1638–1647.
27. Gougeon A. Dynamics of follicular growth in the human: a model from preliminary results. *Hum Reprod* 1986;1:81–85.
28. Zacharias L, Rand WM, Wurtman RJ. A prospective study of sexual development and growth in American girls: the statistics of menarche. *Obstet Gynecol Surv* 1976;31:325–337.

2

PUBERTY AND ITS DISORDERS

EDUCATIONAL OBJECTIVES

Medical Students (1)
APGO Objective No. 46

Physiology of puberty
Physical, emotional, and reproductive
  system maturation
Expected age and sequence of puberty
Abnormalities of puberty

Residents in Obstetrics/Gynecology (2)
CREOG Objective

Diagnosis and management of precocious
  puberty and delayed puberty

Practitioners (3)
ACOG Recommendation

Puberty
Precocious puberty
Delayed puberty

DEFINITION

Puberty involves a sequence of gradual physical, endocrine, reproductive, and emotional maturation changes leading to adulthood.

ENDOCRINOLOGY

The adrenal gland increases its synthesis and secretion of dehydroepiandrosterone between the ages of 6 and 8 years. However, no data are available to support the idea that the adrenal glands are essential in initiating puberty; on the contrary, it has been documented that puberty can be achieved in primary adrenal insufficiency. Evidence strongly suggests that genetic makeup plays a leading role in this event, as well as exposure to light, geographic location, general health, and emotional status (4). When puberty commences, this process usually lasts approximately 4 to 5 years (range 1.5–6 years) (5), culminating in sexual maturity.

Between 10 and 13 weeks of fetal age, the hypothalamus initiates the secretion of gonadotropin-releasing hormone (GnRH), which stimulates pituitary gonadotropins (short hormonal loop). At approximately 20 weeks of gestation, gonadotropins reach their peak (at that time, the hypothalamic–adenohypophysis system's development is considered to be complete), and shortly thereafter, gonadotropin levels decrease. At term and after delivery, gonadotropins increase until 1 to 2 years of age, and they remain in a quiescent, low-level stage until puberty (6). At

the beginning of puberty, a nocturnal luteinizing hormone (LH) pulsatile pattern is established, with daytime activity occurring shortly thereafter. Gonadotropins, upon reaching their expected pulsatile rhythm, stimulate ovarian steroidogenesis (7).

Timing and Pattern of Puberty

Clinically, puberty is divided into the following four stages: (i) thelarche, (ii) menarche, (iii) growth spurt, and (iv) menarche.

Thelarche

Thelarche is the first stage of secondary sex characteristic maturation: the expression and initiation of breast development, which usually manifests between the ages of 9 and 11 years (median age 9.8 years). The interval from the time of breast budding (enlargement of the breast and elevation of the areola and nipples) to the time of a fully-developed, adult-type contour breast is approximately 3 to 3.5 years. Tanner's clinical pubertal sequence classification (4) of breast and pubic hair development has been widely accepted as a means to chart progress and changes during puberty, and those changes are presented in Fig. 2.1.

Additionally, this stage is characterized by increasing vaginal acidity and an increase in the number of Doderlein bacilli (natural vaginal bacterial flora). These changes verify adequate function of the hypothalamic–pituitary–ovarian axis.

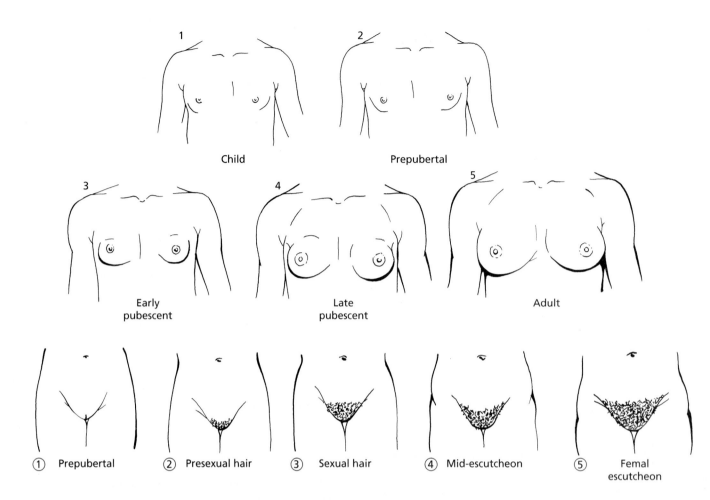

	Breast			Pubic Hair	
Stage	**Description**	**Illustration No.**		**Description**	**Illustration No.**
1	**Prepubertal:** elevation of papilla	1		**Prepubertal:** no pubic hair	1
2	**Breast bud:** elevation of breast and papilla, and areola gets larger; median age 9.8 years	2		**Presexual hair:** lightly distributed, predominantly on the labia majora; long, pigmented hair; median age 10.5 years	2
3	**Early pubescent:** additional breast bulge with no demarcation, division of areola from breast; median age 11.2 years	3		**Sexual hair:** lightly distributed over mons pubis; coarse, curled, dark hair; median age 11.4 years	3
4	**Late pubescent:** secondary elevation of breast, papilla, and areola; median age 12.1 years	4		**Mid-escutcheon:** hair heavily distributed to the mons pubis, adult-type; median age 12.0 years	4
5	**Adult:** adult shape and contour of the breast and recession of the areola; median age 14.6 years	5		**Female escutcheon:** characteristic female adult-type of hair distribution; median age 13.7 years	5

FIGURE 2.1. Tanner staging of puberty.

In general, the sequence of sexual maturation rests upon different, specific hormonal target organ stimulation:

■ Estradiol influences breast budding and vaginal acidity at the age of 9 to 11 years, and it influences menarche at the ages of 11.5 to 13.
■ Androgens stimulate sexual hair growth at the ages 10.5 to 11.5 years and the ages of 13.5 to 16 for adult-type hair.
■ Progesterone promotes adult breast development at the ages of 12.5 to 16 years.
■ Growth hormone takes responsibility for a growth spurt at the ages of 11 to 12 years.

Adrenarche

Adrenarche is the second stage of secondary sex characteristic maturation, in which the development of pubic hair occurs. However, in about 20% of girls, the growth of pubic hair is the first pubertal event, followed by thelarche. Adrenarche is usually noticed between 11 and 12 years of age (median 10.5 years). The occurrence of pubic hair does not coincide with axillary hair growth, which usually presents 2 years later than pubic hair. Axillary hair distribution does not commence until after pubic hair growth is concluded (axillary hair deficiency may be linked to a familial trait and should be recognized clinically). Adrenarche is stimulated by dehydroepiandrosterone sulfate (DHEA-S) that is synthesized and secreted from the adrenal glands. During that period, DHEA-S synthesis and secretion are intensified to support this event. When adrenarche is initiated, it indicates the functional integrity of the hypothalamic–pituitary–adrenal androgen axis.

Growth Spurt

Growth spurt is the growth velocity in centimeters per year, and it is estimated at 6 to 11 cm (2.4–4.3 inches), with an average of 9 cm (8). It occurs approximately between the ages of 11 and 12 years [1 year preceding menarche or after 2 years of stage 2 breast development (breast bud)]. In prepuberty, growth hormone (GH) is secreted from the anterior pituitary gland to maintain child growth at a velocity of 4 cm per year. GH is released from the pituitary in a pulsatile pattern. During puberty, GH secretion intensifies, particularly during sleep, both in amplitude and in the number of pulses. Locally, GH needs insulin-like growth factor-I (somatomedin C) as a mediator; however, GH does not require a mediator in its action on epiphyseal cartilage. Increasing levels of ovarian sex steroids during that period interact with GH by increasing its secretion; at the same time, GH stimulates synthesis and secretion of insulin-like growth factor-I (9). These hormonal interactions are necessary in stimulating and controlling the growth spurt in general, but sex steroids express their ability to act directly and independently on bones (10).

Menarche

The first menses (menarche) in the United States is expected at an average age of 12.8 years (11) (range 11.5–13 years). Recently, the age of menarche has had an upward trend, which has been linked to environmental factors (12). There is a predictable and constant linear growth of approximately 5 cm from the time of the growth spurt to menarche. Subsequently, the menstrual cycle is anovulatory, and an anovulatory cycle may last for 12 to 18 months. After this period of relative sterility, menses is expected to occur in regular intervals, ranging from 21 to 35 days (28 ± 7 days), with a duration of 2 to 8 days (averaging 3–5 days), and an anticipated blood loss of 30 to 50 mL, (blood loss of ≥80 mL per cycle warrants clinical evaluation).

There are equally important, nonhormonal factors that participate in secondary sex characteristic maturation, such as an adequate body weight between 38.8 and 48.08 kg, with body fat being between 16% and 23.5% (13). A critical body weight of 47.8 kg is a prerequisite for inducing ovulation (20%–30% of overweight girls experience menarche earlier than girls of normal weight). Underweight individuals experience delayed menarche (14).

Optic contact with light is considered necessary for the sequential, timely occurrence of secondary sex characteristics. It has been documented that the sleep period is an important aspect of puberty, because GH, follicle-stimulating hormone (FSH), and LH pulsatile secretions increase in amplitude and frequency at that time (4,6).

Emotional and behavioral fluctuation is observed during puberty. The most common emotional events associated with secondary sex characteristic development and maturation are euphoria, depression, mood swings with paradoxical and hysterical reactions, crying with ease, and a negative attitude toward school, possibly resulting in academic and behavioral problems. These psychological, clinical changes eventually subside when maturation is reached, and reassurance about the transitional nature of these disturbances is usually enough to assuage the patient's fears; in extreme cases, however, counseling is advisable. Violent behavior is one of the most difficult sequela, in a social and legal sense, because reassurance, in this instance, is not enough. Those patients who present with violent behavior should receive appropriate counseling. An essential element of providing adequate support is to recognize the early symptoms of violent behavior and to react immediately by providing therapy as needed.

PUBERTAL DISORDERS

An aberration of the chronology of the sequence of secondary sex characteristic development and maturation is cause for clinical concern. It has been established that a majority of girls begin puberty by the age of 13, regardless of race (15). In general, when pubertal changes are clinically manifest before the age of 8 years, it is considered a precocious puberty, whereas no pubertal development occurring by the age of 17 years is regarded as delayed puberty. Of course, there are clinical situations in which the evaluation of an adolescent patient can be initiated before the age of 17.

Clinically, and for practical purposes, pubertal disorders have been divided into precocious puberty and delayed puberty.

Precocious Puberty

Precocious puberty is defined as the clinical manifestation of any secondary sex characteristic development (maturation) before the age of 8 years.

Incidence

In the general population, incidence is estimated at 1 per 5,000 to 1 per 10,000, with a female:male ratio of 4:1 to 8:1 (16).

Classification

Central precocious puberty (CPP) or idiopathic, isosexual precocious puberty, occurs in 80% of all forms of precocious puberty, and it is considered to be complete, isosexual (the sequence of events of secondary sex characteristic development and maturation is preserved), and GnRH dependent.

Peripheral precocious puberty (PPP), or precocious pseudopuberty, is regarded to be incomplete, isosexual or heterosexual, and GnRH independent. Heterosexual precocious puberty is related to excess androgen synthesis and secretion from either ovarian or adrenal gland sources.

Ectopic or extrapituitary precocious puberty depends on the synthesis and secretion of gonadotropins outside of their normal sources. It occurs in less than 0.5% of cases and is GnRH independent.

Etiology

In general, any form of precocious puberty is characterized by premature development of (a) increasing gonadal steroid hormone secretion, (b) development of secondary sex characteristics, (c) increase of height velocity, and (d) maturation of skeletal bones.

The following different mechanisms appear in the different forms of precocious puberty:

■ In GnRH-dependent central precocious puberty (isosexual precocity), the hypothalamus prematurely initiates pulsatile GnRH production and secretion, which, in

turn, stimulates the pituitary gland to release LH with a pulsatile pubertal pattern. The elevated level of LH and FSH influences the ovaries to synthesize and to excrete estrogen. Such a sequence of events triggers precocious puberty.
■ GnRH-independent peripheral precocious puberty (incomplete isosexual precocity or pseudoprecocious puberty) is considered to have an extrapituitary cause, usually an isolated autonomous ovarian tumor (granulosa cell tumor), ovarian cyst (17), or adrenal tumor causing precocious puberty in girls.
■ Extrapituitary gonadotropin (ectopic) secretion is associated with a tumor of the ovary [dysgerminoma or chorioepithelioma, lipid cell tumor of the ovary (18), or ovarian follicle cyst (19)], or liver hepatoblastoma (20), or mediastinal teratoma, leading to precocious puberty (21,22). Hypothalamic hamartomas of the tuber cinereum (a congenital malformation with the ability to secret GnRH in a pulsatile pattern) do not convert to malignancy nor do they enlarge (23).

There are additional reported causes of true precocious puberty, such as traumatic brain injury [usually associated with cerebral atrophy or focal encephalomalatcia (24–26)], encephalitis, brain abscess, central nervous system tuberculosis, static cerebral encephalopathy, or primary hypothyroidism (27). The McCune-Albright syndrome is an inheritable, genetic origin illness. The syndrome clinically manifests with irregularly edged, hyperpigmented café-au-lait skin macules and autonomous gonadal steroid secretion (frequently from the ovaries by tumors such as granulosa cell or functioning luteinized multiple ovarian cysts, or large solitary cysts). A bone disorder such as polyostotic or familial fibrous dysplasia (28,29), fragile X syndrome (30), myelomeningocele (31), hypothalamic glioma (32), hypothalamic astrocytoma (33), intrasellar choriocarcinoma or hydrocephalus (34), craniopharyngioma (35), cranial therapeutic irradiation for tumors (36) or leukemia (37) (radiotherapy also may cause GH deficiency), arachnoid cyst (38), and von Recklinghausen disease (neurofibromatosis type 1) (39) can be associated with precocious puberty.

Diagnosis

The patient's pertinent history of an unexpected development of secondary sex characteristics and a pubertal growth increment before the age of 8 years should be reported. The mother's pregnancy progress and medication history (conventional or alternative/natural medicine), environmental factors influencing the pregnancy outcome, and labor and mode of delivery may provide valuable information.

When a family history of true precocious puberty is identified, this finding will closely correspond to an occurrence of precocious puberty at the age of 8 years (borderline age of precocious puberty). When family history is negative, true precocious puberty can happen at an earlier age.

A history of administering exogenous estrogen or androgen hormones, including but not limited to natural products [phytoestrogens such soybeans, black cohosh, red clover, alfalfa, licorice, dong quai (40,41)], encephalitis, or head trauma, may elicit the cause of this entity.

General physical examination will confirm the presence of secondary sex characteristics. In some cases, precocious puberty mimics the sequence of regular puberty (thelarche, adrenarche, growth spurt, menarche); although in some cases no chronologic sequence is evident and the patients may be in various stages of puberty.

Height, weight, Tanner staging, and phenotype should be documented. General physical examination should rule out or rule in an abdominal mass (adrenal tumor) and any sign of androgenization or virilization (deepening voice, male hair distribution, oily skin, hirsutism) should be noticed. Skin changes such as café-au-lait type pigmentation (27), dry skin or hair, oily skin, or acne also should be noted. The craniofacial region, proximal femur, and pelvic region should be checked for polyostotic fibrous dysplasia associated with McCune-Albright syndrome (27). Visual disturbances resulting from optic nerve compression should be noted.

Because the ovary, brain, adrenal gland, and thyroid gland can be independently involved in the etiology of precocious puberty, particular attention should be given to these organs in the clinical evaluation.

Pelvic Examination

The appearance of the external genitalia (matured vs. childlike), type of hair distribution (female vs. male), enlargement of the clitoris (a possible sign of androgenization or virilization), size of the labia minora (and their thickness and pigmentation), type of vaginal secretions (acidic or otherwise), and any genital trauma, foreign bodies, infections, or vaginal neoplasms should be noted. Bimanual pelvic examination may establish the ratio between the cervix and uterine corpus and may identify an ovarian tumor.

Laboratory Tests

The most common form of precocious puberty is idiopathic (constitutional) in origin. Diagnosis is based on exclusion; consequently, the organs that participate in this medical entity must be tested (the ovary, brain, thyroid gland, and adrenal gland). The following plasma hormonal evaluation is essential in determining the form of precocious puberty: estradiol levels, gonadotropin concentration, and LH feedback levels in a GnRH stimulation test or a measurement of the pulsatile LH pattern, including the

amplitude and frequency (the test is more beneficial when executed at night).

In the past, exploratory laparotomy or laparoscopy was used to establish the differential diagnosis between an ovarian cyst and an ovarian estrogen-secreting tumor. High-resolution ultrasonography replaced this exploratory, invasive operation. Ultrasonography provides the additional information of the prepubertal versus the pubertal size and volume of the uterus and ovary. A uterine length of 3.5 cm is recognized as the prepubertal limit, and a uterine volume of greater than 1.8 mL is considered to be an unambiguous parameter for the onset of puberty, and is a more accurate marker than ovarian volume (42).

To simplify the clinical management of precocious puberty, the following questions should be answered:

- Is this isosexual precocious puberty? This usually reflects premature activation of the hypothalamus and the pituitary gland.
- Is this heterosexual precocious puberty? This is related to excess ovarian or adrenal androgen secretion.
- Is this premature thelarche? Premature breast development and no other clinical manifestations of secondary sexual maturation other than breast estrogenation (cervical mucus production, thickening of the vaginal mucosa, and growth of the labia minora) occurs in 60% of patients between the ages of 6 months and 2 years, with an incidence of 21.2 per 100,000 early in life. This situation is self-limiting and progresses to normal puberty with no influence on fertility (43,44). In unilateral thelarche, other conditions, such as fibroadenoma, should be kept in mind; thus, breast ultrasonography is of diagnostic value (45).
- Is this premature adrenarche? This usually occurs as transient, early pubic hair growth with increasing adrenal androgens (androstendione, DHEA, DHEA-S). Upon the exclusion of adrenal 21-hydroxylase or 11-deoxycortisol enzyme deficiency (see table on page 8), observation with reassurance of the patient is recommended for management, because premature adrenarche will not have significant influence on future puberty, fertility, or final height (46).
- Is this premature isolated menarche? The absence of other secondary sex characteristics (thelarche, adrenarche, growth spurt) due to causes such as a foreign body, trauma, infection, or neoplasms should be ruled out. This is a transient, self-limiting disorder with no effect on future development, fertility, or growth (47).

It has been documented that, with the new supersensitive serum gonadotropin assays, central precocious puberty can be reliably established with the GnRH stimulation test (a single subcutaneous dose of 100 μg of GnRH is administered, and after 40 minutes the LH serum level is determined). When LH levels exceed ≥8 IU/L, a diagnosis of central precocious puberty is made (48). Other than the GnRH stimulation test, randomly spontaneous LH elevation has a highly predictive volume, because basal serum LH is considered abnormal during the prepubertal period. It is a simple test for central precocious puberty with 100% specificity when LH levels exceed 0.3 IU/L, and 94% sensitivity and 88% specificity when spontaneous LH level reaches 0.1 IU/L (49).

In premature thelarche, the FSH pattern increases, and in precocious puberty, the LH puberty pattern is observed. The LH:FSH ratio 30 minutes after the GnRH stimulation test is less than 1 in patients with premature thelarche and greater than 1 in patients with precocious puberty. Age is accelerated by at least 18 months in precocious puberty, and a corresponding chronologic bone age or an even slightly accelerated one is identified in premature thelarche (50).

Differential Diagnosis

- Adrenal disorder,
- Central nervous system disorder,
- Gonadotropin-producing tumor,
- Hypothyroidism,
- Iatrogenic condition(s),
- Ovarian tumors.

Therapy

Conventional Therapy

In general, the objective for the treatment of precocious puberty is to abort development of secondary sex characteristics and to arrest the progress of the premature closure of the epiphyses. Because there are different types of precocious puberty, selection of a therapy should be based on underlying etiology.

All types of precocious puberty express growth acceleration, with an eventually premature fusion of the epiphyseal cartilage, which is responsible for the paradoxical occurrence of a tall girl and a short adult stature woman.

Isosexual precocious (or central precocious) puberty is characterized by a premature functionally active GnRH pulse generator, and it presides over the pulsatile and feedback regulation of the pituitary–ovarian axis.

GnRH agonists (synthetic analogues of the amino acid sequence of the natural GnRH decapeptide) express their effectiveness at about 15 to 20 times the potency of the natural GnRH neurohormone. GnRH agonists are safe, with few adverse reactions, and they demonstrate long activity (51) and are considered to be the effective first line of therapy for this type of premature puberty. It also has been postulated that GnRH agonists are effective in treating precocious puberty caused by organic etiology (51).

The continuous administration of a GnRH agonist decreases gonadotropin secretion; however, for a few days at first, gonadotropin secretion increases (52).

GnRH agonists also have the selective ability to suppress gonadotropin secretion from the pituitary without compromising the release of other pituitary gland hormones.

GnRH demonstrates the ability to transitionally delay secondary sex characteristics, bone age, and growth rate; however, such treatment decreases growth velocity (53). Randomized studies have documented that adding growth hormone (GH) to the GnRH analogue significantly improves growth rate when compared with a GnRH group alone. These studies also noted that adult height was greater by 2.7 cm in favor of the GH/GnRH group (53).

GnRH agonists can be administered via the nostril on a daily basis, or subcutaneously or intramuscularly in a long-acting, depot form. Transnasal administration (Buserelin) appears to be the least effective form of administration when compared with the subcutaneous or intramuscular routes (54,55). The U.S. Food and Drug Administration has approved leuprolide acetate depot, a super-long-acting GnRH agonist, for administration every 28 days (56,57).

Close monitoring is required for GnRH agonist therapy, and the following approach is suggested:

- Follow-up at 1- to 3-month intervals
- Clinical evaluation of secondary sex characteristics (their maturation stage and growth increment)
- Radiologic evaluation of bone age
- Pelvic ultrasonographic evaluation of ovarian texture and uterine volume (both ovarian size and uterine volume should decrease with adequate GnRH agonist dose therapy)
- Magnetic resonance imaging as an optional study, which documents polycystic ovarian images, corresponding to appropriate GnRH agonist treatment (58)
- Measuring the serum estradiol level and maintaining it under 10 pg/mL (36 pmol/L) to adjust the dose of GnRH agonist
- Basal gonadotropins or LH secretion determined by supersensitive assays
- Growth hormone level

It takes approximately 6 months of initial therapy to notice clinical improvements such as breast involution, menses cessation, and pubic hair reduction, and ultrasonographic studies document appreciative ovarian size and uterine volume reduction (44).

GnRH agonist therapy is continued until the patient's chronologic age matches her expected biologic age of female puberty, or until the epiphyses are fused (59). It is an established fact that children need a higher dose of GnRH agonist than adults to reach therapeutic levels. Use of a GnRH agonist is effective in central precocious puberty treatment, but ineffective in peripheral precocious puberty management (60). However, in select cases such as congenital adrenal hyperplasia or McCune-Albright syndrome associated with precocious puberty, GnRH agonists can be used as a form of treatment (61). Medroxyprogesterone, testolactone, spironolactone, or ketoconazole can be used in these cases (60). Testolactone, in the dose of 40 mg/kg/day, inhibits steroid aromatase activity and is an effective therapy for GnRH-independent precocious puberty in girls with McCune-Albright syndrome, although some patients experience relapse 1 to 3 years after initiation of therapy (62).

Heterosexual precocious puberty treatment is directed toward its underlying cause, which is related to the overproduction of androgens either from adrenal or ovarian tumors (Sertoli-Leydig cell tumor, lipoid cell tumor, or Sertoli cell tumors). The primary clinical approach in either case is surgery.

Congenital adrenal hyperplasia responds to the conservative medical therapy of glucocorticoids. When congenital adrenal hyperplasia is associated with salt wasting, mineralocorticoids should be administered.

Ovarian cysts present a clinical challenge in determining whether the cyst is the result of gonadotropin stimulation or whether it is independent of gonadotropin (autonomous) secreting estrogens. The GnRH stimulation test is useful in making a distinction between autonomous ovarian cysts and ovarian cysts secondary to premature gonadotropin secretion. Multiple bilaterally located ovarian cysts are usually the result of premature pituitary gonadotropin secretion and ovarian stimulation. When an isolated, autonomous ovarian follicular cyst is identified, cystectomy is advised. In the case of recurrent ovarian cysts, conservative medical management is required (63). It has been recommended that in a premenarcheal girl, asymptomatic simple cysts of 3 to 5 cm may be followed up closely with ultrasonography (64).

In primary *hypothyroidism*, the thyroid gland fails to secret thyroid hormones; diagnosis is documented by decreased serum thyroxine and increased serum thyroid-stimulating hormone (TSH), cholesterol, creatinine phosphokinase, lactic dehydrogenase, and characteristic changes in electrocardiographic results. Thyroid hormone replacement therapy is recommended to restore euthyroidism, determined by appropriate clinical and laboratory values. Levothyroxine is a very effective treatment. Pediatric dosage is based on the patient's age, and the dose is adjusted on the basis of clinical response and laboratory tests. In adults, the initial dose is 25 μg per day. The initial dose is increased by 25 to 50 μg per day after 2 to 3 weeks of treatment. The dose is adjusted until serum TSH is established within the normal, expected range, and satisfactory clinical response is noted. Such treatment arrests precocious puberty resulting from this medical condition.

Ectopic or extrapituitary sources of human chorionic gonadotropin lead to precocious puberty. A gonadotropin-secreting tumor in different locations (ovary, liver, mediastinum, and central nervous system) is a primary clinical consideration. Upon adequate location and identification of the tumor, resection is usually recommended. When the lesion is not resectable and a tissue histology is obtained, chemotherapy alone is curative in most instances of intracranial choriocarcinoma (65). Successful GnRH agonist therapy has been reported in hamartomas of the hypothalamus (66).

Thelarche, adrenarche, or menarche can each exist as isolated premature conditions that do not require any specific therapy. One can be reassured that expected puberty will eventually occur, and no adverse effect on reproduction is anticipated. A close clinical follow-up is recommended.

Behavioral and social competency problems in girls with precocious puberty have been reported, particularly in those who experience dysphoric adjustments to the condition of precocious puberty. Elevated levels of sex steroids may directly contribute to aggressive or hyperactive behavior; however, environmental and social factors also may play a significant role (67). To modify such behavioral or social competency problems, it is necessary to control excessive steroid production with parallel psychological counseling. This dual clinical approach will maximize the final clinical outcome.

Complementary Therapy

Reviewing existing data failed to identify any specific therapeutic approaches for any form of precocious puberty in the fields of acupuncture, transcutaneous electrical nerve stimulation, exercise, heat, hypnosis, manipulative (chiropractic) therapy, therapeutic massage, therapeutic touch, biofeedback therapy, imagery, or meditation.

Natural Alternative Therapy

Electronic systems were used in addition to a manual search to identify sources for specific natural alternative therapy. A natural alternative therapy for hypothyroidism was used in place of general therapy, and no specific aspect in precocious puberty was recognized.

Homeopathic treatment does not directly target precocious puberty; it is aimed at the symptomatology associated with precocious puberty (68). When a patient presents symptoms such as sensitivity to cold air, digestive system problems, physical and mental exhaustion, a lapse of menstrual bleeding when bathing in cold water, breast nipple discharge (galactorrhea), hot flashes, headaches (as a result of congestion), and heart palpitations, medication is prescribed to rebalance calcium levels or to correct any malfunctions in calcium metabolism:

Calcarea carbonica 9cH, one dose, administered on the 7th day of the menstrual cycle

15cH, one dose, administered on the 8th day of the menstrual cycle

30cH, one dose, administered on the 9th day of the menstrual cycle

This mode of therapy is offered monthly (68).

For the treatment of precocious puberty whose predominant characteristics are increment growth, mental and physical weakness (particularly in the morning), slowness in learning, lapses in concentration, slowness in walking, growing pains, and weak neck accompanied by neck pain, the suggested remedy is calcarea phosphorica or phosphorous:

Calcarea phosphorica, 15cH, five granules, one dose, three times per week, in the morning or 30cH, one dose every 15 days

Phosphorous, 15cH, one dose every week or every 15 days (68)

Additionally, homeopathic treatment classifies precocious puberty in girls into two phenotypes, male and female.

A girl of male phenotype is slim and flat-chested, and may experience periods of rapid, increasing growth along with periods of equally fast arrest of growth; she also may have oily skin, an increased tendency toward heavy perspiration, and a dark complexion.

A girl of female phenotype has short extremities, a slow growth pattern, and menarche that is later than expected in accordance with other secondary sex characteristics.

The same treatment is offered regardless of the subtype of precocious puberty: sepia officinalis (sepia), 15cH, one dose per week.

Patient Education

General information should be provided about hormonal imbalance. In addition, food allergies, vitamin B, iron, and digestive enzyme deficiency, liver disease, and parasite infestation must be considered and presented before any therapy is implemented. The patient also should be advised to avoid antihistamine medications and sulfa drugs, which exacerbate hypothyroidism.

Diet

Diet should exclude consumption of vegetables such as cabbage, broccoli, brussels sprouts, kale, cauliflower, mustard greens, turnips, spinach, peaches, and pears because they have a capacity to bind the iodine necessary for thyroid hormone synthesis. Diet should include foods containing high concentrations of iodine (fish, kelp, potatoes), high concentrations of vitamin B complex (whole grains, raw nuts, and seeds), and high concentrations of vitamin A (dark green and yellow vegetables).

Nutritional therapy is recommended as follows (69): (a) thyroid glandular; (b) tyrosine amino acid; (c) iodine; (d) vitamin A and B complex; (e) calcium, magnesium, and zinc supplementation; and (f) essential fatty acids.

DELAYED PUBERTY

Absence of secondary sex characteristics by the age of 13.4 years is considered delayed puberty (70).

Incidence

The incidence is unknown, and it is a rare occurrence.

Classification

Two categories of delayed puberty are identified (64): hypogonadal delayed puberty (decreased ability or lack of functional activity of gonads) and eugonadal delayed puberty (preserved gonadal steroidogenesis).

Etiology

Hypogonadal Delayed Puberty

Hypogonadal delayed puberty may be accompanied by either hypergonadotropism (excessive secretion of FSH/LH) or hypogonadotropism (deficiency of FSH/LH).

Hypergonadotropic hypogonadism is the most common form of delayed puberty, accounting for 43% of cases. This type of delayed puberty encompasses ovarian failure with either normal (46,XX) or abnormal prevention or deletion of X chromosome material such as 45,X; 46,X; del X (70).

Ovarian failure with the 46,XX karyotype (chromosomally competent ovarian failure) may result from *in utero* or childhood viral infections, or it can be related to a mutation of the beta subunit of gonadotropins, or faulty gonadotropin receptors. Ovarian failure can occur in association with isolated autoimmune ovarian disorders; multiglandular immunologic disorders; ovarian torsion; galactosomia (defective galactose metabolism, an autosomal-recessive disorder); postradiation or chemotherapy ovarian failure;17 alpha-hydroxylase deficiency in steroidogenesis synthesis; single-gene, autosomal-recessive familial gonadal dysgenesis; and resistant ovarian syndrome (Savage syndrome, in which either follicles are resistant to gonadotropins or gonadotropin receptors are defective) (70,71).

Ovarian failure also may result from abnormal karyotype, otherwise known as chromosomally incompetent ovarian failure. Abnormal prevention or deletion of X chromosome material (such as 45,X; 46,X; del X) is responsible for chromosomally incompetent ovarian failure (70).

Occasionally, Swyer syndrome with abnormal 46,XY karyotype is responsible for ovarian failure and sexual infantilism (70).

Hypogonadotropic hypogonadism is considered a lack of transient or permanent ability to secret GnRH [the arcuate nucleus does not secrete GnRH; therefore, the pituitary secretion of FSH/LH (short hormonal loop)] is not initiated and ovarian steroidogenesis cannot commence], and it is divided into two types: reversible and irreversible.

Reversible medical conditions advance the puberty sequence process with implementation of adequate therapy. The following medical entities may induce hypogonadotropic hypogonadism:

- Physiological delay (nonpathologic constitutional delay), in which maturation is shifted from actual age to that of a normal younger girl
- Congenital adrenal hyperplasia
- Excessive weight reduction or very low body mass condition associated with anorexia nervosa, malnutrition, malabsorption, or vigorous athletic exercise
- Cushing's disease or syndrome
- Primary hypothyroidism
- Diabetes
- Infection
- Prolactinomas
- Emotional or psychosomatic condition
- Use of marijuana (blocks the release of GnRH from the hypothalamus) (72)

Irreversible medical conditions of hypothalamic–pituitary origin responsible for delayed puberty are:

- GnRH deficiency, which can exist as an isolated form or can be associated with an impaired sense of smell (inherited Kallmann syndrome that results from the lack of migration of GnRH neurons from the olfactory placode to the hypothalamus. It occurs at about 19 weeks of gestation and consists of a genetic lack of production of adhesion molecules coded by the KAL gene, located at Xp22.3) (73).
- Pituitary insufficiency.
- Pituitary neoplasms (craniopharyngioma or prolactinoma).

Eugonadal Delayed Puberty

Eugonadal delayed puberty is characterized by preserved gonadal steroidogenesis with the timely sequential development of secondary sex characteristics and an absence of menarche within the expected period.

The following causes are considered:

- Müllerian structure agenesis (Mayer-Rokitansky-Küster-Hauser syndrome exhibiting delayed menarche and congenital absence of the vagina and the uterus, and often associated with congenital urinary tract abnormalities)
- Low genital tract obstruction (transverse vaginal septum or imperforate hymen)
- Vaginal agenesis linked with renal anomalies and skeletal defects
- Primary prolactinemia
- Androgen insensitivity syndrome (testicular feminization is a male type of pseudohermaphroditism)
- Immature, inappropriate positive feedback mechanism that preserves pulsatile LH secretion

Diagnosis

Pertinent medical history may consist of a lack of initiation of the sexual maturation process, with no breast budding or pubic hair growth present by age 13, no breast bud development within 6 to 9 months of adrenarche, or an absence of menarche by age 18. A family history of delayed puberty may be present.

General physical examination demonstrates an absence of secondary sex characteristics or presence of pubic hair for 6 to 9 months as well as an absence of breast budding. Height, weight, and Tanner staging is necessary for documentation. A neurologic examination is necessary when a headache is reported, and an ophthalmologic evaluation should be performed when scotoma or diplopia is present.

Short stature, webbed neck (pterygium colli), shield chest with wide distance between nipples, bilateral cubitus valgus (an increased carrying angle of the elbows), and sexual infantilism may all indicate Turner syndrome.

An absence of pubic hair in an otherwise female genotype, along with an absence of menarche in the patient's medical history, suggests testicular feminizing syndrome.

Pelvic examination reveals childlike appearance of the external genitalia and an absence of pubic hair; if pubic hair is present, it is the only sign of secondary sex characteristic maturation. Bimanual rectovaginal examination is essential for ruling out imperforate hymen or mechanical blockade of outflow. Furthermore, the ratio between the cervix and the uterine corpus and uterine size corresponds to that during childhood.

A female phenotype with an underdeveloped labia minora, blind vaginal canal, absence of the uterus, inguinal hernias, absence or sparseness of pubic hair, large breasts with underdeveloped nipples and pale areolas, and possible eunuchoidal appearance (large hands and feet and long arms) are indicative of testicular feminization syndrome. Complete androgen insensitivity and müllerian agenesis should be kept in mind and clinical difference noticed (in müllerian agenesis, female pubic hair distribution, a normally developed labia minora, and ovaries are present, along with absence of the vagina and uterus; occasionally the uterus is present without a cervical canal).

Laboratory Tests
The initial laboratory and radiographic studies for delayed puberty include:

- Screening for systemic disease
- Radiography to determine bone age, and anterior-posterior-lateral skull radiographs to screen for intracranial lesions or calcification
- Serum LH and FSH levels
- Prolactin level
- Thyroxine, triiodothyronine, resin uptake, thyroid stimulating hormone
- Serum estradiol
- Serum androstendione, DHEA-S, and testosterone (if serum DHEA-S or androstendione and 17-hydroxyprogesterone are elevated, 21-hydroxylase deficient adrenal

hyperplasia is diagnosed; when serum 11-deoxycortisol is elevated, 11-hydroxylase–deficient adrenal hyperplasia is documented)

■ Radiography to determine bone age and to document advancement of fusion process of epiphyses; anterior-posterior-lateral skull radiographs to screen for intracranial lesions or calcification (which are present in >70% of cases) (72). These initial X-ray results may justify obtaining a CT or MRI study to rule out a suprasellar neoplasm.

Interpretation of initial results serves as a vehicle for arriving at a diagnosis and lays a foundation for further, more focused, evaluation. It is important to perform a karyotype study on each patient presenting with elevated gonadotropin levels regardless of phenotype characteristics.

When screening for systemic disease indicates one or more complex systemic medical conditions, such as diabetes or sickle cell disease (in which about 20% of patients will have delayed puberty), the patient will require additional specific evaluation to confirm the diagnosis.

HYPERGONADOTROPIC HYPOGONADISM

A single FSH hormone elevation (>40 mIU/mL, post-menopausal level) in view of a low or undetectable estradiol level and an absence of menarche indicates a hypergonadotropic hypoestrogenic condition. An FSH level elevated to the postmenopausal value warrants a karyotype evaluation to rule out gonadal dysgenesis.

A karyotype study determines different types of gonadal dysgenesis and can lead to different forms of clinical management. Karyotype 45,X (absence of a single cell line of an X sex chromosome and no presence of Barr bodies), otherwise known as Turner syndrome, pure gonadal dysgenesis, or chromosomally incompetent ovarian failure, is characterized by hypergonadotropic (FSH level >30 IU/L and LH level >40 IU/L) hypoestrogenic disorder, female phenotype, and sexual infantilism. This syndrome often presents with a high incidence of cardiovascular disease and, for the most part, coarctation of the aorta. Renal anomalies are also linked to this condition.

Chromosome-banding techniques do not detect characterization of point mutation or small deletions of the X chromosome; therefore, DNA probe technology must be used to determine these abnormalities (64). The short arm on an X chromosome is responsible for genetic somatic information, and the long arm carries genetic information for ovarian follicle maturation and regression (partial deletions of the X chromosome long arm lead to premature ovarian failure at different ages, an absence of the long arm leads to premature ovarian failure before puberty, and a fragmentary loss of the long arm results in

premature ovarian failure sometime in reproductive age) (72).

Karyotype 46,XX, otherwise known as chromosomally competent ovarian failure, presents with high gonadotropin levels (FSH levels >30 IU/L and LH levels >40 IU/L), a normal karyotype, and an absence of menarche. Savage syndrome, or resistant ovary syndrome, is another condition in this group, characterized by (a) gonadotropin elevation, (b) the absence of menarche, (c) the presence of ovarian follicles, and (d) the absence of autoimmune disease.

A definitive diagnosis is established by conducting an ovarian tissue histology study, which documents the presence of follicles and the absence of lymphocytic infiltration, both of which are characteristics of autoimmune disease. To avoid patient exposure to laparotomy, a new laparoscopic technique of full-thickness (from antimesenteric to mesenteric) ovarian slice biopsy was developed. This technique allows a definitive diagnosis to be established in a highly select group of patients with premature ovarian failure versus resistant ovary syndrome (74). Pure gonadal dysgenesis (gonadal streaks), 46,XX karyotype, and delayed puberty can be placed in this group.

A hypergonadotropic patient with a 46,XX karyotype, elevated blood pressure, increased serum progesterone levels, delayed sexual development and steroid synthesis is compromised due to a 17-alpha-hydroxylase deficiency.

Karyotype 46, XY (Swyer syndrome) presents as a female phenotype, with an absence of secondary sex characteristics, müllerian structures, and the presence of gonadal streaks. Gonadectomy should be performed under the following circumstances when a Y chromosome composition is present in a karyotype: (a) a 20% chance of malignant neoplasia (gonadoblastoma, dysgerminoma) is present, and (b) the testicular tissue component within the gonad promotes virilization (approximately 70% of patients in this group will be affected) due to heterosexual development.

Prophylactic gonadectomy is performed as soon as the diagnosis is established and the procedure is usually executed through laparotomy (64). A laparoscopic technique has been developed to avoid laparotomy, and it appears to be a very successful mode of treatment (75).

HYPOGONADOTROPIC HYPOGONADISM

When the initial laboratory study results of LH and FSH reveal levels less than 5 IU/L, it denotes a hypogonadotropic state:

■ Hypothalamic origin [Kallmann syndrome; neoplasms (craniopharyngioma, congenital hypothalamic malformation-hamartoma), anorexia nervosa, malabsorption, inflammatory disorders, renal disease, regional ileitis, strenuous exercise, stress, marijuana, and constitutional (physiologic) delayed puberty]. It has been postulated that superactive GnRH agonists can be used to differentiate hypogonadotropic hypogonadism from physiologic (constitutional) delayed puberty. In hypogonadotropic hypogonadism, the response to GnRH is low and in physiologic delayed puberty, the response is high (44).

- Pituitary origin [hyperprolactinemia, tumors (craniopharyngioma is a tumor of the Rathke pouch of the pituitary stalk, and it is the most frequent tumor associated with delayed puberty), adenoprolactinoma]
- Eugonadism (müllerian structure agenesis or androgen insensitivity syndrome)

Therapy

Conventional Therapy

Physiologic (constitutional) delayed puberty does not require any treatment. Reassurance of the patient and the anticipation of the normal sequences of puberty later on constitute an acceptable plan for patient management. Some authorities advocate pulsatile GnRH therapy for 1 year when confronted with this entity (76). Such a treatment is started with the subcutaneous administration of 1 to 2 µg of GnRH per pulse, with pulsatile intervals every 90 minutes. Initially, the therapy occurs only at night, and, only later, over 24 hours. This is a very effective mode of therapy, but it is very regimented and demanding, which makes it almost impractical (76). In general, when delayed puberty is associated with systemic disease, the therapy for specific illness should be instituted.

In the case of a 46,XY karyotype, the presence of Y-chromosomal material mandates surgical removal of the streaked gonads (the gonad without follicles); gonadectomy is executed upon diagnosis. If a female phenotype is considered necessary, shortly after the operation, estrogen/progesterone hormonal replacement therapy is initiated.

Hormonal replacement therapy in delayed puberty is commenced with conjugated estrogen in a low dose of 0.3 mg (Premarin) or estradiol (Estrace) at a dosage of 0.5 mg per day in a continuous manner for 6 months to 1 year. Breast budding is noticed soon after the estrogen/progesterone therapy begins. Initially, a low dose of estrogen is required to maximize the patient's adult height. After this initial, continuous therapy, a sequential mode of treatment is started. The dose of conjugated estrogen is increased to 0.625 mg per day, or estradiol 1 mg daily, and is continued for 26 days. Progestin, such as medroxyprogesterone acetate (Provera), is added at a dosage of 5 to 10 mg daily at the 14th or 16th day of estrogen therapy and continued for 10 or 12 consecutive days. Upon completion of the 26th day

of therapy, regular monthly bleeding is expected (usually bleeding occurs within 3 days of ingestion of the last tablet of estrogen and progestin), and progress in the sequence of puberty should be noticed. A new, sequential therapy starts on the 5th day of bleeding each month.

Sequential estrogen/progestin therapy can be administered in another manner: the estrogen can be administered daily (one dose), and progestin can be administered for the first 10 to 12 days of each month. This mode of treatment seems more effective, because hypoestrogenism is the dominating causative factor in hypogonadotropic delayed puberty.

Such therapy promotes (a) development of secondary sex characteristics, (b) maximum growth potential, (c) prevention of osteoporosis, and (d) monthly bleeding. A hypogonadic hypoestrogenic state generally requires hormonal replacement therapy as described above.

Hypothalamic or pituitary neoplasms (craniopharyngioma, congenital hypothalamic malformation-hamartoma, adenoprolactinomas) may require neurosurgical therapy, if conservative medical treatment is not indicated, or if it fails to reverse delayed puberty. Irradiation therapy may be indicated in select cases, such as in order to shrink large tumors or when medical treatments fail.

The following scenarios in delayed puberty can induce hyperprolactinemia:

- Central nervous system without the complement of the pituitary gland, such as trauma, tumors, infections, infiltrative disease, cavernous sinus thrombosis, and temporal arteritis
- Pituitary gland trauma, prolactinoma, functional disorders
- Thyroid gland dysfunction (hypothyroidism)
- Body or chest trauma, burn, surgery, abdominal surgery, hysterectomy, oophorectomy
- Medications such as tranquillizers, antidepressants, antihypertensive, steroidal hormones, antituberculins

These conditions require specific therapy or the discontinuation of a drug to control excessive prolactin secretion.

In general, conservative medical therapy is satisfactory in hyperprolactinemia (77). Functional hyperprolactinemia and micro- and macroadenoma can be successfully treated with 2-bromo-alpha-ergocriptine (Parlodel), which is started in a low dose: half of a 2.5-mg tablet at night, and then gradually increasing the dose until the full tablet of 2.5 mg twice daily. If gastrointestinal symptoms or hypotension with syncope occur, a vaginal route of administration of one tablet daily is advisable. The surgical management of macroadenomas has a high rate of recurrence (80%), morbidity, and mortality; therefore, surgery should be preserved for a select group of patients. Surgical treatment of microadenoma is associated with a 40% rate of recurrence. Radiotherapy has a limited application in this situation.

A eugonadal condition (e.g., a transverse vaginal septum and an imperforate hymen) can be treated surgically to correct these anatomic defects and restore outflow. There are two medical entities, Mayer-Rokitansky-Küster-Hauser syndrome and complete androgen insensitivity syndrome, in which the uterus is absent and either absence of the vagina or vaginal hypoplasia is encountered. In both instances, the vagina can be created surgically. Testicular feminization syndrome has Y-chromosomal material; however, gonadectomy and inguinal mass resection can be postponed until after the development of puberty (surgery can be performed between the ages of 16 and 18, because gonadal malignant neoplasms infrequently happen before 25 years of age, and due to the absence of reaction to androgen no virilization takes place) (78).

Prepubertal children who have abused marijuana may experience delayed puberty (44). Therefore, when necessary, adequate drug rehabilitation therapy should be implemented. Such treatment restores the normal sequence of pubertal development with no reproductive sequelae.

Complementary Therapy

Analyzing the existing English-language literature on delayed puberty, it appears that only homeopathic methods of therapy are addressed. A natural medicine approach to this condition was not identified. The search established the presence of information related to the treatment of such conditions as amenorrhea, ovarian failure, hyperprolactinemia, and hypoestrogenic states. Because these conditions are related to delayed puberty, the natural medicine approach is presented in other related sections.

Patient Education
The patient is provided with an education program so that she or he may become familiar with the holistic approach of natural medicine. The patient is encouraged to actively participate in his or her clinical management. Information on mind/spirit/body as one unit, diet, exercise, weight reduction, natural supplements, minerals, vitamins, herbal medicine, meditation, and the effect of stress on the particular medical condition is presented.

Diet

In select cases, it may be advisable to prescribe a diet high in calories, cholesterol, and fats in order to induce weight gain or to prescribe decreased exercise when a patient's weight is below the pubertal range for any reason, particularly when due to malnutrition, crash dieting, or anorexia nervosa.

In obesity, a low-fat and low-calorie diet, with increased fiber and fluid intake, as well as exercise are recommended. When indicated, nutritional counseling is advised (79).

In ovarian failure, an appropriately balanced diet for this condition is advised: plenty of grains, beans [especially soy beans, fruits, vegetables (particularly dark leafy greens, nuts and seeds, especially flax seeds), and fish (salmon, tuna, halibut, sardines) (79)].

In a hypoestrogenism diet, generally it is advisable to increase calories by increasing protein, fat, and carbohydrate consumption. Regular, whole-food meals, increased soy foods and flax seeds, and abstention from dieting should be recommended (79).

Exercise
In ovarian failure, exercise is designed to build muscular mass with aerobic physical activity and weight-bearing exercise on a regular basis for 30 to 60 minutes 4 to 7 days per week. In hypoestrogenic states, reduction of vigorous to moderate exercise is suggested (79).

Stress Reduction
Providing direction to stress reduction management, tonifying-nutritive support for the reproductive system, as well as for the general constitution of the patient. Counseling should be requested from specialists as needed (79).

Supplements (79)
Mineral and vitamin supplementation is offered in an identical manner for both ovarian failure and hypoestrogenism:

- Calcium. In the hypoestrogenic state, the daily requirement of calcium increases (80), so daily intake should be in the following range (79): calcium carbonate, 1,200 to 1,500 mg per day; calcium citrate, 600 to 750 mg per day. For a variety of foods containing calcium, the reader is referred to the U.S. Agricultural Handbook No. 456 (USDA nutritive value of American foods in common units).
- Magnesium. Magnesium citrate/malate in the dose of 200 to 400 mg/day is considered an important supplement in increasing bone density (81).
- Manganese. In a dose of 15 to 30 mg per day, manganese assists in stimulating mucopolysaccharides, a necessary component of bone calcification (82).
- Zinc. In a dose of 15 to 20 mg per day, zinc is a necessary component for bone osteoblast and osteoclast formation (83).
- Copper. In a dose of 1.5 to 3.0 mg per day, copper may inhibit bone resorption (79).
- Boron. In a dose of 3 to 5 mg per day, boron participates in calcium and magnesium metabolism, and increases the serum concentration of estradiol. Through these mechanisms boron prevents bone loss (84).
- Vitamin D in a dose of 400 to 800 IU per day increases bone density (it has been documented that bone density

increased within 2 years in postmenopausal women treated with 400 IU of vitamin D₃, when compared with the placebo group, the bone density decreased) (85).

- Vitamin K, in a dose of 150 to 500 μg per day, is a necessary component in the production of osteocalcin (the protein matrix that promotes bone mineralization, which is part of the bone remodeling and bone repair process). Vitamin K is considered to be a preventive factor in the formation of osteoporosis (79).

Natural Hormonal Replacement

For natural hormonal replacement therapy, the same formula is used in both ovarian failure and hypoestrogenic states. This recipe consists of a combination of three estrogens in the following amounts: estriol, 1 mg; estradiol, 0.125 mg; estrone, 0.125. This formula is administered orally, one capsule, two times daily for 25 days per month. On the 16th day of estrogen therapy, 100 mg of micronized natural progesterone, twice daily, is added and continued for 10 days. Such a mode of treatment should induce endometrial bleeding each month and should be repeated monthly.

In addition to this formula, a standardized extract of black cohosh, 40 to 80 mg, twice per day, is implemented for both conditions (79).

Hyperprolactinemia may respond to natural therapy with capsules, tincture, and tea from the Chaste tree (other names: agneau chaste, chaste tree berry, gatillieris, gatillier, hemp tree, keushchbaum, and monk's pepper); in this way, it may help to reverse delayed puberty. A 20-mg capsule is taken orally, twice daily (85). When extract is prescribed, 40 drops of standardized extract is taken per day (79). The capsule dosage can be increased up to 175 mg per day (79).

Chaste tree derivatives are contraindicated during pregnancy and breast-feeding (85,86). It is possible that this herbal medication may interfere with the efficacy of birth control pills because of its ability to act like a hormone (86).

Homeopathic Therapy

For the treatment of delayed puberty, homeopathy classifies patients into two morphologic types: type I is a slim, short girl, with soft skin and long, blond, thin, silklike, fragile hair; type II is a girl that tends to be overweight with fluid retention (edema), has dark hair, bruises with ease, and has vein stasis in her lower extremities. Menarche is delayed in both types and therapy is offered with:

- *Anemone pulsatilla* or pulsatilla [other names: crowfoot, Easter flower, kubjelle, meadow, anemone, pasque flower, praire anemone, *Pulsatille herba,* smell fox, stor, and windflower (85)] is administered in a dose of 15cH in granule, 5 granules daily, and when symptoms improve, every other day (68). The potential for kidney

side effects may outweigh the known therapeutic effects, and because there is a lack of clinical studies to determine the safety and effectiveness of pulsatilla, caution must be exercised in its use (85).

- Senecio is given in a dose of 5cH in granule, 5 granules twice daily (68).
- Cyclamen is given in a dose of 9cH in granule, 5 granules once daily, and when psychological symptoms occur shortly before menses, one dose of 30cH is administered.

REFERENCES

1. Association of Professors of Gynecology and Obstetrics. *Medical student educational objectives,* 7th ed. Washington, DC: 1997.
2. Council on Resident and Gynecology (CREOG). *Educational objectives core curriculum for residents in obstetrics and gynecology,* 5th ed. Washington, DC: CREOG, 1996.
3. American College of Obstetrician and Gynecologists (ACOG). Technichal bulletin No. 201. Washington, DC: ACOG, 1995.
4. Tanner JM. *Growth at adolescence,* 2nd ed. Oxford, UK: Blackwell Scientific, 1962.
5. Lee PA. Normal ages of pubertal events among American males and females. *J Adolesc Health Care* 1980;1:26–29.
6. Kaplan SL, Grumbach MM, Aubert ML. The ontogenesis of pituitary hormones and hypothalamic factors in the human fetus: maturation of central nerves system regulation of anterior pituitary function. *Recent Prog Horm Res* 1976;32:161–243.
7. Oerter KE, Uriarte MM, Rose SR, et al. Gonadotropin secretory dynamics during puberty in normal girls and boys. *J Clin Endocrinol Metab* 1990;71;1251–1258.
8. Fried RI, Smith EE. Postmenarcheal growth patterns. *J Pediatr* 1962;61:562–566.
9. Mansfield MJ, Rudlin CR, Crigler JF, et al. Changes in growth and serum growth hormone and plasma somatomedin-C levels during suppression of gonadal sex steroid secretion in girls with central precocious puberty. *J Clin Endocrinol Metab* 1988;66:3–9.
10. Attie KM, Ramierez NR, Conte FA, et al. The pubertal growth spurt in eight patients with true precocious puberty and growth hormone deficiency: evidence for a direct role of sex steroids. *J Clin Endocrinol Metab* 1990;71:975–983.
11. Zacharias L, Rand WM, Wurtman RJ. A prospective study of sexual development and growth in American girls: the statistics of menarche. *Obstet Gynecol Surv* 1976;31:325–337.
12. Dann TC, Roberts DF. Menarcheal age in University of Warwick young women. *J Biosoc Sci* 1993;25:531–538.
13. Maclure M, Travis LB, Willett W, et al. A prospective cohort study of nutrient intake and age at menarche. *Am J Clin Nutr* 1991;54:649–656.
14. Frisch RE. Body fat, puberty and fertility. *Biol Rev Camb Philos Soc* 1984;59:161–168.
15. Harlan WR, Harlan EA, Grillo GP. Secondary sex characteristics of girls 12 to 17 years of age: the US health examination survey. *J Pediatr* 1980;96:1074–1077.
16. Laufer MR, Goldstein DP. Pediatric and adolescent gynecology. In: Ryan KJ, Berkowitz RS, Barbieri RL, eds. *Kistner's gynecology principles and practice.* St. Louis: Mosby-Year Book, 1995: 571–632.
17. Rodriguez-Macias KA, Thibaud E, Houang M, et al. Follow up of precocious pseudopuberty associated with isolated ovarian follicular cyst. *Arch Dis Child* 1999;81:53–56.

18. Dengg K, Fink FM, Heitger A, et al. Precocious puberty due to a lipid-cell tumor of the ovary. *Eur J Pediatr* 1993;52:12–14.

19. Taulier-Raybaud C, Morel Y, La Selve H, et al. Ovarian follicle cysts and precocious puberty. *Pediatrie* 1986;41:607–616.

20. Navarro C, Correster JM, Sancho A, et al. Paraneoplastic precocious puberty. Report of a new case with hepatoblastoma and review of the literature. *Cancer* 1985;56:1725–1729.

21. Kaul TK, Bakran A. Endocrine secreting malignant mediastinal tratoma. *Thorac Cardiovasc Surg* 1990;38:251–253.

22. Porcelli F, Barbareschi M, Mosca L, et al. Pseudo-precocious puberty associated with mediastinal teratoma and polycystic ovary. *Helv Paediatr Acta* 1985;40:75–82.

23. Romner B, Trumpy JH, Marhaug G, et al. Hypothalamic hamartoma causing precocious puberty treated by surgery: case report. *Surg Neurol* 1994;41:306–309.

24. Shaul PW, Towbin RB, Chernausek SD. Precocious puberty following severe head trauma. *Am J Dis Child* 1985;139:467–469.

25. Sockalosky JJ, Kriel RL, Krach LE, et al. Precocious puberty after traumatic brain injury. *J Pediatr* 1987;110:373–377.

26. Blendonohy PM, Philip PA. Precocious puberty in children after traumatic brain injury. *Brain Injury* 1991;5:63–68.

27. Pringle PJ, Stanhope R, Hindmarsh P, Brook CG. Abnormal pubertal development in primary hypothyroidism. *Clin Endocrinol (Oxf)* 1988;28:479–486.

28. Yavuzer R, Khilnani R, Jackson IT, et al. A case of atypical McCune-Albright syndrome requiring optic nerve decompression. *Ann Plast Surg* 1999;43:430-435.

29. Prasher VP. Familial precocious puberty in girls. *J R Soc Med* 1993;86:61.

30. Moore PS, Chudley AE, Winter JS. True precocious puberty in girl with the fragile X. *Am J Med Genet* 1990;37:265–267.

31. Proos LA, Dahl M, Ahlsten G, et al. Increased perinatal intracranial pressure and prediction of early puberty in girls with myelomeningocele. *Arch Dis Child* 1996;75:42–45.

32. Baba H, Ryu N, Mori K, et al. Hypothalamic glioma with diencephalic syndrome and following precocious puberty: a case report. *No To Shinkei* 1989;41:1029–1035.

33. Tashiro T, Aida T, Sugimoto S, et al. A case of hypothalamic astrocytoma with precocious puberty. *No Shinkei Geka* 1992; 20:61–65.

34. Brauner R, Rappaport R, Nicod C, et al. True precocious puberty in non-tumor hydrocephalus. An analysis of 16 cases. *Arch Fr Pediatr* 1987;44:433–436.

35. Ogilvy-Stuart AL, Clayton PE, Shalet SM. Cranial irradiation and early puberty. *J Clin Endocrinol Metab* 1994;78: 1282–1286.

36. Giuffre R, Di Lorenzo N. Evolution of a primary intrasellar germinomatous teratoma into a choriocarcinoma. Case report. *J Neurosurg* 1975;42:602–604.

37. Rappaport R, Brauner R. Growth and endocrine disorder secondary to cranial irradiation. *Pediatr Res* 1989;25:561–567.

38. Kaplan SL, Crumbach MM. The neuroendocrinology of human puberty: an ontogenic perspective. In: Grumbach MM, Sizonenko PC, Aubert ML, eds. *The control of the onset of puberty.* Baltimore: Williams & Wilkins, 1999:1–68.

39. Listernick R, Charrow J, Greenwald M, et al. Natural history of optic pathway tumors in children with neurofibromatosis type 1: a longitudinal study. *J Pediatr* 1994;125:63–66.

40. Costell C. Estrogenic substance from plants. *J Am Pharm Assoc (Wash)* 1950;39:177–180.

41. Holt S. Phytoestrogens for healthier menopause. *Altern Ther Health Med* 1997;1:187–193.

42. Ivarsson SA, Nilsson KO, Persson PH. Ultrasonography of the pelvic organs in prepubertal and postpubertal girls. *Arch Dis Child* 1983;58:352–354.

43. Van Winter JT, Noller KL, Zimmerman D, et al. Natural history of premature thelarche in Olmsted County, Minnesota. 1940–1984. *J Pediatr* 1990;116:278–280.

44. Styne DM. New aspects in the diagnosis and treatment of pubertal disorders. *Pediatr Clin North Am* 1997;44:505–529.

45. Boothroyd OB, Carty H. Breast masses in childhood and adolescence: a presentation of 17 cases and review of the literature. *Pediatr Radiol* 1994;24:81–84.

46. Ibanez L, Virdis R, Potau N, et al. Natural history of premature pubarche: an auxological study. *J Clin Endocrinol Metab* 1992; 74:254–257.

47. Murram D, Dewhurst J, Grant DB. Prematur menarche: a follow-up study. *Arch Dis Child* 1983;58:142–143.

48. Eckert KL, Wilson DM, Bachrach LK, et al. A single-sample, subcutaneous gonadotropin-releasing hormone test for central precocious puberty. *Pediatrics* 1996:97:517–519.

49. Neely EK, Wilson DM, Lee PA, et al. Spontaneous serum gonadotropin concentrations in the evaluation of precocious puberty. *J Pediatr* 1995;127:47–52.

50. Pohlenz J, Habermehl P, Wemme H, et al. The differentiation between premature thelarche and pubertas praecox on the basis of clinical, hormonal and radiological findings. *Dtsch Med Wochenschr* 1994;119:1301–1306.

51. Conn PM, Crowley WF. Gonadotropin-releasing hormone and its analogs. *Annu Rev Med* 1994;45:391–405.

52. Knobil E. The endocrine control of the menstrual cycle. *Rec Prog Horm Res* 1980;36:53–88.

53. Tuvemo T, Gustafsson J, Proos LA. Growth hormone treatment during suppression of early puberty in adopted girls. Swedish Growth Hormone Advisory Group. *Acta Paediatr* 1999;88: 928–932.

54. Heinrichs C, Craen M, Vanderschueren-Lodeweyckx M, et al. Variations in pituitary-gland suppression during intranasal buserelin and intramuscular depot-triptorelin therapy for central precocious puberty. Belgian Study Group for Pediatric Endocrinology. *Acta Paediatr* 1994;83:627–633.

55. Stasiowska B, Vannelli S, Benso L. Final height in sexually precocious girls after therapy with an intranasal analoque gonadotropin-releasing hormone (buserelin). *Horm Res* 1994;42:81–85.

56. Carel JC, Lahlou N, Guazzarotti L, et al. Treatment of central precocious puberty with depot leuprorelin. French Leuprorelin Trial Group. *Eur J Endocrinol* 1995;132:699–704.

57. Tanaka T, Hibi I, Kato K, et al. A dose finding study of a super long-acting luteinizing hormone-releasing hormone analog (leuprolide acetate depot, TAP-144-SR) in the treatment of central precocious puberty. The TAP-144-SR CPP Study Group. *Endocrinol Jpn* 1991;38:369–376.

58. Ambrosino MM, Hernanz-Schulman M, Genieser NB, et al. Monitoring of girls undergoing medical therapy for isosexual precocious puberty. *J Ultrasound Med* 1994;13:501–508.

59. Jay N, Mansfield MJ, Blizzard RM, et al. Ovulation and menstrual function of adolescent girls with central precocious puberty after therapy with gonadotropin-releasing hormone agonists. *J Clin Endocrinol Metab* 1992;75:890–894.

60. Wheeler MD. Update on therapy for precocious puberty. *Compr Ther* 1994;20:351–355.

61. Pescovitz OH, Comite F, Cassorla F, et al. True precocious puberty complicating congenital adrenal hyperplasia: treatment with a luteinizing hormone–releasing hormone analog. *J Clin Endocrinol Metab* 1984;58:857–861.

62. Feuillan PP, Jones J, Cutler GB Jr. Long-term testolactone therapy for precocious puberty in girls with the McCune-Albright syndrome. *J Clin Endocrinol Metab* 1993;77:647–651.

63. Rodriguez-Macias KA, Thibaud E, Houang M, et al. Follow up of precocious pseudopuberty associated with isolated ovarian follicular cyst. *Arch Dis Child* 1999;81:53–56.

64. The American College of Obstetricians and Gynecologists

(ACOG). Precis V. An Update in Obstetrics and Gynecology. Washington, DC: ACOG, 1994:259, 389.

65. Massie RJ, Shaw PJ, Burgess M. Intracranial choriocarcinoma casing precocious puberty and cured with combined modality therapy. *J Paediatr Child Health* 1993;29:464–467.

66. Mahacholertwattana P, Kaplan S, Grumbach MM. The luteinizing hormone–releasing hormone-secreting hypothalamic hamartoma is a congenital malformation: natural history. *J Clin Endocrinol Metab* 1993;77:118–121.

67. Sonis WA, Comit F, Blue J, et al. Behavior problems and social competence in girls with true precocious puberty. *J Pediatr* 1985; 106:156–160.

68. Holtzscherr A, Legros AS. *Pratique homeopathique en gynecologie.* Boiron, France: Centre d'Enseignement et de Developpement de l'Homeopathie, 1994.

69. Chopra D, ed. *Alternative medicine. The definitive guide.* Tiburon, CA: Future Medicine, 1997:936–937.

70. Albanese A, Stanhope R. Investigations of delayed puberty. *Clin Endocrinol (Oxf)* 1995:43:105–110.

71. Reindollar RH, Tho SPT, McDonough PG. Delayed puberty: an updated study of 326 patients. *Trans Am Gynecol Obstet Soc* 1989;8:146–151.

72. Beckman CRB, Ling WNP, Herbert WP, et al. *Obstetrics and gynecology,* 3rd ed. Baltimore: Williams & Wilkins, 1998: 430–435.

73. Schwanzel-Fukuda M, Bick D, Pfaff DW. Luteinizing hormone-releasing hormone (LHRH)-expressing cells do not migrate normally in an inherited hypogonadal (Kallmann) syndrome. *Mol Brain Res* 1989;6:311–326.

74. Ostrzenski A. A new laparoscopic full-thickness slice ovarian biopsy (from antimesenteric to mesenteric margin). *J Gynecol Surg* 1995;11:109–112.

75. Ostrzenski A, Homa T, Klimek M, et al. Video laparoscopic gonadectomy in Swyer's syndrome. *Pol Ginecol* 1995;66(suppl): 178–180.

76. Stanhope R, Pringle PJ, Brook CGD, et al. Induction of puberty by pulsatile gonadotropin releasing hormone. *Lancet* 1987;2: 552–555.

77. Vance ML, Cragun JR, Reimnitz C, et al. CV205-502 treatment of hyperprolactinemia. *J Clin Endocrinol Metab* 1989;68:336–339

78. Manuel M, Katayama KP, Jones HW Jr. The age of occurrence of gonadal tumors in intersex patients with a Y chromosome. *Am J Obstet Gynecol* 1976;124:293–300.

79. Hudson T. *Women's encyclopedia of natural medicine. Alternative therapies and integrative medicine.* Lincolnwood, IL: Keats, a Division of NTS/Contemporary Publishing, 1999:15–27.

80. Heaney R. Nutritional factors and estrogen in age related bone loss. *Clin Invest Med* 1982;43:79–81.

81. Abraham G, Greawl H. A total dietary program emphasizing magnesium instead of calcium. Effect on the mineral density of calcaneous bone in postmenopausal women on hormonal therapy. *J Reprod Med* 1990;35:503–507.

82. Leach R Jr, Meunster A, Wien E. Part I. Studies on the role of manganese in bone formation. Part II. Effect upon chondroitin sulfate synthesis in chick epiphyseal cartilage. *Arch Biochem Biophys* 1969;133:22–28.

83. Nielsen F. Boron: an overlooked element of potential nutritional importance. *Nutr Today* 1988;1/2:4–7.

84. Ooms ME, Roos JC, Bezemer PD, et al. Prevention of bone loss by vitamin D supplementation in elderly women: a randomized double-blind trial. *Clin Endocrinol Metab* 1995;80:1052–1058.

85. Fetrow CW, Avila JR. The compete guide to herbal medicines. Springhouse, PA: Springhouse Corporation, 1999:126–127, 396–397.

86. McGuffin M, Hobbs C, Upton R, et al., eds. *Botanical safety handbook.* Boca Raton, FL: CRC Press, 1997.

3

MENSTRUAL CYCLE AND MEDICAL DISORDERS

EDUCATIONAL OBJECTIVES

Medical Students *APGO Objective*	*Residents in Obstetrics/Gynecology* *CREOG Objective*	*Practitioners* *ACOG Recommendation*
No specific recommendation	No specific recommendation	No specific recommendation

A menstrual function is a complex mechanism that requires the synchronized and sequential interaction of the hypothalamic-pituitary-ovarian axis, the healthy endometrium, and a patent uterine-cervical-vaginal canal. In addition, several other organs, such as the central nervous system, adrenal glands, thyroid gland, liver, and kidneys, influence the function of menstrual cycle. Naturally, each disorder related to these organs or emotional stress may interrupt this multifaceted and sensitive mechanism. Systemic illness may affect the menstrual cycle and the menstrual cycle may influence the course of medical disorders. It is an observable fact that conjunction of exacerbation of the same systemic illnesses at the different phases of the menstrual cycle occurs. Menstrual function, on the other hand, can be affected either by endocrinologic disorder or by organic conditions of the specific organ.

EFFECT OF MEDICAL DISORDERS ON THE MENSTRUAL CYCLE

Malnutrition eventually will cause cessation of menses, leading to infertility. A mild reduction in caloric intake does not significantly affect the menstrual cycle in otherwise healthy women (1). An acute malnutrition effect on the menstrual cycle is a reversible process, and recovery may be expected when adequate nutrition is reestablished (2).

Whatever the cause (diet, starvation, exercise, illness, or compromised intestinal absorption), weight loss may lead to an aberration in gonadotropin secretion (particularly luteinizing hormone), and the change in gonadotropin secretion influences menstrual dysfunction (3). The younger the patient or the greater the weight loss, the lower the serum hormone concentrations will be (4). Weight loss of 10% to 15% of expected weight for height will interfere with menstrual function and will result in secondary amenorrhea (5,6).

Malabsorption associated with systemic disease may negatively disturb the menstrual cycle function. Common medical conditions that may cause malabsorption are listed as follows (7):

- Bile salt deficiency resulted from bile salt binders (cholestyramine, calcium carbonate, neomycin), small bowel resection, Crohn disease, bacterial overgrowth, intestinal diverticula, blind loop syndrome, cholestasis, and hepatic cirrhosis
- Inadequate absorptive surface (considerable intestinal resection, jejunoileal bypass, gastrocolic fistula)
- Lymphatic obstruction (lymphoma, intestinal lymphangiectasia, Whipple disease)
- Maldigestion (chronic pancreatitis, pancreatic carcinoma, cystic fibrosis)
- Mucosal disease (infection, inflammatory disease, radiation enteritis, ulcerative jejunitis, biochemical disorders) Infiltrative disorders (amyloidosis, scleroderma), endocrine disorders

Liver disease leads to decreased serum estrogen levels due to the diminished capacity of the hydrolysis of biliary estrogen conjugates. Alcoholic or nonalcoholic chronic liver disease may result in amenorrhea, infertility, and loss of libido (8).

The following endocrine disorders affect the menstrual cycle:

- *Hyperthyroidism*, including Graves disease (elevated serum thyroid hormones) may lead to oligomenorrhea, amenorrhea, and infertility. *Hypothyroidism* (including Hashimoto disease) may cause delayed puberty, precocious puberty, menorrhagia, metrorrhagia, and infertility.
- *Cushing syndrome* is associated with amenorrhea, acne, and hirsutism. *21-hydroxylase* and *17-hydroxyprogesterone* deficiency induces amenorrhea and virilization.

Adrenal gland insufficiency (Addison disease) also produces amenorrhea.

■ *Autoimmune endocrinopathy* may cause premature ovarian failure as an isolated condition (autoimmune oophoritis), in which specific antiovarian antibodies are produced. In many instances other autoimmune disorders are linked to premature ovarian failure (autoimmune adrenal insufficiency, autoimmune thrombocytopenia, juvenile onset of diabetes mellitus, hypoparathyroidism, hypothyroidism, myasthenia gravis, pernicious anemia, rheumatoid arthritis, systemic lupus erythematosus).

■ Diabetes mellitus is associated with oligomenorrhea or amenorrhea in about 30% of treated patients. Menstrual dysfunctions are not directly related to diabetes mellitus, but increased hypothalamic dopaminergic activity causes menstrual function derangement. In general, functional hypothalamic-pituitary menstrual dysfunction is postulated (9,10).

Kidney disorders linked to chronic renal insufficiency induce amenorrhea when serum creatinine levels are elevated between 5 and 10 mg/dL. Hemodialysis usually does not regulate the abnormal menstrual cycle. In the majority of cases, shortly after successful kidney transplantation the regular ovulatory menstrual cycle resumes (11). Approximately 50% of women on hemodialysis demonstrate elevated serum prolactin levels that are refractory to either to l-dopa or dopamine suppression (12). Patients who undergo hemodialysis therapy routinely receive heparin and anticoagulants, placing such a patient at high risk for severe, heavy endometrial bleeding or intraabdominal bleeding due to rupture of an ovarian cyst, and such an event may result in a life-threatening condition. These potential complications in both instances can be prevented with a low-dose oral contraceptive (8).

Other conditions negatively affect the menstrual cycle, such as *galactosemia*. Amenorrhea resulting from hypergonadotropic hypogonadism may be caused either by liver damage, which is usually present along with cataracts and mental retardation, or direct ovarian toxicity by galactose or its metabolites, leading to ovarian atrophy (13). *Betathalassemia* may lead to amenorrhea brought on by iron overload, which has a damaging effect on both the pituitary and gonadal systems (14).

EFFECT OF MENSTRUAL CYCLE ON MEDICAL DISORDERS

Systemic illnesses may worsen during a specific phase of the menstrual cycle and subside during other phases indicate the influence of menstrual cycle hormone fluctuation on the particular disease. The following systemic disease symptoms may remain under the menstrual cycle influence.

Menstrual migraine headaches (vascular headaches are caused by the initial vasoconstriction phase and followed by the vasodilatation phase) increase in frequency and intensity shortly after menarche and are estimated to be in the range of 8% to 14% (15). Improvement of migraine headaches is observed during pregnancy in up to 90% of affected women, and headaches intensify in the postpartum period (16). During the climacteric period, menstrual headaches may improve or worsen when on estrogen replacement therapy (ERT) (17). The usual contraindications to hormone replacement therapy (HRT) may be applied to women with migraines (18). Similar effects are observed when oral contraceptives are administered (19). The treatment of menstrual headaches falls into three categories, as described below (20).

Avoidance of migraine trigger factors can be achieved by changes in life-style. Foods containing tyramine, such as aged cheese, chocolate, yogurt, yeast, beer, wine, alcohol, monosodium glutamate, or sodium nitrate, should be restricted. Psychological stress, fatigue, visual stimuli, or weather changes also may trigger the migraine attack (21).

Prophylaxis is indicated when treatment for menstrual migraine headaches is not successful. A preventive treatment should decrease the frequency, intensity, and duration of the acute attack. However, it is a known phenomenon that a preventive therapy for menstrual migraine headaches will not eliminate headaches associated with menses. The following therapeutic agents may be used for prevention (20,22):

■ Ergotamine (dihydroergotamine) is effective in both prevention and acute attack management when taken once or twice daily (20,23).

■ Transdermal or oral estrogen started just before menstruation or ovulation time and continued for 3 to 6 days may prevent induction of menstrual migraine (23). Estradiol 1 mg sublingually immediately at the onset of headaches may disrupt the acute attack of menstrual migraine headaches (24).

■ Prostaglandin inhibitors, particularly nonsteroidal anti-inflammatory drugs, administered just before the time of headaches may prevent attack or reduce the severity of headaches (23,25).

■ Calcium channel blockers

■ Beta-blockers

■ Tricyclic antidepressant

■ Anticonvulsant

Symptoms of the acute attack may be treated with either a single agent or a combination of ingredients. The newer selective serotonin agonists (e.g., Sumatriptan) have been very effective in the treatment of both nonmenstrual and menstrual migraine (20). All the medications listed above can be used successfully for the treatment of the acute attack. Gonadotropin suppression medication (gonadotropin-releasing hormone [GnRH] agonists) combined with low-dose ERT is a very effective form of treatment. Hysterectomy with bilateral oophorectomy followed by low-dose ERT is an effective method of management of menstrual migraine headaches (23), although it is rarely indicated. In postmenopausal migraine headaches related to HRT it is helpful to administer estrogen continuously rather than via the cyclic method. Additionally, changing the route of administration of estrogen may reduce migraine headaches (22).

Asthma, seemingly as menstrual migraine headaches, is more often observed after menarche (26). It has been documented that asthma symptoms become worse shortly before menses (27,28). Exacerbation of premenstrual asthma may be caused by a cyclic administration of oral contraceptive or other exogenous sex hormones (29). There are other asthma-predisposing factors, such as cold air, exercise, pollutants, irritants, reflux esophagitis, histamine, and other pharmacologic agents (aspirin, nonsteroidal antiinflammatory drugs, cholinergic agonists). Asthmatic symptoms such as wheezing, dyspnea, paroxysmal nonproductive or productive cough, and chest tightness are common clinical findings. Clinical signs include expiratory or inspiratory wheezes, pulsus paradoxus, widened pulse pressure, and, in severe cases, a quiet chest. Therapy for asthma, such as theophylline, antibiotics, beta-adrenergics, anticholinergics, and corticosteroids, can be administered for asthma exacerbation premenstrually (30). Ovarian function suppression with long-acting gonadotropin-releasing hormone agonists (GnRH-agonists) (31); danazol, and depoprovera, demonstrates the same clinical potential and can be used in the treatment of this medical entity (24,30).

Aphthous ulcers or Mikulicz oral aphthae are a well-documented condition in conjunction with the menstrual cycle (32,33). Clinically, this condition is characterized by a clustering of one to five 2- to 10-mm, moderately painful lesions with oral mucosal paresthesia and erythematous, papular, necrotic, oval ulceration, surrounded by a bright red halo. They heal in 1 to 2 weeks without scarring. The symptoms usually occur in the luteal phase of menstrual cycle or with the onset of menses (30). The cause of this condition remains unknown, but immunologic and emotional disturbances have been implicated. The therapeutic approach has not been definitively established. Regardless of the lack of convincing evidence, hormonal therapy for aphthous ulcers is usually offered. Either the estrogens or progesterone therapies are prescribed with variable effectiveness. Estrogen pellet implants are also suggested for treatment (30). An oral suspension of sucralfate (an antacid solution) is the safe and effective treatment modality for recurrent aphthous ulcers. It significantly reduces the duration of pain, healing time, and duration of remission, as has been documented in a prospective randomized, double-blind, placebo-controlled, cross-over clinical trial (34).

Because emotional disturbances have been implicated as one of the pathogenetic hypotheses, the effects of relaxation/imagery approach have been clinically tested. This study has found little support for the role of high hypnotic therapeutic value in the treatment of recurrent aphthous stomatitis (35).

Dermatoses can get worse in the luteal phase and during menses. Acne, atopic dermatitis, autoimmune progesterone dermatitis, aphthous stomatitis, dermatitis herpetiformis, hereditary angioedema, lichen planus, lupus erythematosus,

mycosis fungoides, and rosacea demonstrate premenstrual exacerbation (30). The therapeutic approach is directed to the underlying skin disorder, and suppression of ovarian steroidogenesis may be helpful.

Diabetes may deteriorate during the luteal phase of the menstrual cycle, although improvement has been observed as well (36). Fluctuation in carbohydrate metabolism during the menstrual cycle is well documented; however, the means by which the hormonal ambience of the menstrual cycle affects glucose homeostasis is not completely understood (24). Diabetic ketoacidosis, severe insulin reaction, and a hypoglycemic state are often observed close to expected menses, and ovarian suppression with GnRH agonists has been postulated in such cases (37). In addition to an appropriate diet, insulin dosages need to be adjusted in order to control diabetes.

Rheumatoid arthritis symptoms such as joint pain and morning stiffness are intensified during menses and early in the proliferative phase of the menstrual cycle (38,39). Estrogen therapy (40), oral contraceptives (41), and HRT (42) provide relief from the symptomatology of rheumatoid arthritis, but these therapeutic paradigms can not prevent its occurrence (24). Estrogen and progesterone not only have regulatory menstrual cycle capacities but also demonstrate antiinflammatory action, and both of these components of pharmacologic actions are used in easing arthritis symptoms (43).

Catamenial epilepsy is defined as a seizure exacerbated by menstruation or occurring during menses. Such a broad definition leads to difficulty in establishing the prevalence of this condition, which is estimated between 10% and 70% (24,30). When catamenial epilepsy is limited to the 10-day time frame (4 days before and 6 days after menses), in which epilepsy occurs, prevalence is about 12.5% (44). Because the diagnosis of catamenial epilepsy has implications for its management, a standardized definition is needed.

The full scope of catamenial epilepsy has yet to be addressed sufficiently. Therefore, optimal management strategies are difficult to outline for this condition (45). Charting seizures in reference to menses and determining 22-day serum progesterone levels should be sufficient to establish the diagnosis (46). The addition of acetazolamid (125–500 mg/day, 5 to 7 days prior to and through menses) to anticonvulsant therapy (phenytoin, phenobarbital, primidone, and carbamazine) may be beneficial in some cases (30). Progesterone (50–400) mg twice daily in the form of vaginal suppositories is available (oral micronized natural progesterone probably is equally effective); however, its effectiveness has not been clinically proven. Progestin (e.g., medroxyprogesterone acetate 10 mg orally two to four times daily) or one dose of depo-provera 120–150 mg intramuscularly every 6–12 weeks (47) combined with an anticonvulsant is often used in the management of catamenial epilepsy, and this regimen appears to reduce the frequency of seizures (24,47). If oral contraceptives are chosen, they should be administered in a continuous pattern to avoid exacerbation of seizure on pill-free days (47). It is worthwhile to mention that anticonvulsant agents amplify metabolism of oral contraceptives, so a contraceptive agent should contain a higher dose of estrogen the component (50 μg), or an alternative method of contraception should be used, such as a barrier technique (24,30).

Myasthenia gravis is a neuromuscular disorder resulting in weakness and fatiguability of skeletal muscles, caused by an autoimmune-mediated decrease in acetylcholine receptors at the neuromuscular junction (7). Symptoms of myasthenia gravis worsen progressively through the follicular-ovulatory-luteal phases of the menstrual cycle and then improve shortly before menses and throughout the bleeding phase. Such improvement occurs in approximately 25% to 50% and this remission is considered to be the result of hormone-induced changes in acetylcholinesterase enzyme activity (48). It has been determined that the amount of medicine controlling symptoms must be increased two- to threefold in the luteal phase over what is is necessary in the follicular phase. In general, a hormonal manipulation is not an effective approach in the management of this condition, although oral micronized estradiol alone in an interrupted mode has been reported to be beneficial (endometrial hyperplasia can result from such approach). When oral medroxyprogesterone was added to micronized estradiol, the myasthenia gravis profoundly worsened. Therefore, the patient should be monitored cautiously regardless of oral contraceptive or HRT administration (30).

Irritable bowel syndrome (IBS) is clinically characterized by irregular bowel movement habits and recurrent abdominal pain (bowl movement will relieve pain), and has no identifiable organic underlying cause. IBS may differ in symptomatology, and three groups can be identified:

- Chronic, recurrent abdominal pain with constipation (spastic colon)
- Chronic, recurrent abdominal pain and altering constipation with diarrhea
- Chronic, recurrent abdominal pain and painless diarrhea (7,49)

Women are more affected than men (3–20 times), and worsening symptoms are often observed at the time of ovulation throughout the luteal phase (progesterone dominant) with loss stool or diarrhea shortly before menses.

Treatment of symptoms with an antispasmolitic, bulk-forming laxative, and promotility medications are available. Some clinicians suggest using prostaglandin synthesis inhibitors (24). GnRH agonist treatment is a beneficial modality in the management of IBS (50).

Other medical conditions with a low clinical prevalence are also influenced by the menstrual fluctuating function:

- Anaphylaxis-like reaction (anaphylactoid attack) is a potentially life-threatening medical entity, related either to progesterone sensitivity or hypersensitivity to some

metabolic substance in menstrual fluid. Independently, it has been documented by different investigators that suppression of the ovarian steroidogenesis function (either by GnRH agonist administration or oophorectomy) prevents anaphylactoid attacks (51–54). A clinical picture is consistent with urticaria, angioedema, hypotension, laryngeal edema, and shock (52). A randomized, double-blind clinical trial of GnRH agonists and placebo documented that all patients experienced remission on this agent (53). Taking potential serious sequelae of this condition both therapies hysterectomy with bilateral salpingo-oophorectomy (surgical permanent castration) and GnRH agonist (medical transient castration) are beneficial in women with recurrent, cyclic anaphylaxis associated with the menstrual function. Oral contraceptives appear to be contraindicated in this condition (30).

- Behçet syndrome distinguishes itself clinically by the presence of the triad of ophthalmia, oral ulceration, and genital ulceration. Blindness is the most serious sequelae of this syndrome. Cyclic exacerbation is observed in the luteal phase and becomes worse shortly before menses. Improvement is noticeable in the follicular phase of the menstrual cycle (55). The therapy may include hormonal manipulation, transfer factor (in the absence of severe ophthalmologic or neurological manifestation) (55), corticosteroid agents, and colchicines (30).

- Endocrine allergy to steroid hormone is a known clinical occurrence. Urticaria, erythema multiforme, and the development of dyshidrosiform lesions 5 to 10 days prior to menstrual bleeding are clinical manifestations of this condition, and the symptoms subside with the onset of menses (56). Progesterone is the most common hormone indicated in endocrine sensitivity (57). Suppression of ovarian function with oral contraceptives or estrogen alone can be beneficial (30).

- The homeopathic dilution technique, with extremely low doses of progesterone (ranging from 0.0016 to 2.5 mg), appears to be successful in the majority of patients (58).

- Hereditary angioedema is an autosomal dominant disorder, although it can be an acquired disorder. This condition is characterized by upper respiratory obstruction, severe abdominal colic pain, and skin angioedema. These symptoms, in some patients, occur at the beginning of menses or in other women when taking oral contraceptives or estrogens alone, or during the latter half of pregnancy (59). Methyltestosterone, danazol, oxymethalone, and stanozolol (anabolic steroid) yield a beneficial effect (30,60).

- Porphyrias (abnormality associated with heme biosynthesis) attacks demonstrate the association with estrogens or menses (61). Prophylaxis of acute intermittent porphyria is advocated with hematin or hemin. Estrogens and oral contraceptives may precipitate attacks of acute and intermittent porphyria and therefore should be used with caution (61). GnRH agonists prevent cyclical, neurovisceral attacks of acute intermittent porphyria; however, the drawback of this treatment involves the potential for osteoporosis occurring secondary to hypoestrogenism induced by the GnRH agonists (62–64).

A detailed discussion of medical systemic illnesses, diagnosis, and conventional-complementary-alternative natural therapies associated with menstrual function is beyond the scope of this chapter. For more information, other appropriate publications should be consulted (7).

REFERENCES

1. Pirke KM, Schweiger U, Lemmel W, et al. The influence of dieting on the menstrual cycle of healthy young women. *J Clin Endocrinol Metab* 1985;60:1174–1179.
2. Smith CA. The effect of wartime starvation in Holland upon pregnancy and its product. *Am J Obstet Gynecol* 1947;53:599–602.
3. Travaglini P, Bech-Peccoz P, Ferrari C, et al. Some aspects of hypothalamic-pituitary function in patients with anorexia nervosa. *Acta Endocrinol (Copenh)* 1976;81:252–262.
4. Schweiger U, Laessle R, Pfister H, et al. Diet-induced menstrual irregularities: effect of age and weight loss. *Fertil Steril* 1987;48:746–751.
5. Sanborn CF, Martin BF, Wagner WW. Is athletic amenorrhea specific to runners? *Am J Obstet Gynecol* 1982;143:859–861.
6. Abraham SF, Beumont PJV, Fraser IS. Body weight, exercise and menstrual status among ballet dancers in training. *Br J Obstet Gynecol* 1982;89:507–510.
7. Fauci AS, Braunwald E, Isselbacher KJ, et al. *Harrison's principles of internal medicine.* New York: McGraw-Hill, 1998.
8. Steinkampf MP. Systemic illness and menstrual dysfunction. *Obstet Gynecol Clin North Am* 1990;17:311–319.
9. Djursing H, Nyholm HC, Hagen C, et al. Depressed prolactin levels in diabetic women with anovulation. *Acta Obstet Gynecol Scand* 1982;61:403–406.
10. Djursing H. Hypothalamic-pituitary-gonadal function in insulin treated diabetic women with and without amenorrhea. *Dan Med Bull* 1987;34:139–147.
11. Bierman M, Nolan GH. Menstrual function and renal transplantation. *Obstet Gynecol* 1977;49:186–189.
12. Lim VS, Kathpalia SC, Frohman LA. Hyperprolactinemia and impaired pituitary response to suppression and stimulation in chronic renal failure: reversal after transplantation. *J Clin Endocrinol Metab* 1979;48:101–107.
13. Kaufman FR, Hogut MD, Donnell GN, et al. Hypergonadotropic hypogonadism in female patients with galactosemia. *N Engl J Med* 1981;304:994–998.
14. De Sanctis V, Vullo C, Katz M, et al. Hypothalamic-pituitary-gonadal axis in thalassemic patients with secondary amenorrhea. *Obstet Gynecol* 1988;72:643–647.
15. Nattero L. Menstrual headaches. *Adv Neurol* 1982;33:215–226.
16. Stain GS. Headaches in the first postpartum week and their relationship to migraine. *Headaches* 1981;21:201–205.
17. Kaiser HJ, Meienberg O. Deterioration or onset of migraine under oestrogen replacement therapy in the menopause. *J Neurol* 1993;240:195–196.
18. Fettes I. Migraine in the menopause. *Neurology* 1999;53(suppl 1):29–33.
19. Silberstein SD. The role of sex hormone in headaches. *Neurology* 1992;42(suppl 2):37–42.
20. Bartleson JD. Treatment of migraine headaches. *Mayo Clin Proc* 1999;74:702–708.
21. Van den Bergh V, Amery WK, Waelkens J. Trigger factors in migraine: a study conducted by the Belgian Migraine Society. *Headache* 1987;27:191–196.
22. Silberstein SD, Merriam GR. Estrogens, progestins, and headaches. *Neurology* 1991;41:786–793.
23. Boyle CA. Management of menstrual migraine. *Neurology* 1999;53(suppl 1):14–18.
24. Case AM, Reid RL. Effect of the menstrual cycle on medical disorders. *Arch Intern Med* 1998;158:1405–1412.
25. Silberstein SD. Menstrual migraine. *J Womens Health Gend Based Med* 1999;8:919–931.
26. Dawson B, Horobin G, Illsley R, et al. A survey of child hood asthma in Aberdeen. *Lancet* 1969;1:827–830.
27. Gibbs CJ, Counts II, Lock R, et al. Premenstrual exacerbation of asthma. *Thorax* 1984;39:833–836.
28. Ensom MH, Chong E, Carter D. Premenstrual symptoms in women with premenstrual asthma. *Pharmacotherapy* 1999;19:374–382.
29. Derimanov GS, Oppenheimer J. Exacerbation of premenstrual asthma caused by an oral contraceptive. *Ann Allergy Asthma Immunol* 1998;81:243–246.
30. Boggess KA, Williamson, Homm RJ. Influence of the menstrual cycle on systemic disease. *Obstet Gynecol Clin North Am* 1990;17:321–342.
31. Murray RD, New JP, Barber PV, et al. Gonadotrophin-releasing hormone analogues: a novel treatment for premenstrual asthma. *Eur Respir J* 1999;14:966–967.
32. Dolby AE. Recurrent Mikulicz's oral aphthae: their relationship to the menstrual cycle. *Br Dent J* 1968;124:359–360.
33. Ferguson MM, McKay Hart D, Lindsay R, et al. Progesterone therapy for menstrually related aphthae. *Int J Oral Surg* 1978;7:463–470.
34. Rattan J, Schneider M, Arber N, et al. Sucralfate suspension as a treatment of recurrent aphthous stomatitis. *J Intern Med* 1994;236:341–343.
35. Andrews VH, Hall HR. The effect of relaxation/imagery training on recurrent aphthous stomatitis: a preliminary study. *Psychosom Med* 1990;52:526–535.
36. Widom B, Diamond MP, Simonson DC. Alternations in glucose metabolism during menstrual cycle in women with IDDM. *Diabetes Care* 1992;15:213–220.
37. Letterie GS, Fredlund PN. Catamenial insulin reactions treated with a long-acting gonadotropin-releasing hormone agonist. *Arch Intern Med* 1994;154:1868–1870.
38. Latman NS. Relation of menstrual cycle phase to symptoms of rheumatoid arthritis. *Am J Med* 1983;74:957–960.
39. Rudge SR, Kowanko IC, Drury PL. Menstrual cyclicity of finger joint size and grip strength in patients with rheumatoid arthritis. *Ann Rheum Dis* 1983;42:425–430.
40. Mueller MN, Kappas A. Sex hormone in experimental and human arthritis. *Proc Inst Med Chicago* 1963;24:303–304.
41. Wingrave SJ, Kay CR. Reduction in incidence of rheumatoid arthritis associated with oral contraceptives. *Lancet* 1978;1:569–571.
42. Da Silva JAP, Hall GM. The effects of gender and sex hormones on the outcome in rheumatoid arthritis. *Clin Rheumatol* 1992;6;196–219.
43. Persellin RH. The effect of pregnancy on rheumatoid arthritis. *Bull Rheum Dis* 1977;27:922–927.
44. Duncan S, Read CL, Brodie MJ. How common is catamenial epilepsy? *Epilepsia* 1993;34:827–831.
45. Zahn C. Catamenial epilepsy: clinical aspects. *Neurology* 1999;53(suppl 1):34–37.

46. Herzog AG, Klein P, Ransil BJ. Three patterns of catamenial epilepsy. *Epilepsia* 1997;38:1082–1088.
47. Zimmerman AW. Hormones and epilepsy. *Neurol Clin* 1986;4: 853–861.
48. Vijayan N, Vijayan VK, Dreyfus PM. Acetylcholinesterase activity and menstrual remission in myasthenia gravis. *J Neurol Neurosurg Psychiatry* 1977;40:1060–1065.
49. Schuster M. Diagnostic evaluation of IBS. *Gastroenterol Clin North Am* 1991;20:269–278.
50. Wood JD. Efficacy of leuprolide in treatment of the irritable bowel syndrome. *Dig Dis Sci* 1994;39:1153–1154.
51. Maggs WJ, Pescovitz OH, Metcalfe D, et al. Progesterone sensitivity as a cause of recurrent anaphylaxis. *N Engl J Med* 1984; 311:1236–1238.
52. Basomba A, Guerrero M, Camos A, et al. Grave anaphylactic-like reaction in the course of menstruation. *Allergy* 1987;42: 477–479.
53. Slater JE, Raphael G, Cutler GB Jr, et al. Recurrent anaphylaxis in menstruating women: treatment with a luteinizing hormone-releasing hormone agonist [SC] a preliminary report. *Obstet Gynecol* 1987;70:542–546.
54. Burstein M, Rubinow A, Shalit M. Cyclic anaphylaxis associated with menstruation. *Ann Allergy* 1991;66:36–38.
55. Wolf RE, Fudenberg HH, Welch TM, et al. Treatment of Behçet's syndrome with transfer factor. *JAMA* 1977;238: 869–871.
56. Hart R. Autoimmune progesterone dermatitis. *Arch Dermatol* 1977;113;426–429.
57. Jones WN, Gordon VH. Auto-immune progesterone eczema. *Arch Dermatol* 1969;169:57–59.
58. Mabray CR, Burditt ML, Martin TL, et al. Treatment of common gynecologic-endocrinologic symptoms by allergy management procedures. *Obstet Gynecol* 1982;59:560–564.
59. Warine RP, Cunliffe WJ, Greaves MW, et al. Recurrent angioedema: familial and estrogen-induced. *Br J Dermatol* 1986; 115:731–734.
60. Sheffer AL, Fearon DT, Austen KF. Clinical and biochemical effects of stanozolol therapy for hereditary angioedema. *J Allergy Immunol* 1981;68:181–187.
61. Perlroth MG. The porphyrias. In: Rubenstein E, Federman DD, eds. *Scientific American medicine.* New York: Scientific American, 1976.
62. Anderson KE, Spitz IM, Sassa S, et al. Prevention of cyclical attacks of acute intermittent porphyria with a long-acting agonist of luteinizing hormone-releasing hormone. *N Engl J Med* 1984;311:643–645.
63. Anderson KE, Spitz IM, Bardin CW, et al. A gonadotropin releasing hormone analogue prevents cyclical attacks of porphyria. *Arch Intern Med* 1990;150:1469–1474.
64. Yamamori I, Asai M, Tanaka F, et al. Prevention of premenstrual exacerbation of hereditary coproporphyria by gonadotropin-releasing hormone analogue. *Intern Med* 1999;38:365–368.

4

GENETIC DISORDERS AND CONGENITAL MALFORMATION IN GYNECOLOGY

EDUCATIONAL OBJECTIVES

Medical Students *APGO Objective*	*Residents in Obstetrics/Gynecology* *CREOG Objective*	*Practitioners* *ACOG Recommendation*
No specific recommendation	No specific recommendation	No specific recommendation

This chapter is limited to the gynecologic genetic disorder and congenital developmental abnormalities with emphasis on pragmatic aspects; therefore, basic genetic terms and its understanding are essential. In 1956, 46 human chromosomes were identified (1). Since that time, significant progress in human genetics has been made. Some basic terminology commonly used in describing gynecologic genetic disorders is presented below (2):

- *Genotype* is the individual genetic makeup.
- *Phenotype* is the clinical expression of results of interaction between genotype and environmental factors (expression of a gene or genes).
- *Allele* is an alternative form of a gene (a DNA sequence, at a given locus).
- *Genetic locus* is a precise location on a chromosome.
- *Homozygous* refers to identical alleles at the locus (an individual is homozygous).
- *Heterozygous* refers to different alleles at the locus (an individual is heterozygous).
- *Autosomal trait* is a phenotype expression of heterozygotes (one copy of a mutant allele and one normal copy) by genes on one of the 22 pairs of nonsex chromosomes (autosomes).
- *Recessive trait* is a phenotype expression of homozygotes for the mutant allele (a double dose of abnormal genes).
- *X-linked trait* (not sex-linked) is a phenotype expression by a mutant gene on the X chromosome.
- *Compound heterozygotes* refers to two different alleles at a given locus.
- *Double heterozygotes* refers to one allele at two different loci.
- *Mutation* is a change in the genetic material.
- *Euploid* is the number of chromosomes in a haploid gamete (N).
- *Diploid* is the number of chromosomes in a somatic cell (2N).
- *Aneuploid* is any number of chromosomes that are non-euploid (i.e., monosomy or trisomy).
- *Meiosis* is a process by which recombination of gene location and reduction from the diploid (2N) number of chromosomes to the haploid number of chromosome (N) in a gametal cell occur.

Meiosis is categorized as follows:

In reduction division–I, a DNA replica is developed and two identical chromatids are fused at the centromere, which will remain intact in this phase until ovulation. This stage may last for several years.

Reduction division–II is triggered by fertilization, and no DNA synthesis is involved. Chromosomal disjunction produces 23 chromosome pairs: one set of 23 chromosomes is transmitted to the second polar body, and the other set remains in the cell.

Mitosis is a process by which nuclear DNA is copied and transmitted to an offspring cell. It is executed in four phases:

- Prophase
    Arrangement of paired chromosomes
    Vanishing of nuclear membrane
    Emergence of the achromatic spindle
    Creation of polar bodies
- Metaphase
    Arrangement of chromosomes in the equatorial plane of the spindle to form monaster
    Division of chromosomes in halves
- Anaphase
    Formation of the diaster
- Telophase
    Formation of two daughter cells

Upon completion of the meiotic process, each daughter nucleus receives 23 chromosomes (haploid number), half the number of chromosomes.

A chromosome is a structure within the animal cell's nucleus containing double-stranded DNA, which contains 1,000 to 2,000 genes and five subtypes of the histones (proteins). The double-stranded DNA is coiled and binds by histones, creating subunits called nucleosomes, which are essential in the condensation process of chromosomes and participate in gene transcription. DNA is responsible for transmitting genetic information (2).

Karyotyping (or karyotype analysis) is a clinical study determining the number and structure of chromosomes. It can be done from any nucleated human cell. Most commonly it is performed from a peripheral blood lymphocyte. A lymphocyte culture is arrested in the metaphase of mitosis. The results present 23 pairs of chromosomes systematically arranged from the largest to the smallest and position centromere pair of chromosomes. A lymphocyte culture is usually aligned and depicted in an organized form, allowing a clinical interpretation. A chromosome is recognized by its size, shape, and specific banding characteristics. The centromere is the point where two sister chromatids are connected and evaluation of the short arm (named p) and long arm named (q) is performed. Based on the distance of chromosome arms from a centromere, three categories are recognized: metacentric (equal length from a centromere), submetacentric (short length from a

centromere), acrocentric (absent or significantly decreased length of short arms) (Fig. 4.1). Chromosomal aberration can be identified from the number of chromosomes or the structure of a chromosome and accordingly is analyzed as follows (2).

A numerical chromosomal abnormality results in some form of aneuploidy or polyploidy and is a consequence of nondisjunction (failure of a chromosome to split during the meiotic or mitotic process).

Structural abnormality may affect a single chromosome, with an aberration such as a deletion, duplication of part of a chromosome, pericentricity (involving the centromere), paracentricity (not involving centromere), or inversion. Many chromosomes also may be affected by structural defects, such as insertion (genetic material from one chromosome into another), translocation [reciprocal translocation (exchange of chromosomal material) or Robertsonian translocation (centric fusion)]. A carrier of translocation is not clinically affected, albeit offspring may display clinical abnormalities as a result of unbalanced chromosomes.

SEX CHROMOSOMES

In gynecologic genetic disorders, particular interest is focused on sex chromosomes. The X and Y chromosomes are responsible for many genetic disorders. Sexual differentiation into female or male is determined by the presence or

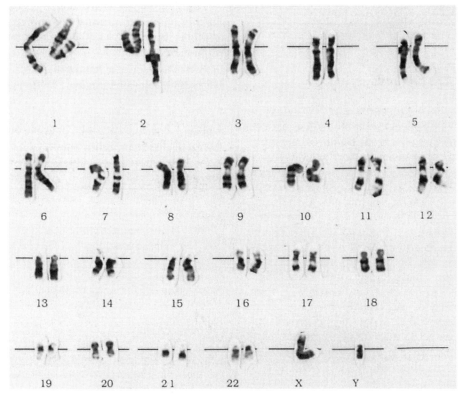

FIGURE 4.1. Normal human karyotype (46,XY).

absence of the Y chromosome. The sexual differential process evolves in subsequent stages (2).

From the time of conception until about 4 weeks of human embryonic life, the gonad remains in the undifferentiated stage. At 6 to 7 weeks, the undifferentiated gonad initiates sexual differentiation. In the absence of a Y chromosome, an XX female gonad will develop. When a Y chromosome is present, the short arm contains a DNA sequence, recognized as the sex-determining region of Y (SRY), which induces the synthesis of a testicular-determining factor responsible for development of the testes. The H-Y antigen is located on the short arm and is accountable for development of seminiferous tubules within the testes. The gonad will be converted into the testes, which produce testosterone and Müllerian inhibitory factor (MIF), or else is recognized as antimüllerian hormone (AMH), which is produced in the Sertoli cells. Testosterone stimulates the Wolffian duct to grow, and MIF is responsible for regression of the müllerian duct structure (the fallopian tubes, uterus, and the upper one third of the vagina). Failure to produce MIF results in the development of müllerian duct structures despite the presence of an XY karyotype. Wolffian duct development will lead to internal male structures (vas deferens, epididymis, and seminal vesicles). Testosterone by itself is incapable of masculinizing the urogenital sinus. Locally, testosterone is converted to dihydrotestosterone in the presence of 5-alpha-reductase. Dihydrotestosterone induces virilization, leading to penis and scrotum development. Therefore, a Y chromosome is responsible for sex determination.

SEX CHROMOSOME ABERRATION

Gonadal dysgenesis refers to sex chromosome abnormalities (45,X, 46,XX, or 46,XY karyotype, and mosaicism) by which ovarian tissue is replaced with streak gonads (connective tissue depraved germ cells). A 45,X karyotype is often diagnosed (40%) among gonadal dysgenesis (3). The chromosomal X short arm is responsible for somatic changes, and the long arm provides information for ovarian development (2).

Turner syndrome or monosomy X (Bonnevie-Ullrich syndrome) was first described in 1938 (4) and usually refers to young women with somatic changes attributed to this syndrome and sexual infantilism. Ullrich gave a similar description of the syndrome in 1930. These two conditions are distinguished by a lack of sexual infantilism in pediatric patients, as described by Ullrich (4). In this syndrome a second X chromosome is absent, leading to follicular maturation failure and massive oocyte atresia.

Definition

A female phenotype is associated with sexual infantilism (immaturity) and gonadal dysgenesis. The gonads of a patient with Turner syndrome, contain oocytes during fetal life; however, they vanish by the age of 2 years. In a healthy woman, oocytes vanish during menopause; in patients with Turner syndrome, oocytes disappear before menarche (menopause occurs before menarche) (2).

Incidence

Turner syndrome occurs in about 1 in 5,000 live births or 1 in 2,500 female births (6).

Classification

Turner syndrome (young women)
Bonnevie-Ullrich syndrome (female pediatric patients)

Etiology

Sex chromosome aberration.

Diagnosis

A medical history should elicit the following information:

- Absent secondary sex characteristics (insufficient estrogen/androgen ovarian production)
- No puberty changes
- Primary amenorrhea
- Short stature observed at birth
- Reported somatic abnormalities
- Infertility

Physical Examination

A general physical examination may reveal numerous somatic abnormalities that may correspond to a clinical picture of Turner syndrome. In general, the uterus, fallopian tubes, vagina, and female external genitalia are not affected directly by gonadal dysgenesis, although lack of sex hormonal stimulation will not induce transformation to a mature state. The only undeveloped genital organs are the ovaries; therefore, a hypoestrogenic clinical picture dominates. Lack of appropriate sex hormone concentration leads to an infantile appearance of the external genitalia, no menses, lack of breast development, and decreased or absent pubic and axillary hair. Occasionally, elevated blood pressure of idiopathic origin and diabetes mellitus may be present. Clinical findings in Turner syndrome are presented in Table 4.1.

Pelvic examination confirms the presence of infantile external female genitalia and the underdeveloped vagina with flat fornices, hypoplastic cervix, and uterus. Ovaries are not palpable bilaterally.

Laboratory studies should specifically target the dominant symptomatology to verify presumptive clinical diagnosis. Pertinent tests are listed in Table 4.2.

Other Studies

- Ultrasonography demonstrates severe hypoplastic gonads with a few oocytes present, or undetected gonads
- Magnetic resonance imaging (MRI) may help document streak gonads or severe hypoplastic gonads

TABLE 4.1. CLINICAL CHARACTERISTIC (STIGMATA) OF TURNER SYNDROME ABNORMALITIES

Organ	Manifestation
Phenotype	Female
Stature	Short (≤150 cm or ≤60 inches), often from birth
Face	Narrow maxilla and small mandible bones
Mouth	Straight lower lip and curve upper lip, imitating sharklike appearance
Eyes	Epicanthic folds
Neck	Short, webbing of the posterior neck (50%), low posterior hairline
Chest	Shieldlike shape (>80%)
Breast	Underdeveloped with pale areolae and widely spaced
Heart	Coarctation of the aorta (about 35%)
Upper extremities	Elbow abnormality such as cubitus valgus; short fifth finger

Differential Diagnosis

Other forms of gonadal dysgenesis

Conventional Therapy

■ Upon 45,X/46,XY karyotype determination, gonadectomy is recommended due to the increased risk of developing bilateral gonadoblastoma or dysgerminoma or even embryonal carcinoma (7) [malignant transformation is a little lower (15%–30%) than in Swyer syndrome with a 46,XY karyotype]. Gonadectomy can be executed either via a classic laparotomy approach or via a laparoscopic approach (8). With the availability of assisted reproductive technology today, the uterus and fallopian tubes should be preserved because pregnancy and live birth have been achieved via ovum donation, *in vitro* fertilization, and

embryo transfer (IVF-ET). Exogenous hormonal therapy is required and is coordinated with IVF-ET (9–11).

Turner syndrome or Bonnevie-Ullrich syndrome in each karyotypic form requires the following therapeutic consideration. Stimulation of growth in a pediatric group of patients is recommended, although the optimal timing of commencing long-term growth hormone therapy must be established. Growth retardation begins *in utero* and continues throughout childhood, resulting in a short adult stature (average 143 cm) (12). The growth range has been increased by 10.6 to 17.2 cm. However, when growth hormone therapy (50 μg/kg per day) was initiated late (12.9 ± 2.2 years) the final height increased by only 3.7 to 4.7 cm (13). It is necessary to bear in mind that exogenous estrogens influence both growth and maturation of the bone epiphyseal plates. Teenagers with this syndrome who have received growth hormone treatment did

TABLE 4.2. SPECIFIC LABORATORY TESTS FOR TURNER SYNDROME

Test	Confirmatory Results
Buccal mucosal cells	Chromatin (Barr body) negative
Karyotype	45,X (monosomic aberration for the X chromosome >50%)
	46,XX (46 X structural abnormal X such as isochromosome-X[46,X,i(Xq)]; deletion of portion of the X chromosome [46,XXp–]; or ring chromosome; and chromatin-positive (Barr body present; in about 15% among Turner syndrome patients)
	Mosaicism (nondisjunction in a mitosis phase after fertilization and occurs in about 15% of Turner syndrome cases; in mosaicism with a normal 46,XX cell line, puberty, menarche, menses, and pregnancy can occur)
	45,X/46,XX or
	45,X/46,XY, or
	45,X/46,X, abnormal X, or
	45,X/47,XXX, or
	45,X/46,XX/47,XXX
Roentgenograms	Dysplasia of long bones and fourth and fifth metacarpals (positive metacarpal sign may be present)
	Hypoplasia of sacral wings and lateral ends of clavicles can be identified.
Ultrasonography	May determine the hypoplastic cervix and uterus and the absence of ovaries.

Reprinted from Gelehrter TD, Collins FS, Ginsburg D. *Principles of medical genetics,* 2nd ed. Baltimore: Williams & Wilkins, 1998; with permission.

not lose bone mineral density; therefore, it is recommended that estrogen therapy not be initiated until after growth hormone therapy (14). The single most important factor in determining height gain is the number of years of growth hormone therapy prior to beginning estrogen therapy. A randomized, controlled study revealed that when estrogen therapy was given at the age of 15 years, the girls were significantly taller as adults, as compared with commencing estrogen at the age of 12 years (15).

Stimulation of maturation of external and internal genital organs and breast with hormonal therapy can occur, including endometrial bleeding. Essentially, sequential estrogen-progesterone hormonal replacement therapy is needed. Equivalent or conjugated equine estrogen at a dose of 0.625 mg continuously with last 12 days micronized natural progesterone 200 mg or medroxyprogesterone 10 mg or other progestin is recommended. Hormone replacement therapy is discussed in more detail in Chapter 12.

Prevention of illnesses associated with hypoestrogenism, such as osteoporosis and coronary artery disease, is advocated. A combination of estrogen/progesterone replacement therapy with calcium and vitamin D supplementation is recommended.

Assisted reproduction as it relates to Turner syndrome falls into two categories:

■ Oocyte cryopreservation for later IVF-ET is suggested. If the early diagnosis of gonadal dysgenesis is established, full-thickness (antimesenteric to mesenteric) ovarian slice biopsy to retrieve ovarian tissue containing an oocyte is worthwhile in selected patients, if performed in a timely fashion. The presence of an oocyte should be determined before surgery. Ovarian biopsy can be executed via laparotomy or via a laparoscopic approach (16).

■ Ovum donation and IVF-ET requires exogenous hormonal treatment before IVF-ET and for the initial 100 days of *in utero* pregnancy (10,11). The pregnancy rate per transfer in Turner syndrome patients with the 45,X karyotype is about 30% and approximately 25% in patients with the 46,XX karyotype (9).

Complementary Therapy

The mean verbal IQ in Turner syndrome patients is within normal limits; however, the mean performance IQ is approximately 10 points below average (17). Hence, complementary therapy may assist in improving specific space/form perception and visual-motor deficiency. Through specially designed programs, such skill enhancement can be achieved.

Alternative Therapy

No published data are available addressing Turner syndrome management with a complementary alternative approach. Natural hormonal replacement therapy can be recommended in the same manner as for menopause or premature ovarian failure; however, there are no published data to support such an approach. Homeopathic-specific therapy recommendations have not been addressed. The same principals and remedies can be applied as for menopause.

OTHER FORM OF GONADAL DYSGENESIS
Swyer Syndrome (46,XY)

Swyer syndrome presents with a female phenotype and a male 46,XY karyotype. Patients may or may not demonstrate Turner syndrome somatic characteristics (Turner stigmata) (18), which are listed in Table 4.1. This syndrome may correspond clinically and biochemically to abnormalities associated with a 46,XX karyotype of gonadal dysgenesis. Potential transformation (20%–30%) of intraabdominal testicular tissue to bilateral gonadoblastoma, dysgerminoma, or embryonal carcinoma calls for surgical removal of streak gonads as early in life as possible [HY antigen positivity is often present in association with these malignancies (19)]. It also has been pointed out that multiple family members have been affected by XY chromosomal aberration (20). In partial gonadal dysgenesis, some patients may demonstrate external genitalia masculinization.

Diagnosis

Pertinent medical history usually refers to delayed pubertal development.

General physical examination identifies no breast development or minimal enlargement. Occasionally, Turner syndrome stigmata are present (Table 4.1).

Pelvic examination may document external genitalia masculinization with a different degree of clitoromegaly. Hypoplastic genitalia (external genitalia, the vagina, cervix, and the uterus) are present.

Laboratory tests may reveal (a) elevated serum gonadotropins, (b) low serum estrogen levels, (c) normal serum androgen levels, and (d) 46,XY karyotype.

Other Studies

■ Ultrasonography demonstrates severe hypoplastic gonads with a few oocytes present, or undetected gonads.

■ Magnetic resonance imaging (MRI) may document streak gonads or severe hypoplastic gonads

Differential Diagnosis

Other forms of gonadal dysgenesis

Conventional Therapy

Conventional therapy can be instituted in the following steps:

1. Surgical extirpation of gonads is advised as early in life as possible, with preservation of the uterus and fallopian tubes.
2. Estrogen/progesterone sequential therapy is prescribed in a mode similar to that used to treat Turner syndrome.
3. Ovum donation and IVF-ET with exogenous hormonal treatment before and for the initial 100 days of *in utero* pregnancy. It has been reported that the pregnancy rate per embryo transfer was approximately 75% for a patient with a 46,XY karyotype (9).

Complementary and Alternative Therapies

There are no specific data available in reference to complementary and alternative therapies for this genetic abnormality, but natural hormonal therapy can be suggested.

Familial Gonadal Dysgenesis (46,XX)

Familial gonadal dysgenesis is a female phenotype with a normal female 46,XX karyotype. It may result either from cytogenetically invisible sex chromosome rearrangement or gene mutation (17).

Pertinent Medical History

- Deafness is often reported.
- Short stature is observed in some patients, but it is not a distinct feature in familial gonadal dysgenesis (21).

General Physical Examination

- Normal stature (mean height 165 cm or 66 inches)
- No Turner syndrome stigmata present
- Absence of secondary sex characteristics

Pelvic examination (21) is similar to that described for patients with gonadal dysgenesis associated with abnormal karyotypes.

Laboratory

- Endocrine profile: elevated gonadotropin, hypoestrogenism, normal low or low level of androgens
- 46,XX karyotype (21)

Other Studies

- Ultrasonography demonstrates severe hypoplastic gonads with absent or few oocytes present, or undetected gonads.

- MRI may document streak gonads, or severe hypoplastic gonads with or without oocytes present.

Conventional Therapy

A therapeutic approach similar to that used for other forms of gonadal dysgenesis is used.

Complementary and Alternative Therapy

There are no specific data available for this genetic abnormality.

Mosaicism (Mixed Gonadal Dysgenesis)

Mosaicism occurs in an individual with two cell lines where one line is 45,X and the second line is 46,XX, 46,XY, or 47,XXX. Mosaicism may incorporate a structural abnormality on either chromosome X or chromosome Y. Approximately 50% of patients with Turner syndrome have a mosaic pattern of chromosomal aberration (6). Diagnosis of and therapy for mosaic conditions are similar to those presented above.

The clinically recognizable conditions are described as follows. Individuals with the 45,X/46,XX cell lines reach normal adult height in about 75% of patients; Turner syndrome stigmata occur less frequently. Secondary sex characteristics develop in about 18%; among them, 12% report menses (approximately 3% of patients with a 45,X karyotype experience menses) (21). Other forms of mosaicism include 46,X/47,XXX and 45,X/46,XX/47,XXX, but these variations occur infrequently.

HERMAPHRODITISM

Hermaphroditism occurs in an individual with both genders' external genitalia (ambiguous external genitalia).

Classification

True hermaphroditism is the presence of both gonadal tissues (ovarian and testicular tissue) and ambiguous external genitalia; the majority of patients present with a normal female 46,XX karyotype, and a minority have both the XX and XY sex chromosomes.

Female pseudohermaphroditism is characterized by the presence of ovaries, masculinization of the female external genitalia, and a female 46,XX karyotype.

Male pseudohermaphroditism is defined as the presence of testes, ambiguous external genitalia, a male 46,XY karyotype, and wolffian derivatives (vasa differentia, seminal vesicles, epididymides).

Etiology

True hermaphroditism is caused by either translocation of the Y chromosome to autosomal genes expressing sex reversal or fusion between two zygotes (chimerism) (22). Ovaries and testes may be present as two separate organs or as one organ (ovotestes) in which both ovarian and testicular tissues are harbored.

Female pseudohermaphroditism may result from endogenous or exogenous androgen exposure. The endogenous excess androgen synthesis can be associated with adrenogenital syndrome or congenital adrenal hyperplasia (genetically transmitted in an autosomal-recessive mode), which may result from multiple congenital enzyme deficiencies responsible for cholesterol pathway transformation to cortisol. Clinically, 21-hydroxylase with or without sodium wasting, 11-beta-hydroxylase, and 3-beta-ol-dyhydrogenase [affecting only dehydroepiandrosterone (DHEA), a weak androgen] are significant contributors to this syndrome, and in only about 5% of patients is congenital adrenal hyperplasia (CAH) a cause of female pseudohermaphroditism (23). Adrenal cortisol synthesis is reduced, triggering increased adrenocorticotropic hormone (ACTH) secretion that cannot be inhibited through a negative feedback mechanism due to lack of the ability of adrenal gland cortisol synthesis. By this mechanism, elevated ACTH levels stimulate to synthesize steroid precursors for excess androgen production. Adrenal gland function begins at 8 to 9 weeks' gestation. From that time, a fetus *in utero* is exposed to excess androgen. Virilization of sensitive tissue of external genitalia results in expression of the genital ambiguity. Because neither ovaries nor müllerian ducts are androgen dependent, they proceed with their natural development.

Maternal administration of testosterone, norethindrone, norethindrone acetate, or other synthetic progestins during pregnancy may induce female fetal virilization *in utero* (24,25). Maternal androgen-secreting tumors such as luteoma of pregnancy, arrhenoblastoma, Krukenberg tumor, or Leydig cell tumor during pregnancy can virilize a female fetus (26,27).

Male pseudohermaphroditism is characterized either by complete testicular feminization syndrome (also known as androgen insensitivity syndrome) or partial testicular feminization syndrome (Reifenstein syndrome). Both of these entities involve a male 46,XY karyotype, with testes located intraabdominally or in the inguinal canal or labioscrotal fusion. Lack of pubertal virilization is present. This unnatural location of the testes may predispose to neoplastic malignant transformation (testicular carcinomas). Testicular carcinomas in this syndrome usually occur in the second or third decade of life and occur in 5% of patients (28). It is believed that this syndrome is caused by end-organ androgen insensitivity (the absence of functional receptors) with normal levels of serum testosterone. Complete testicular feminization syndrome is an X chromosome recessive

inherited condition (29). The difference between these two syndromes is in the extent of mesonephrotic development of the structures (wolffian differentiation).

Partial testicular feminization syndrome (Reifenstein syndrome) is inherited in the X-linked recessive mode and presents as male ambiguous external genitalia (phallic enlargement and partial labioscrotal fusion) at birth; at puberty, female secondary sex characteristics developed. Male pseudohermaphroditism also may be caused by 5-alpha-reductase deficiency.

Diagnosis

True hermaphroditism diagnosis is reached as follows:

- A pertinent medical history of ambiguous external genitalia with different degrees of virilization is reported. Some patients may report the presence of menses.
- General physical examination may reveal the presence of secondary sex characteristics with ambiguous external genitalia in some patients. When breast development is present, there is enough ovarian tissue to produce estrogens. Short adult stature is usually observed.
- Pelvic examination may show ambiguous external genitalia. The uterus, fallopian tubes, ovaries (fallopian tubes and ovaries can be palpated as one adnexal unit), and upper vagina are usually present (paramesonephrotic origin); when the uterus is absent, it may indicate the presence of ovotestes or testes. The presence of external genitalia demonstrates labioscrotal fusion, displacement of the urethral orifice (imitating a male location), scrotal hyperpigmentation (significant diagnostic meaning in 21- or 11-beta-hydroxylase deficiency), and clitoromegaly. If the diagnosis is missed at birth, pubic hair distribution may occur at about 2 years of age. Wolffian derivatives or mesonephric derivatives (vasa differentia, seminal vesicles, epididymides) are usually not identified.

To establish a diagnosis of true hermaphroditism, ruling out female pseudohermaphroditism is essential.

Laboratory

A 46,XX karyotype and other XY or XX cell lines are present.

FEMALE PSEUDOHERMAPHRODITISM

21-Hydroxylase deficiency without sodium wasting can be diagnosed by establishing (a) virilization of female external genitalia and (b) occasional sodium wasting. The clinical characteristics of 21-hydroxylase deficiency with sodium wasting are the same.

Laboratory

- Increased serum androgen levels
- Elevated serum 17-alpha-hydroxyprogesterone, DHEA, and testosterone
- Increased 24-hour urine collection of 17-ketosteroids, pregnanetriol, and pregnanetriolone

MALE PSEUDOHERMAPHRODITISM

Pertinent medical history usually is consistent with pubertal feminization, primary amenorrhea, and ambiguous external genitalia. These patients demonstrate female psychosexual orientation and behavior.

General examination may reveal a female phenotype with long upper and lower extremities and large hands and feet. Well-developed breast tissues (ductal and glandular) and large breasts are present, but the areolas are poorly developed and pale. Axillary and pubic hair are absent or scant.

Pelvic examination shows the absence or scanty hair distribution and ambiguous external genitalia, as well as absence of the uterus, fallopian tubes, and the upper part of vagina (müllerian paramesonephrotic structures). The vagina ends blindly and is commonly shorter than normal—merely a dimple, or 1 to 2.2 cm long. Inguinal hernia is often present (in about 50%), and normal-sized testes reside in the hernial sac, testes are palpable in the inguinal canal, or labioscrotal fusion is present bilaterally. In some patients, testes are identified intraabdominally. Despite feminization, a patient with incomplete testicular feminization will present with clitoromegaly and labioscrotal fusion.

Laboratory results for both complete and incomplete androgen insensitivity syndromes are similar:

- Serum testosterone, DHEA, and androstenedione levels are elevated
- Serum follicle stimulating hormone is within normal limits or elevated; luteinizing hormone (LH) is elevated (abnormal gonadal–hypothalamic–pituitary feedback mechanism)
- High levels of serum estradiol
- 46,XY karyotype

Differential Diagnosis

A typical female phenotype with the absence of the uterus suggests the possibility of two other medical entities: testicular feminization syndrome and Mayer-Rokitansky-Küster-Hauser syndrome (müllerian agenesis).

Clinically distinguishing between these two conditions is relatively simple. Testicular feminization syndrome (androgen insensitivity syndrome) presents with the absence of pubic and axillary hair distribution and a 46,XY karyotype. In contrast, müllerian agenesis demonstrates the presence of pubic and axillary hair and a normal female 46,XX karyotype. In Reifenstein syndrome (incomplete androgen insensitivity syndrome), a female phenotypic spectrum is less accentuated than in complete androgen insensitivity syndrome.

Therapy

21-Hydroxylase Deficiencies

If the prenatal diagnosis establishes 21-hydroxylase deficiencies, oral maternal therapy with dexamethasone can be initiated, although this form of therapy is still considered experimental (23).

If the diagnosis is established prior to 2 years of age, surgical reconstruction should be undertaken before 4 years of age (30). Such timing assists an affected child in developing a female psychosexual orientation.

Upon reaching the diagnosis, cortisol treatment should be initiated to balance fluid and electrolytes.

Male Pseudohermaphroditism Therapy

In complete testicular feminization, due to the low malignancy risk prior to age 25 to 30 years, prophylactic gonadectomy (orchiectomy) should be performed shortly before that age to preserve hormonal synthesis and full development of feminization. Benign tubular adenomas (Pick adenomas) are frequent events, probably due to increased LH levels. After orchiectomy, hormonal replacement therapy is recommended (see Chapter 12).

Partial testicular feminization gender assignment may constitute a dilemma due to the ambiguity of external genitalia. When female gender is selected early, gonadectomy should be performed, and hormonal replacement therapy should be initiated at the anticipated beginning of puberty.

5-ALPHA-REDUCTASE DEFICIENCY

Due to a lack of 5-alpha-reductase, the penis, scrotum, and virilization fail to develop in an individual with a 46,XY karyotype and male internal genitalia. This medical entity is inherited as an autosomal-recessive disorder (31–33).

Diagnosis

Pelvic examination reveals female external genitalia, an enlarged phallus, and a blindly ending vagina. In some patients testes are palpable in the scrotum or the inguinal canal and others have testes located intraabdominally.

Laboratory

- High normal serum testosterone levels

- Normal or low serum dihydrotestosterone levels
- Elevated basal ratio testosterone/dihydrotestosterone in the postpubertal period
- Analysis of ratios of etiocholanolone to androsterone in urine is a confirmatory test

Therapy

If female gender is assigned at birth, the testes should be extirpated before puberty, followed by estrogen replacement therapy. Reconstructive external genitalia surgery should be performed at the time that will not profoundly affect development of psychosexual orientation.

CONGENITAL MALFORMATION IN GYNECOLOGY

In the absence of a Y chromosome, the undifferentiated gonad progresses to ovaries at 8 to 9 weeks' gestation, and in with lack of müllerian inhibitor, the müllerian duct is transformed into the uterus, fallopian tubes, cervix, and upper one third of the vagina. Without cloacal virilization, the urogenital sinus develops and connects the mesonephrotic ducts and bladder by creating the vestibule (female external genitalia, lower two thirds of the vagina).

Urogenital Sinus Congenital Malformations

Developmental abnormalities related to urogenital sinus congenital malformations most commonly seen in gynecologic practices fall into two categories.

Labia minora fusion results either from an inflammation (34) or from a developmental abnormality that occurs during the embryonic period (35,36). It has been documented that the majority of patients with inflammatory labia minora fusion experience concomitant urinary tract infections with positive urine cultures. Obtaining a urine culture and performing a sensitivity assay will assist in selection of the appropriate antibiotic and in clinical management of the inflammatory cause of the labia minora fusion (34). Congenital labia minora fusion is commonly first noted during puberty, when abnormal menses and dysmenorrhea are the dominant complaints. Physical examination, ultrasonography, intravenous pyelography, and laboratory tests are within normal limits. Surgical correction should be considered to prevent the development of symptoms associated with menarche and menses (36).

Imperforate hymen occurs in 1 in 2,000 girls. Mucus or menstrual flow accumulates behind the imperforate hymen and may cause mucocolpos or hematocolpos, respectively (37,38). In addition, distal mucocolpos and proximal hematocolpos may be present (39). At birth, the presence of mucocolpos may lead to diagnosis; nevertheless, the diagno-

sis is usually reached after puberty, when initial menstrual flow causes hematocolpos followed by retrograde menstruation with stretching of the uterine cavity (hematometrocolpos). The fallopian tubes cause not only cyclical abdominal distention, pain, and often urinary retention (40,41), but also bilateral hematosalpinx that may be responsible for signs and symptoms of acute abdomen. A ruptured hematosalpinx may create a life-threatening situation that requires surgical exploration of the abdominopelvic area (40).

Diagnosis

Pertinent medical history is characteristic for complaints of cyclic abdominopelvic pain at early puberty.

Pelvic examination may disclose the hymen bulging as the bluish membrane at the peritoneum. This classic sign is essentially diagnostic. In the absence of such a sign, however, rectal ultrasonography is a useful diagnostic tool in imperforate hymen (42).

Therapy

Therapy consists of making a cruciform or star-shaped hymenal incision. Caution should be exercised to avoid inadvertent injury to the urethral meatus or the Bartholin gland orifices (38).

Müllerian Duct Abnormalities

Müllerian duct (paramesonephric duct) abnormalities may clinically express as congenital anomalies of the vagina, uterus, and fallopian tubes.

Vaginal developmental abnormalities are observed in the various forms of pseudohermaphroditism. Here the consideration is given to the abnormal vaginal conditions in women with intact external female genitalia. Müllerian duct fusion occurs during embryologic development. Vaginal developmental abnormalities can be differentiated as follows.

Vaginal aplasia, or the congenital absence of the vagina (Mayer-Rokitansky-Küster-Hauser syndrome), is associated with paramesonephrotic duct aplasia (müllerian aplasia or failure of the müllerian ducts to develop) (43). In this condition, urinary tract abnormalities often coexist. The syndrome is characterized not only by the absence of the vagina but also by the fallopian tubes and uterus (rudimentary uterine horns are may be located on the pelvis side walls). The ovaries and their functions are preserved.

Incidence is about 1 in 4,000 female births, and among first-degree relatives it occurs in approximately 1% to 5% (44).

Diagnosis

Pertinent medical history includes primary amenorrhea with the inability to have vaginal sexual intercourse.

The general *physical examination* shows that after puberty a normal female phenotype with secondary sex characteristics is usually present.

Pelvic examination reveals that the vulva usually contains the short, blindly ending vagina. The uterus is absent, or rudimentary uterine horns are present and can be palpated bilaterally on the pelvic walls.

Laboratory

- Gonadotropins and sex hormones are within normal limits.
- Ultrasonography or MRI may be used to determine the extent of genital tract congenital anomalies and whether both kidneys are present. Rudimentary horns may contain functional endometrial tissues leading to cyclic hematometra and occasionally may cause cyclic pelvic pain. Leiomyomata may grow and create pelvic discomfort.
- Intravenous urography should be performed because urinary tract abnormalities are present up to 15% of patients (45).
- Radiography of the skeleton may document abnormalities of the hand, foot, spine, or other bones (46,47).

Therapy

Therapy generally falls into three categories.

Psychotherapy is essential to cope with this condition. It is devastating for a young woman to learn that she cannot have vaginal intercourse and cannot bear children. The feeling of femininity can be severely compromised, and profound depression with suicidal tendency may occur. The girl's parents also may require emotional support therapy. Familiarizing patients with therapeutic options, prospective marriage, and having a child (a patent's own oocyte can be used) through reproductive technology and surrogacy or adoption are very helpful parts of the management.

Conservative, not surgical, management involves creating a *de novo* vagina (nonsurgical vaginoplasty) by gradual dilatation and stretching of the vagina [Frank procedure (48)]. This is achieved via intermittent pressure with progressive increases in the width and length of vaginal dilators. Patient cooperation and compliance is essential. It has been reported that a vagina up to 85% functional can be created with no surgery (50).

Surgical management involves extirpation of the rudimentary horns, if they cause symptoms. Surgical vaginoplasty also should be offered to patients who failed nonsurgical management. Several surgical techniques have been developed that range from skin grafting through the parietal peritoneum, to the intestine (ileum, colon, cecum, or sigmoid colon) being used for forming a neovagina (50). When the intestine is used to line the neovaginal space, a laparotomy or laparoscopic approach can be applied (51).

Vaginal atresia is the reflection of the urogenital sinus not contributing to the development of the distal two thirds of the vaginal length. The upper one third of the vagina, and the cervix and corpus uterus may be well developed. Vaginal atresia occurs in about 10% to 20% of patients with absence of the vagina (49). This condition also can be associated with other anomalies.

Surgical correction consists of creation of a *de novo* vaginal canal that connects the upper part of the existing vagina.

Transverse Vaginal Septa

Transverse vaginal septa are the result of failure of vaginal canal formation by 20 weeks of fetal development and may present as complete or incomplete:

- The low location has a clinical course similar to that observed in imperforate hymen with hematocolpos formation. It is thinner than in a high location.
- The mid-location is situated at the junction of the lower third and upper two thirds of the vagina and is usually less than 1 cm thick (50).
- The high location is the most common transverse form of this condition. It usually is located at the junction of the lower two thirds and upper one third of the vagina. A high location of transverse septa limits menstrual flow collection in the upper vagina. Because the capacity of the upper vagina is small, retrograde menstruation not only predisposes to more severe and early occurrence of symptoms during menses, but also may result in pelvic endometriosis (50,51).

Diagnosis

Ultrasonography or MRI establishes the diagnosis and documentation of transverse septa.

Therapy

A reconstructive operation is essential because endometriosis may compromise fertility. When the vagina is constricted, excision of the septa with vaginal wall advancement and approximation of the ends may be necessary. Occasionally, postoperative application of vaginal dilators is recommended. It is important to remember that an incomplete septal excision may result in constrictive vaginal walls, and such an occurrence may have life-long consequences in sexual function, because it is very difficult to overcome this problem with repeated reconstructive surgery. An abdominal and transvaginal approach may be needed in such a location. Laparoscopy has been applied with good results (52). If vaginal stenosis is significant and the vaginal walls are not suitable for substantial advancement, vaginal dilatation immediately postsurgery may be the only option for a successful outcome. The location of transverse septa influences the fertility rate, even if reconstructive surgery creates a fully functional vagina [the pregnancy rate is about 25% for patients with an affected upper vagina and approximately 43% when the middle third is affected (53)].

Longitudinal vaginal septa occasionally cause symptoms such as dyspareunia or failure of penetration. It has been reported that longitudinal vaginal septa are associated with an autosomal-dominant syndrome expressed by urinary stress incontinence, longitudinal vaginal septa, and hand abnormalities (54).

Surgical intervention to completely remove the septum is indicated only when clinical symptomatology is present.

Congenital Cervical Abnormalities

A congenital cervical abnormality is a rare condition. Approximately 48% of patients have isolated congenital cervical atresia with a normal vagina; 52% of patients have either complete or partial vaginal atresia (55). The presence of a normal uterus and vagina with the absence of significant cervical hypoplasia is rare (50). This condition clinically manifests as:

- The presence of a fibrous cord with endocervical gland islands
- Cervical aplasia is the absence of cervical stroma

Diagnosis is based on clinical findings, such as the absence of the cervix with a normal vagina and uterine corpus or partial atresia (short, blindly ending vagina), or vaginal agenesis (absence of the vagina). Verification of clinical findings can be substantiated either by ultrasonography or MRI. Urinary tract abnormality should be excluded by intravenous pyelography.

Therapy is difficult and requires a surgical approach that can be categorized as follows:

- Hysterectomy or uterine fundus extirpation is the definitive therapy for this condition to relieve severe cyclic pelvic pain and avoid additional surgery (53). It is important to recognize the emotional aspect of hysterectomy, particularly in teenage girls. Such definitive surgery may leave profound psychological scars, particularly in reference to the aspect of decreased femininity (50,56,57).
- Hysterectomy can be accomplished via laparotomy, transvaginally, or by a laparoscopic approach (58).
- Uterovaginal anastomosis creates a fistula communication between the functioning endometrial cavity and the vagina with or without vaginoplasty. This type of procedure is indicated in patients associated with the complete congenital absence of the cervical stroma (55,59,61).
- Utero-cervico-vaginal cannulation is preserved for the patient with a fibrous cervical cord (59). This operation carries the risk for severe infection, sepsis, and death.
- Preservation of the uterus may sustain reproductive capacity, especially using assisted reproductive technology (50,62).

Congenital Uterine Anomalies

Uterine developmental abnormality during embryonic life results from müllerian faulty fusion or absorption.

Incidence

The prevalence of uterine anomalies is estimated to be approximately 0.04% to 0.13% in the general population; in women with a history of reproductive abnormalities, the prevalence is about 10% to 15% (63).

Classification

Congenital uterine anomalies have been classified by the American Fertility Society into the following categories (64).

Class I: Hypoplasia/Agenesis
The absence of the fallopian tubes, uterus, cervix, and vagina is associated with paramesonephrotic or müllerian duct aplasia. It may present clinically as the complete absence of the uterus or with only the presence of rudimentary uterine horns, no cervix, and no vagina. This medical condition is also known as Mayer-Rokitansky-Küster-Hauser syndrome. The clinical presentation and its management are described in the earlier section on vaginal agenesis.

Class II: Unicornuate Uterus
A unicornuate uterus (about 2%) is the result of failure of one of the müllerian ducts to develop, leading to half of a uterus with a single fallopian tube being connected, and with a functional endometrium present. A unicornuate uterus may be sufficient to maintain pregnancy to term in about 66%, but spontaneous abortion occurs in 34%, and premature delivery in 29% (45).

Infertility is not an issue with this condition, but first trimester spontaneous abortion (about 50%), second trimester abortion, stillbirth, and preterm delivery (about 15%) are associated with unicornuate uterus.

Urinary tract abnormalities, particularly ipsolateral renal agenesis, are encountered in this condition (about 70%).

If a nonfunctional symptomatic rudimentary uterine horn is present, extirpation should be performed. Prophylactic cervical cerclage may be helpful in pregnancy salvage.

Class III: Uterus Didelphys
Uterus didelphys is the duplication of the uterus that results from division of the paramesonephrotic ducts in the embryonic stage. In some cases, two separate uteruses, two cervices, and two fallopian tubes may develop. The complete failure of müllerian ducts to fuse results in uterus duplex didelphys (uterus duplex separatus), with one Fallopian tube connected to the upper segment of each uterus that

can function independently from each other and maintain a normal pregnancy with two independent genital tracts.

The clinical diagnosis is based on the presence of vaginal septa, two cervices, and occasionally two separate uteruses, which may be palpable on pelvic examination. Ultrasonography, MRI, or computed tomography may assist in reaching the diagnosis. Hysterosalpingography provides additional diagnostic information and documentation. Diagnostic laparoscopy is a useful tool for differentiation of the uterus didelphys from the bicollis unicornuate uterus.

Premature labor and delivery occur in approximately 40% of cases and constitute a great clinical challenge; some authorities recommend prophylactic cerclage. Strassman's unification procedure is the operation of choice; although, successful hysteroscopic metroplasty with resection of the dividing wall and preservation of both cervices has been successfully accomplished.

Class IV: Bicornuate Uterus
Bicornuate uterus or uterus duplex bicornis is the result of incomplete müllerian duct fusion, with the development of two uteruses and a mutual medial uterine wall. Two separate uterine cavities with independently functioning endometria and myometria are present. Two cervices and a single vagina develop. On each uterine corner, one fallopian tube is attached.

Bicornuate uterus or uterus bicornis unicollis is an anomaly of partial müllerian duct fusion and occurs at a higher level than uterine duplex bicornis. A single cervix and vagina complete the genital tract. One vagina and one cervix with two uterine cavities constitute this type of uterine anomaly.

Diagnosis

Hysterosalpingography, ultrasonography, MRI, or computed tomography may be used initially for screening; however, the definitive diagnosis is established via laparoscopy, which provides necessary information to set it apart from septate uterus or uterus didelphys. The most frequent clinical symptom is pregnancy loss.

Therapy may require metroplasty either by Strassman's unification procedure, Tompkins' procedure, or Jones' metroplasty, which is indicated for habitual abortions. Cervical cerclage is another therapeutic option and less invasive than metroplasty. Hysteroscopic metroplasty carries a greater risk of perforation than classic metroplasty.

Class V: Septate Uterus
In septate uterus or uterus septus, the uterine cavity is completely longitudinally divided into two compartments by a thin septum. This condition results from failure of septum absorption (the septum is present in all female fetuses and is absorbed at 18 weeks of gestation). To reach the diagnosis and distinguish septate uterus from bicornuate uterus, concomitant laparoscopy and hysteroscopy (or laparoscopy

alone when hysterosalpingography confirms the existence of two uterine compartments) may be used.

Uterus subseptus is a partial longitudinal division of the uterus to a lesser degree than septate uterus.

First trimester spontaneous abortion is associated with septate uterus (about 20%) and is the main clinical challenge.

Therapy

The therapy of choice is hysteroscopic sharp resection of the septum with scissors or contact laser. Transabdominal metroplasty, either by the Strassman, Tompkins, or Jones technique, yields about 80% success. Immediately following metroplasty, estrogen therapy is initiated at the equivalent dose of conjugated equine estrogen (2.5 mg twice daily for 1 month).

Class VI: Arcuate Uterus
A saddle-shaped uterus with a fundal uterine cavity indentation with or without changes of the uterine contour is an arcuate uterus. Such changes are considered as a variant of the normal uterus, and no therapy is required.

Class VII: Diethylstilbestrol-Related Uterine Abnormality
In utero, a female fetus exposed to diethylstilbestrol may produce a T-shaped uterus, which can compromise reproductive capacity due to a small uterine cavity and by a small uterus. Approximately 50% of women with this entity experience first trimester spontaneous abortion, and about 13% to 40% experience premature delivery.

Therapy in most instances involves bed rest and expectant management; surgical intervention is not successful.

REFERENCES

1. Kan YW, Dozy AM. Antenatal diagnosis of sickle-cell anemia by DNA analysis of amniotic-fluid cells. *Lancet* 1978;2:910–912.
2. Gelehrter TD, Collins FS, Ginsburg D. *Principles of medical genetics,* 2nd ed. Baltimore: Williams & Wilkins, 1998.
3. Simpson JL, Golbus MS. *Genetics in obstetrics and gynecology,* 2nd ed. Philadelphia: WB Saunders, 1992.
4. Turner HH. A syndrome of infantilism, congenital webbed neck and cubitus valgus. *Endocrinology* 1938;23:566–571.
5. Urlich P. Turner's syndrome and status Bonnevie-Urlich: a synthesis of animal phenogenetics and clinical observation on typical complex of developmental anomalies. *Am J Hum Genet* 1949;1:179–186.
6. Hook EB, Warburton D. The distribution of chromosomal genotypes associated with Turner syndrome: live birth prevalence rates and evidence for diminished fetal mortality and severity in genotypes associated with structural X abnormalities or mosaicism. *Ann Hum Genet* 1983;64:24–31.
7. Wachtel SS. *H-Y antigen and the biology of sex determination.* New York: Grune & Stratton, 1983.
8. Ostrzenski A. Homa T, Klimek M, et al. Laparoscopic gonadectomy in Swyer's syndrome. *Ginecol Pol* 1995;66(suppl):178–180.

9. Cornet D, Alvarez S, Antoine JM, et al. Pregnancies following ovum donation in gonadal dysgenesis. *Hum Reprod* 1990;5: 291–293.

10. Sauer MV, Lobo RA, Paulson RJ. Successful twin pregnancy after embryo donation to a patient with XY gonadal dysgenesis. *Am J Obstet Gynecol* 1989;161:380–381.

11. Bianco S, Agrifoglio V, Mannino F, et al. Successful pregnancy in a pure gonadal dysgenesis with 46,XY karyotype patient (Swyer's syndrome) following oocyte donation and hormonal treatment. *Acta Eur Fertil* 1992;23:37–38.

12. Lyon Al, Landau H, Chen M, et al. Growth curve for girls with Turner syndrome. *Arch Dis Child* 1985;60:932–937.

13. Van den Broeck J, Van Teunenbroek A, Hokken-Koelega A, et al. Efficacy of long-term growth hormone treatment in Turner's syndrome. European Study Group. *J Pediatr Endocrinol Metab* 1999; 12:673–676.

14. Park E, Bailey JD, Cowell CA. Growth and maturation of patients with Turner's syndrome. *Pediatr Res* 1983;17:1–7.

15. Chernausek SD, Attie KM. Role of oestrogen therapy in the management of short stature in Turner syndrome. *Acta Paediatr Suppl* 1999;88:130–132.

16. Ostrzenski A. A new, laparoscopic full-thickness slice ovarian biopsy (from antimesenteric to mesenteric margin). *J Gynecol Surg* 1995;11:109–112.

17. Nora JJ, Fraser FC, Bear J, et al. *Medical genetics: principles and practice.* Philadelphia: Lea & Febiger, 1994:59.

18. Berkowitz GD, Fechner PY, Zacur HW, et al. Clinical and pathological spectrum of 46,XY gonadal dysgenesis: its relevance to the understanding of sex differentiation. *Medicine (Baltimore)* 1991; 70:375–383.

19. Wachtel SS. *H-Y antigen and the biology of sex determination.* New York: Grune & Stratton, 1983.

20. German JL, Simpson JL, Chaganti RSK, et al. Genetically determined sex-reversal in 46, XY humans. *Science* 1978;202:53–56.

21. Simpson JL. Gonadal dysgenesis and sex chromosome abnormalities. Phenotypic/karyotypic correlations. In: Vallet H, Porter IH, eds. *Genetic mechanisms of sexual development.* New York: Academic, 1979:365.

22. de la Chapelle A. The complicated issue of human sex differentiation. *Am J Hum Genet* 1988;43:1–3.

23. Levine LS, Pang S. Prenatal diagnosis and treatment of congenital adrenal hyperplasia. In: Milunsky A, ed. *The fetus.* Baltimore: John Hopkins University Press, 1993.

24. Grumbach MM, Ducharme JR, Moloshok RE. On the fetal masculinizing action of certain oral progestins. *J Clin Endocrinol Metab* 1959;19:139–176.

25. Simpson JL. *Disorders of sexual differentiation. Etiology and clinical delineation.* New York: Academic, 1976.

26. Verhoeven ATM, Mastboom JL, Van Leusden HAIM, et al. Virilization in pregnancy coexisting with an (ovarian) mucinous cystadenoma: a case report and review of virilizing ovarian tumors in pregnancy. *Obstet Gynecol Surv* 1973;28:597–622.

27. Manganiell PD, Adams LV, Harris RD, et al. Virilization during pregnancy with spontaneous resolution postpartum: a case report and review of the English literature. *Obstet Gynecol* 1995;50: 404–410.

28. Simpson JL. Genetic control of sexual development. In: Teoh ES, Ratnman SS, Goh VHH, eds. *Advances in fertility and sterility: releasing hormones and genetics and immunology in human reproduction.* Lancaster, UK: Parthenon, 1987.

29. Shkolny DL, Brown TR, Punnett HH, et al. Characterization of alternative amino acid substitutions at arginine 830 of the androgen receptor that causes complete androgen insensitivity in three families. *Hum Mol Genet* 1995;4:515–521.

30. Henderen WH, Donahoe PK. Correction of congenital abnormalities of the vagina and perineum. *J Pediatr Surg* 1980;15:751–763.

31. Imperato-McGinley J, Peterson RE, Gautier T, et al. Androgens and the evaluation of male-gender identity among pseudohermaphrodites with 5-alpha-reductase deficiency. *N Engl J Med* 1979;300:1233–1237.

32. Mendez JP, Ulloa-Aguirre A, Imperato-McGinley J, et al. Male pseudohermaphroditism due to primary 5-alpha-reductase deficiency: variation in gender identity reversal in seven Mexican patients from five different pedigrees. *J Endocrinol Invest* 1995; 18:205–213.

33. Mendonca BB, Inacio M, Costa EM, et al. Male pseudohermaphroditism due to primary 5-alpha-reductase 2 deficiency. Diagnosis, psychological evaluation, and management. *Medicine (Baltimore)* 1996;75:64–76.

34. Leung AK, Robson WL. Labial fusion and urinary tract infection. *Child Nephrol Urol* 1992;12:62–64.

35. Simpson JL. Genetic aspect of gynecologic disorders occurring in 46,XX individuals. *Clin Obstet Gynecol* 1972;15:157–182.

36. Evruke C, Ozgunen FT, Kadayifci O, et al. Labial fusion in a pubertal girl: a case report. *J Pediatr Adolesc Gynecol* 1996;9:81–82.

37. Johansen JK, Larsen UR. Imperforate hymen. A simple, but overlooked diagnosis. *Ugeskr Laeger* 1998;160:5948–5949.

38. Salvat J, Slamani L. Hematocolpos. *J Gynecol Obstet Biol Reprod (Paris)* 1998;27:396–402.

39. Ahmed S, Morris LL, Atkinson E. Distal mucocolpos and proximal hematocolpos secondary to concurrent imperforate hymen and transverse vaginal septum. *J Pediatr Surg* 1999;34:1555–1556.

40. Bakos O, Berglund L. Imperforate hymen and ruptured hematosalpinx: a case report with a review of the literature. *J Adolesc Health* 1999;24:226–2268.

41. Hall DJ. An usual case of urinary retention due to imperforate hymen. *J Accid Emerg Med* 1999;16:232–233.

42. Kushnir O, Garde K, Blankstein J. Rectal sonography for diagnosing hematocolpometra. A case report. *J Reprod Med* 1997; 42:519–520.

43. Simpson JL. Genetics of the female reproductive ducts. *Am J Med Genet* 1999;89:224–239.

44. Carson SA, Simpson JL, Malinak LR, et al. Heritable aspects of uterine anomalies. II. Genetic analysis of Müllerian aplasia. *Fertil Steril* 1983;40:86–90.

45. Buttram VC. Müllerian anomalies and their management. *Fertil Steril* 1983;40:159–163.

46. Verp MS, Simpson JL, Elias S, et al. Heritable aspects of uterine anomalies. I. Three familial aggregates with Müllerian fusion anomalies. *Fertil Steril* 1983;40:80–85.

47. Griffin JE, Creighton E, Maddon JD, et al. Congenital absence of the vagina. The Mayer-Rokitansky-Kuster-Hauser syndrome. *Ann Intern Med* 1976;85:224–236.

48. Frank RT. Formation of an artificial vagina without operation. *N Y State J Med* 1940;40:1669–1672.

49. Jones HW Jr, Wheeless CR. Salvage of the reproductive potential of women with anomalous development of the Müllerian ducts: 1868–1968–2068. *Am J Obstet Gynecol* 1969;104:348–364.

50. Edmonds DK. Congenital malformations of the genital tract. *Obstet Gynecol Clin North Am* 2000;27:49–62.

51. Ota H, Tanaka Ji, Murakami M, et al. Laparoscopy-assisted Ruge procedure for the creation of neovagina in patient with Mayer-Rokitansky-Kuster-Hauser syndrome. *Fertil Steril* 2000;73:641–644.

52. Banerjee R, Daufer HR. Reproductive disorders and pelvic pain. *Semin Pediatr Surg* 1998;7:52–61.

53. Haddad B, Barranger E, Paniel BJ. Blind hemivagina: long-term follow-up and reproductive performance in 42 cases. *Hum Reprod* 1999;14:1962–1964.

54. Rock JA, Zacur HA, Dlugi AM. Pregnancy success following surgical correction of imperforate hymen and complete transverse vaginal septum. *Obstet Gynecol* 1982;59:448–451.

55. Edwards JA, Gale RP. Camptobrachydactyly: a new autosomal

dominant trial with two probable homozygotes. *Am J Hum Genet* 1972;24:464–474.

56. Rock JA, Schlaff WD, Zacur HA, et al. The clinical management of congenital absence of the uterine cervix. *Int J Gynecol Obstet* 1984;22:231–235.

57. Ostrzenski A. Laparoscopic panhysterectomy with reconstructive posterior culdoplasty and vaginal vault suspension. Port Washington, NY: IVY, Medical Science Publishing International, 1993:5–15.

58. Ostrzenski A. Psychological impact of pelvic surgery: a comparison of laparoscopy versus laparotomy. In: Grochmal S, ed. *Minimal access gynecology*. Oxford, UK: Radcliffe Medical Press, 1995:16–23.

59. Fujimoto VY, Miller JH, Klein NA, et al. Congenital cervical atresia: report of seven cases and review of the literature. *Am J Obstet Gynecol* 1997;177:1419–1425.

60. Ostrzenski A. New retroperitoneal culdoplasty and colpopexy at the time of laparoscopic total abdominal hysterectomy (L-TAH). *Acta Obstet Gynecol* 1998;77:1017–1021.

61. Farber M, Marchant DJ. Congenital absence of the uterine cervix. *Am J Obstet Gynecol* 1975:121:414–417.

62. Edmonds DK. Diagnosis, clinical presentation and management of cervical agenesis. In: Gidwani G, Falcone T, eds. *Congenital malformation of the female genital tract*. Philadelphia: Lippincott Williams & Wilkins, 1999:169.

63. American College of Obstetrician and Gynecologists (ACOG). Precis V. An update in obstetrics and gynecology. Washington, DC: ACOG, 1994:434–435.

64. American Fertility Society. Classification of adnexal adhesions, distal tubal occlusion, tubal occlusion secondary to tubal ligation, tubal pregnancies, Müllerian anomalies and intrauterine adhesions. *Fertil Steril* 1988;49:944–955.

5

DYSMENORRHEA

EDUCATIONAL OBJECTIVES

Medical Students (1) *APGO Objective No. 50*	*Residents in Obstetrics/Gynecology (2)* *CREOG Objectives*	*Practitioners (3)* *ACOG Recommendations*
Definitions of primary and secondary dysmenorrhea Causes of dysmenorrhea Management strategies	Pertinent history Physical examination Diagnostic studies Diagnosis Management Follow-up	Proper diagnosis Distinguishing primary from secondary dysmenorrhea Differential diagnosis Proper understanding of symptomatology Proper patient consultation and reassurance Specific therapy in primary dysmenorrhea Treatment of the underlying pathology in secondary dysmenorrhea

DEFINITION

Dysmenorrhea is pelvic pain associated with the bleeding phase of the menstrual cycle (painful menses), or soon before menses.

INCIDENCE

Over 50% of menstruating women experience varying degrees of dysmenorrhea. Approximately 10% to 15% of dysmenorrheic women are disabled for 1 to 3 days per cycle, and dysmenorrhea is responsible for the loss of approximately 140 million working hours in the United States. Thirty-eight percent of women regularly use medical therapy to treat their dysmenorrhea (3–5).

CLASSIFICATION

Dysmenorrhea is traditionally classified as either primary or secondary (Table 5.1), based on the absence or presence of identifiable pelvic pathology (3,6).

ETIOLOGY

Primary Dysmenorrhea

In an ovulatory menstrual cycle, progesterone induces an endometrial overproduction of prostaglandin F_{2a} [increas-ing the frequency, duration, and intensity of smooth muscle contractility (5)], leading to an elevation of intrauterine pressure: up to 400 mm Hg, with a baseline intrauterine pressure of up to 50 mm Hg. When pressure increases from 80 to 100 mm Hg during menstruation, a woman may become dysmenorrheic. At the same time, prostaglandin F_{2a} mediates smooth muscle contractility in other parts of the body, producing associated symptoms (8).

Secondary Dysmenorrhea

Painful menstruation is directly related to a clinically demonstrable pelvic pathology (Table 5.1). An existing pelvic pathology may induce painful menstruation through several generally accepted mechanisms: distention, hemorrhage, inflammation, ischemia, pressure, perforation, stretching, and so forth.

DIAGNOSIS

Primary Dysmenorrhea

Diagnosis is based on the exclusion of pelvic disease. The patient's pertinent history (Table 5.2) and physical examination (including a pelvic examination with rectovaginal palpation) are used to rule out pelvic pathology (8,9). When an examination is performed during an acute stage of symptoms, the patient may look pale and trembling. It is a

TABLE 5.1. IDENTIFIABLE PELVIC PATHOLOGY IN DYSMENORRHEA

Pathology	Primary Dysmenorrhea	Secondary Dysmenorrhea
Pelvic	Absent	Acquired uterine outflow obstruction
		Adenomysis
		Adhesions
		Cervical stenosis
		Cervical lesions
		Congenital uterine outflow obstruction
		Endometriosis
		Inflammation
		Infection
		Intrauterine contraceptive device
		Leiomyomata
		Neoplastic tumors
		Nongynecologic etiology
		Polyps of the uterus
		Psychogenic

sanctioned form of practice to initiate therapy for this medical entity with a prostaglandin synthetase inhibitor (see Table 5.4), oral contraceptives, or both for diagnostic purposes as well (9).

Such a clinical test is usually performed for 3 to 4 months; if no improvement is noticed, further evaluation is warranted to distinguish between primary and secondary dysmenorrhea. A definitive diagnosis including (but not limited to) psychogenic factors, cannot be delayed due to a patient's young age (4).

Secondary Dysmenorrhea

A patient's meticulous history and thorough physical examination may show an organic cause, such as uterine malformations, or pathology originating in the endometrium, endometrial cavity, myometrium, or uterine serosa; adnexal pathology (ovarian or tubal in source); adjacent organ pathology (the ureters, bladder, or rectum), pelvic infection, or inflammatory condition; or endometriosis. Acute or fixed uterine retroflexion (12), adenomyosis (13,14), or adenomyomata (15,16) are sometimes identified as the cause (Table 5.3). When a pelvic clinical evaluation identifies existing pathology, further study should be performed without delay, thus allowing for the confirmation of underlying medical conditions and for the implementation of the appropriate therapy. Secondary dysmenorrhea, however, may be present with no demonstrable pelvic pathology by palpation (e.g., adhesions, the early stages of endometriosis, hydrosalpinx, etc.), and those patients should receive the initial therapy for primary dysmenorrhea.

Therapy

Initial therapies should be directed to inhibit prostaglandin production or its effect on the myometrium with nonsteroidal antiinflammatory drugs (NSAIDs) (17) (Table 5.3), and to suppress ovulation with oral contraceptives for at least 3 to 4 months. If this therapy fails, further clinical evaluation must be conducted (Table 5.3), including diagnostic laparoscopy (18,19). A psychogenic cause of the menstrual pain may be presumed when a clinical workup does not identify an organic basis for dysmenorrhea, initial therapy with NSAIDs and oral contra-

TABLE 5.2. SYMPTOM PROFILES OF PRIMARY AND SECONDARY DYSMENORRHEA

Symptoms	Primary Dysmenorrhea	Secondary Dysmenorrhea
Onset	1. Shortly after menarche (within 6–12 mo) 2. Gradual 3. Coincides with menses	1. After age 20 years 2. Gradual 3. Worsens with menses
Occurrence	Hours before or the first 12–72 h of menstrual bleeding	Long before, during, and after menstrual bleeding
Recurrence	Each menstrual cycle	Each menstrual cycle
Severity	Improves with time	Progressively worsens
Pain	Usually during menses	At times other than menses and gets worse during menses
Location	Diffusely located in lower Middle abdomen and suprapubic area	One or both lower abdominal quadrants
Radiation	Back area	Determined by underlying organic processes
Duration	1–3 days	5–7 days
Character of pain	Laborlike (coming and going), cramping, colicky, spasmodic	Same and related to underlying pelvic pathology
Aggravation	Stress, fatigue, pelvic somatization	Stress fatigue, pelvic somatization
Associated symptoms: Nausea, vomiting, diarrhea, nervousness, headaches, dizziness, tiredness	Present	Absent

TABLE 5.3. DIAGNOSIS OF POTENTIAL PELVIC PATHOLOGY OF SECONDARY DYSMENORRHEA, AND ITS CONVENTIONAL THERAPY

Pathology	Diagnosis	Therapy
Adenomyosis	Presumptive diagnosis: a typical history (secondary dysmenorrhea, menorrhagia, deep, midline dyspareunia) Pelvic examination shortly before and/or during menses: enlarged, boggy, and tender uterus. MRI may assist to differentiate from myomata. Ultrasonography will not assist in reaching diagnosis; hysterosalpingography may suggest adenomyosis by demonstrating intramural canals. Definitive diagnosis: histopathology verification.	No satisfactory long-term medical therapy available. Hysterectomy definitive surgical treatment Conservative surgical therapy is not satisfactory. Shortly before menopause, treatment with GnRH agonists may obviate need for hysterectomy. In postmenopausal period, symptoms will subside.
Adenomyomata	MRI	Hysterectomy
Adhesions	Medical history: previous abdominal/pelvic surgery, endometriosis, PID. Pelvic examination: may reveal restricted motion of the uterus. Definitive diagnosis: laparoscopy	Lysis of adhesions when indicated
Adnexal pathology	Ultrasonography	Conservative or definitive surgery when indicated
Cervical stenosis	Clinical cervical canal evaluation	1. Cervical dilatation when indicated (dilation between nos. 11 and 14 Hegar's dilators), and a glass rod should be placed into the cervical canal for 48 h). 2. Cervical dilatation with laminaria (10).
Chronic PID	Pertinent medical history. Pelvic examination may reveal: (a) mucopurulent malodorous discharge from the urethra, Skene's duct, cervix, vagina, anus; (b) adnexal tenderness with cervical and uterine motion, adnexal thickening; (c) Marked increase of inflammatory cells in saline preparation of the cervical secretion; (d) laboratory evidence of elevated WBC, ESR, C-reactive protein, decreased Hb, multiple cervical cultures; (e) Endometrial biopsy evidence of acute or chronic inflammation; (f) Laparoscopy of limited use.	Multiple antibiotic regimen on ambulatory or hospital basis as indicated
Congenital or acquired uterine outflow obstruction	Ultrasonography, hysterosalpingography, MRI	Surgical correction as indicated
Endometrial polyp	Symptoms: Intermenstrual, premenstrual, and postmenstrual. Abnormal, long, heavy with clots, uterine bleeding, low, dull, midline pain.	Surgical removal (via hysteroscopy or curettage. Due to mobility polyps may elude a curette in 25%)
Endometriosis	Medical history (dysmenorrhea, dyspareunia, premenstrual, backache and sometimes abnormal uterine bleeding). Pelvic examination: Posterior cul-de-sac painful nodularity, limited uterine motion, often uterine retroflexion, tender and enlarged adnexa. Direct visualization via laparoscopy or laparotomy (lesion biopsy is recommended for histology verification) and extent of the disease should be determined. Ultrasonography for ovarian endometrioma. MRI or CT has limited application. Laboratory: CA 125 (helpful, but not specific)	Expectant management. Medical (oral contraceptive [pseudopregnancy], progestins, danazol [pseudomenopause], GnRH agonists) Conservative surgery (excision electrocoagulation or laser ablation of lesions, lysis of adhesions, reconstruction of organs when indicated via laparoscopy or laparotomy) with or without extra procedures such as uterine nerve ablation, presacral neurectomy, uterine suspension, or oophoropexy. Combination of medical and conservative surgical approach. Definitive extirpative surgical therapy (total hysterectomy with bilateral salpingo oophorectomy).

(continued)

TABLE 5.3. *(continued)*

Pathology	Diagnosis	Therapy
Intrauterine contraceptive device	Clinical identification	Removal of IUD
Leiomyomata uteri	Medical history: heavy and long menstrual bleeding (menorrhagia is to lose >80 mL of blood during menses), painful menses, pelvic pressure or abdominal/pelvic pain. Abdominal-pelvic examination. Ultrasonography (as a screening tool, descrete <1.5 cm). Myomata may not be detected.	Observation and reassurance with periodic pelvic examination and pelvic ultrasonography to assess of uterine enlargement (if necessary, ruling out ureteral compression causing hydroureter and/or hydronephrosis). Medical approach: intermittent progestin, prostaglandin synthetase inhibitor, or a combination of the two. GnRH analogues (temporary use in selective cases in premenopausal period or before surgery). Surgery: myomectomy (laparoscopic or hysteroscopic, or laparotomy, or transvaginal approach); myolysis (laparoscopic with electrocautery or laser); hysterectomy; myolysis (laparoscopic with electrocautery or laser).
	Hysterosalpingography (occasionally for submucosal myomata). MRI will determine the number, size (including <1.5 cm), and presence of degeneration.	Nonsurgical intervention: arterial embolization.
Pelvic somatization, stress, or fatigue	No pelvic pathology identified. Poor response to the initial therapy. Symptoms of clinical depression or other psychological or psychiatric abnormality present.	Psychotherapy in addition to NSAIDs (OC may aggravate clinical depression).
Uterine retroflexion	Symptoms: dysmenorrhea, dyspareunia, sense of bladder and/or rectal pressure.	Conservative symptomatic medical management; pessary; uterine suspension (retroperitoneal hysteropexy) (12)

GnRH, gonadotropin-releasing hormone; MRI, magnetic resonance imaging; PID, pelvic inflammatory disease; WBC, white blood cell; ESR, erythrocyte sedimentation rate; Hb, hemoglobin; CT, computed tomography; IUD, intrauterine device; NSAID, nonsteroidal antiinflammatory drug; OC, oral contraceptive.

ceptives fail, and symptoms of depression are present (Table 5.3).

DIFFERENTIAL DIAGNOSIS

- Chronic pelvic pain
- Irritable bowel syndrome

THERAPY

Primary Dysmenorrhea

Pretreatment assessment for the severity of pain should be performed. It is highly recommended that the patient maintain a self-assessment pain chart, using a scale of 0 to 10 (0 indicating no pain, and 10 indicating severe, incapacitating pain, confining the patient to bed). For clinical management purposes, pain should be classified as 1 to 3 for mild pain; 4 to 7 for moderate pain; and 8 to 10 for

severe pain. This may assist in the selection of an appropriate mode of therapy and in determining improvement.

Patient education in supportive measures and contributory factors, such as body positioning, anxiety, food, lifestyle, drug interaction, and the control of undesirable side effects, may help to improve symptomatology.

Conventional Therapy

The core of conventional therapy for primary dysmenorrhea is medical management with prostaglandin inhibitors (Table 5.4), low doses of oral contraceptives (20), or a combination of both. If oral contraceptives cannot be used, an oral progestogen (dydrogesterone) is recommended in doses of 10 mg daily between days 5 and 25 of each cycle (21).

Ibuprofen appears to have the most favorable risk:benefit ratio (19). The prostaglandin synthesis inhibitors, however, should be avoided with previously documented hypersensitivity to ibuprofen, other NSAIDs, or aspirin, because severe anaphylactic-like reactions can occur, possibly result-

TABLE 5.4. FDA-APPROVED, NONSTEROIDAL ANTIINFLAMMATORY DRUGS FOR PRIMARY DYSMENORRHEA TREATMENT

Generic Name	Trade Name	Loading Dose	Maintenance Dose
Ibuprofen	Motrin	400 mg	400 mg every 4 h
	Rufen	1,200–1,600 mg	600–800 mg every 4 h
	IBU	1,200–1,600 mg	600–800 mg every 4 h
Naproxen	Naprosyn	500 mg	250 mg every 4–6 h
Naproxen sodium	Aflaxen	550 mg	275 mg every 6–8 h
	Anaprox	550 mg	275 mg every 6–8 h
Meclofenamate	Mecolmen	100 mg	50–100 mg every 4–6 h
Mefenamic acid	Ponstil	500 mg	250 mg every 4–6 h

FDA, U.S. Food and Drug Administration.

ing in death. Undesirable side effects include gastrointestinal irritation, ulceration, nausea, prolonged bleeding, renal papillary necrosis, and decreased renal blood flow.

When there is no relief of dysmenorrhea from initial medical or other treatment, the full extent of clinical evaluation fails to identify pelvic pathology, and incapacitating pain is present, presacral neurectomy should be considered (20).

Complementary Therapy

Patient Education

Providing teaching (audiovisual and reading) resources to familiarize the patient with controlling environment stimuli, positioning the body, preserving energy, self-hypnosis, biofeedback, and any one form of meditation may help to alleviate symptomatology.

Diet

The following foods are recommended: whole grains, legumes, fruits and vegetables, seeds (ground, raw flax seed, pumpkin seed), one glass of blueberry or huckleberry juice daily, and fish (trout, mackerel, salmon). The following foods should be avoided: dairy products, saturated fats, salt, alcohol, sugar, caffeine, and wheat (49).

Acupuncture

The objective of acupuncture therapy is to reestablish or enhance the body's equilibrium of energy flow. Management of primary dysmenorrhea by acupuncture is a particularly effective mode of therapy in preventing and controlling painful menstruation (23–25). Acupuncture is equally useful in decreasing associated symptoms such as nausea, headache, backache, fluid retention, and breast tenderness (23). However, acupuncture should be avoided during the active phase of bleeding, because its application to the pelvic area may disrupt menstrual flow (26,27). Overall acupuncture is a safe mode of therapy; however, both serious and minor complications have been reported (28).

Exercise

Many observational studies suggest that exercise is an effective method in managing primary dysmenorrhea; however, evidence definitively supporting this claim is lacking (29).

Transcutaneous Electrical Nerve Stimulation

Transcutaneous electrical nerve stimulation is a nonpharmacologic modality of transcutaneous nerve stimulation that has been used to relieve pain. It has been documented in randomized studies that this method of therapy is safe and effective in alleviating painful menstruation and associated symptomatology (30,31).

Heat

The description for dysmenorrhea and therapy for this illness using a heat pad (a hot oil–filled animal bladder, applied to the aching lower abdominal area) appeared in ancient literature, dating from the 2nd century, A D. (32). Different forms of superficial heat sources (liquid, electric, sand, solid, etc.) can be used, including microwave diathermy (33).

Hypnosis

By putting the body in a relaxed sate, hypnotherapy allows the subject to be open to suggestions and focus on specific objectives. This mode of a therapy (quieted hypnosis treatment and self-hypnosis) has been successfully applied in the treatment of chronic pain (34–36). However, a well-designed study to support the validity of hypnosis in the treatment of dysmenorrhea is lacking.

Manipulative (Chiropractic) Therapy

The results of an observational case study (35) suggest that manipulation of the spine is a beneficial method for the amelioration of painful menstruation. The safety and effectiveness of spinal manipulation to relieve the pain and distress of primary dysmenorrhea was documented in a randomized study (36,37). It also was established that there is no difference in clinical outcome when a high-force or a low-force spinal manipulation was applied (37).

Therapeutic Massage

Therapeutic massage, in its rubbing form, is one of the oldest medical interventions used to relieve pain, and it was clinically applied until the pharmaceutical revolution of the 1940s (38–40). There has been a long tradition of massage treatment for primary dysmenorrhea with a great deal of anecdotal evidence of its effectiveness; however, there is a lack of scientific data to support its safety and efficacy. Each of the major categories of massage (European, deep tissue, pressure-point, and movement integration) can be used in pain treatment.

Therapeutic Touch

Proponents of this type of medical intervention suggest that it is beneficial in facilitating comfort and healing, but they do so with no scientific support for such a claim (41). In evidence based views, therapeutic touch is considered as a form of placebo effect and can be used as an adjuvant in the nursing approach (43,44). Therapeutic touch is broadly used in pain management, but it is not specifically designated for the treatment of primary dysmenorrhea.

Biofeedback Therapy

Learning how to control specific organ function, usually with electronic equipment (electromyography, electroencephalography, galvanometry, thermistor analysis), is used until a subject familiarizes herself with her symptomatology and behavioral responses in order to eradicate or reduce her symptoms. Observational and case study reports indicate that, with biofeedback therapy, the symptoms of primary dysmenorrhea improved (45–47). The best clinical outcome can be expected when biofeedback treatment is commenced prior to the onset of symptomatology associated with primary dysmenorrhea (45).

Imagery

The therapeutic effect of imagery is accomplished by having the body respond to self-created concrete or symbolic images in the mind. Unlike hypnosis, a therapist does not suggest an image to the patient. Imagery is anecdotally considered to be an effective tool in pain control, but no data are available in reference to the treatment of primary dysmenorrhea.

Meditation

Through the simultaneous process of tranquilizing the mind and bringing it to center on the present, meditation (concentrative, mindfulness, transcendental) is believed to reduce pain perception. Yoga and imagery as adjunctive therapies may have some value (46) in supporting the physical and emotional needs of coping with pain in general, and perhaps in primary dysmenorrhea as well. However, this area requires a well-designed study to determine its clinical applications.

Nutritional Supplements

Minerals

The following minerals are suggested in the treatment of primary dysmenorrhea: calcium, potassium, zinc, and essential fatty acids (49). Magnesium's safety and effectiveness in the treatment of primary dysmenorrhea has been documented in randomized, controlled trials (the dose of Magnesiocard comprised 3×5 mmol granulate; administered orally on the day preceding menstruation and on the first and second day of cycle) (50).

Vitamins

Vitamin B_3 (niacin, niacinamide), when taken with colestipol, which increases its serum level, or isoniazid, which lowers vitamin serum levels (51), and vitamin B_6 (pyridoxine, pyridoxamine, pyridoxal), when taken with oral contraceptives, lowers vitamin serum levels and may interact with other drugs (51). Vitamin C (ascorbic acid), when administered with aspirin, barbiturates, corticosteroids, indomethacin, oral contraceptives, sulfonamides, or tetracycline, lowers vitamin serum levels (51).

Natural Alternative Therapy

Herbal Medicine

Tinctures in equal parts of skullcap, black haw, and black cohosh may be taken as needed (1–2 teaspoons) (52). *Coryaalis ambigua* (*Coryaalis yanhusuo*), in a dose of 5 to 10 g/day of the dried rhizome or 10 to 20 mL/day of a 1:2 extract, is recommended (52). Another recommendation is to take a combination of phytosynergistic composition (53) with 5 mL of the following:

Blue cohosh (*Caulpophyllum thalictroides*) 375 mg
Black cohosh (*Cimicifuga racemosa*) 500 mg
Wild yam (*Dioscorea villosa*) 875 mg
Cramp bark (*Viburnum opulus*) 875 mg
Ginger (*Zingiber officianale*) 125 mg

Such compositions are designed to have antispasmodic, relaxant, antiinflammatory, restorative, and tonifying effects on the uterine muscles (53). It is worthwhile to recognize that different parts of the same plant can yield different therapeutic effects (54).

Craniosacral Therapy

The therapeutic approach for craniosacral therapy is based on the theory that cranial rhythm (increasing and decreasing the cerebrospinal fluid pressure and ranges from 6 to 10 cycles per minute), within a craniosacral system, exists and is independent from the heart and respiratory rhythm (49). By manipulating the skull bones, a therapist is able to remove presumptive resistance to the cerebrospinal fluid flow. It is postulated that this type of treatment is effective in the management of painful menstruation (49). The diagnostic and therapeutic effectiveness of cranial bone motion and craniosacral rhythm are subjects of debate (55–58).

Homeopathy

The fundamental characteristic of clinical applicability of homeopathy is based on the conviction that a substance in a very low dose may cure an illness and in a high dose may become a cause of a sickness. Therefore, from natural resources, such animal, mineral, or plant remedies are prepared in dilution that may stimulate the human body to natural healing process (treating "like with like").

Recently, homeopathy credibility among health providers has become more accepted due to documentation of its safety and effectiveness in clinical scientific research (59). Accordingly, Septia and Lachesis preparations are recommended for dysmenorrhea by homeopathy practitioners (49).

REFERENCES

1. Association of Professors of Gynecology and Obstetrics. *Medical student educational objectives,* 7th ed. Washington, DC: Association of Professors of Gynecology and Obstetrics, 1997.
2. Council on Resident and Gynecology (CREOG). *Educational objectives core curriculum for residents in obstetrics and gynecology,* 5th ed. Washington, DC: CREOG, 1996.
3. American College of Obstetricians and Gynecologists (ACOG). Technical Bulletin No. 68. Washington, DC: ACOG, 1983.
4. Andersch B, Milsom I. An epidemiologic study of young women with dysmenorrhea. *Am J Obstet Gynecol* 1982;144:655–660.
5. Klein JR, Litt IF. Epidemiology of adolescent dysmenorrhea. *Pediatrics* 1981;68:661–664.
6. Ylikorkola O, Dawood MY. New concepts in dysmenorrhea. *Am J Obstet Gynecol* 1978;130:833–847.
7. Pickles VR, Hall WJ, Best FA, et al. Prostaglandins in endometrium and menstrual fluid from normal and dysmenorrheic subjects. *Br J Obstet Gynaecol* 1965;72:185–195.
8. Dawood MY, ed. *Dysmenorrhea.* Baltimore: Williams & Wilkins, 1981.
9. Langlosis PL. The size of the normal uterus. *J Reprod Med* 1970;4:220–228.
10. Ostrzenski A. Resectoscopic cervical trauma minimized by inserting laminaria digitata preoperatively. *Int J Fertil* 1994;39:2:111–113.
11. Chan WY, Dawood MY, Fuchs F. Prostaglandins in primary dysmenorrhea: comparison of prophylactic and non-prophylactic treatments with ibuprofen and use of oral contraceptive. *Am J Med* 1981;70:535–541.
12. Ostrzenski A. Laparoscopic retroperitoneal hysteropexy: a randomized trial. *J Reprod Med* 1998;43:361–366.
13. Kurman RJ. *Blausteins's pathology of the female genital tract,* 4th ed. New York: Springer-Verlag, 1994:518.
14. Ostrzenski A. Extensive iatrogenic adenomyosis after laparoscopic myomectomy. *Fertil Steril* 1998;69,143–145.
15. Quigley JC, Hart WR. Adenomatoid tumors of the uterus. *Am J Clin Pathol* 1981;76:627–635.
16. Rollason TP, Redman CW. Atypical polypoid adenomyomata-clinical, histological, and immunocytochemical findings. *Eur J Gynecol Oncol* 1988;9:444–451.
17. Smith RP. *Gynecology in primary care.* Baltimore: Williams & Wilkins, 1996:398.
18. Goldstein DP, deCholnoky C, Emans SJ, et al. Laparoscopy in diagnosis and management of pelvic pain in adolescents. *J Reprod Med* 1980;24:251–256.
19. Zhang WY, Li Wan Po A. Efficacy of minor analgesics in primary dysmenorrhea: a systematic review. *Br J Obstet Gynecol* 1998;105:780–789.
20. Chen FP, Chang SD, Chu KK, et al. Comparison of laparoscopic presacral neurectomy and laparoscopic uterine nerve ablation for primary dysmenorrhea. *J Reprod Med* 1996;41:463–466.
21. Chamberlain G. ed. *Gynecology by ten teachers,* 16th ed. London: Holder Headline Group, 1995:178.
22. Sundell G, Milsom I, Andersch B. Factors influencing the prevalence and severity of dysmenorrhea in young women. *Br J Obstet Gynecol* 1990;97:588–594.
23. Helms JM. Acupuncture for the management of primary dysmenorrhea. *Obstet Gynecol* 1987;51:51–55.
24. Steinberger A. The treatment of dysmenorrhea by acupuncture. *Am J Chin Med* 1981;9:57–61.
25. Slagoski JE. Resolution of acute dysmenorrhea with one-point therapy. *Int J Chin Med* 1984;1:1–5.
26. Mussat M. *Acupuncture.* Paris: MEDSI, 1980:167–185.
27. Vallette E, Niboyet JEH, Jarricot H. *Gynecologie-obstetrique: therapeutique par acupuncture.* Paris: MEDSI, 1981:9–17.
28. Lao L. Safety issues in acupuncture. *J Altern Complement Med* 1996;2:27–31.
29. Golomb LM, Solidum AA, Warren MP. Primary dysmenorrhea and physical activity. *Med Sci Sports Exerc* 1998;30:906-909.
30. Milsom I, Hedner N, Mannheimer C. A comparative study of the effect of high-intensity transcutaneous nerve stimulation and oral naproxen on intrauterine pressure and menstrual pain in patients with primary dysmenorrhea. *Am J Obstet Gynecol* 1994;170:123–129.
31. Dawood MY, Ramos J. Transcutaneous electrical nerve stimulation (TENS) for the treatment of primary dysmenorrhea: a randomized crossover comparison with placebo TENS and ibuprofen. *Obstet Gynecol* 1990;75:656–660.
32. O'Dowd MJ, Philipp EE. *The history of obstetrics and gynaecology.* New York: Parthenon, 1994:345–347.
33. Vance AR, Hayes SH, Spielholz NI. Microwave diathermy treatment for primary dysmenorrhea. *Phys Ther* 1996;76:1003–1008.
34. Spira JL, Spiegel D. Hypnosis and related techniques in pain management. *Hosp J* 1992;8:89–119.
35. Nickelson C, Brende JO, Gonzalez J. What if your patient prefers an alternative pain control method? Self-hypnosis in the control of pain. *South Med J* 1999;92:96.
36. Lark SM. *Menstrual cramps. A self-help program.* Los Altos, CA: Westchester Publishing, 1993.
37. Liebl NA, Butler LM. A chiropractic approach to the treatment of dysmenorrhea. *J Manipulative Physiol Ther* 1990;13:101–106.
38. Kokjohn K, Schmid DM, Triano JJ, et al. The effect of spinal manipulation on pain and prostaglandin levels in women with primary dysmenorrhea. *J Manipulative Physiol Ther* 1992;15:279–285.
39. Hondras MA, Long CR, Brennan PC. Spinal manipulative therapy versus low force mimic maneuver for women with primary dysmenorrhea: a randomized, observer-blinded, clinical trial. *Pain* 1999;81:105–114.

40. Field TM. Massage therapy effects. *Am Psychol* 1998;53:1270–1281.

41. Goats GC. Massage: the scientific basis of ancient art. Part I. The techniques. *Br J Sports Med* 1994;28:149–152.

42. Goats GC. Massage: the scientific basis of ancient art. Part II. Physiological and therapeutic effects. *Br J Sports Med* 1994;28:153–156.

43. Meehan TC. Therapeutic touch as a nursing intervention. *J Adv Nurs* 1998;28:117–125.

44. Clark PE, Clark MJ. Therapeutic touch: is there a scientific basis for the practice. *Nurs Res* 1984;33:37–41.

45. Balick L, Elfner L, May J, et al. Biofeedback treatment of dysmenorrhea. *Biofeedback Self Regul* 1982;7:499–520.

46. Gimbel MA. Yoga, meditation, and imagery: clinical applications. *Nurse Pract Forum* 1998;9:234–255.

47. Bennink CD, Hulst LL, Benthem JA. The effect of EMG biofeedback and relaxation training on primary dysmenorrhea. *J Behav Med* 1982;5:329–341.

48. Dietvorst TF, Osborne D. Biofeedback-assisted relaxation training for primary dysmenorrhea: a case study. *Biofeedback Self Regul* 1978;3:301–305.

49. Golgberg B, ed. *Alternative medicine.* Tiburon, CA: Future Medicine Publishing, 2001:149, 273, 660–661.

50. Fontana-Klaiber H, Hogg B. Therapeutic effects of magnesium in dysmenorrhea. *Schweiz Rundsch Med Prax* 1990;79:491–494.

51. Brinker F. *Herb contraindications and drug interactions,* 2nd ed. Sandy, OR: Eclectic Medical, 1998.

52. Bone K. *Clinical applications of Ayurvedic and Chinese herbs,* 2nd ed. Warwick, Queensland, Australia: Phytotherapy Press, 1997: 25–28.

53. Bone K, Burgess N, McLeod D. *Phytosynergistic prescribing.* Portland, OR: Health Formulas, 1994:65.

54. Eliopoulos C. *Integrating conventional and alternative therapies.* St. Louis: CV Mosby, 1999.

55. Wirth-Pattullo V, Hayes KW. Interrater reliability of craniosacral rate measurements and their relationship with subjects' and examiners' heart and respiratory rate measurements. *Phys Ther* 1994;74:908–916.

56. Hanten WP, Dawson DD, Seiden IM, et al. Craniosacral rhythm: reliability and relationships with cardiac and respiratory rates. *J Orthop Sports Phys Ther* 1998;27:231–218.

57. Simultaneous palpation of the craniosacral rate at the head and fee: intrarater and interrater reliability and and rate comparisons. *Phys Ther* 1998;78:1175–1185.

58. Rogers JS, Witt PL. The controversy of cranial bone motion. *J Orthop Sports Phys Ther* 1997;26:95–103.

59. Fisher P. The development of research methodology in homeopathy. *Complement Ther Nurs Midwifery* 1995;1:168–174.

6

PELVIC PAIN

EDUCATIONAL OBJECTIVES

Medical Students (1) *APGO Objectives Nos. 43, 39, 40*	*Residents in Obstetrics/Gynecology (2)* *CREOG Objectives*	*Practitioners (3)* *ACOG Recommendations*
Chronic pelvic pain	Chronic pelvic pain	Chronic pelvic pain
Sexually transmitted infection	Endometriosis	Evaluation of pain
Definition	Pelvic inflammatory disease	Physical evaluation
Incidence	History	Gynecologic pelvic pain
Etiology	Physical examination	Nongynecologic pelvic pain
Clinical manifestations	Diagnostic studies	Therapy
Diagnostic procedures	Diagnosis	Multidisciplinary diagnosis
Management	Management	and management
	Follow-up	

CHRONIC PELVIC PAIN

Definition

Chronic pelvic pain is nonacute, constant, or cyclically persistent pain located in the pelvic area for at least 6 months.

Incidence

Incidence for the general population of chronic pelvic pain has not yet been established. In the U.S. population, the prevalence is approximately 15% among women 18 to 50 years of age (4).

Etiology

The etiology of primary chronic pelvic pain is not clearly understood. It is widely believed that the pathogenesis of this condition is psycho-somatic-social in nature (5). One hypothesis that gained broad acceptance is the vascular theory, which suggests the origin of chronic pelvic pain arises from dilated pelvic veins. In dilated veins, blood flow is significantly reduced, and the altered spinal cord and brain processing of stimuli is subsequently affected in women with this condition (6).

Classification

Pelvic pain is classified into two different types:

- Episodic pelvic pain
    Subacute episodic pelvic pain
    Subacute episodic exacerbated pelvic pain
    Acute episodic pelvic pain of gynecologic origin [ectopic pregnancy, tubal torsion, adnexal torsion, acute salpingitis, tuboovarian abscess, acute pelvic inflammatory disease (PID)] or of nongynecologic origin (appendicitis, urinary tract calculi, incarcerated hernia or diverticulitis)
- Chronic pelvic pain
    Primary chronic pelvic pain
    Secondary chronic pelvic pain (pathologic cause is identifiable)

Diagnosis

In the 1990s, clinical investigations established a dichotomy of symptoms (organic and psychogenic in origin) of chronic pelvic pain. Understanding the pathogenesis of this condition has led to the development of multidisciplinary and biopsychological models for evaluation and management of chronic pelvic pain.

Somatic Symptoms

The characteristics and extent of pelvic pain should be established by direct questions concerning pain location, onset (abrupt or gradual), radiation, duration, severity (mild, moderate or severe), character (sharp or dull), causes of aggravation (what makes pain worse), and pain relief remedy or other measures (what eases pain). Pain rating scale questionnaires are available that target a specific area of pain. Pain evaluation and its rating scales can be established in privacy, allowing ample time for a patient to provide answers. For detailed information of questionnaires such as the McGill Pain Questionnaire or the Pain Disability Index, the reader is referred to commercially available publications (7). Questionnaires can assist in measuring quality of life and economic adverse events caused by chronic pelvic pain (6). The questionnaire is limited by its unrestricted answer format, and women who are not fluent in English will have difficulty with the form. To assess individual patients' interpretation of questions and to follow up with clarification is time consuming; such scrutiny occasionally makes a patient uncomfortable as well. Nevertheless, a questionnaire format is commonly used in clinical scientific research.

Associated symptoms such as nausea, vomiting, diarrhea, headaches, and fatigue should be explored, because they may reveal the cause of the chronic pain and point to further clinical investigation.

Psychological Symptoms

Psychological symptoms in chronic pelvic pain are manifest as follows (5,8,9):

- Mood disturbances
- Disruption of daily routine activity
- Compromised interpersonal relationships
- Anxiety related to pain exacerbations
- Depression (evaluation is based on criteria set for diagnosis established by the American Psychiatric Association) (10)

Physical examination should include the following:

- Lower extremity evaluation should incorporate the length of the legs, ability or limitation of motion and abduction at the hip level, strength, sensation conduction, and walking limitation.
- Back examination should determine ability and limitation of back motion in standing and bending positions, and the presence or absence of any deformity in standing and bending positions. Tenderness points or trigger tenderness spine points also should be determined.
- Chest wall trigger points or chest deformity should be identified.
- Abdominal and pelvic evaluation is routinely executed.

A pain map can be created by the patient under direct physician instruction during the physical examination. A female body illustration chart aids in this endeavor, which presents a female image in the front, back, and lateral aspects. A patient is instructed to indicate the pain site in reference to the different phases of the menstrual cycle, routine physical activities, and sexual intercourse. The use of different colors reflecting the type and occurrence of pain associated with different physiologic and environmental conditions is very helpful. Patient-assisted pelvic pain mapping can synchronize pain symptoms with a potential existing pathology.

Laboratory tests are routinely offered for chronic pelvic pain (11). All patients should undergo the following tests:

- Complete blood count with differential
- Urinalysis
- Urogenital testing for sexually transmitted disease, particularly for chlamydia and gonorrhea

Selected patients may undergo the following tests, based on history and physical examination findings:

- Tests for autoantibodies
- Antinuclear antibody
- Rheumatoid factor
- Erythrocyte sedimentation rate
- Vaginal wet smear
- Testing for urinary or gastrointestinal infections

Imaging studies, primarily ultrasonography, are frequently used in the evaluation of chronic pelvic pain. However, transvaginal ultrasonography is unlikely to disclose further pelvic pathology in women with chronic pelvic pain who demonstrated no anatomic abnormalities during routine gynecologic examination (12). It is widely believed, though, that lower abdominal pelvic ultrasonography may add pertinent information when women are evaluated for pelvic pain (11).

Magnetic resonance imaging can assist in reaching a presumptive diagnosis of adenomyosis when medical history or physical examination suggest the presence of this entity. Intravenous pyelography may establish the urologic origin of chronic pelvic pain (11,13).

Endoscopic evaluation is applied for multiple purposes in the assessment of chronic pelvic pain, but it is not necessarily indicated for routine use. Use of endoscopy can be characterized as follows.

Gynecologic endoscopic studies focus predominantly on the use of laparoscopy. Hysteroscopic examination, in selected cases, is also a valuable part of the evaluation of chronic pelvic pain.

Laparoscopy in the evaluation of chronic pain is a recognized and accepted procedure. However, randomized clinical trial results have not proved laparoscopy to be of diagnostic or therapeutic significance when compared with noninvasive approaches (14).

Laparoscopic examination for chronic pelvic pain is performed in over 40% of cases. This form of evaluation should be reserved for those cases in which other noninvasive evaluation failed to identify the pathology responsible for the chronic pelvic pain. It is estimated that approximately 65% of women with chronic pelvic pain have an existing abnormality identified by laparoscopic examination (15).

Hysteroscopic evaluation is indicated when a uterine intracavitary abnormality is a possible cause of chronic pelvic pain. History and pelvic examination as well as other laboratory tests may suggest submucosal fibroid or large endometrial polyps.

Endoscopic approaches may play dual roles in the assessment of chronic pelvic pain: to reach diagnosis and to treat the identified abnormality at the same time.

Urologic endoscopic studies are indicated if urologic symptomatology is present. Cystoscopic examination is performed primarily when interstitial cystitis must be excluded.

Gastrointestinal endoscopic studies are indicated in those cases for which medical history, physical examination, and laboratory tests suggest lower intestinal tract pathology. Proctoscopic, sigmoidoscopic, or colonoscopic evaluation can be offered in such clinical situations.

Differential Diagnosis

The differential diagnosis can be divided into three categories. *The gynecologic causes* of chronic pelvic pain may include the following (6,11):

- Ovarian remnant syndrome
- Ovarian residual syndrome
- Pelvic congestion syndrome
- Endometriosis
- Primary or secondary dysmenorrhea
- PID
- Uterine leiomyomata with or without degenerative process
- Adenomyosis
- Hydrosalpinx

Ovarian remnant syndrome develops when functional ovarian tissue is left *in situ* after failure to remove completely the ovary during bilateral oophorectomy. It is characterized by chronic pelvic pain or dyspareunia. A tender pelvic mass can be identified on bimanual pelvic examination or documented by ultrasonography. Occasionally it is difficult to establish the diagnosis not only due to the small size of the lesion but also due to distorted pelvic anatomy resulting from previous surgery or adhesions. In such a clinical event, an ovarian pharmacologic stimulation agent may facilitate identification of these remnants. The definitive therapy for this condition is surgical extirpation (which can be a difficult procedure). Medical therapy is empiric, and hormonal manipulation may prevent recurrences (16,17).

Ovarian residual syndrome is defined by pathology in the conserved ovary or ovaries. It consists of pelvic pain, pelvic mass, and dyspareunia as a single or a cluster of symptoms (18). The diagnosis is reached by routine pelvic mass evaluation, and therapy depends on identification of definitive

ovarian pathology. This subject is discussed further in Chapter 22.

Nongynecologic causes of chronic pelvic pain have numerous etiologies. The urinary tract is affected by the following conditions (5,11):

- Interstitial cystitis
- Urethral syndrome
- Detrusor dyssynergia
- Chronic calculi

The gastrointestinal system may produce chronic pelvic pain associated with the following conditions (5,6,11):

- Irritable bowel syndrome
- Inflammatory bowel disease
- Diverticulitis

The musculoskeletal system is affected by the following entities (11):

- Arthritis
- Fibromyalgia
- Hernias
- Vertebral disk disorders
- Scoliosis

Psychogenic causes of chronic pelvic pain may include the following clinical entities (5,8,11):

- Physical or sexual abuse
- Clinical depression
- Opioid seeking
- Somatization
- Factitious disorders
- Premenstrual dysphoric disorder
- Hypochondriasis

Conventional Therapy

Upon completion of initial clinical noninvasive evaluation (medical history, physical examination, and laboratory studies), but before diagnostic laparoscopy, conservative medical, empiric treatment for primary chronic pelvic pain is recommended.

Clinical reassurance with *counseling* supported by ultrasonography scanning is associated with significant pain reduction and improvement in mood among patients with chronic pelvic pain. These findings are supported by randomized controlled clinical trials and in many cases may serve as the first line of approach in the management of this condition (6).

Medroxyprogesterone acetate (10–30 mg orally per day) or injectable medroxyprogesterone acetate depot (150–300 mg every 1–3 months) has been proven in randomized controlled clinical trials to be an effective mode of hormonal treatment for chronic pelvic pain. Its benefit may be restricted to the duration of treatment (6,19).

The multidisciplinary approach is an effective paradigm in the management of chronic pelvic pain. The effectiveness and safety of this approach has been well documented in randomized controlled trials (6,20,21).

Oral analgesics such as nonsteroidal antiinflammatory drugs (NSAIDs) are considered the first analgesic line of treatment. NSAIDs provide triple therapeutic actions: analgesic, antiinflammatory, and antiprostaglandin synthesis effects. They should be administered on a scheduled and not as a needed mode of administration (11,22,23). The most commonly prescribed NSAIDs for pelvic pain are presented in Table 6.1.

Ovarian function suppression is recommended when treatment with NSAIDs provides insufficient relief of pain. A low monophasic agent (e.g., 30–35 μg of the ethinyl estradiol component of oral contraceptives) reduces prostaglandin synthesis and suppresses ovarian steroid production. Oral contraceptives for chronic pelvic pain can be administered continuously or cyclically. A 3-month trial of oral contraceptives is recommended. If no satisfactory relief is reported, the course of therapy should be discontinued and further clinical minimally invasive evaluation is warranted (22,23).

As previously discussed, chronic pelvic pain is the clinical entity of dichotomous symptomatology; therefore, both somatic and psychogenic components should be equally addressed in formulating a management model for an individual patient.

Psychotherapy—individual, group, or family therapy—is recommended for those patients who present with mood disorder associated with chronic pelvic pain or for those with a history of sexual abuse or victimization. Such programs can be successful when other therapeutic interventions are included, such as nutrition, eating behavior modification, sleep disorder therapy, hygiene guidance, and physical exercise (23).

Behavioral therapy, particularly cognitive-behavioral therapy, is a useful adjunct to conventional treatments in chronic pelvic pain. Cognitive-behavioral therapy incorporates a patient's thoughts and influence the patient's behavioral affect in relation to the perception of pain intensity, coping mechanism of pain, and effect of pain on daily routine activity. A successful program can reroute a patient's concerns about pain and body image toward identification and management of stressful occurrences. Therefore, treatment may embrace progressive muscle relaxation techniques, stress management strategies, and coping with pain techniques (23,24).

Psychotropic medication can reduce pain, decrease depression and anxiety, and improve sleep patterns. The dose of these agents usually is lower (10–25 mg at the bedtime) than the dose administered for the treatment of depression. Patients with mood disturbance (depression or anxiety) or sleep disorders are good candidates for this therapeutic modality (23).

Upon completion of empiric treatment for the somatic and psychogenic components of pelvic pain, surgical therapy can be considered.

Among conservative *surgical management* options, diagnostic laparoscopy is a useful tool in the armamentarium of treatment of chronic pelvic pain, and it is particularly effective in establishing secondary causes of chronic pelvic pain. Indeed, it can provide the definitive diagnosis in approximately 65% of cases by identifying and mapping an existing pelvic pathology. Endometriosis is diagnosed in one third of chronic pelvic pain cases assessed via diagnostic laparoscopy. Histologic verification of endometriosis is obtained to ensure an accurate diagnosis. Adhesions are established in one fourth of cases of secondary chronic pelvic pain (14).

Operative laparoscopy as a minimally invasive approach can be successful in selected cases of secondary chronic pelvic pain. Surgical extirpation of the ovarian remnant provides not only definitive diagnosis but also definitive treatment for this condition (16,17). Surgical resection of residual ovary pathology or oophorectomy also is performed (18).

Adhesiolysis can be performed through a laparoscopic approach; however, clinical randomized controlled studies did not document improvement of chronic pelvic pain from this procedure (6). Prevention of adhesion formation is more effective than removing or dividing adhesions. Using barrier agents is one option in preventing adhesions following pelvic surgery. Gore-Tex is superior to Intreceed in this regard, yet requires suturing and later removal, there-

TABLE 6.1. SELECTED NSAIDS IN CHRONIC PAIN THERAPY

Generic Name	Trade Name	Loading Dose	Maintenance Dose
Ibuprofen	Motrin	400 mg	400 mg every 4 h
	Rufen	1,200–1,600 mg	600–800 mg every 4 h
	IBU	1,200–1,600 mg	600–800 mg every 4 h
Naproxen	Naprosyn	500 mg	250 mg every 4–6 h
Naproxen sodium	Aflaxen	550 mg	275 mg every 6–8 h
	Anaprox	550 mg	275 mg every 6–8 h
Meclofenamate	Mecolmen	100 mg	50–100 mg every 4–6 h
Mefenamic acid	Ponstil	500 mg	250 mg every 4–6 h

fore limiting its use. Intreceed may significantly reduce adhesion formations. The effectiveness of Seprafilm in preventing adhesion formation could not be supported in randomized controlled clinical trials. Therefore, preventing adhesions by implementing appropriate surgical technique during initial surgery and by using barrier agents as a form of prevention of adhesions may be more effective than performing adhesiolysis (25). All conservative procedures for chronic pelvic pain can be executed either though laparoscopic or laparotomy approaches.

Operative hysteroscopic procedures for presumptive uterine cavity pathology (mainly submucosal uterine leiomyomata or large polyps) may be applied in selected cases.

The definitive surgery for chronic pelvic pain is total hysterectomy. Hysterectomy is effective in easing chronic pelvic pain in approximately 60% of cases. It is imperative to identify potential risk factors for persistent pelvic pain following hysterectomy, because up to 40% of hysterectomized patients may continue to experience long-term pelvic pain (26).

Complementary and alternative therapies are offered in the same categories as for dysmenorrhea, as discussed in Chapter 5.

ENDOMETRIOSIS

Endometriosis (the ectopic endometrium) is the presence of the endometrial tissue or that resembling endometrial tissue outside its natural endometrial cavity location.

Incidence

The true prevalence of pelvic endometriosis cannot be determined with certainty. Only a trial that included a large number of randomly selected women who were subjected to diagnostic laparoscopy could provide any reliable data. Therefore, neither the prevalence (proportion of population affected at any given time) nor the incidence (new cases per annual occurrence) of endometriosis is known. Indirectly, the prevalence of endometriosis has been estimated as follows (27):

- In asymptomatic women, the prevalence is estimated at 2% to 22%, depending on the diagnostic criteria used.
- In dysmenorrheic patients, the prevalence ranges from 40% to 60%.
- Among subfertile women, the prevalence ranges from 20% to 30%.

The peak incidence of endometriosis is at about 40 years of age. The severity of symptoms and probability of this diagnosis increases with age (27).

The overall occurrence among women in the United States is estimated to be approximately 1% to 7% (28). The accurate prevalence of endometriosis among the adolescent population is unknown; nevertheless, the estimated prevalence of endometriosis among girls subjected to laparoscopic evaluation for chronic pelvic pain is about 45% (29).

Etiology

The cause of endometriosis is unknown (27), although this condition was described in Europe over 300 years ago (30). It is considered to be a chronic, progressive disease (estrogen plays an essential role in the progression of endometriosis and pain), with a tendency toward deterioration with time, and may cause infertility and destruction of internal genital organs. The natural history of endometriosis is unpredictable. Frequently there is no direct correlation between the extent of endometriosis and severity of symptomatology. Several classic theories are present and those most often accepted are listed as follows:

- Meyer's theory (circa 1909) is based on metaplasia of the coelomic epithelium, which involves embryologically totipotential cells expressing metaplastic transformation into the functioning endometrial tissue (31).
- Halban's theory (circa 1924) purports the migration of endometrial cells through vascular and lymphatic channels (32).
- Sampson's theory (circa 1927) suggests development of endometriosis via dissemination of the exfoliated endometrium into the peritoneal cavity at the time of menstruation. This theory is also known as the retrograde implantation theory or the transplantation theory of endometriosis (33,34).

Other hypotheses have been advanced more recently:

- Abnormal immune function and inappropriate response of the peritoneal defense system indicate an association between endometriosis and changes in humoral and cell-mediated immunity (35,36). Therefore, immunologic factors may play a key role in determining the development of endometriosis and its heterogenous symptoms (37).
- The angiogenesis theory suggests that angiogenetic factors [e.g., vascular endothelial growth factor (VEGF) from activated macrophages under the influence of ovarian steroids] produce endometriosis tissue. Interleukin-8, expressed in endometrial stromal cells, basic fibroblast groth factor (FGF), expressed in endometriotic tissue, and platelet-derived endothelial cell growth factor (PD-ECGF), expressed in lining epithelial cells independently of the sex steroidal milieu, might contribute to the characteristic advancement of angiogenetic lesions in endometriosis in susceptible individuals (38).
- The genetic susceptibility theory suggests chromosomal instability in the mechanism of endometriosis development (39).

Endometriosis affects women primarily during their reproductive years. However, this condition has been reported in adolescents (40,41) [70% of adolescent girls with chronic pelvic pain unresponsive to medical management have pelvic endometriosis (40)]. Postmenopausal endometriosis has been reported, although endometriosis often becomes quiescent at the time of menopause (42). Symptomatic endometriosis can occur during pregnancy (43).

The predisposing factors for developing endometriosis are categorized as follows:

- The familial risk of endometriosis is increased sevenfold among mothers, sisters, and daughters of affected women (44).
- Menstrual cycle pattern abnormalities such as early menarche, frequent menstruation, or late menopause are frequently associated with endometriosis (27,45).
- Genital tract anomalies such as imperforate hymen, vaginal septum, cervical stenosis or agenesis, and uterine abnormalities can increase the risk for developing endometriosis (46).

Classification

Endometriosis is classified as either pelvic (27) or extrapelvic endometriosis.

Pelvic endometriosis can be further subclassified (47). Superficial endometriosis implantation is considered to be asymptomatic and can lead to adhesions or ovarian cysts (endometrioma). Deep endometriosis implantation can affect retroperitoneal areas and usually involves the posterior cul-de-sac, the rectovaginal septum, and the uterosacral ligament complex. Some clinicians consider adenomyosis to be a form of deep pelvic endometriosis. Deep pelvic endometriosis is associated with severe symptomatology.

Extrapelvic endometriosis may affect any part of the body. The main areas of occurrence include the diaphragm, thoracic cavity, gastrointestinal tract, scarless umbilical area, abdominal and perineal areas, abdominal wall, and incisional implants. It can manifest in an interesting phenomenon of bleeding that occurs from the lungs, bladder, or rectum (sites other than the vagina) during regular menses and is known as *vicarious menstruation* (27,48–53). Bladder endometriosis can present clinically with frequency, urgency, and pain and no documented infection, imitating interstitial cystitis in about 70%. Hormonal therapy for bladder endometriosis may be effective (49). Ureter endometriosis is a rare insidious condition that can evolve into compromise or complete loss of kidney function (51).

The American Society for Reproductive Medicine (ASRM) introduced a system of classification for endometriosis in 1979 to define the extent of endometriosis, pelvic pain characteristics, associated infertility, and morphologic type. The ASRM classification has been revised several times, most recently in 1997 (54). The current version was designed to improve predictions of fertility by adding color photographs (morphologic variations of endometriotic implants) to maintain a level of consistency in describing the clinical appearance of endometriosis and to present changes in the evaluation of posterior cul-de-sac obliteration. Previous versions of ASRM classification better correlated with pain symptoms than fertility outcome; an effort was made to rectify this weakness in the preceding version (55).

The ASRM classification is widely accepted and includes the following categories:

- Pelvic endometriosis extent
- Detailed description of endometriosis location
- Scoring system that provides information in reference to severity by assigning a point score for size and location of endometriosis and associated pelvic adhesions

The ASRM classification system assigns points to the stages of endometriosis as follows:

- Stage I or minimal endometriosis: 1 to 5 points
- Stage II or mild endometriosis: 6 to 15 points
- Stage III or moderate endometriosis: 16 to 40 points
- Stage IV or severe endometriosis: greater than 40 points

For more details on the ASRM classification system, the reader is referred to the ASRM publication (54) or to the commercially available classification form.

Diagnosis

Pelvic endometriosis is surgically diagnosed predominantly via laparoscopy. Histologic verification provides a definitive diagnosis and is the preferable method, although some authorities recommend laparoscopy to further verify the classic appearance of endometriosis (3). Due to the polymorphism of endometriotic implants and the similarity with other conditions such as hemosiderin deposits or hemangioma, histologic confirmation is widely accepted as part of the diagnostic process. Histologic assessment serves not only as a diagnostic tool, but also helps avoid over- or underdiagnosis.

Pertinent medical history for pelvic endometriosis is not specific (56), although the presence of the following symptoms may suggest pelvic endometriosis:

- Dysmenorrhea associated with endometriosis, unlike primary dysmenorrhea, exhibits intensification in pain severity with time. Pain may continue through the cycle, with different degrees of pain noted (40).
- Chronic pelvic pain, particularly that unresponsive to conservative medical therapy, strongly suggests endometriosis (40). However, most women with endometriosis are pain free (56). Chronic pelvic pain associated with endometriosis is usually cyclic (endometriosis is a hor-

monally responsive condition) (57). Nevertheless, some patients may experience acyclic pain with exacerbation at mid-cycle and again shortly before menses (40).

- Infertility in association with pelvic endometriosis is a well-established phenomenon.
- Deep dyspareunia is reported frequently in association with deep pelvic endometriosis located in the posterior cul-de-sac, rectovaginal septum, or uterosacral ligaments.
- Menstrual characteristics suggesting pelvic endometriosis include menarche at less than 12 years of age, interval of menstrual cycle less than 28 days, and heavy flow lasting longer than 5 days. These findings may raise suspicion for endometriosis, but menstrual symptoms are not reliable as indicators of the disease based on observational studies (58).
- Painful defecation can be present when the rectovaginal septum is affected by endometriosis.
- Abdominal enlargement is occasionally reported, when endometriosis is associated with ascites, and must be differentiated from a malignant process (59).

All patients evaluated for abdominopelvic pain should be instructed to maintain a pain diary. A pain diary should include descriptions of the pain itself; the association of pain with the menstrual cycle, defecation, urination, and sexual intercourse; aggravation or relief of pain associated with food, drink, or other other substances; and daily physical and mental activities.

The physical examination usually does not yield any pertinent information, provided the skin is not affected by endometriosis. When the skin or an incisional scar is affected, lesions are usually bluish and can be tender, and size and tenderness may or may not fluctuate with the menstrual cycle.

Speculum examination may reveal small bluish implants (usually 0.5–1 cm in diameter) on the vaginal mucosa or more often on the ectocervix. When examination is performed shortly before menses, blood may be seen oozing directly from the lesions. Such an abnormality can be histologically confirmed, establishing the definitive diagnosis of endometriosis. Speculum examination may establish displacement of the entire cervix lateral to the midline of the vagina and is due to uterosacral ligament scarring (61). External cervical stenosis also may be present in conjunction with chronic pelvic pain and is a common finding associated with endometriosis (62). Some clinicians prefer to perform clinical examination for endometriosis during menstruation.

Bimanual pelvic examination (either vaginoabdominal or rectoabdominal) can confirm lateral cervical displacement. A retroverted or retroflexed uterus with limited mobility (fixed), posterior cul-de-sac nodules, or rectovaginal or uterosacral ligament nodularity can be appreciated in about 36% of all endometriosis cases. Approximately 78% of patients have posterior cul-de-sac tenderness (63). When

ovarian endometrioma is present, an adnexal mass can be identified either unilaterally or bilaterally.

Laboratory tests are not available to establish a definitive diagnosis of endometriosis. In the context of clinical assessment, selective use of the biochemical marker serum CA-125 may assist in determining whether further testing is needed (64) or can be used to determine the responsiveness of endometriosis to treatment or to establish recurrence (65).

Evaluation of infertility in women with endometriosis should include an assessment of autoantibody status. Approximately 30% of women with unexplained infertility have immune changes characteristic of endometriosis (36).

Imaging studies such as ultrasonography or magnetic resonance imaging play a limited role in the diagnosis of endometriosis in selected cases (64) .

Laparoscopic evaluation is the ultimate method for the diagnosis of endometriosis with or without pathologic verification of specimens (preferably with histologic verification that documents the presence of extrauterine glandular and stroma endometrial tissue). At the same time, endometriosis staging and pain mapping can be performed. Negative laparoscopic findings do not exclude pelvic endometriosis, because invisible lesions can be present. Classic or typical endometrial implants that present as blue, gray, or brown (powder burn) lesions are considered diagnostic. The atypical appearance of endometriosis—such as petechial or vesicular, or white, clear, red, flame, reddish brown lesions—are frequently present and can be observed in a cluster (54).

Differential Diagnosis

The differential diagnosis of pelvic endometriosis includes:

- Pelvic inflammatory disease (PID)
- Pelvic splenosis
- Primary dysmenorrhea
- Other than endometriotic causes of secondary dysmenorrhea
- Other than ovarian endometriotic causes of benign and malignant adnexal masses
- Hemangioma

Pelvic splenosis can mimic endometriosis not only symptomatically but also in its laparoscopic appearance. Pelvic splenosis is suspected in women who have sustained splenic trauma or have undergone surgical intervention on the spleen. Patients may be asymptomatic or may express endometriosis-like symptoms. The definitive diagnosis is established intraoperatively by frozen-section microscopic evaluation. Surgical excision either through a laparoscopic approach (by means of excision with scissors or excision/ablation with electrocautery or laser) or via laparotomy. Surgical treatment is indicated when pelvic splenosis causes pelvic pain, hemorrhage, torsion, or adhesions (66).

Conventional Therapy

The objectives of endometriosis treatment are to ameliorate symptoms, to inhibit the natural progress of the disease, and to assist in reproductive goals that this entity may compromise. The initial step of therapy is conservative medical management of symptoms, before subjecting patients to invasive procedures such as laparoscopic diagnosis (under general anesthesia), staining, and therapeutic surgical intervention. It is also important to remember that endometriosis is a self-limiting condition and can regress spontaneously in up to 58% of patients, and considerable placebo benefit has been demonstrated (27,56). No medical or conservative surgical treatment will alleviate pelvic endometriosis completely; all treatments have either risks or side effects, and recurrent symptoms develop in up to 45% of women within 5 years after initial therapy. Therefore, treatment of endometriosis should be offered to those women who demonstrate signs and symptoms of progression, tissue damage, or physiologic disturbances. Treatment for pelvic pain or prophylactic therapy to prevent progression must be considered as empiric and not specific (56).

Pelvic endometriosis management can be compartmentalized into three steps. Step I therapy includes empirical treatment for dysmenorrhea and chronic pelvic pain:

- Nonsteroidal anti–inflammatory drugs (NSAIDs) alone
- Progestin therapy alone
- Oral contraceptives in a cyclic mode alone, preferably monophasic with a progestin-dominant component [some formulations contain a progestin component such as ethynodiol didiacetate, norethindrone, or norgestrel (67)]
- Combination of cyclic oral contraceptives and NSAIDs
- Psychotherapy in combination with any of these drugs

Step I clinical management should be discontinued after 3 months of any course of treatment that has been offered (the most commonly used mode for initial management of chronic pelvic pain and dysmenorrhea in the United States is a combination of oral contraceptives and NSAIDs, although progestins can significantly improve symptoms of chronic pelvic pain).

Step II therapy is laparoscopy, which is designed to provide a definitive diagnosis (preferably with histologic confirmation) and surgical therapy at the same time. Laparoscopic excisional biopsy of any suspicious lesion can be performed and specimens submitted for frozen-section evaluation. Laparoscopic resection of endometriosis by means of excision with mechanical scissors, with electrocautery or with a laser can be executed. Ablation of endometriotic implants can be achieved with electrocautery (unipolar or bipolar electrocautery), laser vaporization, or endocoagulation.

Attention should be directed to removing or obliterating as many endometriotic lesions as possible. Such an approach maximizes the potential for overall outcome. Long-term (5 years after initial operative laparoscopy) pelvic pain reduction in approximately 66% of patients was reported in one study (68), but clinical independent verification of these results is absent. Recurrent pelvic endometriosis following initial laparoscopic surgical intervention occurs in approximately 28% of patients within 18 months and in up to 40% within 9 years (69).

Step III therapy is medical therapy with gonadotropin-releasing hormone (GnRH) agonists following operative laparoscopy. This mode of therapy is considered to be first line in patients over 16 years of age who have completed puberty. GnRH agonists induce a pseudomenopausal and continuous hypoestrogenic state by decreasing secretion from the pituitary gland. By reducing estrogens levels, GnRH agonists inhibit proliferation of endometrial implants. An amenorrheic state ensues owing to endometrial atrophy, which prevents retrograde seeding of the endometrium.

Various routes of administration can be used for GnRH agonists. Nasal spray (Nafarelin) in a dose of one puff twice daily to alternating nostrils (70) should be used for no longer than 6 months (the U.S. Food and Drug Administration has not approved any GnRH agonist for longer use). Results of a prospective randomized double-blind controlled clinical study showed that a 3-month course of Nafarelin provided effective symptom relief for endometriosis with gradual return of symptoms (71).

Intramuscular injection (depot-leuprolide 3.75 or 11.25 mg) is administered every 4 weeks or every 3 months, respectively. It induces hypoestrogenism and amenorrhea (90%) and is as effective as danazol in managing the symptoms of endometriosis and presents fewer undesirable side effects when compared with danazol. The predominant side effects of GnRH agonists include vasomotor menopausal symptoms such as hot flashes, vaginal dryness, heart palpitation, night sweats, and headaches; decreased libido also may be observed (72,73). These symptoms do not have a serious impact on health. The long-term side effect of reducing bone mass (a mean loss of 5.9%–13.8% of the pretreatment vertebral body bone mass after 6 months of treatment with GnRH agonists) presents a much more serious health concern, because bone mass recovery is a very slow process (74). Add-back therapy with estrogen or progestins improves the clinical tolerance (menopausal symptoms) and reduces bone mass loss (75).

Oral contraceptives are particularly useful after diagnostic/operative laparoscopy for patients who have not completed puberty. Epidemiologic data suggest that oral contraceptives are associated with a reduced incidence of endometriosis (76). They should be offered on a continuous basis following initial laparoscopic surgery. A continuous mode of administration can be changed to a cyclic mode; but when endometriosis symptomatology reoccurs, a continuous method should be reinstituted (40). Oral contraceptive treatment (continuous or cyclic) may be continued indefinitely until the patient expresses a desire for fertility. Meta-analysis of randomized studies on the effectiveness of oral contraceptives for pain associated with endometriosis has shown no significant differences between the effectiveness of oral contraceptives and GnRH agonists in relieving dyspareunia or nonmenstrual pain. The use of oral contraceptives in a conventional manner is less effective than a GnRH agonist in the relief of dysmenorrhea (76). Side effects such as headaches, hypertension, fluid retention, nausea, or psychological disturbances may occur.

Subcutaneous injection of GnRH agonists also can be offered.

A second line of medication can be offered upon reaching the definitive diagnosis of endometriosis. Progestin only is recommended in the following forms:

- Medroxyprogesterone acetate is given at a dosage of 30 to 50 mg per day orally.
- Medroxyprogesterone acetate depot (injectable) at a dose of 150 mg is administered intramuscularly every 1 to 3 months. This high dose of progestin can produce side effects that include headaches, fluid retention, psychological disturbances, and endometrial bleeding (77,78).
- Megestrol acetate, 40 mg per day orally for 24 months, can be an effective mode of therapy, although the lack of controlled studies makes its efficacy difficult to quantify (79).

Analysis of observational and randomized placebo-controlled studies indicate the efficacy of progestins for temporary relief of endometriosis-associated pelvic pain is comparable with that of other agents (GnRH agonists or danazol) with less side effect (79).

Danazol is a 17-alpha-ethyl testosterone derivative that expresses its therapeutic effect on endometriosis by increasing androgen levels, which in turn suppresses follicular development and maturation. Such events eventually lead to a hypoestrogenic state that decreases the proliferative ability of endometriosis.

Danazol at a dosage of 800 mg per day in divided doses is recommended. Despite its acceptable efficacy, cosmetically and metabolically intolerable side effects associated with hyperandrogenism (oily skin, acne, hirsutism, voice deepening, abnormal endometrial bleeding, weight gain) make the use of this medication less attractive, particularly because hirsutism and voice deepening are not completely reversible after discontinuation (80). Danazol is now seldom used due to its metabolic and clinical side effects, and the presence of other equally effective medications with fewer complications.

Anastrazole, an aromatase inhibitor, may be administered at 1 mg per day in combination with 1.5 g per day elemental calcium, and *Alendromate* (a nonestrogenic inhibitor of bone resorption) may be given at a dosage of 10 mg per day for 9 months for severe pelvic endometriosis. Preliminary short-time results are very promising in pain elimination and near-complete eradication of implants unresponsive to other standard medication (42). The use of an aromatase inhibitor in unusually aggressive cases of recurrent postmenopausal endometriosis presents a new option for managing resistant, recurrent pelvic endometriosis. However, the absence of controlled study data makes the safety and effectiveness of this approach difficult to quantify.

Surgical management of endometriosis is categorized as conservative, definitive, and radical. Conservative surgical management can avoid the side effects associated with medications and can temporarily reduce or, in a small number of cases, relieve symptomatology associated with endometriosis. As previously indicated, the laparoscopic approach is an effective conservative method for removing or destroying endometriotic implants, either with mechanical instruments (excision), electrocautery (excision or fulguration), or laser instruments (excision or ablation). Operative laparoscopic or laparotomy intervention for chronic pelvic pain and infertility associated with endometriosis yields comparable clinical outcomes (81).

Complementary denervation (interruption of pelvic sensory nerve pathway innervation via uterosacral nerve oblation or presacral neurectomy) is routinely used to reduce midline pelvic pain, mainly for severe primary or secondary dysmenorrhea. However, based on clinical randomized evidence, such procedures cannot be recommended (82,83). Also, there is no consensus on the outcome of adhesiolysis on patients with chronic pelvic pain (82).

Definitive surgical management of endometriosis is hysterectomy with or without bilateral salpingo-oophorectomy. Hysterectomy for chronic pelvic pain of presumed uterine origin consistently demonstrates reduction of relief of pain 1 year after surgery in approximately 83% to 97% of patients (82). Women under the age of 30 years who undergo hysterectomy for pelvic pain associated with endometriosis not only report more frequently residual symptoms than older women but also present emotional disturbances (from hysterectomy itself and pain related) and more disruptive behavior due to pain (84).

Radical surgery for endometriosis consists of significant retroperitoneal dissection to the pelvic floor with maximal resection of endometrial implants and some nonmüllerian structures. Deep symptomatic rectosigmoid endometriosis may require full-thickness segmental rectal or sigmoid or rectosigmoid resection with immediate end-to-end reanastomosis as part of the radical operation. It is recommended for the deep, infiltrative type of endometriosis that involves genital and adjacent pelvic organs. Endometriosis at this location produces severe symptomatology that is usually unresponsive to medical and conservative surgical management (85–87).

Endometriosis associated with a pelvic mass and massive ascites strongly suggests malignant neoplastic disease. Such an occurrence of endometriosis often is unresponsive to standard endometriosis management and may require multiple exploratory laparotomies and possibly thoracotomies for associated pleural and pulmonary involvement (59).

Conventional therapy for infertility associated with endometriosis is discussed in Chapter 11.

Complementary Therapy

Complementary therapy is designed to enhance conventional treatment, not to serve as an independent substitution. The lack of controlled studies makes the efficacy of these traditional approaches difficult to define.

Patient Education

Endometriosis, as a chronic medical entity, is notoriously difficult to manage, and frequent relapses of the disease cause frustration not only to the patient, but also to medical practitioners over the lack of reliable medical or surgical therapy. Education should emphasize the natural potentially progressive course of endometriosis. The disease may affect women of any age, including adolescents and postmenopausal women. However, the majority of the cases become quiescent during the postmenopausal period. Initial diagnosis is clinical, with conservative symptomatic medical management including but not limited to psychotherapy. An initial course of therapy should be offered for no longer than 3 months, if a patient is unresponsive. Cases resistant to the initial treatment should be subjected to diagnostic and operative laparoscopy, with definitive diagnosis preferably reached by histologic verification. Post-laparoscopic medical treatment as an integral part of management should be made clear. A second opinion is desirable for patient reassurance. A patient should know about spontaneous remission of endometriosis. Asymptomatic forms of endometriosis require no therapeutic intervention.

Therapeutic modalities should be clearly presented accordingly to staging and symptomatology of endometriosis. Clinical follow-up with a support group is an effective form of patient reassurance. A support group mediated by a knowledgeable counselor (a gynecologist or other practitioner) should be an integral part of endometriosis management. There is a significant demand for and high patient satisfaction with the concept of integrating a patient support group into the standard model of health care for endometriosis.

Diet

Diet is an important part of the management of endometriosis. Increased consumption of the following foods is recommended (89):

- Vegetables such as cauliflower, Brussels sprouts, and carrots
- Protein from sources such as salmon, turkey, chicken, tofu, beans, and soy nuts in small portions

- Fiber in the form of whole-grain breads, rice, raw vegetables, and flax seeds
- Filtrated water, up to 8 glasses per day

Decreased consumption of the following foods is recommended:

- All animal fats
- All food containing sugar, chocolate, caffeine, and alcohol

The following dietary practices should be avoided:

- Heating food in plastic container
- Consuming foods contaminated with pesticides

Nutritional Supplements

The results from an observational clinical case study suggest that dietary changes and administration of supplements are promising options in managing endometriosis (90). It has been documented that oral beta-carotene can effectively enhance thyroxine plus lymphocytes. The results of this study support the use of beta-carotene for enhancing the immune system (91). Because the hormonally responsive mucosal immune system has been implicated in the pathogenesis of endometriosis (92), enhancing the immune system seems logical. The absence of definitive data on this subject makes clinical recommendation anecdotal at this moment.

Daily supplements are suggested as follows (89):

- Vitamins
  Vitamin C, 6,000 to 10,000 mg
  Vitamin E, 400 to 800 IU
  Vitamin B complex, 50 to 100 mg
- Other supplements
  Gamma-linolenic or alpha-linolenic oil, 300 mg
  Beta-carotene, 50,000 to 150,000 IU
  Selenium, 200 to 400 µg
  Lipotropics, two to four capsules

Alternative Therapy

Alternative therapy is designed to cope with symptomatology and its elimination or reduction in severity. Phytotherapy and micronized natural progesterone are predominantly offered to cope with symptoms.

Herbal Remedies

Herbal remedies in endometriosis are essentially used for pain relief. Methods of treatment for pelvic pain associated with endometriosis and dysmenorrhea (a component of endometriotic symptoms) are similar. The reader is therefore also referred to Chapters 5 and 11.

Botanical agents may be used in the treatment of endometriosis. An herbal remedy for acute pain is composed of a compound tincture of the following substances (89):

Black cohosh, 1 oz
Wild yam, 1 oz
Cramp bark 1 oz
Valerian 1 oz

The tincture is administered in the amount of $\frac{1}{2}$ to 1 teaspoon every 2 to 4 hours in acute phase of pelvic pain.

An herbal remedy for chronic pain is composed of a compound tincture of the following substances (89):

Chaste tree, 1 oz
Dandelion, 1 oz
Prickly ash, 1 oz
Motherwort, 1 oz

The tincture is administered in the amount of $\frac{1}{2}$ teaspoon three times per day.

An extract of Turska's formula (five drops three times daily) is composed of the following substances:

Aconite nappellus (monkshood)
Bryonia alba (bryony)
Gelsemium sempervirens (yellow jessamine)
Phytolacca americana (poke root)

Rhubarb root (*Rheum palmatum L.*) has been tested in open clinical trials, and initial results are promising in reducing the clinical signs and symptoms of endometriosis (93,94).

Natural Progesterone Therapy

Natural progesterone creams are recommended in different regimens to apply on the skin in the following schedules (89):

- Option 1: from days 8 to 28 of the menstrual cycle at a dosage of $\frac{1}{4}$ to $\frac{1}{2}$ teaspoon twice daily
- Option 2: from days 15 to 28 of the menstrual cycle at a dosage of $\frac{1}{4}$ to $\frac{1}{2}$ teaspoon twice daily
- Option 3: from days 22 to 28 of the menstrual cycle at a dosage of $\frac{1}{4}$ to $\frac{1}{2}$ teaspoon twice daily

Lack of controlled clinical trial results of this mode of therapy makes recommendation for its clinical use as a standard management approach difficult.

Homeopathic Therapy

Homeopathic therapy is primary directed toward the symptomatic relief of dysmenorrhea. More information is presented in Chapter 5.

PELVIC INFLAMMATORY DISEASE

The female upper genital tract structures (uterus, fallopian tubes, and ovaries) can be individually infected or as a unit. Therefore, sexually transmitted disease and other causes of gynecologic infection are described in the benign disorders of the vulva, vagina, cervix, uterus, fallopian tubes, and ovaries. Approximately 60% of PID cases can be attributed to a sexually transmitted organism. All sexual partners having sexual contact within 60 days preceding symptoms should be notified and treated (95,96).

Definition

Pelvic inflammatory disease is infection of the upper genital tract and adjacent pelvic structures, and the inflammatory process is not associated with pelvic surgery or pregnancy.

Incidence

The incidence of PID in the United States is unknown but is estimated to account for approximately 5% to 20% of all gynecologic hospital admissions (97).

Etiology

Microorganism pathogens (aerobic bacteria, anaerobic bacteria, mycoplasmas, ureoplasmas, etc.) are responsible for PID, the most commonly identified being *Chlamydia trachomatis* and *Neisseria gonorrhea*. It is a common notion that tubal occlusion (including tubal ligation) protects against PID, but cases have been reported proving otherwise. Tuboperitoneal fistula, spontaneous anastomosis at the occlusion site, spontaneous recanalization, incomplete tubal occlusion due to a faulty surgical technique, rupture of the weakened tubal wall, infection initiated by a surgical procedure itself, systematic infection by hematogenous spread, lymphatic spread, and changes in immunologic status may play a role in the mechanism of PID after tubal sterilization (98).

A complicated clinical course of PID ($\geq$14 days in hospital, therapy requiring surgery or hospital readmission) is affected by older patient age and drug use, which should be identified at the initial evaluation (99).

Classification

Pelvic inflammatory disease is clinically classified as either acute or chronic.

Diagnosis

Clinical diagnosis of PID is limited due to the wide variety of clinical presentations, nonspecific clinical diagnostic criteria, and low sensitivity and poor specificity of laboratory tests (95,100). A high index of suspicious for PID whenever sexually active women have pelvic symptomatology is a secure clinical policy.

Pertinent medical history, although nonspecific, may be presented as follows:

- Constant lower abdominopelvic pain
- Abnormal vaginal discharge
- Irregular endometrial bleeding
- Dyspareunia
- Fever and chills
- Nausea and vomiting

This cluster of symptoms strongly suggests the presence of acute PID.

Physical examination may reveal oral temperature over 101°F (>38.3°C), warmer than normal skin, and diffuse lower abdominopelvic tenderness with or without rebound tenderness.

Speculum examination may or may not reveal vaginal discharge (more frequently vaginal discharge is present). Cervical and adnexal tenderness may be induced by motion. Sometimes *pelvic examination* is difficult to appropriately execute due to severe discomfort, particularly when diffuse pelvic peritonitis is present. An adnexal mass or swelling usually can be appreciated

Imaging studies, particularly ultrasonography, are useful when the pelvic examination is inconclusive or difficult to execute, or tuboovarian abscess is clinically suspected.

Laboratory tests should include the following:

- Pregnancy test in sexually active women and women of reproductive age
- Blood count with differential (leukocytosis is commonly present)
- Erythrocyte sedimentation rate (can be elevated >15 mm/h)
- C-reactive protein (elevation may be observed)
- Gram-stain
- Cervical culture for *Neisseria gonorrhea,* aerobic and anaerobic bacteria, mycoplasma, and ureoplasma
- Cervical *Chlamydia trachomatis* DNA probe [in the absence of the cervix (posthysterectomy), urethral culture and probe can be performed]

The definitive diagnosis is based either on histopathologic verification of endometritis or laparoscopic findings consistent with PID. Histology or laparoscopic confirmation is not frequently recommended.

Laparoscopic criteria for the diagnosis of acute PID are as follows (101):

- Exudate is present at the fimbriated end or on the serosa of the fallopian tubes.
- Erythema of the fallopian tubes can be identified.
- Edema of the fallopian tubes is recognized.

Based on fallopian tube mobility and the presence or the absence of an inflammatory mass, a severity scoring system for PID was formulated (101):

- Mild state is associated with movable and patent fallopian tubes.

- Moderate state is identified when fallopian tubes are not freely movable and tubal patency is uncertain.
- Severe state is identified by the presence of an inflammatory mass.

Differential Diagnosis

The differential diagnosis for PID most commonly includes:

- Ectopic pregnancy
- Appendicitis
- Ovarian cyst
- Adnexal torsion
- Diverticulitis

Conventional Therapy

Conventional therapy for sexually transmitted disease is described in Chapters 15, 17, 19, 23, and 24.

Emerging evidence from randomized controlled clinical trials suggests that selective screening for silent chlamydia infection effectively reduces the incidence of PID (100).

The Centers for Disease Control and Prevention recommend an empiric oral therapy for all sexually active women, including adolescents, who present with presumptive clinical signs and symptoms of PID (102). Within 72 hours of initial therapy, a follow-up visit is advocated to evaluate clinical improvement versus failure of the course of the disease. If oral therapy is not successful, parenteral treatment should be instituted until a patient is symptom free for 24 hours; then oral therapy is readministered with doxycycline 100 mg twice daily for 14 consecutive days (other oral antibiotics can be used as indicated by culture and sensitivity). Clinical retesting should be offered 4 to 6 weeks after the completion of therapy (102).

Possible sequelae of delayed diagnosis or untreated or inadequately treated PID include a decrease in reproductive potential (tubal factor or periovarian factor associated with adhesion as a result of periooophoritis), sterility, tuboovarian abscess, a risk factor for ectopic pregnancy, and chronic pelvic pain (95). The aggressiveness of the causative pathogen and the anatomic location also figure in the severity of complications, which could include septicemia and even death (103).

Complementary Therapy

Complementary and alternative therapies should be considered in addition to conventional therapy with antibiotics or surgery. The following therapeutic suggestions are offered (89).

- Diet
    Vegetable broths, steamed vegetable, salads, and fruits
    Acidophilus yogurt, 4 to 8 oz per day

- Supplements
- Vitamins

   Vitamin A, 25,000 to 50,000 U per day for 2 weeks
   Vitamin C, 1,000 to 2,000 mg three times daily
   Vitamin E, 400 U twice daily
   Zinc, 45 to 60 mg per day

Alternative Therapy

Phytotherapy is recommended as follows (89,104):

- *Echinacea angustifolia* or *Echinacea pallida,* 355-mg capsules or 335-mg tablets every 2 to 3 hours, or liquid extracts ¹/₂ teaspoon every 3 hours during the course of active infection (89,104)
- Garlic, fresh bulb 2 to 5 g, 600-mg tablets, or allicin tablets, total potential 5 mg twice daily

The scarcity of scientific clinical data and lack of controlled clinical trials makes it difficult to quantify the safety and efficacy of complementary and alternative therapies.

REFERENCES

1. Association of Professors of Gynecology and Obstetrics. *Medical student educational objectives,* 7th ed. Washington, DC: Association of Professors of Gynecology and Obstetrics, 1997.
2. Council on Resident and Gynecology (CREOG). *Educational objectives core curriculum for residents in obstetrics and gynecology,* 5th ed. Washington, DC: CREOG, 1996.
3. American College of Obstetrician and Gynecologists (ACOG). Educational Bulletin no. 223. Washington, DC: ACOG, 1996.
4. Zondervan K, Barlow DH. Epidemiology of chronic pelvic pain. *Baillieres Best Pract Res Clin Obstet Gynaecol* 2000;14:403–414.
5. Moore J, Kennedy S. Causes of chronic pelvic pain. *Baillieres Best Pract Res Clin Obstet Gynaecol* 2000;14:389–402.
6. Stones EW, Mountfield J. Interventions for treating chronic pain in women. *Cochrane Database Syst Rev* 2000;2:CD000387.
7. *Clinical practice. A source book.* Vol 11. Sarasota, FL: Professional Resources Press, 1992.
8. Stones RW, Selfe SA, Fransman S, et al. Psychological and economic impact of chronic pelvic pain. *Baillieres Best Pract Res Clin Obstet Gynaecol* 2000;14:389–402.
9. Rosenthal RH. Psychology of chronic pelvic pain. *Obstet Gynecol Clin Noth Am* 1993;20:627–642.
10. American Psychiatric Association (APA). *Diagnostic and statistical manual of mental disorders,* 4th ed. Primary care version. Washington, DC: APA, 1995.
11. Scialli AR, for the Pelvic Pain Expert Working Group. Evaluating chronic pelvic pain. A consensus recommendation. *J Reprod Med* 1999;44:945–952.
12. Stovall DW. Transvaginal ultrasound findings in women with chronic pelvic pain. *Obstet Gynecol* 2000;95(suppl 1):57.
13. Cody RF Jr, Ascher SM. Diagnostic value of radiological tests in chronic pelvic pain. *Baillieres Best Pract Res Clin Obstet Gynaecol* 2000;14:433–466.
14. Peters AA, van Dorst E, Jellis B, et al. A randomized clinical trial to compare two different approaches in women with chronic pelvic pain. *Obstet Gynecol* 1991;77:740–744.
15. Howard FM. The role of laparoscopy as a diagnostic tool in chronic pelvic pain. *Baillieres Best Pract Res Clin Obstet Gynaecol* 2000;14:467–494.
16. Orford VP, Kuhn RJ. Management of ovarian remnant syndrome. *Aust N Z J Obstet Gynaecol* 1996;36:468–471.
17. Price FV, Edwards R, Buchsbaum HJ. Ovarian remnant syndrome: difficulties in diagnosis and management. *Obstet Gynecol Surv* 1990;45:151–156.
18. Rane A, Ohizua O. Acute residual ovary syndrome. *Aust N Z J Obstet Gynaecol* 1998;38:447–478.
19. Prentice A. Medical management of chronic pelvic pain. *Baillieres Best Pract Res Clin Obstet Gynaecol* 2000;14:495–499.
20. Grace VM. Pitfalls of the medical paradigm in chronic pelvic pain. *Baillieres Best Pract Res Clin Obstet Gynaecol* 2000;14:5255–5399.
21. Flor H, Fydrich T, Turk DC. Efficacy of multidisciplinary pain treatment centers: a meta-analytic flow. *Pain* 1992;49:221–230.
22. Hoffman AD. Breast and gynecological disorders. In: Hoffman AD, Greydanus DE, eds. *Adolescence medicine,* 3rd ed. Stamford, CT: Appleton & Lange, 1997:552–565.
23. Reiter RC. Evidence-based management of chronic pain. *Clin Obstet Gynecol* 1998;41:422–435.
24. Steege JF. Basic philosophy of the integrated approach: overcoming the mind-body spilt. In: Steege JF, Metzger DA, Levy BS, eds. *Chronic pelvic pain: an integrated approach.* Philadelphia: WB Saunders, 1998:5–12.
25. Farquhar C, Vandekerckhove P, Watson A, et al. Barrier agents for preventing adhesions after surgery for subfertility. *Cochrane Database Syst Rev* 2000;2:CD000475.
26. Hillis SD, Marchbanks PA, Peterson HB. The effectiveness of hysterectomy for chronic pelvic pain. *Obstet Gynecol* 1995;86:941–945.
27. Farquhar CM. Extracts from the "clinical evidence." Endometriosis. *BMJ* 2000;320:1449–1452.
28. Barbieri RL. Etiology and epidemiology of endometriosis. *Am J Obstet Gynecol* 1990;162:565–567.
29. Laufer MR, Goldstein DP. Pelvic pain, dysmenorrhea and premenstrual syndrome. In: Emans SJ, Laufer MR, Goldstein DP, eds. *Pediatric and adolescent gynecology,* 4th ed. Boston: Little, Brown, 1998:363–410.
30. Knapp VJ. How old is endometriosis? Late 17th- and 18th-century European description of the disease. *Fertil Steril* 1999;72:10–14.
31. Meyer R. Uber entzundliche netrope epithelwucherungen im weiblichen Genetalg ebiet und uber eine bis in die Wurzel des Mesocolon ausgedehnte benigne Wucherung des Dar mepithel. *Virchows Arch Pathol Ant* 1909;195:487–502.
32. Halban J. Hysteroadenosis metastica. *Wien Klin Wochenschr* 1924;37:1205–1228.
33. Sampson JA. Peritoneal endometriosis due to the menstrual dissemination of endometrial tissue into the peritoneal cavity. *Am J Obstet Gynecol* 1927;14:422–469.
34. Sampson JA. The development of the implantation theory for the origin of peritoneal endometriosis. *Am J Obstet Gynecol* 1940;40:549–557.
35. Halme J, Becker S, Haskill S. Altered maturation and function of peritoneal macrophages: possible role in pathogenesis of endometriosis. *Am J Obstet Gynecol* 1987;156:783–789.
36. Dmowski WP. Immunological aspects of endometriosis. *Int J Gynaecol Obstet* 1995;50(suppl 1):3–10.
37. Mulayim N, Arici A. The relevance of the peritoneal fluid in endometriosis-associated infertility. *Hum Reprod* 1999;14(suppl 2):67–76.
38. Fujimoto J, Sakaguchi H, Hirose R, et al. Angiogenesis in endometriosis and angiogenetic factors. *Gynecol Obstet Invest* 1999;48(suppl 1):14–20.
39. Gogusev J, de Joliniere JB, Telvi L, et al. Genetic abnormalities

detected by comparative genomic hybridization in a human endometriosis-derived cell line. *Mol Hum Reprod* 2000;6: 821–827.

40. Propst AM, Laufer MR. Endometriosis in adolescents. Incidence, diagnosis and treatment. *J Reprod Med* 1999;44: 751–758.

41. Emmert C, Romann D, Riedel HH. Endometriosis diagnosed by laparoscopy in adolescent girls. *Arch Gynecol Obstet* 1998; 261:89–93.

42. Takayama K, Zeitoun K, Gunby RT, et al. Treatment of severe postmenopausal endometriosis with and aromatase inhibitor. *Fertil Steril* 1998;69:709–713.

43. Gregora M, Higgs P. Endometriosis in pregnancy. *Aust N Z J Obstet Gynaecol* 1998;38:106–109.

44. Meon MH, Magnus P. The familial risk of endometriosis. *Acta Obstet Gynecol Scand* 1993;72:560–564.

45. Moene MH, Schei B. Epidemiology of endometriosis. *Acta Obstet Gynecol Scand* 1997;76:559–562.

46. Sanfalippo JS. Endometriosis in adolescents. In: Wilson EA, ed. *Endometriosis.* New York: Alan R Liss, 1987:161–172.

47. Querleu D. Pelvic pin and external endometriosis. Physiopathology and treatment. *Contracept Fertil Sex* 1995;23: 29–36.

48. Jubanyik KJ, Comite F. Extrapelvic endometriosis. *Obstet Gynecol Clin North Am* 1997;24:411–440.

49. Westney OL, Amundsen CL, Mc Guire EJ. Bladder endometriosis: conservative management. *J Urol* 2000;163:1814–1817.

50. Demoux R, Lechevallier E, Boubli L, et al. Pelvic endometriosis with urologic involvement. Therapeutic principles: apropos of 2 cases. *Prog Urol* 1999;9:705–755.

51. Rouzier R, Deval B, Muray JM, et al. Ureteral endometriosis: three cases. Diagnostic and therapeutic management. Literature review. *Contracept Fertil Sex* 1998;26:173–178.

52. Daoudi K, Bongain A, Isnard V, et al. Umbilical endometriosis. A case report. *Rev Fr Gynecol Obstet* 1995;90:442–443.

53. Ramsanahie A, Giri SK, Velusamy S, et al. Endometriosis in a scarless abdominal wall with underlying umbilical hernia. *Int J Med Sci* 2000;169:67.

54. American Society for Reproductive Medicine. Revised American Society for Reproductive Medicine classification of endometriosis. *Fertil Steril* 1997;67:817–882.

55. Schenken RS. Modern concepts of endometriosis. Classification and its consequences for therapy. *J Reprod Med* 1998;43 (suppl):269–275.

56. Wardle PG, Hull MG. Is endometriosis a disease? *Baillieres Clin Obstet Gynecol* 1993;7:673–685.

57. Hurd WW. Criteria that indicate endometriosis is the cause of chronic pelvic pain. *Obstet Gynecol* 1998;92:1029–1032.

58. Mahmood TA, Templeton AA, Thomson L, et al. Menstrual symptoms in women with pelvic endometriosis. *Br J Obstet Gynaecol* 1991;98:558–563.

59. Muneyyirci-Delale O, Neil G, Serur E, et al. Endometriosis with massive ascites. *Gynecol Oncol* 1998;69:42–46.

60. Fernandez H, Harmas A. Clinical presentation and natural history of endometriosis. *Rev Prat* 1999;49:258–252.

61. Propst AM, Storti K, Barbieri RL. Lateral cervical displacement is associated with endometriosis. *Fertil Steril* 1998;70:568–570.

62. Barbieri RL. Stenosis of the external cervical os: an association with endometriosis in women with chronic pelvic pain. *Fertil Steril* 1998;70:571–572.

63. Chatman K, Ward A. Endometriosis in adolescents. *J Reprod Med* 1982;27:156–160.

64. Duleba AJ. Diagnosis of endometriosis. *Obstet Gynecol Clin North Am* 1997;24:331–346.

65. Pittaway DE, Fayez JA. The use of CA-125 in the diagnosis and management of endometriosis. *Fertil Steril* 1986;46:790–795.

66. Higgins RV, Crain JL. Laparoscopic removal of pelvic splenosis. *J Reprod Med* 1995;40:140–142.

67. Dickey RP. Biological activity of oral contraceptive components. In: Dickey RP, ed. Managing contraceptive pill patients. Durant, OK, 1991:138–139.

68. Redwine DB. Treatment of endometriosis-associated pain. *Infertil Reprod Med Clin North Am* 1993;3:697–721.

69. Olive DL. Conservative surgery. In: Schenken RS, ed. *Endometriosis: contemporary concept in clinical management.* Philadelphia: JB Lippincott, 1989:213–247.

70. Burry KA. Nafarelin in the management of endometriosis. Quality of life assessment. *Am J Obstet Gynecol* 1992;166: 735–739.

71. Hornstein MD, Yuzpe AA, Burry KA, et al. Prospective randomized double-blind trial of 3 versus 6 months of Nafarelin therapy for endometriosis associated pelvic pain. *Fertil Steril* 1995;63:955–962.

72. Wheeler JM, Knittle JD, Miller JD. Depot leuprolide acetate versus danazol in the treatment of women with symptomatic endometriosis. I. Efficacy results. *Am J Obstet Gynecol* 1992; 167:1367–1371.

73. Wheeler JM, Knittle JD, Miller JD. Depot leuprolide acetate versus danazol in the treatment of women with symptomatic endometriosis: a multicenter, double-blind randomized clinical trial. Assessment of safety. The Lupron Endometriosis Study Group. *Am J Obstet Gynecol* 1993;169:26–33.

74. Dawood MY. Impact of medical treatment of endometriosis on bone mass. *Am J Obstet Gynecol* 1993;168:674–684.

75. Audebert A. Medical treatment of endometriosis. *Rev Part* 1999;49:269–275.

76. Moore J, Kennedy S, Prentice A. Modern combined oral contraceptive for pain associated with endometriosis. *Cochrane Database Syst Rev* 2000;2:CD001019.

77. Luciano AA, Turksoy N, Carleo J. Evaluation of oral medroxyprogesterone acetate in the treatment of endometriosis. *Obstet Gynecol* 1988;72:323–327.

78. Vercellini P, Cortesi I, Crosignani PG. Progestins for systemic endometriosis: a critical analysis of the evidence. *Fertil Steril* 1997;68:393–401.

79. Shlaff WD, Dugoff L, Damewood MD, et al. Megestrol acetate for treatment of endometriosis. *Obstet Gynecol* 1990;75: 646–648.

80. Dmowski WP, Cohen MR. Antigonadotropin (danazol) in the treatment of endometriosis. Evaluation of post-treatment fertility and three-year follow-up data. *Am J Obstet Gynecol* 1978: 130:41–47.

81. Crosignani PG, Vercellini P, Biffignandi F, et al. Laparoscopy versus laparotomy in conservative surgical treatment for severe endometriosis. *Fertil Steril* 1996;66:706–711.

82. Vercellini P, De Giorgi O, Pisacreta A, et al. Surgical management of endometriosis. *Baillieres Best Pract Res Clin Obstet Gynaecol* 2000;14:501–523.

83. Wilson ML, Farquhar CM, Sinclair OJ, et al. Surgical interruption of pelvic nerve pathways for primary and secondary dysmenorrhea. *Cochrane Syst Rev* 2000;2:CD001896.

84. MacDonald SR, Klock SC, Milad MP. Long-term outcome of nonconservative surgery (hysterectomy) for endometriosis-associated pain in women <30 years old. *Am J Obstet Gynecol* 1999;180(part 1):1360–1363.

85. Coronado C, Franklin RR, Lotze EC, et al. Surgical treatment of symptomatic colorectal endometriosis. *Fertil Steril* 1990;53: 411–416.

86. Verspyck E, Lefrance JP, Blondon J. Diagnosis and treatment of rectal and sigmoid endometriosis. *Ann Chir* 1997;51:1106–1110.

87. Niclin JL, Perrin L, Gael P. Radical surgery for endometriosis. *Aust NZ J Obstet Gynaecol* 1999;39:68–74.

88. Wingfield MB, Wood C, Henderson LS, et al. Treatment of endometriosis involving a self-help group positively affects patients' perception of care. *J Psychosom Obstet Gynecol* 1997;18:255–258.

89. Hudson T. *Women's encyclopedia of natural medicine.* Lincolnwood, IL: Keats Publishing, 1999:79–88.

90. Kresch AJ. Combining new immune therapies with traditional endometriosis treatment. *J Am Assoc Gynecol Laparosc* 1996;3(suppl):22.

91. Alexander M, Newmark H, Miller RG. Oral beta-carotene can increase the number of OKT4+ cells in human blood. *Immunol Lett* 1985;9:221–224.

92. Rier SE, Yeaman GR. Immune aspect of endometriosis: relevance of the uterine mucosal immune system. *Semin Reprod Endocrinol* 1997;15:209–220.

93. Wang DZ, Wang ZQ, Zhang ZF. Treatment of endometriosis with removing blood stasis and purgation method. *Chung His I Chieh Ho Tsa Chih* 1991;11:515, 524–526.

94. Bone K. *Clinical applications of Ayurvedic and Chinese herbs,* 2nd ed. Warwick, Queensland, Australia: Phytotherapy Press, 1997:59.

95. Munday PE. Clinical aspect of pelvic inflammatory disease. *Hum Reprod* 1997;12(suppl):121–126.

96. Vermillion ST, Holmes MM, Soper DE. Adolescents and sexually transmissible diseases. *Obstet Gynecol Clin North Am* 2000;27:163–179.

97. Rolfs RT, Galaid EI, Zaidi AA. Pelvic inflammatory disease: trends in hospitalizations and office visits, 1979 trough 1988. *Am J Obstet Gynecol* 1992;166:983–990.

98. Levgur M, Duvivier R. Pelvic inflammatory disease after tubal sterilization: a review. *Obstet Gynecol Surv* 2000;55:41–50.

99. Jamieson DJ, Duerr A, Macasaet MA, et al. Risk factors for a complicated clinical course among hospitalized with pelvic inflammatory disease. *Infect Dis Obstet Gynecol* 2000;8:88–93.

100. Paavonen J. Pelvic inflammatory disease. From diagnosis to prevention. *Dermatol Clin* 1998;16:747–756.

101. Jacobson L. Differential diagnosis of acute pelvic inflammatory disease. *Am J Obstet Gynecol* 1980;138(Part 2):1006–1011.

102. Centers for Disease Control and Prevention. 1998 guidelines for treatment of sexually transmitted diseases. *MMWR* 1998;47:1–2.

103. Nunez Esteban M, Sanchez Fernandez C. Acute pelvic inflammatory disease. *Rev Enferm* 1997;20:17–20.

104. Fetrow CW, Avila JR. *The complete guide to herbal medicines.* Springhouse, PA: Spring Corporation, 1999.

7

PREMENSTRUAL DYSPHORIC DISORDER

Educational Objectives

Medical Students (1) **APGO Objective No. 53**	**Residents in Obstetrics/Gynecology (2)** **CREOG Objectives**	**Practitioners** **ACOG Recommendation**
Definition of PDD Etiology theories Diagnosis Management	Pertinent history (emotional aspect, physical aspect, timing symptoms, severity, associated pathology, medication use) Physical examination Diagnostic studies Diagnosis (psychosis, organic disease, PDD) Management (possible interventions)	No specific recommendation

As the knowledge and understanding of this unique medical entity progresses, the nomenclature of this condition is continually changing. An endocrinologist from New York in 1931 described and termed this condition as premenstrual tension (PMT); in 1953, a new terminology emerged as premenstrual syndrome (PMS); in 1987, the nomenclature was changed to late luteal phase dysphoric disorder; and finally, in 1994, *premenstrual dysphoric disorder* (PDD) was adapted.

DEFINITION

Premenstrual dysphoric disorder (PDD) is affective dysfunction with a cyclic occurrence of psychosomatic symptoms in relation to a premenstrual phase of the menstrual cycle.

INCIDENCE

Premenstrual dysphoric disorder usually affects women of reproductive age, and the prevalence is estimated to be about 40% (3). PDD has a significant impact on a woman's life, altering her normal function in 3% to 8% of cases (4).

ETIOLOGY

The pathogenesis of PDD is unknown, but several etiologic theories have been advanced:

- The hormonal etiology is based on clinical observations of recurrence of psychosomatic symptoms in relation to the luteal phase and the absence of symptoms during the other phases of the menstrual cycle. The absence of symptoms in anovulatory cycles led to the theory that hormonal production in the corpus luteum causes the symptoms (5). It has been postulated that an imbalance between estrogen and progesterone is present during the luteal phase of the menstrual cycle (6). However, such views have not been substantiated in clinical well-designed studies (7,8).
- Neurotransmitter system etiology refers to such transmitters as serotonin (9,10), noradrenaline, or GABA (11).
- Psychoneuroendocrine etiology takes into account interactions of ovarian hormones with neurotransmitters (12).
- Endogenous opioid withdrawal etiology is based on documentation of hypoestrogenism that may induce beta-endorphin deficiency in women with PDD (13) (beta-endorphin can be increased by estrogens). It also has been documented that hot flushes (relative hypoestrogenism)

are present in some women with PDD. This transient low estrogen level triggers low production of beta-endorphin, which may lead to PDD. Abnormal prostaglandin production in women with PDD also may interfere with beta-endorphin synthesis, causing PDD (14).

- The nutritional deficiency etiology is based on cravings for particular foods (sweets, salt, chocolate), experienced by most women with PDD; however, a clinical study cannot substantiate this hypothesis (15).

DIAGNOSIS

The diagnosis of PDD focuses on the psychological and somatic components. Clinical evaluation is required in this regard.

The patient should be instructed to maintain a prospective symptoms diary on a daily basis for 2 to 3 months [retrospective recording of signs and symptoms of PDD or self-diagnosis by a patient is not valuable in clinical standing (16,17)]. It is crucial to establish a correct diagnosis initially to avoid ineffective therapy for PDD and to implement an inadequate treatment for any underlying condition that mimics PDD (perimenopause or menopause, thyroid disease, other medical or psychiatric conditions). A patient whose everyday functioning and occupational performance are distorted by PDD, timely, forceful evaluation to be perused in highly organized and systematic approach. Many diary charts are available, and the PMT-Cator chart was developed to assist in gathering symptoms in a prospective manner (18). Physician knowledge and compassion, patient education, and systematic clinical evaluation are irreplaceable tools in the management of patients with PDD.

Pertinent medical history should be obtained by focusing on the psychosomatic aspect of this condition. It has been established that when specific areas of the medical history were addressed, information emerged that was statistically significant for the diagnosis of PDD (19). Therefore, exploring these areas in systemic order is helpful in PDD determination: (a) postpartum depression, (b) emotional changes after oral contraceptive discontinuation, and (c) alcohol or drug use.

The same study documented patient age, age of menarche, smoking history, and family history of psychiatric disorders of the women with PDD; when compared with controls, the results were similar (19).

Initial medical history requires late-on verification of signs and symptoms by charting them daily.

Step I is to explore the patient's history for evidence of PDD. The following approach is suggested (3,7–9,11,12, 16,17,20):

1. Psychological symptom verification
   a. History of behavioral symptoms
      i. Craving for specific foods such as sweets, salt, chocolate, etc.
      ii. Decreasing coordination ability
      iii. Decreasing enthusiasm and motivation
      iv. Decreasing self-control for overcriticism of others
      v. Increasing valiant behavior and verbal abuse of others
      vi. Increasing social isolation
   b. History of emotional symptoms
      i. Anger
      ii. Anxiety
      iii. Irritability
      iv. Mood swing
      v. Sadness
   c. History of cognitive symptoms
      i. Decreasing concentration ability
      ii. Decreasing memory
      iii. Feeling neglected and out of control
2. Social history
   a. Family conflict or dysfunction
   b. Illness or death in the family
   c. Physical, verbal, or sexual abuse
   d. Financial distress
3. Somatic symptoms
   a. Bloating
   b. Breast tenderness
   c. Constipation
   d. Fatigue
   e. Headaches
   f. Joint pain
   g. Weight gain

Step II is to verify signs and symptoms, and their pattern and severity regarding psychosomatic abnormalities emerging only during the luteal phase of the menstrual cycle. Prospective charting of symptoms and self-rating are practiced for two to three consecutive menstrual cycles. Symptoms occurring in a stable cyclic pattern in the luteal phase should establish the diagnosis of PDD, and documentation that PDD symptoms appear in a stable pattern over time has been verified (21).

The following parameters are used to establish the initial diagnosis of PDD:

- Stable cyclic pattern of psychosomatic symptoms
- Cluster of symptoms occurring only in the luteal phase
- Follicular phase of the menstrual cycle symptom free
- Symptom resolution soon after the onset menses

Step III of the diagnostic approach is to rule out medical conditions mimicking PDD. Further clinical evaluation is warranted when analysis of prospective charting records shows (a) the absence of psychosomatic symptom clustering, (b) the presence of signs and symptoms throughout the menstrual cycle, or (c) exacerbation of symptomatology.

The absence of pathognomonic symptoms, identifiable objective clinical signs, or laboratory tests forces a heavier reliance on the ability of the practitioner and patient to interpret the symptoms charted. To unify the diagnosis of PDD, the American Psychiatric Association established the following diagnostic criteria (22):

1. Markedly depressed mood, feelings of hopelessness, or self-deprecating thoughts
2. Marked anxiety, tension, feeling of being "keyed up" or "on edge"
3. Marked affective lability (e.g., feeling suddenly sad or tearful or increased sensitivity to rejection)
4. Persistent and marked anger or irritability or increase in interpersonal conflicts
5. Decreased interest in usual activities (e.g., work, school, friends, hobbies)
6. Subjective sense of difficulty in concentrating
7. Lethargy, easy fatigability, or marked lack of energy
8. Marked change in appetite, overeating, or specific food cravings
9. Hypersomia or insomnia
10. A subjective sense of being overwhelmed or out of control
11. Other physical symptoms such as breast tenderness or swelling, headaches, joint or muscle pain, a sensation of "bloating" or weight gain

At least one of the symptoms must be 1, 2, 3, or 4, and the presence of more than five symptoms during the last week of the luteal phase that disappear after menstruation constitutes a diagnosis of PDD.

The disturbances must markedly interfere with work or school or with usual social activities and relationships with others (e.g., avoidance of social activities, decreased productivity and efficiency at work or school). The disturbances must not be an exacerbation of the symptoms of another disorder (e.g., major depressive disorder, panic disorder, dysthymic disorder, or a personality disorder).

DIFFERENTIAL DIAGNOSIS

The differential diagnosis should encompass both psychological and somatic aspects of PDD. Because PDD lacks specific pathognomonic symptoms or clusters of symptoms, frequently somatic complaints cannot be documented by objective findings on physical examination. The nonspecific symptoms of PDD may mimic or overlap other medical or psychiatric conditions.

Laboratory tests are obtained only when other medical conditions mimicking PDD must be ruled out:

- Thyroid disease, predominantly hypothyroidism, is ruled out by determining the serum thyroid-stimulating hormone, triiodothyronine, and thyroxine levels [it has been reported that the results of the thyrotropin-releasing hormone stimulating test may be abnormal in women with PDD (23)].

- Perimenopausal or menopausal symptoms require determination of serum follicle-stimulating hormone levels. Many women with PDD exhibit hot flashes in the luteal phase of the menstrual cycle (3,24).
- Galactorrhea itself may mimic PDD, and an elevated serum prolactin level establishes the diagnosis of hyperprolactinemia. It has been documented that prolactin level elevation is not associated with PDD; therefore, bromocriptine treatment without increased prolactin levels is not indicated (3).
- Cushing's syndrome may mimic PDD rarely, with the dominant symptom being depression. Those patients usually have associated elevated blood pressure, obesity, and diabetes. Diagnosis is reached by performing an overnight dexamethasone suppression test (3) .
- Anemia requires the appropriate hematologic evaluation.
- Chronic fatigue syndrome is best evaluated by a practitioner specializing in this field.
- Vascular collagen is best evaluated with a specialist in this field.
- Early diabetes mellitus can be ruled out by a standard glucose tolerance test.
- Dysmenorrhea is the most common gynecologic disorder that should be taken under consideration in the differential diagnosis.

CONVENTIONAL THERAPY

Currently, a variety of therapies are offered for PDD, ranging from self-care methods to surgical removal of the uterus or ovaries, or both. Today, definitive surgical treatment has only historical meaning; however, observations that hysterectomy did not ameliorate this condition laid the foundation for ovulation suppression therapy (medical oophorectomy) in PDD. Some treatments are based on anecdotal data, and some are based on evidence-based controlled studies. The following therapeutic paradigms are recommended for PDD.

Selective Serotonin Reuptake Inhibitors

Among the group of serotonin reuptake inhibitors for PDD treatment, *fluoxetine* (Prozac) is the most tested and used drug. The oral dose of 20 mg daily, intermittently administered during the luteal phase of the menstrual cycle, is a highly effective and safe therapeutic approach for the psychological and physical symptoms of PDD, as several well-designed controlled and open-label clinical trials have documented (25–27). The side effect is usually transient and minor (dizziness, headaches, nausea, and insomnia), and fluoxetine may interact with other antidepressants (monoamine oxydase inhibitors, tricyclic antidepressants) (28). A preliminary clinical controlled study indicates that fluoxetine does not increase teratogenicity when used in first-trimester pregnancy (29). However, no clinical data are available on the long-term effect of fluoxetine on potential developmental teratology. There is less clinical experience with other drugs from this group, such as fluvoxamine, paroxetine, sertraline, and venlafaxine.

The serotonin reuptake inhibitors gained clinical recognition as first-line agents for PDD therapy due to their effectiveness, safety, lack of serious side effects, and ease of administration.

Alprazolam (a benzotaine medication) at a dosage of 0.25 to 5 mg daily is an effective mode of therapy; however, it is highly addictive and must be tapered down by 25% daily shortly after menses to avoid withdrawal side effects (anxiety, palpitations, tremors, and occasionally seizures) (3).

Gonadotropin-Releasing Hormone Agonists

Treatment of PDD with gonadotropin-releasing hormone (GnRH) agonists is clinically accepted and its effectiveness is well documented (30,31). GnRH agonists can be administered intramuscularly (Depo-Lupron), subcutaneously (Lupron), and intranasally (buserelin), and more information is provided in the later section on polycystic ovary syndrome (PCOS). One drawback of this modality is the hypoestrogenic state associated with ovarian suppression (medical oophorectomy) and its sequelae, such as bone demineralization and vasomotor symptoms (menopausal symptoms) (32). In order to counteract these undesirable side effects, particularly osteoporosis, two clinical approaches are suggested: (a) add-back estrogen and progesterone [PDD symptoms will significantly improve but small insignificant increases in daily symptoms may be observed (29)], and (b) GnRH agonists in a low dose [a daily dose of 100 µg buserelin spray administered intranasally is effective treatment for PDD; however, the therapy is prone to induce anovulation, particularly with increasing age (33)].

Progesterone Therapy

Progesterone therapy for PDD has been used for over 60 years (34). Numerous open-label clinical trials of progesterone supplementation in the luteal phase of the menstrual cycle for PDD have been declared successful (35). However, well-designed controlled double-blind clinical studies established that any form or dose of progesterone therapy (vaginal or rectal suppository, oral micronized, or natural transdermal) is not more effective than placebo (36,37). For this reason, the U.S. Food and Drug Administration has not approved progesterone for PDD therapy.

Oral Contraceptive Therapy

The efficacy of oral contraceptive therapy has not been demonstrated despite often being used in the clinical setting.

The capacity for oral contraceptives to suppress ovulation is the primary mechanism used for PDD therapy; it was documented that an improvement was observed in the initial few cycles only (38). Somatic symptoms in women with PDD are not usually dominant (menstrual pain or premenstrual breast tenderness); when present, oral contraceptives provide significant relief for menstrual pain or breast tenderness. Psychological symptoms do not significantly improve, and oral contraceptive treatment shows either a delayed or more prolonged pattern of premenstrual negative mood disorders (39).

It is believed that the estrogen component is the effective agent in PDD therapy (40).

Danazol

Danazol (200 mg twice a day for 3 months given during the luteal phase of the menstrual cycle) is an effective therapy in 43.8% of patients with PDD (8.3% placebo-controlled). Danazol therapy reduced PDD symptoms to asymptomatic levels (41). Another clinical randomized placebo-controlled double-blind study documented that 200 mg daily is the best dosage for relieving PDD symptoms with a few undesirable side effects (42).

Diuretics

Most diuretics (thiazides, ammonium chloride, metolazone, triamterene, chlorthalidone) have been used in the treatment of PDD for some time (35). Diuretics are not effective for the treatment of all symptoms of PDD (psychological and somatic), but they provide some relief from premenstrual weight gain and bloating (43).

Spironolactone at a dosage of 100 mg daily is an exception. A double-blind placebo-controlled cross-over study established that spironolactone is an effective modality for both the negative mood changes and somatic symptom therapy (44).

Prostaglandin Inhibitors

Prostaglandin inhibitors, specifically mefenamic acid (Ponstil at a dosage of 250–500 mg three times daily in the luteal phase), has been studied in several randomized, double-blind, cross-over, placebo-controlled clinical trials. It induced marked improvement in somatic symptoms, such as fatigue, headaches, general aches, and abdominopelvic pains, as well as most mood symptoms. Mood swing improved most significantly, and other symptoms, such as depression, irritability, tension, and poor performance at tasks, significantly improved over placebo controls (45–48).

Psychotherapy

Psychotherapy plays a significant role in PDD management. It has been documented that among the PDD cluster of symptoms, psychological profiles dominate in charted self-reported complaints (49). The effectiveness of this treatment has been documented by randomized clinical trials. Cognitive therapy has been implemented as a psychological therapeutic tool for PDD, and the results unequivocally establish a role for this form of management (50). Participation in a peer support group that provides information on positive concomitants of the menstrual cycle can benefit women with PDD (51). Fostering patient understanding of PDD through patient education, support psychotherapy, caring with compassion may assist in premenstrual symptom reduction.

COMPLEMENTARY THERAPY

Patient Education

Patient education is an essential aspect of treating PDD. Because a patient is an inseparable partner in establishing the diagnosis, education must be emphatically stressed. Unquestionably, PDD exists as a clinical entity without definitive knowledge of its pathogenesis, so no single therapeutic paradigm is available. The complexity of this condition, other overlapping medical entities, variety of symptoms reported (>150), and self-deprecating or lethargic mood of patients makes patients with PDD very apprehensive. The following area of patient education must be addressed when clinical PDD is suspected:

- Cyclic occurrence of psychosomatic symptoms only in the luteal phase of the menstrual cycle. Those symptoms vary in severity and form from patient to patient. There is no single pathognomonic symptom or sign for PDD. Within a few hours of menstrual flow, both psychological and somatic symptoms subside, and patients remain symptom free during the proliferative phase of the menstrual cycle.
- Understanding differences in menstrual molimina (appetite changes, swelling, and menstrual-like cramps) from symptoms of PDD.
- Understanding the diagnostic importance of contemporary, prospective charting of all symptoms on a daily basis for 2 to 3 months.
- Understanding the necessity for life-style changes as indicated.
- Inclusion of a patient's husband, close family or friend in the diagnostic and therapeutic process.
- Reassuring a patient that most women with PDD can be helped.
- No single treatment is available to cure all patients; a trial of therapeutic modality should be continued for two to three menstrual cycles. If necessary, the dose of medication can be adjusted. If signs and symptoms do not subside, another medication or treatment modality should be implemented.

Most women have some knowledge about premenstrual symptoms, but how to associate them with the menstrual cycle is not always clear to them. It has been determined that after observing a videotape describing PDD symptoms and their negative consequences in daily life, women's self-reporting of symptoms were enhanced (52). It is obvious from this study that audiovisual educational material may be a useful tool to properly educate patients about premenstrual dysphoric disorder. Benefits in reaching the definitive diagnosis of PDD with well-educated patients will be an easier task.

Diet

Improper nutritional daily intake has not been linked as a cause to PDD (74), even though natural medicine emphasizes the importance of diet as an integral part of the therapeutic approach (75). There are ample studies to support the view that nutritional imbalance may exacerbate PDD (42,76). PDD symptoms such as irritability, fatigue, craving for sweets and chocolate resemble in many ways hypoglycemic-like symptomatology; however, clinical research has not supported this view (77).

Dietary recommendations includes fresh fruits, vegetables, whole grains, nuts, seeds, legumes, fish and flax oil (75,78).

Acupuncture

A national probability sample study in reference to PDD and remedy use showed that acupuncture is least frequently used by women with PDD (53). In general, most investigators presenting their views on complementary therapies indicate that acupuncture is a helpful part of a comprehensive treatment program. However, a search for acupuncture therapy applicability in the PDD condition using multiprogrammed computerized data bank systems and a manual search failed to identify any study. The National Institutes of Health (NIH) is conducting two studies in this field and results are not available yet (data identified through the NIH computer system). Referring a patient with PDD for acupuncture therapy should be accompanied with an explanation that this type of treatment is based strictly on traditional, anecdotal knowledge with no supporting scientific or control study data available.

It is useful to apprise the patient of the possible complications of acupuncture related to reapplication of reusable needle; use of disposable single-use needles prevents such a complication.

Chiropractic Therapy

A statistically significant higher incidence of spinal dysfunction has been determined in women with PDD when compared with a control group of non-PDD sufferers. Based on this observation, spinal dysfunction was implicated as a causative factor in PDD (54). This hypothesis was clinically tested in a well-designed, multicenter, randomized, placebo-controlled, crossover trial and revealed statistically significant decreased PDD symptom scores in the treatment group (55). Long-term results of chiropractic PDD is lacking at this time.

Exercise

A nation sample study of U.S. women established that exercise is the most frequently (18%) used form of treatment for PDD among complementary therapies. In addition, responders to the survey found alternative approaches to be an effective therapeutic modality (53). Exercise in frequently prescribed as an integral part of a life-style modification program. The evidence supporting exercise treatment effectiveness is largely anecdotal, and it is difficult to conduct such a study due to the lack of dedication and consistency of the PDD participants in such a study (56). Small clinical control studies have documented that moderate exercise decreases premenstrual symptomatology; however, a power study was insufficient for interpretation (57,58).

How exercise affects PDD symptomatology is not definitively determined. The type of exercise (aerobic exercise vs. strength training) was evaluated, and it has been demonstrated that the aerobic exercise group improved on more PDD symptoms than the strength training group (59). Jogging, cycling, or fitness walking for 30 minutes four times weekly appears to be beneficial (3) in improving PDD symptoms. Specific instructions as to the form and extent of exercise must be specified by a practitioner to make exercise effective in the management of PDD (60). It has been established that only a causal relationship exists between exercise and mental health status (61). Because the predominant cluster of symptoms in PDD are psychological in nature, exercise does not have a significant impact on the management of this medical condition. Aerobic exercise significantly improves physical fitness, but no significant changes can be proven in either positive or negative mood changes (62). In most cases, it appears reasonable to encourage women with PDD to exercise regularly and consider exercise as one of the adjunct treatments in management of this entity.

Reflexology Therapy

Reflexology therapy is the application of manual pressure or medical massage to reflex points on the body, such as the ears, hands, and feet (there are somatotopic areas that correspond to a specific organ of the body). Reflexology is thought by many clinicians to be a safe therapy promoting body rebalance of homeostasis and has no side effects (63,64).

Applying reflexology treatment to the ear, hand, and foot demonstrated a significantly greater decrease in premen-strual symptoms than the women subjected to placebo reflexology. Effectiveness of this therapy has been documented in a randomized controlled study (65), and the clinical evidence-based findings make reflexology therapy worthwhile to include in the clinical management of PDD.

Light Therapy

Light therapy is based on the foundation that bright white light influences hormonal changes (e.g., cortisol, prolactin, thyroid-stimulating hormone) and can increase core body temperature amplitude (66). An observational study suggested that all light treatments reduce the depressive rating from baseline levels (67). A randomized, double-blind, counter-balanced, cross-over controlled study of 30 minutes of evening light therapy (10,000 lux cool-white fluorescent light) established that this form of therapy is an effective treatment for PDD (68). Such a treatment is easy to apply and has low potential for side effects, so recommendations for such complementary therapy seem to be rational.

Life-Style Changes

The concept is that PDD is a stress-related disorder (69) [a summation effect of inner and external stress (3)]; therefore, stress reduction should play a role in a therapeutic approach. Some life-style factors have been identified as being most influential on PDD symptomatology: obesity, cigarette smoking, alcohol consumption, and exercise. However, recent published data have not demonstrated consistent associations with obesity, exercise, and alcohol consumption with menstrual symptoms. Cigarette smoking is associated with an increased risk for all menstrual cycle disorders. Life-style is modifiable; however, clinical research suggests that better results are accomplished when clinical interventions are aimed at cigarette smoking. Termination of cigarette smoking may reduce the prevalence of PDD symptoms and optimize the outcome of the treatment of menstrual cycle disorders (70). In a general program of PDD treatment, stress reduction with life-style changes via behavioral modification, diet modification, aerobic exercise regimens are recommended as first-line therapy in the management of PDD.

Relaxation Therapy

Muscle tension (function of sympathetic nerve arousal) increases in the premenstrual phase of the menstrual cycle in women with PDD. This phenomenon has been documented with electromyography; consequently, reducing muscle tension may assist in alleviation of PDD symptoms (71). A clinical observational trial of progressive muscle relaxation exercise followed by guided imagery documented that such mind–body intervention may decrease premenstrual distress significantly (72). A randomized study established that the relaxation response is effective treatment for physical and emotional premenstrual symptoms, even in women with severe symptoms (73).

Nutritional Supplements

There is no scientific evidence to support the notion that nutritional supplements are effective in the treatment of PDD, so such recommendations should be considered empiric (3). Natural supplements (multiple vitamin and minerals) have been prescribed for PDD by natural alternative practitioners for some time. In a double-blind, placebo-controlled, cross-over clinical trial, nutritional supplements were found to be effective in a select group of women with PDD. The study was conducted with the Optivite R formula (multiple vitamin and minerals designed to meet recommended daily allowances; this formula did not satisfy calcium or vitamin D daily recommendations) (79).

In the original classification system, PMT was used (80) and with evolution of knowledge, the nomenclature was changed from PMT to PMS (75). The following four clinical subgroups have been identified (80) in a natural alternative treatment concept:

- In PMT-A or PMS-A, *A* stands for anxiety and is considered to be the most prevalent of the four subgroups. Symptoms occurring in PMS-A include anxiety, irritability, nervous tension, and sometimes emotional lability that is detrimental to a patient, her family, and society. Patients in this group are reported to respond to *vitamin B_6* treatment at a dosage of 200 to 800 mg daily. A patient should be informed about the potential side effect of vitamin B_6 and its sequelae.
- In PMT-C or PMS-C, *C* stands for carbohydrate craving. Symptoms include craving for sweets, increased appetite, indulgence in eating refined sugar, headaches, fatigue, dizziness, and heart palpitations. Adequate replacement of *magnesium* at a dosage of 300 mg one to three times per day may ameliorate the symptoms.
- PMT-D or PMS-D is the least common but the most dangerous subgroup due to the increased risk for suicide. *D* stands for depression. Symptoms include withdrawal, crying with ease, no appetite, insomnia, confusion, and forgetfulness. Treatment for this subgroup should be established with a *psychiatrist*.
- PMT-H or PMS-H is the second most common subgroup. *H* stands for hyperhydration. Symptoms include water and salt retention, weight gain of more than 3 pounds, abdominal bloating, breast tenderness (mastalgia), and edema of the face, hands, or ankles. *Vitamin B_6 and vitamin E are recommended.*

Natural alternative therapists have commonly accepted this classification and use it as clinical guide for management.

Observational clinical research results suggested that a nutritional supplement for women (Optivite, 6–12 tablets daily for 3–6 months) yields satisfactory results [caution must be exercised when 6 tablets daily of Optivite R is administered, because this dosage will accumulate to approximately 300 mg of vitamin B_6 (3)] (81). These results were confirmed by a double-blind controlled longitudinal study, which established that a nutritional supplement may play a role in the management of women with PDD (82).

Vitamin B_6 (pyridoxine) at a dosage of 50 mg two to four times per day is recommended by natural medicine practitioners (75). However, vitamin B_6 at a dosage of 100 mg daily has been found in randomized, placebo-controlled, double-blind, cross-over clinical trial to be an ineffective therapy for PDD (83). An analysis of the literature of randomized, placebo-controlled, clinical trials suggests inconclusively (predominantly due to the lack of an adequate power study) that dosages of vitamin B_6 of up to 100 mg daily are probably beneficial in treating premenstrual symptoms (84,85). The conflicting reports on the effectiveness of vitamin B_6 do not specifically address the pros and cons. Peripheral sensory neuropathy (sensation of tingling, numbness, and reduced sensation in the hands or feet) was observed at a dosage of 150 mg/day during long-term administration (86).

Vitamin E (alpha-tocopherol) 400 to 800 IU daily is suggested for women with PDD (75). It has been postulated, based on a randomized, dose-response study, that vitamin E at dosages of 150, 300, and 600 IU daily may be of value in women with severe PDD symptoms (87).

Essential fatty acid (gamma linolenic acid) at a dosage of 3 to 4 g daily is recommended (75). Treatment with essential fatty acid was documented in a randomized, double-blind, cross-over clinical trial as being ineffective therapy for PDD. Improvement over time was ascribed to a placebo effect (88).

Calcium carbonate is an effective form of PDD therapy at a dosage of 1,200 to 1,600 mg per day (89,90). A well-designed and executed prospective, randomized, double-blind, placebo-controlled, parallel-group, multicenter clinical trial established that calcium supplementation is a simple and effective treatment for negative mood affect, food craving, water retention, and pain associated with PDD symptomatology (89). Analyzing other studies focusing on calcium supplementation in the management of PDD supported the notion of its sound treatment option. A supplemental dose of calcium can be reduced appropriately when a patient consumes a large quantity in her diet (90).

Magnesium levels are decreased in women with PDD throughout the entire menstrual cycle, not just the luteal phase (91). This finding may justify administration of magnesium for women with PDD select cases. However, there is no clear-cut medical evidence that such an approach will provide a beneficial effect. The recommended dose is 300 mg one to three times per day (75).

Other vitamin, mineral, and amino acid deficiencies, such as vitamin A, B complex, zinc, copper, and tryptophan have been suggested to play an important role in PDD symptomatology (78,92). However, there are no convincing scientific data to support supplementation with these nutritional products. It has been established that vitamin A and tryptophan are toxic in high doses (3).

NATURAL ALTERNATIVE THERAPY

Herbal Medicine

Vitex agnus castus (chaste tree berry) at a dose of 40 drops liquid (extract) or 175 mg daily standardized extract is recommended for PDD symptoms (75). There is no strong clinical evidence regarding the effectiveness of the chaste tree berry in the therapy of premenstrual symptoms. The effective dose has not been determined, and the dose quoted above is suggestive. An additional drawback of this form of therapy is that a positive effect may take up to 18 months (93).

Ginkgo (Ginkgo biloba) at a dosage of 80 mg standardized extract twice daily is an effective treatment of congestive symptoms associated with PDD, particularly breast symptoms; psychological symptoms also have improved. The safety and effectiveness of this regimen has been documented by multicenter double-blind, placebo-controlled studies (94).

Other herbal medicines, such as wild yam, licorice root, dong quai, black cohosh, kava extract, St. John's wort, skullcap, dandelion, and cramp bark, are prescribed based on their ability to control an individual symptom. Their clinical use is based largely on tradition and anecdotal data (75,78).

Homeopathy

Homeopathy is a therapeutic approach encompassing three main participants in one unit: a patient (with personality characteristics and a medical condition), a practitioner (with his or her individual concept of treatment approach with critically different educational levels), and a medication (95).

The homeopathic treatment approach in women with PDD depends on the dominant symptomatology (96): congestive symptoms, psychological and behavioral symptoms, and somatic symptoms.

Congestive symptoms include breast tenderness, abdominal bloating, vein congestion, water retention (weight gain of 1 to 7 pounds or 0.5 to 3.0 kg), fatigue, emotional tension, and hypouresis associated with weight gain of 7 to 22 pounds or 3 to 10 kg. The following therapeutic remedies are recommended for this subgroup:

- *Natrium muriaticum,* natural sea or rock salt, in a dilution of 5 to 30 cH every other day from day 7 of the menstrual cycle to the beginning of menses.
- Sepia, made from the fluid produced in the ink sac of the cuttlefish (*Sepia officinalis*), is used at a dosage of 15 or 30 cH on days 5 and 20 of the menstrual cycle; 9 or 15 cH, five granules daily during the luteal phase of menstrual cycle; and in a graduated stepped up dilution: 9 cH on day 19 of the cycle, 15 cH on day 20, and 30 cH on day 21.
- Lachesis, prepared from the venom of the snake *Lachesis muta*, is used in a stepped up dilution dose: 9 cH on day 20 of the cycle, 15 cH on day 21, and 30 cH on day 22.
- Pulsatilla, prepared from the entire plant *Pulsatilla nigricans,* is administered in two formulations: 9 cH dilution, five granules daily from day 14 of the menstrual cycle (when predominantly behavioral symptoms occur, the dilution of 15 cH is used), or the stepped up dilution, 9 cH, 15 cH, and 30 cH on days 20, 21, and 22 of the menstrual cycle, respectively.
- Vazopressine is used in a 15 cH dilution, once daily during the luteal phase of the menstrual cycle.
- *Apis mellifica* (see above).

Psychological and behavioral symptoms include insomnia, tremor, irritability, increased aggressiveness, anxiety, fatigue, lack of concentration, depression, decreased coordination, food craving, and libido changes. In this subgroup, the following recommendations are made:

- Lachesis (see preceding section on congestive symptoms)
- Ignatia amara, made from the fruits of *Strychnos ignatia*
- Nux vomica (see above)
- Chamomilla, made from *Matricaria chamomilla*
- Other remedies: moschus, platina, palladium, tuberculinum, *Ambra grisa*

All these remedies are administered at a dilution of 15 to 30 cH once daily, although the dose can be adjusted and taken only once monthly.

Somatic symptoms include headaches, back pain, nausea, constipation or diarrhea, convulsion, allergy, heart palpitations, and dermatology changes such as acne, oily skin, cold sores, and nail fragility. The following remedies are suggested:

1. Mastalgia
   a. *Bryonia alba* comes from the plants *Bryonia alba* or *Bryonia diocia*.
   b. *Apis mellifica,* made from the entire honeybee body, including the venom, is taken at a dilution of 9 to 15 cH, and the frequency must be adjusted and the dose taken often due to short-lived activity.
2. Abdominopelvic congestion
   a. *Lycopodium clavatum,* made from spores of the ossy plant
   b. Pulsatilla (see earlier section on congestive symptoms)

c. Other remedies such as helonias, palladium, *Actaea recemosa*, *Lilium tigrinum*
3. Vein congestion
   a. Pulsatilla (see earlier section on congestive symptoms), at a dilution of 9 cH, five granules daily
   b. Sepia (see earlier section on congestive symptoms), at a dilution of 9 cH, five granules daily
   c. *Nux vomica,* made from the dried seeds of the plant *Strychnos nux vomica,* the poison nut, at a dilution of 9 cH, five granules daily
   d. *Arnica montana* is made from the whole plant, used at a dilution of 9 or 15 cH, one to three times weekly
   e. Other remedies include aesculus at a dosage of 6 DC, 20 drops twice daily; hamamelis at a dosage of 6 DH, 20 drops twice daily; vipera at a dilution of 5 cH, three granules twice daily.

There are no scientific data available to support homeopathy for PDD, and suggested treatments are based on tradition of clinical experience and anecdotal data. To define the role of homeopathy among other therapies, broader education of all health practitioners in this discipline is needed, clinical research in this field should be developed, and the public must be informed about its availability and the nature of health-care delivery. In addition, easy access to homeopathic remedies is essential for promulgation of this medical discipline.

Ayurvedic Therapy

The ayurvedic therapeutic approach in women with PDD is based on a foundation of imbalance that occurs in three categories, and treatment is addressed according to abnormality identified among these three categories (78): Doshas balance, biological rhythm, and purification.

Doshas balance, or bodily humors, is achieved by actions taken to balance the realms of pata energy, pitta energy, and kapha energy.

Pata energy, according to ayurvedic concept, is necessary for rhythmic endometrial bleeding (menses), and disproportion of energy may lead to symptoms such as emotional lability, anxiety, insomnia, and constipation. To alleviate this imbalance, the following clinical management is recommended:

- Organization of a regular, structured daily routine
- Decreased work-load and increased rest and sleeping time
- Incorporation of one of the forms of meditation
- Change in diet (increased consumption of olive oil, cooked warm foods such as cereal and stews, sweet-tasting foods without refined sugar or salt)

Pitta energy is claimed to be essential in maintaining hormonal ambiance in the menstrual cycle. Changing this energy equilibrium causes symptoms such as irritability, anger, skin rash, and diarrhea to emerge. To balance pitta energy, the following approach is suggested:

- Organization of a regular, structured daily routine
- Incorporation of one of the forms of meditation
- Control of behavioral abnormality
- Reduction of overperformance and overactivity
- Avoidance in the diet of spicy and greasy foods, artificial ingredients, caffeine, chocolate, and alcohol

Kapha energy determines menstrual-effluent components, and derangements may lead to clinical symptoms such as fluid retention, weight gain, breast engorgement, and weariness. It has been suggested that the following approach may help to correct this imbalance:

- Regular exercise with increased intensity
- Diet enhanced with spicy foods and legumes and elimination of sour and sweet foods

Biological rhythm is adopting a concept that the earth's energy positively influences human energy. To benefit from this phenomenon, it is advisable to establish a routine of retiring to bed at 10 p.m.and rising at 6 a.m.

Purification is applied to eliminate waste and impurity (ama) from the body. It can be achieved by:

- Changing the diet (increasing consumption of warm to hot water and avoiding meat, cheese, caffeine, and alcohol)
- Administration of castor oil, 4 to 5 teaspoons in the morning, or senna tea in the morning followed by a light diet for the remainder of the day on day 14 or 15 of the menstrual cycle

REFERENCES

1. Association of Professors of Gynecology and Obstetrics. *Medical student educational objectives,* 7th ed. Washington, DC: Association of Professors of Gynecology and Obstetrics, 1997.
2. Council on Resident and Gynecology (CREOG). *Educational objectives core curriculum for residents in obstetrics and gynecology,* 5th ed. Washington DC: CREOG, 1996.
3. Chihlal HJ. Premenstrual syndrome. *Obstet Gynecol Clin North Am* 1990;17:457–479.
4. Kouri EM, Halbreich U. State and trait serotonergic abnormalities in women with dysphoric premenstrual syndrome. *Psychopharmacol Bull* 1997;33:767–770.
5. Dalton K. *The premenstrual syndrome and progesterone therapy.* William Heinemann, London, U.K.: 1965.
6. Muse KN, Cetel NS, Futterman LA. The premenstrual syndrome effects of "medical ovariectomy." *N Engl J Med* 1984;311: 1345–1349.
7. Rubinow DR, Hoban C, Grover G, et al. Changes in plasma hormones across the menstrual cycle in patients with menstrually related mood disorders and in control subjects. *Am J Obstet Gynecol* 1988;158:5–11.
8. Hammarback S, Ekholm UB, Backstrom T. Spontaneous anovulation causing disappearance of cyclical symptoms in women with the premenstrual syndrome. *Acta Endocrinol (Copenh)* 1991; 125:132–137.

9. Halbreich U, Tworek H. Altered serotonergic activity in women with dysphoric premenstrual syndromes. *Int J Psych Med* 1993; 23:1–27.

10. Kouri EM, Halbreich U. State and trait serotonergic abnormalities in women with dysphoric premenstrual syndromes. *Psychopharmacol Bull* 1997;33:767–770.

11. Halbreich U, Piletz JE, Carson S, et al. Increased imidazoline and alpha2 adrenergic binding in platelets of women with dysphoric premenstrual syndromes. *Biol Psychiatry* 1993;34:676–686.

12. Pearlstein TB. Hormones and depression: What are the facts about premenstrual syndrome, menopause, and hormone replacement therapy? *Am J Obstet Gynecol* 1995;173:646–653.

13. Coung CJ, Couam CB, Kao PC, et al. Neuropeptide levels in premenstrual syndrome. *Fertil Steril* 1985;44:760–765.

14. Brush MG, Watson SJ, Horrobin DF, et al. Abnormal essential fatty acid levels in plasma of women with premenstrual syndrome. *Am J Obstet Gynecol* 1984;150:363–366.

15. Mira M, Stewart PM, Abraham SF. Vitamin and trace element status in premenstrual syndrome. *Am Clin Nutr* 1988;47:636-641.

16. Sampson GA, Prescott P. The assessment of the symptoms of premenstrual syndrome and their response to therapy. *Br J Psychiatry* 1981;38:399–405.

17. Harrison WM, Robkin JG, Endicott J. Psychiatric evaluation of premenstrual changes. *Psychosomatics* 1985;26:789–792, 795, 798–799.

18. Magos AL, Studd JWW. A simple method for the diagnosis of premenstrual syndrome by use of self-assessment disk. *Am J Obstet Gynecol* 1988;158:1024–1028.

19. Chuong CJ, Burgos DM. Medical history in women with premenstrual syndrome. *J Psychosom Obstet Gynecol* 1995;16:21–27.

20. Keye WR. Premenstrual syndrome. In: Holzman GB, Renehart RD, Moghissi KS, eds. *Precis: an update in obstetrics and gynecology. Reproductive endocrinology.* Washington, DC: ACOG, 1998: 51–54.

21. Roca CA, Schmidt PJ, Rubinow DR. A follow-up study of premenstrual syndrome. *J Clin Psychiatry* 1999;60:763–766.

22. American Psychiatric Association (APA). *Diagnostic and statistical manual of mental disorders,* 4th ed. Washington, DC: APA, 1994.

23. Schmidt PJ, Kahn RA, Rubinow DR. Thyroid function in premenstrual syndrome. *N Engl J Med* 1987;317:1537.

24. Casper RF, Graves GR, Reid RL. Objective measurements of hot flushes associated with the premenstrual syndrome. *Fertil Steril* 1987;47:341–344.

25. Wood SH, Mortola JF, Chan Y, et al. Treatment of premenstrual syndrome with fluoxetine: a double-blind, placebo-controlled, crossover study. *Obstet Gynecol* 1992;80:339–344.

26. Pearlstein T, Stone A. Long-term fluoxetine treatment of late luteal phase dysphoric disorder. *J Clin Psychiatry* 1994;55: 332–335.

27. Romano S, Judge R, Dillon J, et al. The role of fluoxetine in the treatment of premenstrual dysphoric disorder. *Clin Ther* 1999; 21:615–633.

28. Gram L. Fluoxetine. *N Engl J Med* 1994;33:1354–1361.

29. Pastuszak A, Schick-Boschetto B, Zuber C, et al. Pregnancy outcome following first-trimester exposure to fluoxetine (Prozac). *JAMA* 1993;269:2246–2248.

30. Hammarback S, Backstrom T. Induced anovulation as treatment of premenstrual tension syndrome. *Acta Obstet Gynecol Scand* 1988;67:159–166.

31. Brown CS, Ling FW, Andersen RN, et al. Efficacy of depot leuprolide in premenstrual syndrome: effect of symptom severity and type in controlled trial. *Obstet Gynecol* 1994;84:779-786.

32. Dawood MY, Lewis V, Ramos J. Cortical and trabecular bone mineral content in women with endometriosis: effect of

33. Sundstrom I, Nyberg S, Bixo M, et al. Treatment of premenstrual syndrome with gonadotropin-releasing hormone agonist in a low dose regimen. *Acta Obstet Gynecol Scand* 1999;78:891–899.

34. Israel SL. Premenstrual tension. *JAMA* 1938;110:1721.

35. Moline L. Pharmacological strategies for managing premenstrual syndrome. *Clin Pharm* 1993;12:181–196.

36. Freeman E. Progesterone therapy for premenstrual syndrome. In: Smith S, Schiff I, eds. Modern management of premenstrual syndrome. New York: Norton, 1993:152–160.

37. Freeman E, Rickels K, Sondheimer SJ, et al. Ineffectiveness of progesterone suppository treatment for premenstrual syndrome. *JAMA* 1990;264:349–353.

38. Backstrom T, Hannson-Malmsttome Y, Lindke BA, et al. Oral contraceptive in premenstrual syndrome. A randomized comparison of triphasic and monophasic preparations. *Contraception* 1992;46:253–268.

39. Bancroft J, Rennie D. The impact of oral contraceptives on the experience of perimenstrual mood, clumsiness, food craving and other symptoms. *J Psychosom Res* 1993;37:195–202.

40. Tiemstra JD, Patel K. Hormonal therapy in the management of premenstrual syndrome. *I Am Board Fam Pract* 1998;11: 378–381.

41. Hahn PM, Van Vugt DA, Reid RL. A randomized, placebo-controlled, crossover trial of danazol for the treatment of premenstrual syndrome. *Psychoneuroendocrinology* 1995;20:193–209.

42. Watts JW, Butt WR, Edwards RL. A clinical trial using danazol for the treatment of premenstrual tension. *Br J Obstet Gynecol* 1987;94:30–34.

43. Barnhart, KT, Freeman EW,Sondheimer SJ. A clinician's guide to the premenstrual syndrome. *Med Clin North Am* 1995;79: 1457–1472.

44. Wang M, Hammarback S, Lindke BA, et al. Treatment of premenstrual syndrome by spironolactone: a double-blind, placebo-controlled study. *Acta Obstet Gynecol Scand* 1995;74:803–808.

45. Mira M, McNeil D, Fraser IS, et al. Mefenamic acid in the treatment of premenstrual syndrome. *Obstet Gynecol* 1986;68: 395–398.

46. Budoff PW. Use of prostaglandin inhibitors in the treatment of PMS. *Clin Obstet Gynecol* 1987;30:453–464.

47. Jakubowicz DL, Godard E, Dewhurst J. The treatment of premenstrual tension with mefenamic acid: analysis of prostaglandin concentration. *Br J Obstet Gynecol* 1984;91:78–84.

48. Wood C, Jakubowicz DL. The treatment of premenstrual syndrome with mefenamic acid. *Br J Obstet Gynecol* 1980;87: 627–630.

49. Gotts G, Morse CA, Dennerstein L. Premenstrual complaints: an idiosyncratic syndrome. *J Psychosom Obstet Gynecol* 1995;16: 29–35.

50. Blake F, Salkovskis P, Gath D, et al. Cognitive therapy for premenstrual syndrome: a controlled trial. *J Psychosom Res* 1998;45: 307–318.

51. Morse G. Positively reframing perceptions of the menstrual cycle among women with premenstrual syndrome. *JOGNN* 1999;28: 165–174.

52. Marvan ML, Escobedo C. Premenstrual symptomatology: role of prior knowledge about premenstrual syndrome. *Psychosom Med* 1999;61:163–167.

53. Singh BB, Berman BM, Simpson RL, et al. Incidence of premenstrual syndrome and remedy usage: a national probability sample study. *Altern Ther Health Med* 1998;4:75–79

54. Walsh MJ, Polus BI. The frequency of positive common spinal clinical examination findings in a sample of premenstrual syndrome suffers. *J Manipulative Physiol Ther* 1999;22:216–220.

55. Walsh MJ, Polus BI. A randomized, placebo-controlled clinical trial on the efficacy of chiropractic therapy on premenstrual syndrome. *J Manipulative Physiol Ther* 1999;22:582–585.

56. Miller MN, McGowen KR, Miller BE, et al. Lessons learned about research on premenstrual syndrome. *J Womens Health Gend Based Med* 1999;8:989–993.

57. Prior JC, Vigna Y, Alojada N. Conditioning exercise decreases premenstrual symptoms. A prospective, controlled three months trial. *Eur J Appl Physiol* 1986;55:349–355.

58. Prior JC, Vigna Y, Sciarretta D, et al. Conditioning exercise decreases premenstrual symptoms. A prospective, controlled 6-month months trial. *Fertil Steril* 1987;47:402–408.

59. Steege JF, Blumenthal JA. The effects of aerobic exercise on premenstrual syndromes in middle-aged women: a preliminary study. *J Psychosom Res* 1993;37:127–133.

60. Chihlal HJ. *Premenstrual syndrome: a clinical manual,* 2nd ed. Dallas: Essential Medical Information Systems, 1989.

61. Glenister D. Exercise and mental health: a review. *J R Soc Health* 1996;116:7–13.

62. Lennox SS, Bedell JR, Stone AA. The effect of exercise on normal mood. *J Psychosom Res* 1990;34:629–636.

63. Shahai IC. Reflexology: its place in modern health care. *Prof Nurse* 1993;8:722–725.

64. Griffiths P. Reflexology. *Complement Ther Nurs Midwifery* 1996;2:13–16.

65. Oleson T, Flocco W. Randomized controlled study of premenstrual symptoms treated with ear, hand, and foot reflexology. *Obstet Gynecol* 1993;82:906–911.

66. Parry BL, Hauger R, Lin E, et al. Neuroendocrine effect of light therapy in luteal phase dysphoric disorder. *Biol Psychiatry* 1994;36:356–364.

67. Parry BL, Mahan AM, Mostofi N, et al. Light therapy of luteal phase dysphoric disorder: an extended study. *Am J Psychiatry* 1993;150:1417–1419.

68. Lam RW, Carter D, Misri S, et al. A controlled study of light therapy in women with late luteal phase dysphoric disorder. *Psychiatry Res* 1999;86:185–192.

69. Deuster PA, Adera T, South-Paul J. Biological, social, and behavioral factors associated with premenstrual syndrome. *Arch Fam Med* 1999;8:122–128.

70. Kritz-Silverstein D, Wingard DL, Garland FC. The association of behavior and lifestyle factors with menstrual symptoms. *J Womens Health Gend Based Med* 1999;8:1185–1193.

71. Coyne C. Muscle tension and its relation to symptoms in the premenstruum. *Res Nurs Health* 19883;6:199–205.

72. Groer M, Ohnesorge C. Menstrual-cycle lengthening and reduction in premenstrual distress through guided imagery. *J Holist Nurs* 1993;11:286–294.

73. Goodale IL, Domar AD, Benson H. Alleviation of premenstrual syndrome symptoms with the relaxation response. *Obstet Gynecol* 1990;75:649–655.

74. Reid RL. Premenstrual syndrome. *Curr Probl Obstet Gynecol Fertil* 1985;8:1–9.

75. Hudson T. *Women's encyclopedia of natural medicine.* Los Angeles: Keats Publishing, 1999:245–255.

76. Abraham G. Nutritional factors in etiology of the premenstrual tension syndrome. *J Reprod Med* 1983;28:446–464.

77. Freeman E, Sondheimer S. Menstrual cycle, diet and premenstrual syndrome. In: *Encyclopedias of food science, food technology and nutrition.* Academic, London, U.K.: 1993:1–5.

78. Golgberg B, ed. *Alternative medicine.* Tiburon, CA: Future Medicine Publishing, 2001:149;662–663.

79. Chakmakijan Z, Higgins C, Abraham G. The effect of a nutritional supplement, Optivite for women, on premenstrual tension syndrome: effect of symptomatology, using a double blind crossover design. *J Appl Nutr* 1985;37:12.

80. Abraham GE. Nutritional factors in the etiology of premenstrual tension syndromes. *J Reprod Med* 1983;446–464.

81. Goei GS, Abraham GE. Effect of a nutritional supplement, Optivite, on symptoms of premenstrual tension. *J Reprod Med* 1983;28:527–531.

82. London RS, Bradley L, Chiamiri NY. Effect of a nutritional supplement on premenstrual symptomatology in women with premenstrual syndrome: a double-blind longitudinal study. *I Am Coll Nutr* 1991;10:494–499.

83. Hagen I, Nesheim BI, Tuntland T. No effect of vitamin B-6 against premenstrual tension. A controlled clinical study. *Acta Obstet Gynecol Scand* 1985;64:667–670.

84. Wyatt KM, Dimmock PW, Shaughn O'Brien PM. Efficacy of vitamin B-6 in the treatment of premenstrual syndrome: systematic review. *BMJ* 1999;318:1375–1381.

85. Kleijnen J, Ter Riet G, Knipschild P. Vitamin B6 in the treatment of the premenstrual syndrome: a review. *Br J Obstet Gynecol* 1990;97:847–852.

86. Cohen M, Bendich A. Safety of pyridoxine: a review of human and animal studies. *Toxicol Lett* 1986;34:129–139.

87. London RS, Sundaram GS, Murphy L, et al. The effect of alpha-tocopherol on premenstrual symptomatology: a double-blind study. *J Am Coll Nutr* 1983;2:115–122.

88. Collins A, Cerin A, Coleman G, et al. Essential fatty acid in the treatment of premenstrual syndrome. *Obstet Gynecol* 1993;81:93–98.

89. Thys-Jacobs S, Starkey P, Bernstein D, et al. Calcium carbonate and the premenstrual syndrome: effects on premenstrual and menstrual symptoms. Premenstrual Syndrome study Group. *Am J Obstet Gynecol* 1998;179:444–452.

90. Ward MW, Holimon TD. Calcium treatment for premenstrual syndrome. *Ann Pharmacother* 1999;33:1356–1358.

91. Rosenstein DL, Elin RJ, Hosseini JM, et al. Magnesium measures across the menstrual cycle in premenstrual syndrome. *Biol Psychiatry* 1994;35:557–561.

92. Chuong CJ, Dawson EB. Zinc and copper levels in premenstrual syndrome. *Fertil Steril* 1994;62:313–320.

93. Klepser T, Nisly N. Chaste tree berry for premenstrual syndrome. *Alternative Med Alert* 1999;5;64–67.

94. Tamborini A, Taurelle R. Value of standardized Ginko biloba extract (EGb 761) in the management of congestive symptoms of premenstrual syndrome. *Rev Fr Gynecol Obstet* 1993;88:447–457.

95. Holtzscher A, Legros AS. *Pratique homeopathique en gynecologie.* Boiron, France: Centre d'Enseignement et de Developpement de l'Homeopathie, 1994.

96. Poitevin B. Integrating homeopathy in health system. *Bull World Health Organ* 1999;77:160–166.

8

HYPERANDROGENISM

EDUCATIONAL OBJECTIVES

Medical Students (1) APGO Objective No. 48	Residents in Obstetrics/Gynecology (2) CREOG Objectives	Practitioners (3) ACOG Recommendations
Definition of: hirsutism, virilization Normal variations of secondary sex 　characteristics Causes: ovarian, adrenal, pituitary, 　pharmacologic (iatrogenic) Patient evaluation	Pertinent history Physical examination Diagnostic studies Diagnosis: hirsutism, hypertrichosis Etiology Management: possible interventions, 　factors influencing decisions regarding 　intervention, potential complications 　of intervention, potential complications 　of nonintervention Follow-up	Physiology Etiology Evaluation Laboratory studies Other diagnostic procedures Treatment

DEFINITION

Hirsutism is the excess growth of an androgen-dependent pattern of terminal hair (coarse, long, pigmented) in the midline of a woman's body.

Hypertrichosis is the replacement of vellus or lanugo hair (fine, short, nonpigmented, unresponsive to hormonal stimulation) with terminal hair, without an increase in the number of hairs.

Virilism is the transformation of the female phenotype toward male phenotypic expression.

Virilization is the expression of male secondary sex characteristics in the female phenotype, and it is clinically manifested by defeminizing signs: hirsutism, decreasing breast size, clitoral enlargement, regression of the temporal hairline, male-type pubic hair distribution, deepening of the voice, and vanishing female body contour.

Hyperandrogenemia is defined as an increase in any or all of the plasma androgens [free testosterone, bound testosterone, dehydroepiandrosterone-sulfate (DHEA-S), dehydrotestosterone, and androstenedione].

INCIDENCE

Androgenic disorders in women are the most common endocrinopathy, and they affect 10% to 20% of women (4).

The prevalence of hirsutism varies from 2% to 8%, with no significant differences between caucasian and African-American women in the United States (5).

PHYSIOLOGY

Two types of body hair have been defined:

- Vellus hairs (lanugo) are soft, short, thin, nonpigmented, and hormone-independent,
- Terminal hairs are coarse, long, pigmented, and hormone dependent, with defined growth stages: anagen (growing phase), catagen (involution phase), and telogen (resting phase).

The hair follicle is a part of a pilosebaceous unit (the hair follicle and sebaceous gland), and it is influenced by several factors.

Genetic composition predetermines the hair type, color, and distribution, and varies in certain ethnic descent characteristics, and it establishes the degree of sensitivity of the pilosebaceous unit to androgens.

In the hormonal milieu, androgens are the principal hormones responsible for the dimorphism of hair distribution in humans. There are three circulating androgens from three different sources. Testosterone is the most potent androgen that is produced by the peripheral conversion of adipocytes (fat cells) from androgen precursors (50%), and 25% is secreted by the ovaries and adrenal glands. The normal expected serum value of total testosterone is 20 to 80 ng/mL (0.7–2.8 nM), and that of free testosterone is 100 to 200 pg/dL (35–700 pM). DHEA, a weak androgen, is secreted 90% by the andrenal glands and 10% by the ovaries, with the serum level in DHEA-S ranging from 80 to 350 μg/dL (2.2–9.5 μM). Androstenedione, a weak androgen, is secreted by the ovaries (50%) and the adrenal glands, with a serum level of 60 to 300 ng/dL (2.1–10. 5 nM).

Ovarian androgen secretion is stimulated and controlled by luteinizing hormone (LH) and adrenal androgens are regulated by adrenocorticotropin (ACTH). Weak androgens (androstenedione and DHEA) must be peripherally converted in cells to dehydrotestosterone (DHT) in the presence of 5-alpha-reductase. Only free testosterone (unbound to sex hormone–binding globulin (SHBG, which is produced by the liver) is a biologically active hormone and has the ability to bind to the receptors. This mechanism may promote the transformation of hairs from the vellus to the terminal form (which will undergo cyclic growth) and requires only some androgen participation. All these parameters together, such as pilosebaceous unit sensitivity, androgen levels, SHBG concentration, 5-alpha-reductase activity (peripheral conversion to testosterone), can lead to acne (sebaceous gland secretion and bacterial contamination), apocrine sweat gland abscesses (hidradenitis suppurativa), hirsutism, or, rarely, virilism.

The postmenopausal period is linked with hair growth on the face, and hair loss may be noticed on the pubic area, extremities, and axillae.

CLASSIFICATION

- Hypertrichosis
- Hirsutism
- Virilism

ETIOLOGY

The etiology of hirsutism falls into the following categories:

- 1. End-organ hypersensitivity to androgens (familial or idiopathic hirsutism)
- 2. Ovarian causes
  - a. Polycystic ovary syndrome
  - b. Hilus cell hyperplasia
  - c. Androgen-producing tumors:
    - i. Sertoli-Leydig cell tumors (androblastoma and androblastoma)
    - ii. Gynandroblastoma
    - iii. Lipid or lipoid cell tumors
    - iv. Hilus cell tumors
    - v. Adrenal rest tumor

- 3. Adrenal causes
  - a. Congenital adrenal hyperplasia
  - b. Noncongenital adrenal hyperplasia (Cushing's sydrome or disease)
  - c. Tumors
    - i. Virilizing adenoma
    - ii. Virilizing carcinoma
- 4. Other sources
  - a. Genetic chromosomal abnormality, 46,XY with incomplete androgen resistance
  - b. Hypothyroidism
  - c. Hyperprolactinemia

It has been documented that, among these large numbers of causes of hirsutism, the following etiologic factors are responsible for over 90% of its occurrences (6):

- Polycystic ovary syndrome (PCOS) is by far the most common cause of excess androgens and hirsutism, occurring in about 74% of cases.
- End-organ hypersensitivity is the cause in about 7%.
- Congenital adrenal hyperplasia is the cause in about 6%.
- Hyperprolactinemia is the cause in about 4%.

Diseases other than these four account for only 10% of the etiology of hirsutism.

End-Organ Hypersensitivity to Androgens

The moniker *end-organ hypersensitivity to androgens* replaced *familial hirsutism* and *idiopathic hirsutism,* which are characterized by the presence of hirsutism and normal androgen levels. The prevalence of this entity is approximately 6% (6). The cause of this condition is linked to increased 5-alpha-reductase activity in the skin, which converts the potent androgen testosterone to an even more potent androgen, dehydrotestosterone (DHT). In circulation and in target tissues, DHT is predominantly derived from peripheral conversion and is considered a paracrine hormone formed in and active in target tissues (7,8). DHT metabolism also occurs in the skin (9). This conversion ratio is significantly higher in hirsute women with normal androgen levels when compared with hirsute patients with elevated androgen levels in PCOS (10,11). The excessive sensitivity of the pilosebaceous unit to normal levels of androgen stimulates hair growth in a cyclic pattern, eventually leading to hirsutism. This group of hirsute women may experience a regular ovulatory menstrual cycle.

It has been postulated that the skewing of X-chromosome inactivation is associated with end-organ hypersensitivity to androgens (nonhyperandrogenic hirsutism). The androgen receptor gene is located on the X chromosome, and the skewing of the X chromosome may increase in androgen receptor-mediated sensitivity of the hair follicle (12).

POLYCYSTIC OVARY SYNDROME

Polycystic ovary syndrome [first called Stein-Leventhal syndrome in 1935 (13), also known as functional ovarian hyperandrogenism (14)] is considered a complex-heterogeneous condition. In 1990, at the consensus conference of the National Institutes of Health (15), PCOS was comprehensively defined as incorporating the following clinical parameters:

- History of chronic ovulatory dysfunction
- Clinical evidence of peripheral hyperandrogenism and/or biochemical assays of circulating androgens (hyperandrogenemia)
- Exclusion of other causes mimicking PCOS

The prevalence of PCOS is estimated to be approximately 4.6%; although, it could be as low as 3.5% and as high as 11.2%, with no significant difference in prevalence noted between white and black women (16). The trend is to distinguish between PCOS and polycystic ovaries, in which essentially healthy women with no symptoms of PCOS have ultrasonographically determined polycystic ovaries. It has been established that the prevalence based on transvaginal sonography of polycystic ovaries is approximately 14.2% (17); however, the rate varies and can be as high as 27% (18).

When oligomenorrhea is present, the prevalence of PCOS among caucasian women is 4.4% to 7.4% (19); among Pima Indians the rate is 21% (20). When oligomenorrhea is associated with hyperandrogenism, the prevalence is 3.4% to 9%, depending on ethnicity and race (5,21). However, the scientific data also suggest that 74% of hyperandrogenic women present with normal menses and have documented PCOS (22). Incidence data for PCOS have not been presented in the literature.

The underlying primary cause of PCOS is unknown; although, there is a growing consensus that multiple pathophysiologic mechanisms play a role (23,24). First, an intrinsic alternation between GnRH and LH leads to sustained LH secretion and FSH deficiency in relation to LH levels. Also, androgen excess [(which in PCOS increases secretion of androstenedione and 17-beta-hydroxyprogesterone from the ovaries in response to tonic LH release (25)] in the serum shows a correlation with hyperinsulinemia through the insulin-resistance mechanism in PCOS, particularly in obese patients (26). Chronic hyperandrogenemia in PCOS is often clinically expressed either by hirsutism or virilism; therefore, a clinical effort is made to decrease androgen levels. However, it has been documented that such an approach does not reduce hyperinsulinemia (27) nor does increasing insulin sensitivity decrease androgen levels (28).

Such scientific data have very practical clinical implications, not only from the amelioration of reproductive dysfunction but also from the metabolic abnormalities and their medical consequences, such as type 2 diabetes mellitus, hypercholesterolemia, hypertension, and cardiovascular disease. The hormonal imbalance in PCOS also may be linked to a serious risk for endometrial, breast, or ovarian cancer (29).

Insulin resistance (hyperinsulinemia) in some PCOS patients has a unique underlying pathophysiology that distinguishes this form from other insulin resistance cases (30). Women with PCOS are powerless to defeat peripheral insulin resistance. Increasing insulin production and secretion leads to an occurrence of either non–insulin-dependent diabetes mellitus (NIDDM) or glucose intolerance (31) in approximately 40% of patients [with 5% in the general premenopausal population (32)]. Such resistant hyperinsulinemia exacerbates reproductive abnormalities of PCOS and results in insulin resistance in more than 50% of obese patients (33). Insulin resistance with compensatory hyperinsulinemia is considered the principal metabolic aberration of PCOS and can be expressed as insulin insensitivity or insulin action defect, which is evident in NIDDM (34). Furthermore, a defect in insulin-mediated activation of glucose transporter proteins and glucose transport into the cells is at the postreceptor level (23,35). Because insulin receptors and insulin binding are normal (36), this mechanism is at the level of autophosphorylation (37).

Relative risk for coronary heart disease that eventually may lead to myocardial infarction is predicted as increasing by 7.4% in patients with PCOS [the risk factor model was based on age, hypertension, diabetes mellitus, central obesity (increased waist-to-hip ratio), and serum triglyceride concentration and was clinically applied to women with PCOS and an age-matched control group] (38). However, epidemiologic data to support this predicted coronary heart disease risk are currently lacking. Women with PCOS do not have markedly higher than average mortality rates from circulatory disease, and the characteristically unopposed estrogen milieu in PCOS may in fact play a protective role against cardiovascular disease (39).

Type 2 Diabetes Mellitus

It has been established that women with PCOS have higher glucose levels and more frequent glucose intolerance than healthy women (40).

The prevalence of impaired glucose tolerance is 31.1%, and that of type 2 diabetes mellitus is 7.5%. These rates indicate that women with PCOS are at a significantly increased risk for impaired glucose tolerance and type 2 diabetes mellitus. In addition, these risks are distributed among all body weights at a young age. PCOS itself may be more of a risk factor than ethnicity or race for glucose intolerance in young women (41).

Among women with PCOS and diabetes, the mortality rate is significantly higher, with diabetes being a contributing factor to death (39).

Lipid Abnormalities

Lipid abnormalities are persistently abnormal in patients with PCOS, even when an adjustment for body mass index (BMI) is made. For practical purposes, these abnormalities can be gathered into two groups to emphasize the dynamics of changes when compared with those of healthy women (42,43):

■ Abnormally elevated [total cholesterol, low-density lipoprotein (LDL) cholesterol, very low-density lipoprotein cholesterol, ratio of cholesterol to high-density lipoprotein (HDL) and of LDL to HDL, and triglycerides]
■ Lower levels of HDL and HDL2.

Hypertension

Existing data from the literature are misleading and conflicting. Preliminary results indicate that hypertension was present in up to 39% of patients with PCOS (38); however, when an adjustment for BMI was made, this finding was not substantiated (42).

Cancer

Polycystic ovary syndrome predisposes patients to malignant neoplasia. The relative risk for *endometrial cancer* in patients with PCOS is estimated to be about 3.1% (44) and may be induced by the following features observed in PCOS:

■ Obesity (45)
■ Type 2 diabetes mellitus (46)
■ Hyperinsulinemia (47)
■ Unopposed levels of endogenous estrogen (48)

The fact that young women with PCOS may be affected by endometrial cancer implies that PCOS is a risk factor (48,49). Among women with PCOS and associated endometrial hyperplasia, progress to cancer is expected in about 25% of patients (48). In women with unopposed endogenous estrogen, the administration of progesterone or progestin significantly decreases the development of endometrial cancer.

Epithelial ovarian cancer and its relationship with the hormonal ambiance in women with PCOS, featuring abnormal patterns of gonadotropin release in lean women, may be a mitigating factor for an observed association between PCOS and ovarian cancer. The risk for ovarian cancer may increase to 2.5-fold and is stronger among women who never used oral contraceptives (51). According to epidemiologic data and laboratory results, and on theoretical grounds, infertile women have an increased lifetime risk for gynecologic cancer (52).

A low risk for breast cancer is expected among patients with PCOS (53,54).

Diagnosis of Polycystic Ovary Syndrome

The principal objectives in the diagnosis of PCOS involve verifying various clinical signs and symptoms, excluding mimicking disorders, and determining coexisting medical entities that resulted from either PCOS or concomitant conditions. Due to long-term health consequences associated with compensatory hyperinsulinemia in PCOS, it is advisable to determine insulin levels once a PCOS diagnosis is reached. An evaluation of insulin resistance does not provide pertinent information in the diagnostic process of PCOS. A synchronized clinical effort is essential in the diagnosis of PCOS because there is no standard test to confirm this condition.

Pertinent Medical History

Assessing a patient's medical history is paramount in reaching the diagnosis of PCOS. There are four distinct components in the evaluation of PCOS:

■ Menstrual dysfunctions
■ Reproductive capacity
■ Cosmetic aspects (hirsutism, acne, and alopecia)
■ Metabolic abnormality such as glucose intolerance or type 2 diabetes mellitus (NIDDM)

A systematic arrangement of the patient's medical history is helpful for practical implementation of treatment. Menstrual dysfunction in PCOS begins with a normal onset of menarche followed shortly afterward by erratic menstrual bleeding that is characteristic of anovulation (a chronic absence of progesterone and presence of long-standing unopposed estrogen). The occurrence of unpredictable, irregular menses (absence of premenstrual molimina), ranging from oligomenorrhea (more frequent than amenorrhea) to secondary amenorrhea, and often menorrhagia [caused by endometrial hyperplasia due to unopposed estrogens (increased estrogen levels result from peripheral androgen conversion)], have been reported. Oligomenorrhea is considered a functional marker for PCOS. When concomitant symptoms are seen, along with laboratory documentation of elevated ratios of LH/FSH and estrogen status, oligomenorrhea is present in about 90% of patients with PCOS (29).

Usually this cluster of symptoms develops perimenarcheally, frequently in concomitance with obesity and a gradual onset of symptoms. However, normal duration, amount, and regularity of menses, as well as normal weight among women, do not eliminate the possibility of the likelihood of PCOS.

Another possible symptom is infertility, which is encountered in approximately 40% of women with PCOS (55).

Hyperandrenalism

Hirsutism can be traced to the peripubertal period, and the rate of hair growth, for clinical purposes, may be divided into (a) gradual onset and hair growth over time and (b) rapid onset and hair growth over time that may suggest an androgen-producing tumor of either ovarian or adrenal origin.

Acne (excessive sebum production) in young women, particularly of the severe cystic type, is quite frequently observed in PCOS. In fact, severe acne among adolescent women is one of the best predictors of PCOS (56). There is a relationship between the levels of DHEA-S and the severity of cystic acne (57), but plasma-free testosterone does not have any correlation with the severity of acne (58).

Alopecia (hair loss without regrowth) in PCOS is associated with both hyperandrogenism and the effect of dehydrotestosterone on the pilosebaceous unit. Alopecia in patients with PCOS is usually one component of clusters of hyperandrogenic symptoms. The prevalence of alopecia is estimated to occur in less than 10% of patients with PCOS (56). About 60% of women with diffuse alopecia are diagnosed with PCOS (59).

Virilization with defeminization strongly suggests the presence of an androgen-producing tumor. Changes reported by patients include clitoral enlargement, decreased breast size, severe hirsutism, acne, alopecia, brownish black skin discoloration in the genital, anal, upper thigh, and axilla areas (suggesting the presence of acanthosis nigricans), deeper voice, enhanced libido, and amenorrhea.

Obesity becomes apparent with the commencement of menstrual cycle dysfunction and affects approximately 50% of patients with PCOS (60). It is a known phenomenon among clinicians that weight loss is difficult with diet and exercise alone and that resulting obesity is probably a clinical expression of "slow metabolism" (23); contrary to this belief, however, research has documented that obesity occurs due to an excess of caloric intake (61). Android-type body fat distribution may be reported by patients. Abdominal fat deposition is considered a male or android pattern (apple pattern), versus female-type obesity, in which hip and thigh fat distribution (pear pattern) is observed (61,62).

Other causes of hyperandrogenism, such as adrenal hyperplasia, hyperprolactinemia, hypo- and hyperthyroidism, and Cushing disease or syndrome, must be carefully evaluated. Iatrogenic causes of exogenous androgen intake also must be considered when evaluating for PCOS.

Physical Examination

Upon physical examination, the following abnormalities may be identified.

Elevated Blood Pressure

Preliminary data indicate that approximately 39% of patients with PCOS take medication for hypertension (63). In addition, it has been postulated that a long (>40 days) and irregular menstrual cycle increases the risk for hypertension twofold (29). Statistically significant elevated systolic blood pressure also has been reported; however, upon correction to include BMI, there is no longer any statistical significance (64).

Android Obesity

Android obesity with central body fat distribution (apple pattern) and an increased waist-to-hip ratio (>0.80 in women) was observed in PCOS patients (56). Such an increase of the waist-to-hip ratio appears to be a better marker than BMI, and it is associated with a significantly increased mortality rate in older women (64).

Skin Changes

Hirsutism and its degree should be semi-quantified (the standardized Ferriman and Gallwey scoring system can be applied) (76). A score of greater than 8 indicates the presence of hirsutism and a score of less than 8 indicates an absence of hirsutism.

There are other forms of clinical assessment of hair distribution, namely by means of determining the extent of facial hair (Table 8.1.) (67). Computerized assessment of facial hair growth has been introduced, but a scoring system based on this type of assessment has not yet been generated (68).

Oily, shiny skin with inflamed, erythematous follicular papules and pustules of various size may occur. A cystic form at the base of acne is the most common type associated with PCOS (56).

Alopecia in patients with PCOS infrequently manifests in a male-patterned form with bi-temporal hairline recession (temporal balding). Alopecia associated with clinical conditions may be caused by virilization (56), although virilization is not a typical finding in PCOS patients.

Acanthosis nigricans is a clinical sign, often indicating PCOS. In its classic appearance, diffused brownish black or gray skin discoloration occurs in the nape of the neck or axilla, umbilicus, or genital, anal, groin, or upper inner thigh areas. Fibrous papillomata (skin tags) frequently accompany acanthosis nigricans (69).

Breast examination may reveal nipple discharge associated with PCOS in about 10% of patients (56). It may also reveal dark aureoles or the abnormal presence of hairs.

Pelvic Examination

External genitalia may exhibit skin discoloration associated with acanthosis nigricans. Clitoromegaly may be observed,

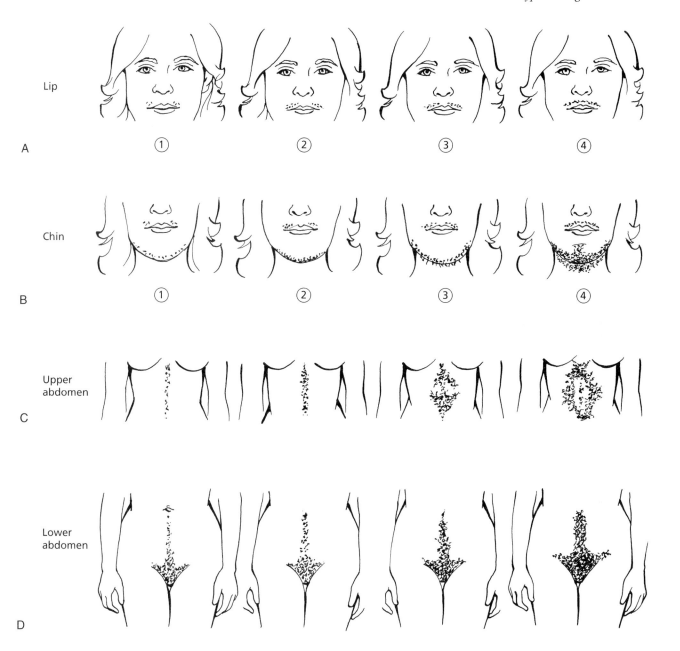

	Lip			
A	①	②	③	④

	Chin			
B	①	②	③	④

Upper abdomen

C

Lower abdomen

D

TABLE 8.1. ASSESSMENT OF HIRSUTISM

Illustration	Side	Grade	Definition
A	Upper lip	1	A few hairs at outer margin
		2	A small moustache at outer margin
		3	A moustache extending halfway from outer margin
		4	A moustache extending to midline
B	Chin	1	A few scattered hairs
		2	Scattered hairs with small concentration
		3 & 4	Complete coverage, light and heavy
C	Upper abdomen	1	A few midline hairs
		2	Rather more, still midline
		3 & 4	Half and complete coverage
D	Lower abdomen	1	A few midline hairs
		2	A midline streak of hairs
		3	A midline band of hair
		4	Inverted V-shaped hair growth

(continued)

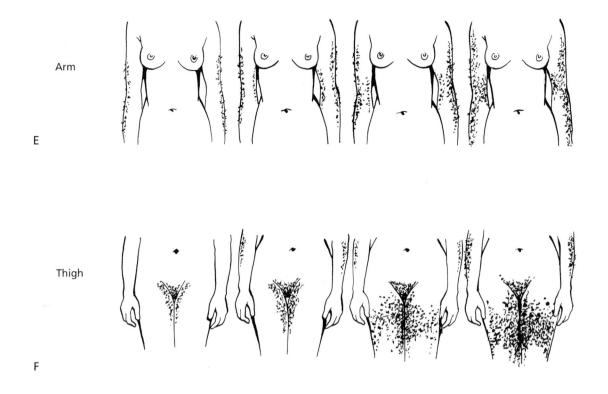

Arm

E

Thigh

F

TABLE 8.1. *(continued)*

Illustration	Side	Grade	Definition
E	Arm	1	Sparse growth affecting no more than one fourth of the limb surface
		2	More hair growth but coverage still incomplete
		3 & 4	Complete coverage light and heavy
	Forearm	1, 2, 3, 4	Complete coverage of dorsal surface: two grades of light and two grades of heavy growth
F	Thigh	1, 2, 3, 4	Same as for arm
	Leg	1, 2, 3, 4	Same as for arm

(continued)

although it is a part of virilization. Cervical mucus has persistently been present, and ovaries are enlarged bilaterally in approximately 40% to 50% of patients (56).

Laboratory

Hormonal Determinations
The LH:FSH ratio traditionally has been used for PCOS diagnosis verification. However, it has been documented that the sensitivity of this test was approximately 44%, and only 20% of patients with PCOS presented with an LH:FSH ratio greater than 3. As a result of this low LH:FSH ratio sensitivity, a suggestion was made to abandon this test as a biochemical criterion for the diagnosis of PCOS (70).

In an oligomenorrheic patient, timing between day 15 after menstruation and day 21 before the next menstruation (labeled as the specific oligomenorrheic phase), LH concentrations were significantly higher than during other phases of an amenorrheic menstrual cycle. For the accurate interpreta-

tion of these measurements, the dates of menstruation both before and after the blood sample should be known (71). Preliminary results suggest taking four samples every 10 minutes to avoid missing a single LH determination level (72).

Luteinizing hormone and FSH serum determination became very popular and an almost mandatory method for PCOS diagnosis. Recent research data indicate that LH pulsatile secretive frequency from the pituitary gland is rapid when compared with that of a healthy control group of women; although, these changes cannot always be measured in peripheral blood samples. Therefore, approximately one third of patients with PCOS demonstrate normal LH levels. Today, FSH assays are more sensitive than those of previous techniques (the upper limit is about 10 mIU/mL), but LH assays have not been modernized (the upper limit is 20–25 mIU/mL) (73–75). Therefore, in this scenario, the LH:FSH ratio will be elevated, at least between 2.0 and 2.5. Thus, using this test in everyday practice would be meaningless.

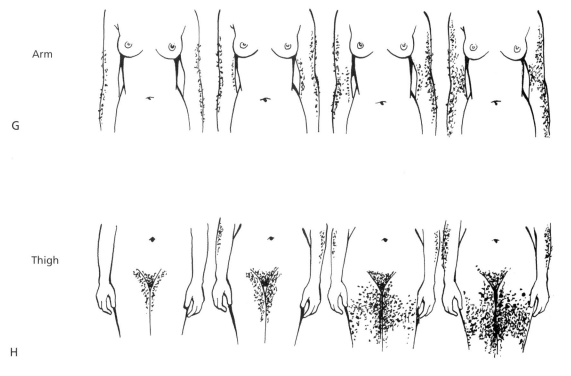

TABLE 8.1. *(continued)*

Illustration	Side	Grade	Definition
G	Upper back	1	A few scattered hairs
		2	Rather more, still scattered
		3 & 4	Complete coverage, light and heavy
H	Lower back	1	A sacral tuft of hairs
		2	Hairs with some lateral extension
		3	Three-fourths coverage
		4	Complete coverage

Adapted from Ferriman A, Gallwey JD. Clinical assessment of body growth in women *J Clin Endocrinol Metab* 1961;21:1440–1447; with permission. Modified from Gorden MC. Menstrual disorders in adolescents. Excess androgens and polycystic ovary syndrome. *Pediatr Clin North Am* 1999;46:519–543; with permission.

The LH:FSH ratio, together with documentation of increased androstenedione levels in serum, are effective markers for PCOS diagnosis. These two combinations of hormone determinations yield the greatest diagnostic sensitivity and specificity for PCOS (76).

When total testosterone (normal range in serum is 20–80 ng/dL) is elevated between 85 and 150 ng/dL (moderate hyperandrogenemia), an ultrasonographic image of the ovaries is compatible with the typical appearance of PCOS, and oligomenorrhea or hirsutism is clinically documented, the total testosterone level appears to be the best single biochemical marker (70%) for PCOS (70). Both the clearance and bioavailability of testosterone are dependent on the serum concentration of sex hormone-binding globulin, whose production is controlled by insulin (74).

Additionally, total testosterone elevation in the serum of greater than 200 ng/dL may indicate the presence of ovarian or androgen-producing neoplasms (73).

Dehydroepiandrosterone sulfate (normal range in serum is 80–350 µg/dL) is another marker of an androgen-producing tumor, and when the threshold serum level reaches 700 µg/mL, an adrenal gland neoplasm is suspected (73).

When the 17-alpha-hydroxyprogesterone serum level is less than 3 ng/mL during the follicular phase of the menstrual cycle, it eliminates the possibility of late-onset (nonclassic) congenital adrenal hyperplasia due to 21-hydroxylase deficiency. Values greater than 3 ng/mL necessitate performing an ACTH stimulating test (73).

Prolactin and growth hormone levels are increased in PCOS (up to 30% of patients with PCOS demonstrate prolactin level elevation). Coexisting prolactinoma is rarely observed in PCOS (75,77). Growth hormone secretion has been documented in obese patients with PCOS and is considered an accompanying parameter of PCOS (78).

Estrogen determination in the diagnostic process of PCOS is not advisable as long as otherwise indicated. However, there are important consequences of acyclic, abnormal estrogen secretion, and it is worthwhile to remember the following:

- Estradiol serum concentrations in PCOS remain at the levels corresponding to the early follicular and mid-follicular phase of the normal menstrual cycle.
- An acyclic pattern of estradiol secretion and an absence of the typically increased level in the preovulatory or mid-luteal phase may be present.
- Peripheral conversion in adipose tissue (extragrandular) from androgens to estrone is more significant when the patient is obese.
- Tonic LH secretion is caused by abnormal estrogen production and a lack of sufficient amounts of progesterone (in the normal menstrual cycle, LH is released cyclically, not constantly).
- Unopposed estrogen may predispose a patient not only to erratic menses and abnormal endometrial bleeding, but also to endometrial adenocarcinoma.

Insulin secretion may be assessed as follows:

- A standard 75-g oral glucose tolerance test or an intravenous (IV) glucose tolerance test may be used. According to the new American Diabetes Association criteria, diabetes is established when a fasting glucose level is greater than 126 mg/dL. However, there is evidence in the literature that this approach is inadequate to diagnose glucose intolerance and diabetes in women with PCOS (41). The World Health Organization criteria for impaired glucose tolerance are 2-hour glucose levels greater than 139 mg/dL, and for type 2 diabetes mellitus are 2-hour glucose levels greater than 200 mg/dL.
- Glycosylated hemoglobin levels may be assessed.
- Glucose-to-insulin ratio may be assessed. Fasting glucose-to-insulin ratio measurements are a highly specific and sensitive test for insulin-resistant PCOS patients. In addition, this test may be a clinically useful indicator for selecting women with PCOS, who are most likely to respond to therapy for improving insulin sensitivity (33).

Ultrasonography

Ultrasonography captures an image of ovarian morphologic details in a noninvasive way. Initially, a transabdominal transducer was used to establish diagnostic criteria for PCOS, and the presence of at least five follicles in each ovary indicated a positive diagnosis of PCOS (79). A classical PCOS ultrasonographic image depicts bilateral ovarian enlargement, increased proportion of the stroma, and a variety in the number and sizes of cysts. Because the transabdominal approach was neither technically satisfactory in its imaging nor suitable for all patients, particularly those with obesity, the transvaginal ultrasonographic study was introduced. Recently, it has been suggested that when 15 or more small follicles are present, the diagnosis of PCOS can be made with confidence (80). The appearance of polycysts (follicles) within the ovary is a sign of functional disruption of the hypothalamic–pituitary–ovary axis and is not a cause of PCOS. Therefore, any woman with a dysfunctional menstrual cycle may present with polycysts in the ovary. There is ample clinical sonographic evidence that the appearance of the ovary in healthy women with normal, regular menstrual cycles may correspond to that of women with PCOS (81–83).

Histologic Evaluation

Histologic evaluation of a polycystic ovary is performed only occasionally on biopsy specimens. Ovaries in patients with PCOS present as thick, hypocellular, and fibrotic and may resemble capsules. Hyperplasia and luteinization of the theca interna are also present. Normal follicularity is observed with an increased number of follicles, and the stroma may contain luteinized stromal cells (84).

In summary, there is no standard approach or test to determine PCOS. Confounding and sometimes conflicting tests are suggested, and in view of multiple abnormal hormonal ambiances and a broad clinical picture associated with this condition; therefore, appropriate management of PCOS remains a clinical challenge. However, in most instances, hirsutism and anovulation and their interactions are present. In the past, menstrual dysfunction in adolescents was considered a stage in the physiologic maturation of the hypothalamic–pituitary–ovarian axis, and a clinical evaluation was postponed until after this maturation process was completed. Today, an early clinical investigation for PCOS and the possibility of therapeutic intervention are advocated for any patients exhibiting menstrual dysfunction, including the adolescent population showing symptoms of PCOS (85).

In a clinical PCOS evaluation, the following approach may assist in *initial determination*. When mild *hirsutism* is observed with a gradual onset of terminal hair growth in reproductive age, along with an *erratic menstrual cycle* (most commonly oligomenorrhea) and no plan for immediate conception, adequate medical history and physical examination may establish the diagnosis of PCOS. In such a clinical scenario, an androgen-secreting tumor is a remote possibility; therefore, determining total testosterone and DHEA-S levels in the serum will not clarify the case. A link between such cases and adrenal 21-hydroxylase (CAH) is difficult to assess based solely on clinical judgment, and testing for 17-alpha-hydroxyprogesterone may be helpful, although the usefulness of this test in everyday practice has not been well established.

When *moderate to severe hirsutism* is observed with a rapid onset of terminal hair growth, along with *menstrual dysfunction*, the total testosterone and DHEA-S levels should be determined and are essential to rule out or rule in an ovarian or adrenal androgen-producing tumor. When the total testosterone level in serum is greater than 200 ng/dL or the DHEA-S level is greater than 700 µg/mL, an ultrasonographic or magnetic resonance imaging (MRI) study may identify the location of the tumor. Occasionally, ovarian or adrenal vein catheterization is performed to reach an appropriate diagnosis (86).

When *virilization* is observed with a sudden and progressive development of virilizing signs and symptoms, a normal menstrual cycle, a short high, and a similar course of the condition in the family history, a 17alpha-hy-deoxyprogesterone level of greater than 3 ng/dL may imply CAH.

It has been postulated that determining total testosterone, DHEA-S, and 17-hydeoxyprogesterone levels in the serum are sufficient studies for an initial screening of PCOS (73).

In addition, a diagnostic armamentarium should incorporate the following elements (23):

- Screening for glucose intolerance, when a patient presents risk factors such as obesity, acanthosis nigricans, or a family history of diabetes (determining the fasting glucose level with the standard 75-g oral glucose tolerance test)
- Determining baseline fasting lipid levels, when a patient is obese

Differential Diagnosis of Polycystic Ovary Syndrome

The following conditions are taken into consideration in the differential diagnosis of PCOS.

Functional Disorders

- *Ovarian hyperthecosis*: bilateral noncystic ovarian enlargement, and slow and gradual onset of symptoms with acanthosis nigricans and insulin-resistance are often present (also called insulin-resistant acanthosis nigricans syndrome, which may result from genetic defects) (56).
- *Congenital adrenal hyperplasia*: 17-alpha-hydroxyprogesterone of greater than 3 ng/dL warrants an ACTH stimulation test, and when responses are greater than or equal to 10 ng/mL, a 21-hydroxylase enzyme defect is established (73).
- *Cushing syndrome*: 1 mg of dexamethasone is administered overnight, and the fasting cortisol level in the serum is determined in the morning. The normal response is less than 5 µg/dL (a response between 5 and 10 µg/dL requires that the test be repeated). A response greater than 10 µg/dL is abnormal and is followed by low-dose, high-dose dexamethasone suppression tests, as well as imaging evaluation to rule out or rule in adrenal hyperplasia, Cushing disease, adrenal adenoma, or an ectopic ACTH production site (73).

Androgen-Producing Tumors

Androgen-producing tumors of the ovary or adrenal gland are a possibility, when the serum's total testosterone levels are greater than 200 ng/dL or DHEA-S levels are greater than 700 µg/mL.

Conventional Therapy for PCOS

Treatment modes for PCOS depend on whether a patient desires immediate fertility. When an underlying cause of PCOS is determined, therapeutic priority should be given to the cause to prevent long-term consequences of the syndrome. Therefore, clinical approaches can be simplified as follows.

If Fertility Is Not Desired

If fertility is not desired, the therapeutic objectives fall into two groups: (a) symptom management (hirsutism, acne, irregular menses, etc.) and (b) health risk management associated with PCOS (diabetes, cardiovascular, etc.). The following treatment may be offered.

Progesterone Therapy
Progesterone therapy alone may be given, if a patient is not sexually active and presents with mild hirsutism:

- Micronized progesterone (Prometrium) alone can be administered orally at the dosage of 100 to 200 mg daily, for a 12-day course each month.
- Progesterone in oil (Lipolutin) can be administered as a 50- to 100-mg intramuscular (IM) injection each month.
- Vaginal gel (Crione 4% or Crione 8%) can be applied every other day for a 12-day course each month.
- Progesterone vaginal effervescent tablets can be administered at the dosage of 100 mg daily for 12 days.

Progestin Therapy
Progestin therapy may be given, although there is some concern about the androgenic potential effect of 19-nortestosterone derivatives and progestins (norethindrone and norgestrol) decreasing SHBG and increasing LDL cholesterol.

- Provera (10- to 20-mg oral tablet) can be administered daily for a 12-day course each month.
- Norlutate (5- to 10-mg oral tablet) can be administered daily for a 12-day course each month.
- Norlutin (5- to 10-mg oral tablet) can be administered daily for a 12-day course each month.

Oral Contraceptive Treatment
Oral contraceptive treatment can be used to reduce the following (87):

- Androgen levels (possible mechanisms include increased synthesis of SHBG in the liver, partial inhibition of 5-

alpha-reductase and androgen receptor binding ability, and suppression of LH levels)
- Exposure time to unopposed estrogens
- Endometrial proliferation
- Incidence of ovarian cancer
- Endometrial cancer

There are some concerns that using oral contraceptives in patients with PCOS may result in the following:

- Increased insulin resistance state
- Increased risk for diabetes
- Increased risk for cardiovascular disease
- Increased serum triglyceride level

The results of clinical scientific research revealed; however, that the management of PCOS with oral contraceptives is not associated with marked risks, such as the potential risks presented above (88).

Oral contraceptive therapy alone for the treatment of hirsutism associated with PCOS is associated with a success rate of greater than 10%. Combining oral contraceptives with antiandrogens is effective in the treatment of hirsutism, mild to moderate acne, and alopecia. Oral contraceptives alone frequently are an effective treatment for acne (89).

Combination of Oral Contraceptives and Antiandrogen Therapy

So far, the U.S. Food and Drug Administration (FDA) has not approved a drug for hirsutism therapy; therefore, medicines approved for other conditions are used. The antiandrogen blocking mechanism that inhibits growth of the hair follicle is expressed by means of either impeding the conversion of testosterone to dehydrotestosterone (a 5-alpha-reductase inhibitor) or preventing testosterone or dehydrotestosterone binding to the androgen receptors. The following antiandrogens are currently being used.

Spironolactone is recommended, starting with a dosage of 50 mg twice daily, and if there is no improvement within 6 months, the dose can be doubled. Dosages of 100 and 200 mg daily were tested, and both dosages significantly reduced hirsutism (90). Cyclic administration of spironolactone for 21 days per month has been tested, but there is no conclusive evidence available that such a mode of therapy is better than one of continuous administration (38,91). Spironolactone is an aldosterone antagonist originally approved for hypertension therapy. It is a weak progestin agent and a weak testosterone inhibitor, competitively inhibiting DHT by binding to its intracellular androgen receptors, and by suppressing the biosynthesis of androgens (38). Spironolactone is often combined with oral contraceptives, which should have a nonandrogenic progestin component.

Unarguably, *cyproterone acetate* as a progestin component in oral contraceptives (Diane) yields the best results for hirsute women with PCOS. When spironolactone is added to Diane, the pills exhibit a synergistic effect in the usual dose, although hirsutism is not improved significantly as compared with the effect of Diane alone (92). Spironolactone alone increases the frequency of menses (polymenorrhea) in approximately 20% to 80% of patients, but the addition of oral contraceptives regulates menstruation. In addition, oral contraceptives provide ovarian suppression, which reduces ovarian androgen production. Administering spironolactone during pregnancy should be avoided. Diabetic patients, elderly patients, and patients on other medications, particularly drugs that may increase the serum potassium level, also should be administered with caution. When using spironolactone monotherapy in women of reproductive age, other forms of contraception should be advised, and pregnancy should be avoided for at least 4 months after the termination of spironolactone (38). Additional minor side effects such as salt depletion, mastodynia, light-headedness, lethargy, polyuria, gastrointestinal disturbance, fatigue, and breast tenderness are usually transitional and self-limited (38,89).

Flutamide is a nonsteroidal antiandrogen that expresses its antiandrogen mechanism by inhibiting nuclear binding of androgens in target tissues (38). It is administered at the dosage of 125 to 250 mg twice daily in combination with or without oral contraceptives, and the effectiveness of flutamide is superior to that of spironolactone in the treatment of female hirsutism and its related androgen-dependent signs and symptoms (91). Fulminant liver failure with potentially fatal consequences (approximately 0.5%) has been reported in patients on flutamide (93,94). Serial blood aminotransferase levels should be monitored during the first few months of flutamide treatment, and the course of the therapy must be discontinued immediately when any episode of nausea, vomiting, fatigue, or jaundice is reported (95). There are no data on flutamide safety during pregnancy. Due to its potential hepatotoxicity, drug administration is questionable and should only be considered for women with PCOS who are resistant to other antiandrogenic treatment (38,89).

Cyproterone acetate (not approved by the FDA) for the treatment of hirsutism is recommended at the dosage of 25 to 50 mg daily for 10 days each month. Its mechanisms incorporate an antigonadotropic effect, blocking the binding of DHT to its cytoplasmatic receptor, decreasing 5-alpha-reductase activities, and interfering with androgen steroidogenesis. Side effects include depression, decreased libido, light-headedness, fluid retention, weight gain, hepatotoxicity, and adrenal insufficiency; however, when given in a cyclic mode for 10 days, complications are observed infrequently. In combination with oral contraceptives, cyproterone acetate is an effective treatment for hirsutism (38,89).

Finasteride (which is not an antiandrogen, because it does not directly bind to androgen receptors) is recommended at the dosage of 5 mg daily for women with hirsutism, and is as effective as 100 mg spironolactone but lacks the significant side effects. Finasteride is a 5-alpha-reductase inhibitor that expresses its mechanism by inhibiting the conversion of testosterone to dehydrotestosterone, which stimulates hairs follicles to grow (96). Occasionally minimal gastrointestinal side effects have occurred, but no menstrual dysfunction has been observed (38).

Ketoconazole, an antifungal medication, is relatively effective at the low dosage of 400 mg daily (98); however, potential hepatotoxicity should be considered (99).

Cimetidine, a histamine type 2 blocker, at the dosage of 300 mg four times daily, was tried and appeared to be ineffective in the treatment of hirsute women (100).

Gonadotropin-Releasing Hormone Agonists

Gonadotropin-releasing hormone agonists (a depot of 3.75 mg IM every 28 days reduces androgen concentrations) are an effective treatment for hirsutism and improve insulin sensitivity (101). Preliminary data indicate that combining GnRH with spironolactone may effectively prevent the bone loss so often associated with GnRH monotherapy. Such dual therapies improve hirsutism and are bone sparing (as documented by biochemical and bone mineral density) (102).

Antiandrogen therapies in PCOS are frequently successful in the treatment of hirsutism; however, upon cessation of medication, hirsutism recurred within 1 year (103).

Electrolysis

Electrolysis, a mechanical hair removal process, can be used for hirsute women with PCOS, but the underlying cause will remain unaddressed. Therefore, it is necessary for conservative medical antiandrogen therapy for hirsutism to continue indefinitely (104).

Laser Therapy

Laser, when applied locally, significantly improves facial hirsutism, but it may be necessary to repeat the procedure. Hyperpigmentation resolves, as do depressions in the skin, but hypopigmentation may persist (105,106).

If Fertility Is Desired

When fertility is desired, an induction of ovulation is indicated in PCOS. The initial infertility workup (at least tubal patency and semen count with morphology assessment) should be conducted. An induction of ovulation can be achieved as follows.

Medical Induction of Ovulation

Clomiphene citrate is a nonsteroid, weak estrogenic and powerful antiestrogenic agent, and is structurally linked to tamoxifen and stilbestrol. In 1967, the FDA approved clomiphene citrate for ovulation induction. The principal mechanism of clomiphene citrate is largely unknown, but it is probably effective through its affinity to estrogen and its ability to bind to estrogen receptors in the hypothalamus.

The hypothalamic site of action for clomiphene citrate probably induces an increase in the frequency of GnRH pulsatile secretion (107). A prerequisite for successful induction of ovulation with clomiphene citrate is an intact hypothalamic–pituitary axis and an adequate level of FSH, estrogen, and prolactin levels. Customary clomiphene citrate treatment is commenced at a dose of 50 mg on the 5th day of spontaneous or progesterone-induced endometrial bleeding, and is continued for 5 consecutive days through the 9th day of the cycle. If ovulation is not achieved, the initial clomiphene citrate dose can be increased by 50-mg increments up to 150 mg as indicated (150 mg is the highest dose recommended by the FDA). When the optimal minimal dose of clomiphene citrate is determined, it should be maintained for four to six consecutive menstrual cycles, and ovulation is expected between 5 and 10 days of the last dose of clomiphene citrate. If pregnancy occurs, it usually happens within a 4- to 6-month period, as found in over 90% of patients. Although, the highest clomiphene citrate dose recommended by the FDA is 150 mg, there is ample evidence that in select cases a dose of 200 mg or higher is necessary to induce ovulation (108). In the majority of cases, a failure to induce ovulation with the 150-mg dose warrants further infertility evaluation. Approximately 80% of patients ovulate in response to the clomiphene citrate therapy, but only 40% of these patients conceive. Due to the established clomiphene citrate safety record, the initiation of ovulation induction is acceptable without completing an infertility workup (109).

The combination of clomiphene citrate and dexamethasone or prednisone is an effective method for the induction of ovulation, particularly when the serum DHEA-S level is greater than 200 μg/dL. Dexamethasone tablets are recommended at a dose of 0.25 to 0.5 mg (or prednisone tablets at a dose of 5–7.5 mg) taken at bedtime 2 weeks before the beginning of menses and continued throughout menstrual cycles together with clomiphene citrate. The combination of these two drugs allows for a decrease in the clomiphene citrate dose and an improvement in ovulation (38,110,111). A glucocorticosteroid therapy paradigm should be discontinued when the patient conceives, and clinical monitoring is a sufficient method for follow-up (38).

There are some *concerns* about clomiphene citrate therapy. Twin gestation occurs in 6.25% to 12.8% of patients; spontaneous abortion occurs in 26.5% of patients; and postclomiphene birth defects occur in 3.1% of patients (this is the same expected rate of birth defects in the population at large) (109,112).

About 15% of patients being treated with clomiphene citrate develop scant and poor-quality cervical mucus. Such an event may prevent conception and may be the cause of low genital tract (including the endometrium) atrophy. Vasomotor hot flashes, nervousness, insomnia, breast tenderness, abdominopelvic discomfort, and residual ovarian enlargement occasionally occur. Ovarian hyperstimulation is often observed when clomiphene citrate treatment is implemented for a long time or when a combination of clomiphene citrate and human chorionic gonadotropin (hCG) (at the dose of 5,000–10,000 IU) is administered IM to trigger ovulation. Five to seven days after the last dose of clomiphene citrate, an hCG injection can be given (based on clomiphene citrate stimulation of follicle growth), when the dominant follicle reaches at least 18 mm in diameter, which is determined by transvaginal ultrasonography (113). The optimal time for conception should be discussed with a patient (often beginning 5 days after the last day of clomiphene citrate, for 1 week).

Contraindications for administering clomiphene citrate are pregnancy, preexisting ovarian cysts, and posttreatment residual ovarian enlargement (109).

Human menopausal gonadotropin (hMG) treatment requires a very experienced clinician to recognize, in timely fashion, when and how to adjust the dose to stimulate follicles, when to add hCG to trigger ovulation, and when to abort the treatment to avoid ovarian hyperstimulation. In addition, the clinician must be familiar with hormonal and ultrasonographic monitoring, as well as the diagnosis and clinical management of ovarian hyperstimulation in different stages of this complication. In PCOS patients, those who did not ovulate on a clomiphene citrate regimen or who failed to conceive following six consecutive, documented ovulatory cycles with the clomiphene citrate therapy. Because patients with PCOS are usually neither hypoestrogenic nor hypogonadotropic, the pregnancy rate is lower (about 30%–40%) than in patients with low estrogen and low gonadotropins levels (the pregnancy rate is greater than 90% for women under 35 years of age in hypoestrogenic-hypogonadotropic patients) (109).

The hMG initial IM dose is 75 to 150 IU daily, and if there is no follicular response for the first 4 days, the dose can be increased by 75 to 150 IU increments daily. The dose is continually increased every 4 days until the follicles respond. When signs of ovarian stimulation become apparent, serum estradiol levels should be determined. When the serum estradiol level reaches 100 pg/mL, transvaginal ultrasonography is begun to provide an image of and to measure the ovarian size, as well as to determine the number of follicles. Upon establishing a serum estradiol level between 500 and 2,000 pg/mL and a dominant follicle size of 16 to 20 mm in diameter 24 hours after the last dose of hMG, a single dose of hCG of 5,000 to 10,000 IU is injected IM. Ovulation is expected within 36 hours. This mode of therapy may result in ovarian hyperstimulation or multiple gestation (109).

Purified FSH, Urofollitropin (Metrodin; an ampule contains 75 IU of FSH and less than 1 IU of LH), is prepared for IM injection. The initial dose of purified FSH is 75 IU daily and can be increased by 37.5 IU (half an ampule) every 7 days as indicated. One dose of hCG of 5,000 to 10,000 IU is administered (the hMG/hCG ovulation induction rule of monitoring by hormonal titer and ultrasonography guidelines is applicable). Such a clinical protocol is associated with a high incidence of single dominant follicles and a low multiple pregnancy rate (114,115).

The newest FSH is human recombinant FSH (rFSH is a DNA recombinant technology), a completely pure form of FSH. rFSH at the initial dosage of 50 IU daily can be used successfully to stimulate follicular growth (116) and yields compatible results with hMG (117).

GnRH agonists, which are synthetic peptides, can be administered at the dose of 20 μg per bolus in 90-minute cycles subcutaneously. No serious side effects occur, and no monitoring with estradiol or ultrosonography is necessary. The ovulation rate per cycle is about 90%, the pregnancy rate per ovulatory cycle is about 30%, and the rate of spontaneous abortion is about 18.5% (118).

Intravenous administration of 5 μg per bolus in 90-minute cycles regulated by a GnRH pump is also a safe and effective approach (119). GnRH agonist therapy via the IV pump has the following characteristics:

- Safety: very few cases of allergy to GnRH have been reported. Local reaction to needle insertion and multi-pregnancy have occurred in only about 5% of patients, and there is a near zero risk for ovarian hyperstimulation.
- High rate of success: in properly selected patients, the cumulative conception rate is approximately 93%, with a mean conception rate of 22% per cycle (119). In clomiphene-resistant PCOS women, the ovulation rate is 56% to 67% (120,121), and the IV pulsatile GnRH agonists are more likely to succeed than those administered subcutaneously in this group of patients) (121).

Indications for GnRH therapy include the following clinical conditions (119–121):

- Normogonadotropic or hypogonadotropic amenorrhea
- Idiopathic hypogonadotropic hypogonadic amenorrhea
- Functional hypothalamic amenorrhea
- Normoandrogenic oligomenorrhea
- PCOS

Bromocriptine (a dopamine receptor agonist) is indicated for patients with PCOS associated with hyperprolactinemia in a divided dose of 5 to 7.5 mg daily. In order to downgrade side effects (such as nausea, dizziness, or hypotension), bromocriptine can be commenced in a gradual step-up dose method and taken with meals. Such therapy may regulate menstrual cycles in PCOS patients (122); however, in cases where hyperprolactinemia is absent, this mode of treatment is not effective (123).

Surgical Induction of Ovulation

Surgical induction of ovulation is achieved via an ovarian wedge resection via a laparotomy or a laparoscopy approach.

Ovarian Wedge Resection. The laparotomy approach has been used for over six decades (in 1935, PCOS and its surgical treatment was described (13), and it was enthusiastically accepted and widely used as a result. A drawback of this technique is morbidity associated with the laparotomy itself as well as abdominopelvic adhesion formation, which may result in the creation of a mechanical cause of infertility or may lead to chronic pelvic pain (124).

Laparoscopic ovarian wedge resection can be executed with either mechanical instruments or a laser.

In the mechanical method of ovarian wedge resection, the thick ovarian tunica albuginea and existing polycysts are removed in a wedge shape with 5-mm laparoscopic scissors. In this technique, no thermosources (such as electrocautery or laser) are used (125). This simple, bloodless procedure can be accomplished within a few minutes, and it eliminates the possibility of thermodamage to the reproductive cells.

Carbon dioxide laser ovarian wedge resection in clomiphene-resistant PCOS patients appears to be superior to electrocautery due to its ability to provide controllable power density, desirable depth of penetration, and predictable thermodamage of surrounding tissue. In addition, the laparoscopic CO_2 laser technique provides a unique opportunity to directly observe the opening process of polycysts. This therapeutic paradigm successfully induces ovulation in 92% of patients, with a crude conception rate of 75%, a 67% rate of healthy baby delivery at term, and an 8% rate of adhesion formation determined by second-look laparoscopy (126,127). However, randomized clinical trials are needed to establish the safety and effectiveness of this modality.

Multiple-Point Ovarian Biopsies. Multiple-point ovarian biopsies can be performed with 5-mm laparoscopic mechanical punch biopsy forceps; however, the clinical application of this technique is not popular, and randomized controlled studies are lacking (128).

Laparoscopic Ovarian Drilling Technique. The laparoscopic ovarian drilling technique can be accomplished with either electrocautery or laser. Translaparoscopic ovarian electrocautery and laser drilling are conceptually linked to the multiple-point ovarian biopsy method, in which mechanical biopsy forceps are substituted with either electrocautery (129,130) or laser (141). The simplicity of ovarian electrocoagulation makes this method easy to learn, and the equipment is standard in every operating room. This approach yields results similar to those of ovarian wedge resection. However, electrothermal penetration in the ovarian cortex exposes reproductive cells to potential damage.

Laparoscopy is a more attractive approach than laparotomy for managing clomiphene-resistant PCOS because it eliminates laparotomy complications, decreases the risk for postoperative adhesions when compared with laparotomy, maintains postoperative repetitive ovulation occurrence for some time, avoids the risk for ovarian hyperstimulation, has no effect on the rate of multiple pregnancies, and does not increase the spontaneous abortion rate. In general, laparoscopy reduces the time of hospitalization and

recovery, decreases postoperative pain and work absenteeism, and results in a highly acceptable abdominal scar cosmetic outcome. Laparoscopic management of PCOS is based on observational studies, and the lack of a controlled randomized study drastically decreases the value of this method in view of evidence-based medicine (132).

Insulin-Sensitizing Agents

Insulin-sensitizing agents (those that improve insulin action) in the management of metabolic aspects of PCOS are becoming an integral part of treatment paradigms of the syndrome, when impaired glucose tolerance or type 2 diabetes mellitus (NIDDM) is present. Before beginning insulin-sensitizing agent therapy, patients should establish a weight reduction program on an individual basis. Obese women with PCOS with no evidence of impaired glucose tolerance or type 2 diabetes will reduce the risk for longterm benefit from weight reduction.

Increased ovarian insulin sensitivity at the level of granulosa cells is mediated through insulin receptors. Such a mechanism enhances the response of human granulosa cells to LH (133,134) and therefore increases ovarian responsiveness to LH. The presence of insulin increases androgen synthesis, which leads to hyperandrogenism. Peripheral insulin resistance is encountered (for the most part in the skeletal muscles and adipose tissue) in patients with PCOS, and increasing the insulin levels enhances ovarian insulin sensitivity (135).

The following oral antihyperglycemic agents are recommended.

Troglitazone is part of the thiazolidinedione class and has demonstrated the ability to increase peripheral insulin sensitivity, ovulation rate (particularly when added to clomiphene citrate), and SHBG levels. This agent decreases insulin resistance, hepatic gluconeogenesis, hyperinsulinemia, plasma androgens in hyperandrogenic patients (mainly total and free testosterone in patients with PCOS), LH levels, estrogen levels, and plasminogen activator inhibitor-1 (a fibrinolytic factor that exhibits the potential for an increased risk for cardiovascular and insulin-resistant syndrome) (136,137). These changes have no influence on body mass or circulating leptin concentrations (138).

Troglitazone is administered at a dosage of 400 mg daily to women with PCOS and impaired glucose tolerance. It ameliorates the metabolic and hormonal derangements associated with this condition. It can be considered as the adjunctive or primary mode of therapy for the syndrome (136,137).

Troglitazone is contraindicated for patients with liver disease, and it should not be administered during pregnancy. A liver function test should be performed monthly to detect early stages of potential hepatotoxicity when troglitazone is administered. The drug also may increase fluid volume (38).

Metformin belongs to the biguanide class and has demonstrated the primary ability to suppress gluconeogenesis in the liver, insulin resistance, hyperinsulinemia, and hyperandrogenism (predominantly total and free testosterone). It increases peripheral tissue sensitivity to insulin without inducing a hypoglycemic state, and it improves menstrual regularity (139,140). Initial therapy is usually commenced with a dose of an 850-mg tablet daily in the morning, and if a patient tolerates it well, the dosage is increased to 1,700 mg daily (850 mg twice daily every 12 hours) (38,139). Side effects are mainly related to gastrointestinal problems such as nausea, vomiting, diarrhea, bloating, and flatulence. Patients with renal impairment may experience lactic acidosis, but metformin has not been reported to be teratogenic (38). Metformin significantly enhances the effectiveness of clomiphene citrate in obese women with PCOS, as compared with clomiphene citrate therapy alone (139,141).

Complementary Therapy for Polycystic Ovary Syndrome

Patient Education

Appropriate instruction about existing management options in conventional-complementary-alternative therapies for PCOS is paramount. Patients' understanding of the nature of PCOS, the nature of a therapy's benefits and risks, and long-term health consequences and their prevention will help patients to manage this condition. Therefore, the management of PCOS should routinely include a patient educational program in the following areas:

- Life-time therapeutic commitment to prevent the following risky PCOS health consequences: menstrual disorders and hirsutism, infertility, galactorrhea, glucose intolerance or diabetes mellitus (NIDDM), cardiovascular risk and hypertension, hyperlipidemia, and risk for endometrial cancer
- Available diagnostic tools
- Optimal medical management incorporating conventional-complementary-alternative treatments and the ways in which the patients' expectations can be matched
- Life-style modification as a form of prevention [gradual weight reduction, appropriate nutrition, exercise, stress-control program (a spirit-mind-body behavioral modification), cessation of cigarette smoking, and moderation in alcohol consumption]

Diet

Some types of diet and the regulation of caloric intake are important components in the clinical management of women with PCOS and obesity (BMI >25 kg/m²). There is a correlation between obese women with PCOS and a higher prevalence of anovulation and hirsutism; additionally, free testosterone (148) and SHBG levels are significantly lower (149) than those of nonobese women with PCOS. A short-term (4 weeks) very low calorie diet (149) [330 kcal/day (Cambridge diet)] and a long-term (6–7

months) low-calorie diet (148) (1,000 kcal/day) led to an improvement of menstrual function and fertility, corresponding with the hormonal changes presented above (148,149). Based on these data, it is apparent that diet should be an integral part of a life-style modification program for obese patents with PCOS. It is worthwhile to remember that very low calorie and low-calorie diets reduce more muscle mass than adipose mass; therefore, moderation should be advised with regard to life-style modifications (diet, exercise, stress reduction, alcohol consumption in moderation, no tobacco or addictive substance use, and regular implementation of spirit-mind-body programs).

Weight Reduction

Weight reduction and maintenance are the essential part of clinical PCOS management. A correlation between obesity [definition based on U.S. weight guidelines for healthy adults (142) from a BMI (expressed in kg/m²), which is determined by weight (kg)/height (m)²] and PCOS has been documented and is estimated to be in the range of 55% to 70% (38).

The first line of PCOS management should incorporate *behavioral eating habit modifications*, an individualized exercise program, weight control, and stress reduction techniques. The first line of therapy for PCOS was presented above. Weight reduction may significantly regulate menstruation, increase the ovulation rate, decrease hyperandrogenism, reduce insulin levels, and normalize gonadotropin pulsatile secretion and its LH:FSH ratio (143,144). A low-calorie diet (1,000–1,500 kcal/day) for 4 to 5 months, together with an appropriate exercise program, may reduce body fat by 13% in obese patients with PCOS (145). Moderate weight loss of more than 5% with long-term calorie restriction is associated with marked clinical improvement (144). Therefore, a closely coordinated effort between an exercise physiologist, nutritionist, and physician will provide the best management outcome in obese women with PCOS.

Recent clinical research data indicate that *life-style modification* without rapid weight loss leads to a reduction of central fat and improves insulin sensitivity, which may restore ovulation in overweight women with PCOS. A life-style modification program (not only emphasizing weight reduction but also other factors) with a reduction of 11% of central body fat improves insulin sensitivity by 71% according to an insulin sensitivity index, leads to a 33% decrease in fasting insulin levels, and causes a 39% reduction in LH levels. In view of this information, it is worthwhile to commence management of obese women with PCOS by designing an appropriate life-style modification program that improves reproductive capacity and prevents long-lasting health sequelae of metabolic derangements associated with this syndrome and obesity (147).

Exercise

Exercise is an important part of life-style modification (146), particularly with today's often sedentary life-style and unlimited food supplies in the United States and other developed countries. In general, exercise itself, without behavioral and life-style modifications, increases concentrations of adrenaline, noradrenaline, 3,4-dihydroxy-phenylglycol, glucose, and insulin; however, exercise-induced hormonal responses in women with PCOS present little, if any, difference when compared with those of a control group. There is a significant decrease in the GH concentration response to exercise in women with PCOS and obesity (147).

Stress-Control Therapy

Stress-control therapy (meditation, hypnosis, biofeedback, etc.) may assist to some extent in reversing chronic anovulation (150,151), although no data are available that specifically refer to PCOS.

Acupuncture and Electroacupuncture

Based on observational clinical trials, classic acupuncture or electroacupuncture is an effective mode of therapy to induce ovulation (152–155). It has been hypothesized that the acupuncture mechanism influences some gene expressions that may normalize the secretion of GnRH, LH, and estradiol (153). However, there are no data available to determine a role for acupuncture in women with PCOS and whether these patients will respond to this treatment.

Nutritional Supplements

There are no specific recommendations established for PCOS therapy.

Natural Alternative Therapy for PCOS

Herbal Medicine

Sairei-to (chan ling-tang; chai-ling-tang, a Saiko agent; tsumura sairei-to) a Chinese herbal medicine, appears to have a steroidal effect in anovulatory PCOS patients, and clinical observational trials documented that the serum LH levels were reduced and the LH:FSH ratio was significantly decreased. Serum testosterone levels were not significantly changed. Sairei-to can induce ovulation in approximately 70.6% of women with PCOS (156).

Vitex agnus castus (Chaste tree), at the dosage of a 20-mg capsule taken orally twice daily, demonstrates the potential to develop multiple follicles, and it influences gonadotropin and ovarian hormone secretions. In addition, it has the ability to cause mild ovarian hyperstimulation syndrome. Side effects include:

- Abdominal pain, cramping, and diarrhea
- Headaches
- Rash and itching
- Increased menstrual flow

Vitex agnus castus has not been specifically clinically tested in women with PCOS (157). *Vitex agnus castus* is contraindicated during pregnancy and lactation (158).

Initial animal results indicate that *Vitex agnus castus* expresses dopaminergic effects in hyperprolactinemia and significantly reduces prolactin secretion (159). This traditional Chinese medicine (TMC) was clinically tested in observational studies in patients with hyperprolactinemia, and its phytotherapeutic ability was demonstrated with negligible side effects (160). Because hyperprolactinemia is often associated with PCOS, it is worthwhile to recommend such an alternative therapy (for select patients) with caution until a controlled study becomes available.

In a case in which oligomenorrhea is associated with PCOS, natural progesterone is recommended (161):

- Natural progesterone cream should contain at least 400 mg progesterone per ounce and half a teaspoon should be applied one to two times daily, from days 7 to 14 of the menstrual cycle, or half a teaspoon one to two times daily, from days 15 to 26. Thus far, no controlled study has documented this therapy's effectiveness.
- Natural progesterone tablets (Prometrium) may be given at the dosage of 100 mg twice daily for 7 to 12 days per month.
- Natural progesterone sublingual tablets may be given at the dosage of 50 to 75 mg twice daily for 7 to 12 days per month.

This type of clinical approach has not been specifically clinically tested for the treatment of oligomenorrhea in PCOS.

Homeotherapy

There are no data available addressing homeotherapy for patients with PCOS.

HIRSUTISM THERAPY

The treatment of hirsutism may frequently be a life-long therapy, and it appears to be effective in the majority of cases. Progression of hirsutism may be inhibited or prevented, and a cure is observed in some patients. A timely initial therapeutic intervention in young mildly hirsute adolescents with a strong family history of hirsutism is advisable. In general, hirsutism itself best responds to agents that block androgens; however, when an ovarian (elevated testosterone) component is present, a suppressive ovarian therapy produces better results than an androgen blocker. It is not true, however, in a case in which an adrenal component, such as late-onset adrenal hyperplasia, contributes to hirsutism; in such a case, antiandrogen treatment generates better results for hirsutism with fewer side effects than glucocorticoids, due to the peripheral receptivity of androgens in the clinical expression of hirsutism (161).

Any mechanical technique of hair removal by itself or in combination with medical treatment appears to be successful, and a combination of two provides faster results. In brief, hirsutism therapy can be divided into two major categories:

Medical Therapy
>   Ovarian suppression
>   GnRH agonists/antagonists
>   Oral contraceptives
>   Cyproterone acetate
>   Androgen receptor blockers
>   Spironolactone
>   Cyproterone acetate
>   Flutamide
>   5-Alpha-reductase inhibitors
>   Finasteride
>   Androgen suppression
>   Glucocorticoids

Mechanical Hair Removal Techniques
- Laser
- Electrolysis
- Shaving
- Plucking

Alternative Therapy

There is no alternative therapy clinical data available for the management of hirsutism.

ACNE

Acne is a common event in women and is due to:

- Elevated serum levels of androgens (hyperandrogenemia)
- Abnormal pattern of hair follicular keratinization, which blocks the skin pores
- Presence of bacteria within hair follicles such as *Staphylococcus epidermidis, Propionibacterium acnes,* and *Pityrosporum ovale*

As a result of the above mechanisms, comedones (small cysts formed within the hair follicle, a characteristic clinical sign) are formed and are often accompanied by inflammation, creating papules, pustules, or nodules. Acne formation may lead to skin scarring, which usually has a profoundly negative cosmetic effect with psychological disturbances. Therefore, any delay of diagnosis and therapy may have negative cosmetic, and psychological effects and should be avoided.

Conventional Therapy for Acne

Acne treatment can be categorized as either topical therapy or systemic therapy.

Topical Therapy

Topical therapy focuses on at least one of the four main factors promoting acne formation: hyperkeratosis, microbacterial colonization, immune responses, and inflammatory responses.

Topical antibiotics, such as tetracycline, erythromycin, and clindamycin, have been used for a long time; however, bacterial resistance is emerging as a significant therapeutic problem. Azelaic acid, benzoil peroxide, and retinoic acid are also often prescribed for acne (162,163).

Tazarotene gel is composed of retinoids that reverse the abnormal pattern of keratinizations through local receptors, and it is effective in about 68% of patients when administered at a concentration of 0.01%. The effectiveness is reduced to 51% when the gel concentration is 0.05%. It should be applied topically in noninflammatory, mild-to-moderate facial acne vulgaris, once daily for 12 weeks (164).

Isotrexin, a combination of isotretinoin (0.05%) and erythromycin (2%), is an effective treatment in the reduction of total lesions and inflamed acne (165).

In polymorphic acne, applying *retinaldehyde 0.1%,* in combination with erythromycin 4%, is a valuable therapeutic paradigm with minimal side effects (166).

A *topical antiandrogen* therapy, which plays a role in seborrhea, is currently being tested as an acne therapy.

Systemic Therapy

It is a clinical conviction that for patients in a hyperandrogenic state, sources should be determined when considering any systemic treatment.

Antibiotics such as *tetracycline, erythromycin, and clindamycin* administered orally are recommended for acne. *Isotretinoin* (Accutane) is indicated for recalcitrant nodular severe acne that is unresponsive to conventional topical or systemic antibiotics. A recommended dose is between 0.5 and 2 mg/kg, given in two divided doses for 15 to 20 weeks (with an initial dose of 0.5–1 mg daily) (167). A single course of therapy is usually effective; although, in some cases a second course of treatment may be necessary (the second course is often commenced after 8 weeks of completing the first course). This drug is absolutely contraindicated in cases of pregnancy and allergies.

An antiandrogenic therapy requires the establishment of possible sources of hyperandrogenism (ovarian, adrenal, idiopathic, and drug), which predetermines a clinical approach. In ovarian or adrenal sources, in most instances a suppression therapy is in order, and in the case of an androgen-producing tumor, surgery is indicated. In an idiopathic form, an antiandrogen treatment is advisable.

Systemic and topical therapies for acne are often combined, particularly oral antibiotics with a topical agents. In addition, an antiandrogen therapy may be combined with topical or oral antibiotics when inflamed acne is present.

Acne scars are a cosmetic dilemma. They are difficult to correct effectively by a single therapeutic modality due to the variety in the depth and width of the scars involved. A three-stage operation has proven to be effective in the treatment of various degrees of acne scars. The following stages were developed to complete acne scar removal:

- Initially, a focal chemical peeling followed by a CO_2 laser scar excision.
- Secondly, skin punched grafts for deep scars.
- Lastly, dermabrasion for any remaining scars

Such a step-by-step approach had a success rate of 75%. It appears to be a promising approach (167), but this observational clinical study has not been evaluated in randomized controlled clinical trials.

Acne may be a clinical manifestation of adverse reactions to the following medications (168):

- Anabolic and androgenic steroids
- Glucocorticoids
- Oral contraceptives
- Danazol
- Bromides
- Iodides
- Isoniazid
- Troxidone

Acne that results from exposure to these medications is usually self-limited some time after discontinuation of use.

Alternative Therapy for Acne

Homeopathy

Homeopathic therapy is essentially directed for acne associated with puberty, and the mode of treatment depends on the type of acne appearance or the time in which acne occurs (169):

- Inflammatory process present with pus secretion
    Pyrogenium (Pyrogen) in a 9 to 15 cH dilution once or twice daily
    Hepar sulphuris calcareum in a 9 to 15 cH dilution once or twice daily
    Sulphur in a 9 to 15 cH dilution once or twice daily
- Noninflammatory acne appearance
    Kalium bromatum in a 9 to 15 cH dilution once or twice daily
    Calcarea sulphurica in a 9 to 15 cH dilution once or twice daily
- Occurring before menses
    Eugenia jambosa in a 9 to 15 cH dilution once or twice daily
- Occurring in association with male-type hair distribution
    Cortico surrenale in a 9 to 15 cH dilution once or twice daily

These medical claims are made based on clinical tradition in homeopathic practice; however, there is a lack of well-designed clinical study to support such therapeutic modalities.

ALOPECIA

Alopecia or female androgenic alopecia, or female pattern baldness, is diffuse hair loss in women with excess androgens with an individual's genetic susceptibility. This condition also has been observed in the absence of detectable levels of circulating androgens in association with hypopituitarism (170). In addition, female patients with diffuse alopecia may demonstrate hyperandrogenism, even without hirsutism, oligomenorrhea, or amenorrhea, and the most common endocrine entity associated with this type of hair loss is PCOS (171). It is also postulated that enhanced 5-alpha-reductase activity occurs in androgenic alopecia, and a disorder of androgen binding may play a role in scalp hair loss (172). Besides these findings, it appears that multiple hormone interactions in a broad range play a role in androgenic hair loss (173). This medical entity may potentially cause adverse psychological sequelae due to diminished body image satisfaction, deleterious effect on self-esteem, and a modest negative effect on social perceptions (174).

Diagnosis of Alopecia

The clinical evaluation of patients with alopecia may require a multiple-step approach: detailed medical history, complete general physical examination, and directed laboratory tests as indicated. The appearance of female androgenic alopecia differs from the classic male pattern. The female pattern is more diffuse, and the frontal hairline is preserved. When necessary, specialized tests are performed, such as a cut-and-plucked hair evaluation, and/or a scalp biopsy to establish the cause of secondary hair loss; even when characteristic histopathologic changes are present, they are rarely helpful in diagnosis (175–177).

Differential diagnosis takes the following into account: a diversified etiologic hyperandrogenism of central and peripheral origins, thyroid dysfunction, diabetes mellitus, drug side effects, alopecia associated with neoplasia [breast cancer, gastric cancer (erythematous alopetic plaque develops approximately 10 months before scalp metastasis) (178)], and microbial infection (179).

Conventional Therapy for Alopecia

Treatment of alopecia includes systemic administration of oral contraceptives, low-dose glucocorticoids, or antiandrogens. A selection of the type of medication is based on the androgen sources (180).

Topical 2% minoxidil (nonhormonal hair growth stimulation) twice daily with a systemic administration of antiandrogen (spironolactone, finasteride, or cyproterone acetate) appears to have some effect in the treatment of alopecia. Alopecia treatment by conservative medical combinations of topical and systemic therapy, hair transplantation, or other forms of surgical techniques, has not been very successful (180,181). Antiandrogen therapy may improve hair growth in up to 50% of patients within 6 to 12 months of therapy, although in everyday practice, hair loss progresses and very little, if any, new hair growth occurs (177). Therefore, reassuring patients that they will not go totally bald immediately may be the most effective type of management, and in combination with medical treatments, it appears to carry some psychological efficacy (174,181). Psychological adjustments have a more noticeable effect among women than men (174).

Drug-induced alopecia is the result of undesirable, adverse side effects of a medicine, and it clinically manifests in a diffused nonscarring form. It is a self-limited, progressively reversible process (only one of the four phases of the hair growth cycle is affected by drugs), which usually begins to reverse upon discontinuation of the drugs. There are drugs such as *antimitotic agents*, often used in gynecology, that almost always cause transitional hair loss. Any unpredictability of other drugs inducing alopecia is usually encountered as an isolated clinical case. The following categories of drugs commonly appear in the literature and may cause alopecia:

- Oral contraceptives, either when on pills or after discontinuation
- Antihypertensive drugs (beta-adrenoreceptor agonists)
- Anticonvulsant agents (mainly valproic acid derivatives)
- Antithyroid medications
- Anticoagulant drugs (all of them)
- Salicylates or nonsteroidal analgesics (very small percentages)
- Cytotoxics
- Psychotropic drugs (tricyclic antidepressants, and up to 15% lithium)
- Hypocholesterolemic agents (few isolated cases)
- Antiinfectious agents (few isolated cases)
- Ethionamide

There is also a long list of medications that occasionally may cause diffuse alopecia, among which are *cimetidine, retinoids, amphetamines, bromocriptine,* and *levodopa.* It has been reported by the Pharmacovigilance Foundation that *antimalarials, sex hormones, acetylcholinesterase inhibitors,* and *angiotensin II antagonists* also may cause alopecia.

Diagnosis of drug-induced alopecia is difficult and is usually confirmed when clinical improvement in hair growth is observed after discontinuation of medications (168,182,183).

Complementary Therapy for Alopecia

Acupuncture

Animal (184) and human clinical observation trials to apply acupuncture as an alopecia treatment claim improvements to some degree (185); however, these observations lack a well-designed evidence-based method of clinical trial. It is paramount for a modern practitioner to recognize the public phenomenon of seeking some type of nonconventional therapeutic paradigm [about 40% of Americans in 1997 (186)]. Acupuncture is one of the primary requested treatment modalities among various complementary therapies. Until a bridge is established between the applicability of acupuncture in female androgenic alopecia and an appropriate clinical evidence-based study, allopathic practitioners may be reluctant to consider it a viable treatment option . Contemporary acupuncture interpretation of the healing mechanism lies in trying to establish an understanding of the problem as a clinical scientific category and at the same time, as an ancient Chinese physiopathologic concept ("yin-yang," "meridians," "energies," etc.). It has been postulated that acupuncture, from a clinical point of view, may act in the following ways (187):

- Striated muscle relaxation
- Antiinflammatory action on the ligaments
- Antidepressant
- Anxiolytic action

Such a cluster of potential acupuncture mechanisms clarifies the reason for its applicability in a clinical setting and brings a practitioner into the familiar territory of clinically adopted expressions.

Reflexotherapy

Reflexotherapy (treatment by irritation of any area of the body distant from the lesion) is suggested for alopecia. The mechanism, which supposedly stimulates hairs to grow, occurs by increasing the microcirculation status of the skin (188). Ischemia as a probable cause of alopecia has been reported (289); therefore, the use of reflexotherapy, in this scope of interpretation, makes sense. In addition, clinical documentation exists to support the notion that reflexotherapy produces a favorable effect on peripheral circulation (190).

Reflexotherapy can be induced by different means, such as acupuncture or electron-ion reflexotherapy, or by using an acoustic device, which also appears to have practical value in determining a specific topography for the distribution of active points of acupuncture, thus improving its efficacy (191). The clinical study, in the best form for scientific assessment purposes, is a randomized double-blind controlled study, and such a model for reflexotherapy was developed successfully (192). At this time, only observational clinical trials are ongoing, and controlled study data to support this claim are lacking.

Patient Education

Patient education should include the following areas:

- Nature of female androgenic alopecia
- Available resources for diagnosis
- Available modes of therapy (conventional, complementary, natural alternative) and surgical treatments

- Success rates of therapy and reassurance of the patient as a part of management

Diet

The following diet recommendation is offered for hair loss (193,194):

- A whole-food diet with skins of cucumbers, potatoes, green and red peppers, and sprouts (high in silicon), green peas, lentils, oats, soybeans, sunflower seeds, and walnuts (high in biotin)
- Lean meats and brown raisins (high in iron)
- Sea vegetables, such as kelp
- Goat's milk
- Juices (carrot, beet, spinach, nettle, alfalfa, and the addition of a little onion juice to the vegetable juices)
- Avoiding foods containing raw eggs (high in avidin, a protein that binds biotin and prevents biotin from being absorbed)

Supplements

The following supplements are recommended (193,194):

- Flax seed oil (improves hair texture)
- Biotin (50 mg three times daily; deficiency may cause hair loss)
- Inositol (100 mg twice daily; vital for hair growth)
- Zinc (50–100 mg daily; stimulates hair growth)
- Iron (combats anemia)
- Copper (3 mg daily; promotes hair growth)
- Amino acid blends (improve hair growth)
- Vitamins: vitamin B complex with vitamin B_3–niacin (50 mg, three times daily), vitamin B_5–pantothenic acid (100 mg, three times daily), vitamin C (3,000–10,000 mg daily), vitamin E (initial dose of 400 IU daily and gradually increasing dose to 800–1,000 IU daily), coenzyme Q_{10} (60 mg daily; improves scalp circulation). In view of the existing medical scientific literature, diffuse female alopecia may result from vitamin deficiency (195).
- Kelp (500 mg daily; supplies minerals)
- Dimethylglycine (100 mg daily; improves scalp circulation)

Natural Alternative Therapy for Alopecia

A search of the literature with the appropriate terms selected from the medical subject headings and applied in a search through augmented Medline and the ACOGNET computerized data bank, as well as a manual search of bibliographies, failed to identify any information related to alternative therapy for female androgenic alopecia. The presentation here is based on existing general therapeutic paradigms applied to alopecia. There is no specific or separate treatment that addresses either universal, total, areata, or androgenic alopecia. Today, a practitioner may be con-

fronted with a natural alternative therapy for alopecia and its drug interactions. Because all forms of alopecia are treated the same way, it is worthwhile to present a brief, general approach to alopecia treatment.

Cell Therapy

Raw glandular thymus, 500 mg daily, stimulates immune function (193).

Self-Care

The following self-care steps for hair growth can be taken (193,194):

- Reclining the head down for 15 minutes daily (increases peripheral blood flow in the scalp)
- Massaging the scalp with fingers and oil (mix two parts almond oil and one part rosemary oil) or without oil
- Applying warm bhringaraj or brahmi oil,
- Using all-natural hair-care products, letting the hair dry naturally, and using a pick and not comb to put hair in place
- Rubbing vitamin E oil into scalp nightly: castor oil, olive oil, and germ oil is rubbed into the scalp for ten minutes, followed by the application of a hot, damp towel for 30 minutes. A plastic shower cap is then placed over the scalp, and the next morning the residue is washed out. After a one-night break, the cycle is repeated.
- Rinsing the scalp daily with double-strength herbal sage tea, and rinsing the scalp daily with apple cider vinegar

Aromatherapy for Alopecia

Recently, randomized controlled independent clinical trials of aromatherapy for alopecia areata revealed that this mode of treatment is significantly more effective when compared with the control group. A mixture of essential oils, such as *thyme, rosemary, lavender,* and *cedar*, are massaged into the scalp daily. This mode of therapy is effective and safe, and it is well documented in a high-ranking evidence-based clinical study (196). It is too soon to say whether or not this therapy can be successfully administered to female androgenic alopecia patients, because this distinct group of women with this diffuse form of alopecia has yet to be tested.

Herbal Therapy for Alopecia

An ayurvedic herb such as ashwagandha (*Withania somnifera* root or Wintwer charry, or Indian ginseng) is anecdotally effective in the treatment of alopecia (194). This remedy is contraindicated in pregnancy due to its abortifacient potential, and it should be used with caution when combined with sedative medications, because it has the ability to increase the tranquilizing effect of the sedative (197).

Licorice [Bio Rizin at a dosage of 100 to 520 mg in oral capsules daily or as a tea (2–4 g of licorice in cup of boiling water to simmer for 5 minutes)] is used three times daily (158,193). It is contraindicated in kidney insufficiency, high blood pressure, low serum potassium levels, pregnancy, liver cirrhosis, and diabetic bile stenosis, and it should not be used for prolonged periods of time. The remedy interacts with digitalis, diuretics (thiazides), aldactone, lanoxin, and antihypertensive drugs (158,197).

Homeopathic Therapy for Alopecia

The following remedy is suggested for the treatment of alopecia (194):

- Sepia in a 15 cH dilution; one dose weekly
- *Arnica montana* in 9 or 15 cH dilutions, once or twice daily

HYPERTHECOSIS

Stromal hyperthecosis [luteinized stromal cells that are not in close proximity to follicles; stromal hyperplasia is usually present (198)] clinically manifests with hirsutism, which may progress to virilization. High circulating levels of androgens, bilateral ovarian enlargement, absent ovarian polycysts, and the lack of a distinct lesion to justify hyperandrogenism can suggest a diagnosis of stromal hyperthecosis. Quite often, acanthosis nigricans, insulin-resistant diabetes, hypertension, and/or obesity accompany this condition (73). Hyperthecosis is predominantly seen during the reproductive years. Some authorities considered hyperthecosis a more severe form of PCOS (199), although the hypothalamic-pituitary physiology in hyperthecosis is different from that in PCOS (200). In hyperthecosis, endometrial hyperplasia or a well-differentiated adenocarcinoma is frequently observed (201). Differential diagnosis of this condition should include pregnancy luteoma and androgen-producing tumors.

Stromal hyperplasia is a condition, in which benign proliferation of the ovarian stroma takes place, in addition to androgen overproduction and secretion (198,201). Commonly, this entity is observed in postmenopausal women and may be associated with endometrial hyperplasia and carcinoma (198).

HAIR-AN SYNDROME

HAIR-AN Syndrome [hyperandrogenism (HA), insulin-resistant (IR), acanthosis nigricans (AN)] is clinically characterized by the presence of masculinization with disproportionate androgen levels (202). The syndrome's pathophysiologic phenomena are insulin resistance and hyperandrogenism, whereas acanthosis nigricans is an epiphenomenon, secondary to HA and IR. It appears that,

physiologically, a vicious cycle or positive feedback mechanism occurs in which the hyperinsulinemic state promotes ovarian androgen production (by two mechanisms—insulin-like growth factor, located in ovarian stroma, and enhanced LH secretion from the pituitary) and the hyperandrogenic state increases insulin-resistance. Acanthosis nigricans occurs in response to these primary physiologic imbalances. HAIR-AN syndrome may be prevalent in up to 5% of women with hyperandrogenism (203). It is important to determine testosterone concentration, which may increase 49- to 250-fold in this syndrome (200,203).

Conventional Therapy for Ovarian Stromal Hyperthecosis, Stromal Hyperplasia, and HAIR-AN Syndrome

Two therapeutic modalities are used: medically conservative GnRH agonist therapy, to suppress ovarian androgen biosynthesis and secretion (205) (insulin-influenced ovarian androgen synthesis is LH dependent), combined with estrogen replacement therapy or oral contraceptive therapy as a preventive modality for osteoporosis (206). Also, oral contraceptives decrease androgen levels by increasing SHBG levels, which can bind free testosterone. The dose and administration of GnRH agonists was discussed earlier in the section on PCOS. A nasal solution (a metered spray pump delivers 200 µg of nafarelin per spray) is administered at the total dose of 1,000 µg daily (207). Hyperthecosis is refractory to oral contraceptive treatment alone, and induction of ovulation with clomiphene citrate usually fails (200). Therefore, hyperthecosis and HAIR-AN syndrome can be effectively managed with long-term GnRH agonist therapy, combined with either estrogen replacement therapy or oral contraceptives.

Surgical treatment by means of a bilateral ovarian wedge resection is rarely successful (205). Bilateral oophorectomy in patients with HAIR-AN syndrome will reduce androgen levels, but it has little, if any, impact on insulin resistance (208).

There are no available *complementary or natural alternative* therapeutic modes for the treatment of these conditions.

ANDROGEN-PRODUCING TUMORS

Androgen-producing tumors may originate from the following ovarian sites (see also Chapters 24 and 25):

- Leydig cell tumors or hilus cell tumors (located in the ovarian hilus); are usually small (<5 mm in diameter). In about 80% of cases, virilization is present; in the remaining cases, hyperestrogenism and its clinical sequelae are present. They are usually benign and unilateral (sporadically bilateral or malignant). The histologic landmark is the presence of a Reinki crystal (small lipid-containing vacuoles), which differentiates this tumor from lipid cell lesions (209–211).

- Sertoli-Leydig cell tumors (arrhenoblastoma or andro-blastoma) contain Sertoli and Leydig cells and fibrob-lasts; approximately 40% of patients display hyperandro-genism or virilization. It is always unilateral; in 97.5% of cases, the diagnosis is reached at stage 1. All well-differ-entiated tumors are benign (211).
- Gynandroblastomas contain both morphologically ovar-ian (granulosa stromal cells) and testicular type cells (tubu-lar Sertoli stromal cells) within the ovarian tumor (both granulosa and arrhenoblastoma tissue). A tumor may pro-duce androgens in excess, causing masculinization, whereas estrogens produce an estrogenizing effect. They characteristically display Call-Exner bodies. Gynandrob-lastoma is a rare, sex cord stromal tumor (212).
- Luteinized thecomas may cause androgenic changes in about 11% of cases (50% will be hyperestrogenic mani-festations with their sequelae, whereas the tumor is hor-monally inactive in 39%). They occur at an average age of 46 years. The size of the tumor varies from small to 10 cm (213).
- Gonadoblastomas contain germ cell and sex cord deriva-tives. They almost always occur in women with gonadal dysgenesis in which a Y chromosome is present. In approximately 60% of cases, clinical virilization is mani-fested. It is a solid tumor that is not considered to be a true neoplasm, but rather a hamartomatous malforma-tion of testicular tissue (211).
- Dysgerminomas are germ cell neoplasias, which occa-sionally display androgenic activity in association with gonadoblastoma, in patients with pure or mixed gonadal dysgenesis (214).
- Luteomas result from stromal cell luteinization and hyperplasia. They are tumorlike (uncapsulated mass) and they may cause virilization during pregnancy or puer-perium and may cause masculinization of the female fetus. Luteomas are self-limited and progressively regress after delivery (209,211).

Diagnosis of Ovarian Androgen-Producing Tumors

Among all ovarian neoplasms, androgen-producing tumors occur in less than 1% and are clinically suspected, when a medical history of sudden onset and rapidly progressive masculinization is reported. Physical examination reveals progressive hirsutism with signs of virilization; in many instances, a tumor can be palpable on bimanual pelvic examination.

Laboratory

A total serum testosterone level of more than 7 nM (the nor-mal range is 0.7–2.8 nM) is present. To differentiate between

ovarian versus adrenal glands as the source of hyperandro-genism, the following laboratory studies are recommended: total serum testosterone, DHEA-S, androstenedione, SHBG, 17-alpha-hydroxyprogesterone, LH, FSH, and prolactin. When DHEA-S or 17-alpha-hydroxyprogesterone is ele-vated, it suggests an adrenal origin of the tumor, congenital adrenal hyperplasia, or Cushing syndrome.

Imaging Studies

Imaging studies (209), such as ultrasonography, magnetic resonance imaging (MRI), or computed tomography (CT), of the ovaries and adrenal glands are valuable, and one or more of them is warranted when the total serum testosterone level exceeds 7 nM. Occasionally (more often in the past than presently), adrenal and ovarian vein catheterization is performed to diagnose localized, small, androgen-producing tumors. Currently, highly sophisticated technology is able to detect small tumors. The procedure that is performed is usu-ally either fluoroscopically guided percutaneous retrograde femoral catheterization of the ovarian and adrenal veins (bilaterally) or intraoperatively, although in both instances it is technically difficult and not without risk (215,216).

Conventional Therapy for Androgen-Producing Tumors

Androgen-producing tumor therapy is divided into two cat-egories: surgical therapy and conservative management.

Surgical therapy and its extent depends on the patient's age and parity. At reproductive age, a full-thickness ovar-ian biopsy, incorporating the ovarian hilar area, may rule out a neoplasm on frozen-section examination [the surgery can be executed either via laparotomy or via laparoscopy (217)]. If a neoplasm is histologically verified as a stromal-type tumor (granulosa cell tumors, granulosa-thecal tumors, Sertoli-Leydig cell tumors), and it is con-fined to one ovary, unilateral oophorectomy is recom-mended (218). Malignant potential in this group is directly related to the degree of differentiation: well, moderately, and poorly differentiated. In the postmenopausal period, a bilateral oophorectomy should be executed when clinical evidence exists for a neoplasm, even if the tumor is not identified (211).

In general, histologic determination of the tumor type dictates the surgical management approach. Today, the rule in oncology is to perform a total abdominal hysterectomy with bilateral salpingo-oophorectomy and full surgical stag-ing in postmenopausal patients. If preservation of child-bearing capacity is desired, unilateral salpingo-oophorec-tomy with full staging is recommended (218). More details concerning oncology are discussed Chapter 25.

Medical conservative management is based on two assumptive principles that ovarian androgen-producing tumors are (a) usually benign or of low malignant potential and (b) gonadotropin dependent (219,220). Taking these theories into account, *GnRH agonists* and hormonal replacement therapy is administered. Practically, such an approach can be contemplated with a patient in a medically compromised condition that prohibits surgical therapy, and in a patient who exhibits masculinization (216).

There is no available data on *complementary or natural-alternative therapies* for ovarian androgen-producing tumors.

ADRENAL ANDROGEN-PRODUCING TUMORS

Steroidogenic adrenal gland tumors cause virilization, and diagnosis is based on medical history, such as virilization or abrupt-onset hirsutism, and confirmed by physical examination, which may reveal a mixed clinical picture of a cushingoid appearance with virilization, or present only with virilization. Laboratory tests demonstrate an elevation of DHEA-S greater than 8 μg/mL, and 17-alpha-hydroxyprogesterone early morning concentrations greater than 2 to 3 ng/mL. Further testing is indicated (at <2 ng/mL, Cushing syndrome is ruled out). Elevation of these two hormones is only indicative of adrenal hyperandrogenism, and they do not indicate a specific condition such as congenital adrenal hyperplasia, Cushing syndrome, or an adrenal tumor. Although testosterone is considered an ovarian marker, an adrenal adenoma may produce it instead of DHEA-S, and in such an event, an image study of the ovaries (normal ovaries) assists in differentiating between ovarian and adrenal origin. When 3-alpha-androstenediol glucoronide is elevated, it indicates peripheral sources of excess androgens.

Because an adrenal androgen-secreting adenoma appears to be an autonomous tumor, without ACTH regulation, an ACTH stimulation test is useless. The lack of adrenal androgen-producing response to ACTH stimulation is caused by a deficiency of ACTH receptor expression (221). An adrenal dexamethasone suppression test will not influence adrenal adenoma secretions. Therefore, stimulation or suppression tests cannot reliably differentiate adrenal androgen-producing tumors from adrenal hyperplasia (221,222). It is important to remember that adrenal androgen-producing tumors can derive from sources other than the adrenal glands, such as the ovaries, central nervous system, liver, and pituitary gland (223).

The value of image studies for diagnosing adrenal adenomas is well established; however, these tumors are often quite small, and conventional imaging modalities are unable to identify them. Contrast material–enhanced CT or MRI is a more precise technique for identifying small adrenal adenomas (224). It is important to stress that adrenal cancer may cause virilization (225).

Conventional Therapy for Adrenal Androgen-Producing Tumors

Adrenal adenomas must be removed surgically. Reaching a diagnosis of an adrenal androgen-secreting tumor and its localization presents a clinical challenge, but early diagnosis and extirpation of an adrenal tumor promises complete remission of signs and symptoms. Postsurgical hormonal follow-up is necessary in determining adequate adrenal tumor resection.

Complementary and natural-alternative treatment paradigms are not available.

REFERENCES

1. Association of Professors of Gynecology and Obstetrics. *Medical student educational objectives,* 7th ed. Washington, DC: Association of Professors of Gynecology and Obstetrics, 1997.
2. Council on Resident and Gynecology (CREOG). *Educational objectives core curriculum for residents in obstetrics and gynecology,* 5th ed. Washington DC: CREOG, 1996.
3. American College of Obstetrician and Gynecologists (ACOG). Technical Bulletin No. 202. Washington, DC: ACOG, 1995.
4. Redmond GP. Androgens and women's health. *Int J Fertil Womens Med* 1998;43:91–97.
5. Knochenhauer ES, Key TJ, Kahsar-Miller M, et al. Prevalence of the polycystic ovary syndrome in unselected black and white women of the Southeastern United States: a prospective study. *J Clin Endocrinol Metab* 1998;83:3078–3082.
6. Carmina E. Prevalence of idiopathic hirsutism. *Eur J Endocrinol* 1998;139:421–423.
7. Benjamin F, Deutsch S, Saperstein H, et al. Prevalence of and markers for attenuated from of congenital adrenal hyperplasia and hyperprolactinemia masquerading as polycystic ovarian disease. *Fertil Steril* 1986;46:215–221.
8. Horton R. Dihydrotestosterone is a peripheral paracrine hormone. *J Androl* 1992;13:23–27.
9. Duffy DM, Legro RS, Chang L, et al. Metabolism of dihydrotestosterone to 5 alpha-androstane-3 alpha, 17 beta-diol glucoronide is greater in the peripheral compartment than in the splanchnic compartment. *Fertil Steril* 1995;64:736–739.
10. Serafini P, Lobo RA. Increased 5 alpha-reductase activity in idiopathic hirsutism. *Fertil Steril* 1985;43:74–78.
11. Mowszowicz I, Melanitou E, Doukani A, et al. Androgen binding capacity and 5 alph-reductase activity in pubic skin fibroblasts from hirsute patients. *J Clin Endocrinol Metab* 1983;56:1209–1213.
12. Vottero A, Stratakis CA, Ghizzoni L, et al. Androgen receptor-mediated hypersensitivity to androgens in women with nonhyperandrogenic hirsutism; skewing of X-chromosome inactivation. *J Clin Endocrinol Metab* 1999;84:1091–1095.
13. Stein IF, Leventhal ML. Amenorrhea associated with bilateral polycystic ovaries. *Am J Obstet Gynecol* 1935;29:181–191.
14. Ehrmann DA, Barnes RB, Rosenfield RL. Polycystic ovary syndrome as a form of functional ovarian hyperandrogenism due to deregulation of androgen secretion. *Endocr Rev* 1995;16:322–353.
15. Zawadzki JK, Dunaif A. Diagnostic criteria for polycystic ovary syndrome: towards a rational approach. In: Dunaif A, Givens JR, Haseltine F, Merriam GR, eds. *Polycystic ovary syndrome.* Boston: Blackwell Scientific, 1992:377–384.
16. Koivunen R, Laatikainen T, Tomas C, et al. The prevalence of

polycystic ovaries in healthy women. *Acta Obstet Gynecol Scand* 1999;78:137–141.

17. Polson DW, Wadsworth J, Adams J, et al. Polycystic ovaries: a common finding in normal women. *Lancet* 1988;1:870–872.

18. Farquhar CM, Birdsdall M, Manning P, et al. Transabdominal versus transvaginal ultrasound in the diagnosis of polycystic ovaries of randomly selected women. *Ultrasound Obstet Gynecol* 1994;4:54–59.

19. Petterson F, Fries H, Nillius SJ. Epidemiology of secondary amenorrhea. *Am J Obstet Gynecol* 1973;117:80–86.

20. Roumain J, Charles MA, de Courten MP, et al. The relationship of menstrual irregularity to type 2 diabetes in Pima Indian women. *Diabetes Care* 1998;21:346–349.

21. Diamanti-Kandarakis E, Kouli CR, Bergiele AT, et al. A survey of the polycystic ovary syndrome in the Greek island of Lesbos: hormonal and metabolic profile. *J Clin Endocrinol Metab* 1999; 84:4006–4011.

22. Carmina E, Lobo RA. Do hyperandrogenic women with normal menses have polycystic ovary syndrome? *Fertil Steril* 1999; 71:319–322.

23. Taylor AE. Understanding the underlying metabolic abnormalities of polycystic ovary syndrome and their implications. *Am J Obstet Gynecol* 1998;179(suppl):94–100.

24. Dunaif A. Hyperandrogenic anovulation (PCOS): a unique disorder of insulin action associated with an increased risk of non-insulin-dependent diabetes mellitus. *Am J Med* 1995;98(suppl 1A):33–39.

25. Kissebah AH, Vydelingum N, Murray R, et al. Relation of body fat distribution to metabolic complication of obesity. *J Clin Endocrinol Metab* 1982;54:254–260.

26. Pasquali R, Casimirri F, Cantobelli S, et al. Insulin and androgen relationship with abdominal fat distribution in women with and without hyperandrogenism. *Horm Res* 1993;39:179–187.

27. Hartz AJ, Rupley DC, Rimm AA. The association of girth measurements with disease in 32,856 women. *Am J Epidemiol* 1984; 119:71–80.

28. Haffner SM, Fong D, Hazuda HP, et al. Hyperinsulinemia, upper body adiposity, and cardiovascular risk factors in non-diabetics. *Metabolism* 1988;37:338–345.

29. Solomon CG. The epidemiology of polycystic ovary syndrome. *Endocrinol Metab Clin North Am* 1999;28:247–263.

30. Dunaif A, Xia J, Book CB, et al. Excessive insulin receptor serine phosphorylation in cultured fibroblasts and in skeletal muscle: a potential mechanism for insulin resistance in the polycystic ovary syndrome. *J Clin Invest* 1995;96:801–810.

31. Legro RS, Dodson WC, Dunaif A. PCOS: a reservoir of reproductive age glucose intolerance poorly detected by fasting blood glucose levels (abstract OR41-3). Proceedings of the Endocrine Society 80th Annual Meeting. New Orleans, LA, June 24–28, 1998.

32. Harris MI, Hadden WC, Knowler WC, et al. Prevalence of diabetes and impaired glucose tolerance and plasma glucose levels in US population aged 20–74 yr. *Diabetes* 1987;36:523–534.

33. Legro RS, Finegood D, Dunaif A. A fasting glucose to insulin ratio is a useful measure of insulin sensitivity in women with polycystic ovary syndrome. *J Clin Endocrinol* 1998;83: 2694–2698.

34. Shoupe D, Kumar DD, Lobo RA. Insulin resistance in polycystic ovary syndrome. *Am J Obstet Gynecol* 1983;147:588–592.

35. Dunaif A, Segal KR, Shelley DR, et al. Evidence for distinctive and intrinsic defects in insulin action in polycystic ovary syndrome. *Diabetes* 1992;41:1257–1266.

36. Ciaraldi TP, El-Roeiy A, Madar Z, et al. Cellular mechanisms of insulin resistance in polycystic ovary syndrome. *J Clin Endocrinol Metab* 1992;75:577–583.

37. Talbot JA, Bicknell EJ, Rajkhowa M, et al. Molecular scanning of the insulin receptor gene in women with polycystic ovary syndrome. *J Clin Endocrinol Metab* 1996;81:1979–1983.

38. Dahlgren E, Jansen S, Lapidus L, et al. Polycystic ovary syndrome and risk for myocardial infarction: evaluation from a risk factor model based on a prospective population study of women. *Acta Obstet Gynecol Scand* 1992;71:599–604.

39. Pierpoint T, McKeigue PM, Isaacs AJ, et al. Mortality of women with polycystic ovary syndrome at long-term follow-up. *J Clin Epidemiol* 1988;51:581–586.

40. Dunaif A, Graf M, Mandeli J, et al. Characterization of groups of hyperandrogenic women with acanthosis nigricans, impaired glucose tolerance, and/or hyperinsulinemia. *J Clin Endocrinol Metab* 1987;65:499–507.

41. Largo RS, Kunselman AR, Dodson WC, et al. Prevalence and predictors of risk for type 2 diabetes mellitus and impaired glucose tolerance in polycystic ovary syndrome: a prospective, controlled study in 254 affected women. *J Clin Endocrinol Metab* 1999;84:165–169.

42. Talbott E, Guzick D, Clerici A, et al. Coronary heart disease risk factors in women with polycystic ovary syndrome. *Arterioscler Thromb Vasc Biol* 1995;15:821–826.

43. Wild RA, Bartholomew MJ. The influence of body weight on lipoprotein lipids in patients with polycystic ovary syndrome. *Am J Obstet Gynecol* 1988;159:423–427.

44. Coulam CB, Annegeres JF, Kranz JS. Chronic anovulation syndrome and associated neoplasia. *Obstet Gynecol* 1983;61: 403–407.

45. Folsom AR, Kaye SA, Potter JD. Association of incident carcinoma of the endometrium with body weight and fat distribution in older women: early findings of the Iowa Women's Health Study. *Cancer* 1989;49:6828–6831.

46. Weiderpass E, Gridley G, Persson I, et al. Risk of endometrial and breast cancer in patients with diabetes mellitus. *Int J Cancer* 1997;71:360–363.

47. Gamyunova VB, Bobrov YF, Tsyrlina EV, et al. Comparative study of blood insulin levels in breast and endometrial cancer patients. *Cancer Res* 1989;49:6828–6831.

48. Hammond CB, Jelovsek FR, Lee KL, et al. Effect of long-term estrogen replacement therapy. II. Neoplasia. *Am J Obstet Gynecol* 1979;133:537–547.

49. Chamlian DL, Taylor HB. Endometrial hyperplasia in young women. *Obstet Gynecol* 1970;36:659–665.

50. Parham KJ. Adenocarcinoma of the endometrium associated with Stein-Leventhal syndrome. *Am J Obstet Gynecol* 1969;105:113–115.

51. Schildkraut JM, Schwingl PJ, Bastos E, et al. Epithelial ovarian cancer risk among women with polycystic ovary syndrome. *Obstet Gynecol* 1996;88:554–559.

52. Meirow D, Schenker JG. The link between female infertility and cancer: epidemiology and possible aetiologies. *Hum Reprod Update* 1996;2:63–75.

53. Gammon MD, Thompson WD. Polycystic ovaries and the risk of breast cancer. *Am J Epidemiol* 1991;134:818–824.

54. Anderson KE, Sellers TA, Chen PL, et al. Association of Stein-Leventhal syndrome with the incidence of postmenopausal breast carcinoma in large prospective study of women in Iowa. *Cancer* 1997;79:494–499.

55. Franks S. Polycystic ovary syndrome. *N Engl J Med* 1995;333: 853–861.

56. Futterweit W. Polycystic ovary syndrome: clinical perspectives and management. *Obstet Gynecol Surv* 1999;54:403–413.

57. Marynik SP, Chakmakjian ZH, McCaffree DL, et al. Androgen excess in cystic acne. *N Engl J Med* 1983;308:981–986.

58. Slayden SM, Azziz R. The role of androgen excess in acne. In: Azziz R, Nestler JE, Dewailly D, eds. *Androgen excess disorder in women.* Philadelphia: Lippincott-Raven, 1997:131–140.

59. Futterweit W, Dunaif A, Yeh HC, et al. The prevalence of hyperandrogenism in 109 consecutive female patients with diffuse alopecia. *J Am Acad Dermatol* 1988;19:831–816.

60. Segal KR, Dunaif A. Resting metabolic rate and postprandial thermogenesis in polycystic ovary syndrome. *Int J Obes* 1990; 14:559–567.

61. Vague J. The degree of masculine differentiation of obesities: a factor determining predisposition to diabetes, atherosclerosis, gut, and uric calculous disease. *Am J Cin Nutr* 1956;4:20–34.

62. Krotkowski M, Bjorntorp P, Sjostrom L, et al. Impact of obesity on metabolism in men and women: importance of regional adipose tissue distribution. *J Clin Invest* 1983;72:1150–1162.

63. Dahlgren E, Johnsson S, Lindstedt G, et al. Women with polycystic ovary syndrome wedge resected in 1956 to 1965: a long-term follow-up focusing on natural history and circulating hormones. *Fertil Steril* 1992;57:505–513.

64. Folsom AR, Kaye SA, Sellers TA, et al. Body fat distribution and 5-year risk of death in older women. *JAMA* 1993;269:483–487.

65. Ferriman A, Gallwey JD. Clinical assessment of body growth in women. *J Clin Endocrinol Metab* 1961;21:1440–1447.

66. Gorden MC. Menstrual disorders in adolescents. Excess androgens and polycystic ovary syndrome. *Pediatr Clin North Am* 1999;46:519–543.

67. Bardin CW, Lipsett MB. Testosterone and androstenedione blood production rates in normal women and women with idiopathic hirsutism or polycystic ovaries. *J Clin Invest* 1967; 46:891–897.

68. Gruber DM, Berger UE, Sator MO, et al. Computerized assessment of facial hair growth. *Fertil Steril* 1999;72;737–739.

69. Futterweit W. *Clinical features of polycystic ovarian syndrome.* New York: Springer-Verlag, 1987:83–95.

70. Robinson S, Rodin DA, Deacon A, et al. Which hormone tests for the diagnosis of polycystic ovary syndrome? *Br J Obstet Gynecol* 1992;99:232–238.

71. von Hooff MH, van der Meer M, Lambalk CB, et al. Variation of luteinizing hormone and androgens in oligomenorrhea and its implications for the study of polycystic ovary syndrome. *Hum Reprod* 1999;14:1684–1689.

72. Collet C, Lecomte P, Guilloteau D, et al. Luteinizing hormone measurement in polycystic ovary syndrome. *Eur J Endocrinol* 1999;141:225–230.

73. Chang JR, Katz SE. Diagnosis of polycystic ovary syndrome. *Endocrinol Metab Clin North Am* 1999;28:397–408.

74. Franks S. Polycystic ovary syndrome: a changing perspective. *Clin Endocrinol (Oxf)* 1989;31:87–120.

75. Arroyo A, Laughlin GA, Morales AJ, et al. Inappropriate gonadotropin secretion in polycystic ovary syndrome: influence of adiposity. *J Clin Endocrinol Metab* 1997;82:3728–3733.

76. Koskinen P, Penttila TA, Anttila L, et al. Optimal use of hormone determinations in the biochemical diagnosis of the polycystic ovary syndrome. *Fertil Steril* 1996;65:517–522.

77. Taylor AE, McCourt B, Martin KA. et al. Determinants of abnormal gonadotropin secretion in clinically defined women with polycystic ovary syndrome. *J Clin Endocrinol Metab* 1997; 82:2248–2256.

78. Slowinska-Srzednicka J, Zgliczynski W, Makowska A, et al. An abnormality of growth hormone/insulin-like growth factor-I axis in women with polycystic ovary syndrome due to coexistent obesity. *J Clin Endocrinol Metab* 1992;74:1432–1435.

79. Yeh HC, Futterweit W, Thornton JC. Polycystic ovarian disease: US features in 104 patients. *Radiology* 1987;163:111–116.

80. Fox R. Transvaginal ultrasound appearance of the ovary in normal women and hirsute women with oligomenorrhea. *Aust N Z J Obstet Gynecol* 1999;39:63–68.

81. Adams J, Franks S, Polson DW, et al. Multifollicular ovaries:

82. Polson DW, Wadsworth J, Adams J, et al. Polycystic ovaries a common finding in normal women. *Lancet* 1988;1:870–872.

83. Botsis D, Kassanos D, Pyrgiotis E, et al. Sonographic incidence of polycystic ovaries in a gynecological population. *Ultrasound Obstet Gynecol* 1995;6:182–185.

84. Lunde O, Hoel PS, Sandvik L. Ovarian morphology in patients with polycystic ovaries and an age-matched reference material. *Gynecol Obstet Invest* 1988;25:192–201.

85. van Hoof MH, Voorhorst FJ, Kaptein MB, et al. Endocrine features of polycystic ovary syndrome in a random population sample of 14–16 year old adolescents. *Hum Reprod* 1999;14: 2223–2229.

86. Marshall LA. Facial hair on a woman: diagnosis and treating a pathological twist on a common problem. *Medscape Womens Health* 1997;2:3.

87. Burkman RT. The role of oral contraceptives in the treatment of hyperandrogenic disorders. *Am J Med* 1995;98(suppl 1A): 130–136.

88. Korytkowski MT, Mokan M, Horowitz MJ, et al. Metabolic effects of oral contraceptives in women with polycystic ovary syndrome. *J Clin Endocrinol Metab* 1995;80:3327–3334.

89. Rittmaster RS. Medical treatment of androgen-dependent hirsutism. *J Clin Endocrinol Metab* 1995;80:2559–2563.

90. Lobo RA, Shoupe D, Serafini P, et al. The effects of two doses of spironolactone on serum androgens and anagen hair in hirsute women. *Fertil Steril* 1985;43:200–205.

91. Cusan L, Dupont A, Gomez JL, et al. Comparison of flutamide and spironolactone in the treatment of hirsutism: a randomized control trial. *Fertil Steril* 1994;61:281–287.

92. Kelestimur F, Sahin Y. Comparison of Diane 35 and Diane 35 plus spironolactone in the treatment of hirsutism. *Fertil Steril* 1998;69:66–69.

93. Andrade RJ, Lucena MI, Fernandez MC, et al. Fulminant liver failure associated with flutamide therapy for hirsutism. *Lancet* 1999;353:983.

94. Wysowski DK, Fourcroy JL. Safety of flutamide? *Fertil Steril* 1994;62:1089–1090.

95. Wysowski DK, Fourcroy JL. Flutamide hepatotoxicity. *J Urol* 1996;209–212.

96. Faloia E, Filipponi S, Mancini V, et al. Effect of finasteride in idiopathic hirsutism. *J Endocrinol Invest* 1998;21:694–698.

97. Crosby PD, Rittmaster RS. Predictors of clinical response in hirsute women treated with spironolactone. *Fertil Steril* 1991;55:1076–1081.

98. Gokman O, Senoz S, Gulekli B, et al. Comparison of four different treatment regimens in hirsutism related to polycystic ovary syndrome. *Gynecol Endocrinol* 1996;10:249–255.

99. Isik AZ, Gokman O, Zeyneloglu HB, et al. Low dose ketoconazole is an effective and safe in the treatment of hirsutism. *Aust N Z J Obstet Gynecol* 1996;36:487–489.

100. Golditch IM, Price VH. Treatment of hirsutism with cimetidine. *Obstet Gynecol* 1990;75:911–913.

101. Dahlgren E, Landin K, Krotkowski M, et al. Effects of two antiandrogen treatments on hirsutism and insulin sensitivity in women with polycystic ovary syndrome. *Hum Reprod* 998;13: 2706–11.

102. Moghetti P, Castello R, Zamberlan N, et al. Spironolactone, but not flutamide, administration prevents bone loss in hyperandrogenic women treated with gonadotropin-releasing hormone agonist. *J Clin Endocrinol Metab* 1999;84:1250–1254.

103. Yucelten D, Erenus M, Gurbuz O, et al. Recurrence rate of hirsutism after 3 different antiandrogen therapy. *J Am Acad Dermatol* 1999;41:64–68.

104. Rittmaster RS. Antiandrogen treatment of polycystic ovary syndrome. *Endocrinol Metab Clin North Am* 1999;28:409–421.

105. Sommer S, Render C, Sheehan-Dare R. Fascial hirsutism treated with the normal-mode ruby laser: results of a 12-month follow-up study. *J Am Acad Dermatol* 1999;41:974–979.

106. Litter CM. Hair removal using an Nd:YAG laser system. *Dermatol Clin* 1999;17:401–430.

107. Kerin JF, Liu JH, Phillipou G, et al. Evidence for hypothalamic site of action of clomiphene citrate in women. *J Clin Endocrinol Metab* 1985;61:265–268.

108. Gorlitsky GA, Kase NG, Speroff L. Ovulation and pregnancy rates with clomiphene citrate. *Obstet Gynecol* 1978;51: 265–269.

109. The American College of Obstetricians and Gynecologists (ACOG). Technical Bulletin No. 197. Washington, DC: ACOG, 1994.

110. Daly DC, Walters CA, Soto-Albors CE, et al. A randomized study of dexamethasone in ovulation induction with clomiphene citrate. *Fertil Steril* 1984;41:844–848.

111. Singh KB, Dunnihoo DR, Mahajan DK, et al. Clomiphene-dexamethasone treatment of clomiphene-resistant women with and without the polycystic ovary syndrome. *J Reprod Med* 1992; 37:215–218.

112. Adashi EY, Rock JA, Sapp KC, et al. Gestational outcome of clomiphene-related conceptions. *Fertil Steril* 1979;31:620–626.

113. O'Herlihy C, Pepperell RJ, Robinson HP. Ultrasound timing oh human chorionic gonadotropin administration on clomiphene stimulated cycle. *Obstet Gynecol* 1982;59:40–45.

114. Grigoriou O, Antomiou G, Antonaki V, et al. Low-dose follicle-stimulating hormone treatment for polycystic ovarian disease. *Int J Gynecol Obstet* 1996;52:55–59.

115. Shoham Z, Patel A, Jacobs HS. Polycystic ovarian syndrome: safety and effectiveness of stepwise and low-dose administration of purified follicle-stimulating hormone. *Fertil Steril* 1991;55: 1051–1056.

116. Hayden CJ, Rutherford AJ, Balen AH. Induction of ovulation with the use of starting dose of 50 units of recombinant human follicle-stimulating hormone (Puregon). *Fertil Steril* 1999;71: 106–108.

117. Jansen CA, van Os HC, Out HJ, et al. A prospective randomized clinical trial comparing recombinant follicle stimulating hormone (Puregon) and human menopausal gonadotrophins (Humegon) in non-down-regulated *in vitro* fertilization patients. *Hum Reprod* 1998;13:2995–2999.

118. Skarin G, Ahlgren M. Pulsatile gonadotropin releasing hormone (GnRH)-treatment for hypothalamic amenorrhea causing infertility. *Acta Obstet Gynecol Scand* 1994;73:482–485.

119. Braat DD, Schoemaker R, Schoemaker J. Life table analysis of fecundity in intravenously gonadotropin-releasing hormone-treated patients with normogonadotropic and hypogonadotropic amenorrhea. *Fertil Steril* 1991;55:266–271.

120. Mais V, Melis GB, Strigini F, et al. Adjusting the dose to the individual response of the patient during the induction of ovulation with pulsatile gonadotropin-releasing hormone. *Fertil Steril* 1991;55:80–85.

121. Saffan DS, Seibel MM. Value of subcutaneous pulsatile gonadotropin releasing hormone in polycystic ovary syndrome. *J Reprod Med* 1992;37:545–551.

122. Buvat J, Buvat-Herbaut M, Marcolin G, et al. A double blind controlled study of the hormonal and clinical effect of bromocriptine in the polycystic ovary syndrome. *J Clin Endocrinol Metab* 1986;63:119–124.

123. Polson DW, Maso HD, Franks S. Bromocriptine treatment of women with clomiphene-resistant polycystic ovary syndrome. *Clin Endocrinol (Oxf)* 1987;26:197–203.

124. Toaff R, Roaff ME, Peyser MR. Infertility following wedge resection of the ovaries. *Am J Obstet Gynecol* 1976;124:92–96.

125. Ostrzenski A, Poreba R, Micinski P, et al. Translaparoscopic modified technique of ovarian wedge resection in PCOD. *Clin Perinatol Gynecol* 1996;16:154–156.

126. Ostrzenski A. Endoscopic carbon dioxide laser ovarian wedge resection in resistant polycystic ovarian disease. *Int J Fertil* 1992; 37:295–299.

127. Ostrzenski A. Endoscopic carbon dioxide laser ovarian wedge resection in resistant polycystic ovarian disease. In: Mishell DR, Lobo RA, Sokol RZ, eds. *The yearbook of infertility.* St. Louis: CV Mosby, 1993:153–154.

128. Cohen J. Laparoscopic procedures for treatment of infertility related to polycystic ovarian syndrome. *Hum Reprod Update* 1996;2:337–344.

129. Gjonnaess H. Polycystic ovarian syndrome treated by ovarian electrocautery through the laparoscope. *Fertil Steril* 1984;41: 20–25.

130. Ostrzenski A, Klimek M, Wojtys A. Videolaparoscopic treatment of resistant polycystic ovaries using monopolar coagulation. *Ginecol Pol* 1992;63:369–370.

131. Huber J, Hosmann J, Spona J. Polycystic ovarian syndrome treated by laser through the laparoscopy. *Lancet* 1988;2:215.

132. Donesky BW, Adashi EY. Surgically induced ovulation in the polycystic ovary syndrome: wedge resection revisited in the age of laparoscopy. *Fertil Steril* 1995;63:439–463.

133. Willis D, Mason H, Gilling-Smith C, et al. Modulation by insulin of follicle-stimulating hormone and luteinizing hormone actions in human granulosa cells of normal and polycystic ovaries. *J Clin Endocrinol Metab* 1996;81:302–309.

134. Willis D, Franks S. Insulin action in human granulosa cells from normal and polycystic ovaries is mediated by the insulin receptor and the type-I insulin-like growth factor receptor. *J Clin Endocrinol Metab* 1995;80:302–309.

135. Dunaif A. Insulin resistance and the polycystic ovary syndrome: mechanisms and implications for pathogenesis. *Endocr Rev* 1997;18:774–800.

136. Ehrmann DA, Schneider DJ, Sobel BE. Troglitazone improves defects in insulin action, insulin secretion, ovarian steroidogenesis, and fibrinolysis in women with polycystic ovary secretion. *J Clin Endocrinol Metab* 1997;82:2108–2116.

137. Hasegawa I, Murakawa H, Suzuki M, et al. Effect of troglitazone on endocrine and ovulatory performance in women with insulin resistance-related polycystic ovary syndrome. *Fertil Steril* 1999;71:323–327.

138. Mantzoros CS, Dunaif A, Flier JS. Leptin concentrations in the polycystic ovary syndrome. *J Clin Endocrinol Metab* 1997;82: 1687–1691.

139. Diamanti-Kandarakis E, Kouli C, Tsianateli T. Therapeutic effects of matformin on insulin resistance and hyperandrogenism in polycystic ovary syndrome. *Eur J Endocrinol* 1998; 138:269–274.

140. Velazquez E, Acosta A, Mendoza SG. Menstrual cyclicity after metformine therapy in polycystic ovary syndrome. *Obstet Gynecol* 1997;90:392–395.

141. Nestler JE, Jakubowicz DJ, Evans WS, et al. Effects of metformin on spontaneous and clomiphene-induced ovulation in the polycystic ovary syndrome. *N Engl J Med* 1998;338: 1876–1880.

142. Dietary guidelines for Americans. Washington, DC: US Government Printing Office, 1996. (Publication no. 1996-402-519).

143. Pasquali R, Casimirri F, Vicennati V. Weight control and its beneficial effect on fertility in women with obesity and polycystic ovary syndrome. *Hum Reprod* 1997;12(suppl 1):82–87.

144. Kiddy DS, Hamilton-Fairley D, Bush A, et al. Improvement in endocrine and ovarian function during dietary treatment of obese women with polycystic ovary syndrome. *Clin Endocrinol (Oxf)* 1992;36:105–111.

145. Andersen P, Seljeflot I, Abdelnoor M, et al. Increase insulin sensitivity and fibrinolytic capacity after dietary intervention in obese women with polycystic ovary syndrome. *Metabolism* 1995;44:611–616.

146. Huber-Buchholtz MM, Carey DG, Norman RJ. Restoration of reproductive potential by lifestyle modification in obese polycystic ovary syndrome: role of insulin sensitivity and luteinizing hormone. *J Clin Endocrinol Metab* 1999;84:1470–1474.

147. Jaatinen TA, Anttila L, Erkkola R, et al. Hormonal responses to physical exercise in patients with polycystic ovarian syndrome. *Fertil Steril* 1993;60:262–267.

148. Franks S, Kiddy DS, Hamilton-Fairley D, et al. The role of nutrition and insulin in the regulation of sex hormone biding globulin. *J Steroid Biochem Mol Biol* 1991;39:835–838.

149. Kiddy DS, Hamilton-Fairley D, Seppala M, et al. Diet induced changes in sex hormone-binding globulin and free testosterone in women with normal and polycystic ovaries: correlation with serum insulin and insulin-like growth factor-I. *Clin Endocrinol (Oxf)* 1989;31:757–763.

150. The Burton Goldberg Group. *Alternative medicine. The definitive guide.* Tiburon, CA: Future Medicine Publishing, 1997:53–72, 769.

151. Eliopoulos C. Integrating conventional and alternative therapies. Holistic care for chronic conditions. St. Louis: CV Mosby, 1999:83–85, 121–122.

152. Yu J, Zheng HM, Ping SM. Changes in serum FSH, LH and ovarian follicular growth during electroacupuncture for induction of ovulation. *Chung His I Chieh Ho Tsa Chih* 1989;9:195, 199–202.

153. Chen BY, Yu J. Relationship between blood radioimmunoreactive beta-endorphin and hand skin temperature during the electroacupuncture induction of ovulation. *Acupunct Electrother Res* 1991;16:1–5.

154. Mo X, Li D, Pu Y, et al. Clinical studies on the mechanism for acupuncture stimulation of ovulation. *J Trad Chin Med* 1993;13:115–119.

155. Chen BY. Acupuncture normalizes dysfunction of hypothalamic-pituitary-ovarian axis. *Acupunct Electrother Res* 1997;22:97–108.

156. Sakai A, Kondo Z, Kamei K, et al. Induction of ovulation by Sairei-to for polycystic ovary syndrome. *Endocr J* 1999;46:217–220.

157. Cahill DJ, Fox R, Wardle PG, et al. Multiple follicular development associated with herbal medicine. *Hum Reprod* 1994;9:1469–1470.

158. Fetrow CW, Avila JR. The complete guide to herbal medicine. Springhouse, PA: Springhouse Corporation, 1999:126–127, 295–296.

159. Sliutz G, Speiser P, Schultz AM, et al. Agnus castus extracts inhibit prolactin secretion of rat pituitary cells. *Horm Metab Res* 1993;25:253–255.

160. Lei J, Ning J, Guo Z. Advances in TCM treatment of hyperprolactinemia. *J Trad Chin Med* 1998;18:230–234.

161. Spritzer P, Billaud L, Thalabard JC, et al. Cyproterone acetate versus hydrocortisone treatment in late onset adrenal hyperplasia. *J Clin Endocrinol Metab* 1990;70:642–646.

162. Gollnick H, Schramm M. Topical therapy in ace. *J Eur Acad Dermatol Venereol* 1998;11(suppl 1):8–12, 28–29.

163. Brzezinska-Wcislo L. Acne vulgaris as a therapeutic problem. *Wiad Lek* 1999;52:168–173.

164. Shalita AR, Chalker DK, Griffith RF, et al. Tazarotene gel is safe and effective in the treatment of acne vulgaris: a multicenter, double-blind, vehicle-controlled study. *Cutis* 1999;63:349–354.

165. Glass D, Boorman GC, Stables GI, et al. A placebo-controlled clinical trial to compare a gel containing a combination of isotretinoin (0.05%) and erythromycin (2%) with gels containing isotretinoin (0.05%) or erythromycin (2%) alone in the topical treatment of acne vulgaris. *Dermatology* 1999;199:242–247.

166. Morel P, Vienne MP, Beylot C, et al. Clinical efficacy and safety of a topical combination of retinaldehyde 0.1% with erythromycin 4% in acne vulgaris. *Clin Exp Dermatol* 1999;24:354–357.

167. Whang KK, Lee M. The principle of a three-stage operation in the surgery of acne scars. *J Am Acad Dermatol* 1999;40:95–97.

168. Oates JA, Wilkinson GR. Principles of drug therapy. In: Isselbacher KJ, Braunwald E, Wilson JD, et al., eds. *Harrison's principles of internal medicine,* 13th ed. New York: McGraw-Hill, 1994:408.

169. Holtzscherer A, Legros MS. *Pratique homeopathique en gynocologie.* Boiron, France: CEDH, 1994.

170. Orme S, Cullen DR, Messenger AG. Diffuse female hair loss: are androgens necessary? *Br J Dermatol* 1999;141:521–523.

171. Futterweit W, Dunaif A, Yeh HC, et al. The prevalence of hyperandrogenism in 109 consecutive female patients with diffuse alopecia. *J Am Acad Dermatol* 1988;19:831–836.

172. Legro RS, Carmina E, Stanczyk FZ, et al. Alternations in androgen conjugate levels in women and men with alopecia. *Fertil Steril* 1994;62:744–750.

173. Schmidt JB. Hormonal basis of male and female androgenic alopecia: clinical relevance. *Skin Pharmacol* 1994;7:61–66.

174. Cash TF. The psychological consequences of androgenic alopecia: a review of the research literature. *Br J Dermatol* 1999;141:398–405.

175. Hordinsky MK. General evaluation of the patient with alopecia. *Dermatol Clin* 1987;5:483–489.

176. Nielson TA, Reichel M. Alopecia: diagnosis and management. *Am Fam Physician* 1995;51:1513–1522, 1527–1528.

177. Callan AW, Montalto J. Female androgenic alopecia: an update. *Aust J Dermatol* 1995;36:51–55.

178. Alopecia neoplastica in a patient with gastric carcinoma. *Br J Dermatol* 1999;141:1122–1124.

179. Cherif-Cheikh JL. Diffuse alopecia. *Rev Prat* 1993;43:2349–2353.

180. Rosenfield RL, Lucky AW. Acne, hirsutism, and alopecia in adolescent girls. Clinical expressions of androgen excess. *Endocrinol Metab Clin North Am* 1993;22:507–532.

181. Rubin MB. Androgenic alopecia. Battling a losing proposition. *Postgrad Med* 1997;102:129–131, 136.

182. Llau ME, Viraben R, Montastruc JL. Drug-induced alopecia: review of the literature. *Therapie* 1995;50;145–150.

183. van den Bemt PM, Brodie-Meijer CC, Krijnen RM, et al. Drug induced alopecia. *Ned Tijdschr Geneeskd* 1999;143:990–994.

184. Waters KC. Acupuncture for dermatologic disorders. *Probl Vet Med* 1992;4:194–199.

185. Ge S. Treatment of alopecia with acupuncture. *J Trad Chin Med* 1990;10:199–200.

186. Cadwell V. A primer on acupuncture. *J Emerg Nurs* 1998;24:514–517.

187. Faust S. For an updated acupuncture. *Rev Med Brux* 1998;19:290–295.

188. Abramov SN, Zen'kevich AP, Shinaev NN. Status of the microcirculation of the skin in patients undergoing reflexotherapy for alopecia. *Vestn Dermatol Venereol* 1984;1:60–63.

189. Wiles JC, Hansen RC. Postoperative (pressure) alopecia. *J Am Acad Dermatol* 1985;12(part 2):195–198.

190. Nikolaev NA. Changes in peripheral hemodynamics in patients with vertebrogenic pain syndromes during reflexotherapy. *Zh Nevropatol Psikhiatr Im SS Korsakova* 1982;82:45–49.

191. Novikov II, Novinskii GD, Vlasov VB. Clinico-morphologic aspects of the active skin points of the upper extremities and their importance in reflexotherapy. *Zh Nevropatol Psikhiatr Im SS Korsakova* 1987;87:58–61.

192. Ceccherelli F, Ambrosio F, Manani G, et al. Proposed method for double-blind study of reflexotherapy phenomena. *Minerva Med* 1980;71:919–922.

193. Balch J, Balch PA. *Prescription for nutritional healing,* 2nd ed. Garden City Park, NY: Avery Publishing, 1997:294–295.

194. The Burton Goldberg Group. *Alternative medicine. The definitive guide.* Tiburon, CA: Future Medicine Publishing, 1997:925–926.

195. Diffuse alopecia in women: classification and views of etiopathogenesis. *Wiad Lek* 1999;52:386–392.

196. Hay IC, Jamieson M, Ormerod AD. Randomized trial of aromatherapy. Successful treatment for alopecia areata. *Arch Dermatol* 1998;134:1349–1352.

197. McGuffin M, Hobbes C, Upton R, et al., eds. *Botanical safety handbook.* Boca Raton, FL: CRC Press, 1997.

198. Boss JH, Scully RE, Wegner KH, et al. Structural variations in the adult ovary clinical significance. *Obstet Gynecol* 1965:25: 747–763.

199. Beckman CRB, Ling FW, Herbert WNP, et al., eds. *Obstetrics and gynecology.* Baltimore: Williams & Wilkins, 1998:442.

200. Nagamani M, Lingold JC, Gomez LG, et al. Clinical and hormonal studies in hyperthecosis of the ovaries. *Fertil Steril* 1981; 36:326–332.

201. Abraham GE, Buster JE. Peripheral and ovarian steroids in ovarian hyperthecosis. *Obstet Gynecol* 1976;47:581–586.

202. Dunaif A, Hoffman AR, Scully RE, et al. Clinical, biochemical, and ovarian morphologic features in women with acanthosis nigricans and masculinization. *Obstet Gynecol* 1985;66:545–552.

203. Barbieri RL, Ryan KJ. Hyperandrogenism, insulin resistance, and Acanthosis nigricans: a common endocrinopathy with distinct pathophysiologic features. *Am J Obstet Gynecol* 1983; 147:90–101.

204. McNatty KP, Smith DM, Makris A, et al. The intraovarian sites of androgen and estrogen formation in women with normal and hyperandrogenic ovaries as judged by in vitro experiments. *J Cin Endocrinol Metab* 1980;50:755–763.

205. Steingold KA, Judd HL, Nieberg RK, et al. Treatment of severe androgen excess due to ovarian hyperthecosis with a long-acting gonadotropin-releasing hormone agonist. *Am J Obstet Gynecol* 1986;154:1241–1248.

206. Adashi EY. Potential utility of gonadotropin-releasing hormone agonists in the management of ovarian hyperandrogenism. *Fertil Steril* 1990;53:765–779.

207. Nagamani M, Van Dinh T, Kelver ME. Hyperinsulinemia in hyperthecosis of the ovaries. *Am J Obstet Gynecol* 1986;154: 384–389.

208. Andreyko JL, Monroe SE, Jaffe RB. Treatment of hirsutism with a gonadotropin-releasing hormone agonist (nafarelin). *J Clin Endocrinol Metab* 1986;63:854–859.

209. Fox H, Buckley CH. *Pathology for gynecologists,* 2nd ed. London: Edward Arnold, 1991:192–213, 218.

210. Russel P, Bannatyne P. *Surgical pathology of the ovaries,* 1st ed. London: Churchill Livingstone, 1989:346–365, 375–378.

211. Moore A, Permezel M, Mulvany N, et al. Hilus cell tumor of the ovary in a virilized women. Case report and review of hyperandrogenism of ovarian origin. *Aust N Z J Obstet Gynecol* 1999; 30:75–78.

212. Chalvardijan A, Derzko C. Gynandroblastoma. Its ultrastructure. *Cancer* 1982;50:710–721.

213. Zhang J, Young RH, Arseneau J, et al. Ovarian stromal tumors containing lutein of Leydig cells (luteinized thecomas and stromal Leydig cell tumors) a clinicopathological analysis of fifty cases. *Int J Gynecol Pathol* 1982;1:270–285.

214. Talerman A. Germ cell tumors of the ovary. In: Kurman RJ, ed. *Blaustin's pathology of the female tract,* 4th ed. New York: Springer-Verlag, 1994:849–914.

215. Farber M, Mananes A, O'Brian DS, et al. Asymmetric hyperthecosis ovarii. *Obstet Gynecol* 1981;57:521–525.

216. Lee WL, Wang PH, Tseng HS, et al. Managing a patient with presumed testosterone-secreting ovarian tumor. *Gynecol Oncol* 1999,75:175–177.

217. Ostrzenski A. A new, laparoscopic full-thickness slice ovarian biopsy (from anti- mesenteric to mesenteric margin). *J Ginecol Surg* 1995;11:109–112.

218. Hoskins WJ. Cancer of the ovary and uterine tube. In: Holzman GB, Rinehart RD, DiSaia PJ, eds. *Precis: un update in obstetrics and gynecology. Oncology.* Washington, DC: American College of Obstetrician and Gynecologists, 1998:48–50.

219. Kennedy L, Traub AI, Atkinson AB, et al. Short term administration of gonadotropin-releasing hormone analog to a patient with a testosterone-secreting ovarian tumor. *J Clin Endocrinol Metab* 1987;64:1320–1322.

220. Pascale MM, Pugeat M, Roberts M, et al. Androgen suppressive effect of GnRH agonist in ovarian hyperthecosis and virilizing tumors. *Clin Endocrinol (Oxf)* 1994;41:571–576.

221. Imai T, Tobinaga J, Morita Matsuyama T, et al. Virilizing adenocortical adenoma: in vitro steroidogenesis, immunohistochemical studies of steroidogenic enzymes, and gene expression of corticotropin receptor. *Surgery* 1999;125:396–402.

222. Sorano D, Prasad V, David R, et al. Hypertension and virilization caused by a unique desoxycorticosterone- and androgen-secreting adrenal adenoma. *J Pediatr Endocrinol Metab* 1999;12: 215–220.

223. Masiakos PT, Flynn CE, Donahoe PK. Masculinizing and feminizing syndromes caused by functioning tumors. *Semin Pediatr Surg* 1997;6:147–155.

224. Kawashima A, Sandler CM, Fishman EK, et al. Spectrum of CT findings in nonmalignant disease of the adrenal gland. *Radiographics* 1998;18:393–412.

225. Beckers A, Parotte MC, Gaspard U, Khalife A. Hyperandrogenism: clinical aspects, investigation and treatment. *Rev Med Liege* 1999;54:274–282.

226. Sherman Al, Brown S. The precursors of endometrial carcinoma. *Am J Obstet Gynecol* 1979;135:947–956.

9

ABNORMAL ENDOMETRIAL BLEEDING

EDUCATIONAL OBJECTIVES

Medical Students (1)
APGO Objective No. 47

Definition of: primary amenorrhea, secondary amenorrhea, oligomenorrhea, polymenorrhea
Causes of amenorrhea
Evaluation methods
Treatment options

Residents in Obstetrics/Gynecology (2)
CREOG Objectives

Pertinent history
Physical examination
Diagnostic studies
Diagnosis: ovarian failure, hypothalamic disorders, chronic anovulation, pituitary disorders, thyroid disorders, adrenal disorders, intrauterine synechiae, tumors
Management: possible interventions, factors influencing decisions regarding intervention, potential complications of intervention, potential complications of nonintervention
Follow-up

Practitioners (3–5)
ACOG Recommendations

Diagnosis
Differential diagnosis
Physical findings
Endometrial sampling
Laboratory studies
Management

DEFINITION

Menstrual and nonmenstrual bleeding disturbances can be attributed to the endometrium and, in general, can be categorized as follows:

- Interval too short (polymenorrhea) or too long (oligomenorrhea/amenorrhea)
- Duration too short (hypomenorrhea) or too long (hypermenorrhea)
- Amount too little (hypomenorrhea) or too much (menorrhagia)

Each category is defined as follows:

- Polymenorrhea is defined as episodes of endometrial bleeding that occur with intervals of 21 days or less.
- Oligomenorrhea is defined as episodes of endometrial bleeding that occur with intervals of 35 days or more [some clinicians consider 40 days to be the cut-off point (6)].
- Primary amenorrhea is defined as follows:
    Absence of menarche, secondary sexual characteristics, and pubertal growth velocity by 14 years of age

    Absence of spontaneous menarche by 16 years of age despite development of secondary sexual characteristics and an adequate growth pattern
- Secondary amenorrhea is defined as follows:
    Cessation of menses for at least three consecutive menstrual cycle intervals
    Absent of menses for 6 months
    Absent of menses for 12 months, or at least six menstrual effluents missed when prior oligomenorrhea was present (7)
- Hypomenorrhea (cryptomenorrhea) is either reflection of duration or amount of menstrual bleeding:
    Duration fewer than 2 days (expected duration is 2–8 days)
    Amount of blood loss during menses is less than 30 mL (8) (the normal volume of blood loss is 30–80 mL).
- Hypermenorrhea (menorrhagia) is defined as regular menses intervals with excessive blood loss (>80 mL) or duration longer than 8 days.
- Metrorrhagia is defined as irregular menses intervals with both excessive blood loss (mt>80 mL) and duration longer than 8 days.

- Menometrorrhagia consists of menorrhagia and metrorrhagia, in which menses cannot be determined.

INCIDENCE

Overall, it is estimated that 15% to 20% of women will experience one or another form of abnormal endometrial bleeding (7). The prevalence of secondary amenorrhea is estimated in the range of 0.3% (9) to 4.9% (10), and oligomenorrhea 6.7% (9). The most common cause of secondary amenorrhea is pregnancy, followed by hypothalamic origin.

CLASSIFICATION

Abnormal endometrial bleeding is classified as follows:

- Polymenorrhea
- Oligomenorrhea
- Amenorrhea (primary or secondary)
- Hypomenorrhea (cryptomenorrhea)
- Menorrhagia (hypermenorrhea)
- Metrorrhagia
- Menometrorrhagia

ETIOLOGY

The etiology of polymenorrhea, oligomenorrhea, primary amenorrhea, hypomenorrhea, hypermenorrhea, metrorrhagia, menometrorrhagia, and exercise-induced menstrual abnormalities, as well as menstrual physiology, are discussed in the Chapters 1, 2, and 10. Therefore, only secondary amenorrhea will be discussed here.

In most cases, secondary amenorrhea has either a physiologic cause or a pathologic cause. The physiologic causes include the following:

- Prepuberty
- Pregnancy
- Lactation
- Menopause
- Constitutionally delayed puberty

Pathologic causes are discussed in the following sections.

Hypothalamic-Pituitary Causes

- Functional hypothalamic amenorrhea is the most common form of hypothalamic origin. Emotional or physical stress, social adaptation problems, and diet may contribute to secondary amenorrhea.
- Changes in neurotransmitter secretion or its metabolism may result in secondary amenorrhea.

- Alternation in hypothalamic–pituitary–ovarian axis feedback
- Tumor compression in the vicinity of the hypothalamic–pituitary portal plexus compromises circulation.
- Chronic illness, exercise-induced amenorrhea, weight reduction, eating disorders (anorexia nervosa, bulimia nervosa)
- Hypogonadotropic causes: Congenital and acquired forms of secondary amenorrhea and hypergonadotropic primary amenorrhea are discussed in Chapter 2.
- Pituitary disorders: Hyperprolactinemia due to the presence of a small pituitary adenoma (prolactinoma) induces hypogonadotropic secondary amenorrhea. Prolactin directly reduces both amplitude and frequency of gonadotropin-releasing hormone (GnRH) pulsatile secretion from the hypothalamus. Hyperprolactinemia is responsible for up to 20% of secondary amenorrhea.

Adenoma and craniopharyngioma tumors may compress, leukemia may inflame with lymphocytes, sarcoidosis may infiltrate and infarction (Sheehan's syndrome or panhypopituitarism or hypophyseal infarction) of the pituitary gland many occur. Brain injury (either secondary to head trauma or neurosurgery) may also result in secondary amenorrhea (7).

Ovarian Disorders

Premature ovarian failure is defined as cessation of ovarian function before 35 years of age according to the American College of Obstetricians and Gynecologists (ACOG) (12); a textbook for students defines it as cessation of ovarian function before 40 years of age (6). It is an idiopathic condition in 52.5% of patients (13). In the vast majority, it is considered an irreversible condition; although, ovarian function has been restored in some cases (13).

Ovarian abnormalities have an immunologic cause in 17.4% (13) to 45% (11) of patients; that is, an immune mechanism obstructs the gonadotropin receptors (defective receptors) (13). The presence of antinuclear antibodies plays a role in premature ovarian failure and constitutes a clinically distinct group (14). Spontaneous pregnancies during estrogen therapy for this condition have been documented. It has been suggested that ovarian antibodies may act as a practical marker for diagnosis, prognosis, and treatment (15). Premature ovarian failure may coincide with other endocrine gland autoimmune disorders, such as thyroid disease, type I diabetes, and Addison disease (7).

X-chromosome genetic mutations (both familial and nonfamilial) have been identified in women with premature ovarian failure: 46,Xi(Xq); 45,X/46XX mosaic; 46,X,der(X)t(X;Y)(q28;q12) mat; and 46,X,t(X;5)(q22;q11.2) mat (16).

Hyperandrogenism of ovarian origin (e.g., polycystic ovary syndrome) is the most common hyperandrogenic cause of secondary amenorrhea. PCOS is characterized by a euestrogenism state, chronic anovulation, and an increased ratio of luteinizing hormone (LH) to follicle-stimulating hormone (FSH) (ratio ≥2:1) (7,12).

Hyperthecosis or ovarian stromal hypertrophy by autonomously secreting androgens interferes with the hypothalamic–pituitary–ovarian axis, leading to secondary amenorrhea (7).

Radiation therapy or *chemotherapy* (particularly cytostatic drugs such as cyclophosphamide (7) can contribute to secondary amenorrhea. Myelocytic leukemia also can be a cause (17).

Anatomic Disorders of the Genital Tract

Congenital disorders are discussed in Chapter 2. Anatomic disorders of the genital tract include *Asherman syndrome*, which is characterized by intrauterine adhesions, intrauterine synechiae, and endometrial scarring. Ovarian function is intact and intrauterine adhesions may affect all or part of the uterine cavity or cervical canal, causing atresia or stenosis and possibly causing hematometria, recurrent abortion, hypomenorrhea, and dysmenorrhea.

Asherman syndrome may result from the following mechanisms:

- Previous postpartum curettage (in 39% of infertile patients who undergo hysterosalpingography, about 5% of patients with a history of recurrent abortion, and 1.5% of infertile women) (18)
- Previous uterine surgery (cesarean section, myomectomy, metroplasty) (19)
- Severe pelvic infection [rarely tuberculosis (20–22) and schistosomiasis are implicated, particularly among patients from underdeveloped countries (18)]
- Cervical stenosis usually follows a cervical conization procedure (18).
- Vaginal stricture or obstruction secondary to bone marrow transplantation for acute myelocytic leukemia, which causes ovarian failure (17)

Other Hormonal Disorders

Thyroid dysfunction [*hypothyroidism* associated with galactorrhea (nipple discharge)] may cause secondary amenorrhea. Hashimoto thyroiditis (chronic lymphocytic thyroiditis) is an autoimmune condition with a high titer of thyroid antimicrosomal antibody, which is considered a diagnostic tool. This entity also may induce amenorrhea. Recently, it has been documented that hypothyroidism in women is less frequently associated with menstrual disturbance than was previously considered. Menstrual irregularities tend to be more frequent in severe hypothyroidism, and oligomenorrhea and menorrhagia are the most common menstrual disturbances (23).

Hyperthyroidism in both forms (Graves disease or toxic diffuse goiter, and Plummer disease or toxic nodular goiter) may cause secondary amenorrhea. However, it is difficult to predict the type of menstrual disorder that may occur, such as oligomenorrhea, amenorrhea, or hypomenorrhea (17). Rarely does thyroid neoplasia itself, or as a part of multiple endocrine neoplasia type IIA and type IIB, (in association with pheochromocytoma and hyperparathyroidism or ganglioneuromatosis, and marfanoid habitus) cause secondary amenorrhea (24).

Adrenal gland disorders, such as late-onset congenital hyperplasia, can result in hyperandrogenism, which induces secondary amenorrhea. The 21-hydroxylase-enzyme defect is the most common form of this functional disorder (7) (see Chapters 2, 8, and 10 for more information.

Exercise, weight reduction, eating disorders, and obesity can lead to secondary amenorrhea. Systemic diseases also can be the cause.

DIAGNOSIS

History

Medical history should establish the following:

- Previous menstrual patterns (intervals, duration, amount of menstrual effluent)
- Pregnancy (amenorrhea related to dilatation and curettage for postpartum hemorrhagia; postpartum endometritis)
- Nipple discharge (galactorrhea)
- Presence or absence of premenstrual molimina (usually present with lower genital tract obstruction and amenorrhea)
- Presence or absence of symptoms suggesting pregnancy: missed periods, frequent urination, fatigue, breast tenderness, nausea and/or vomiting
- Body weight and nutrition pattern (±15% changes from ideal body weight may cause secondary amenorrhea)
- Eating disorders: anorexia nervosa induces hypogonadotropic hypogonadic amenorrhea (25), and bulimia nervosa (26) induces amenorrhea in 36% of patients. Oligomenorrhea, defective luteal phase, or a normal menstrual cycle may be observed in 45% of patients (26,27). Preliminary results suggest that clinical menstrual dysfunctions may be more common in vegetarians (28).
- Intense and sustained strenuous exercise may have a negative effect on interrelated conditions, including eating disorders, osteopenia, and psychosocial disorders.
- In primary and secondary amenorrhea, suppression of LH and FSH hormones is demonstrated, most likely as a result of both hypothalamic–pituitary–ovarian axis and hypothalamic–pituitary–adrenal axis malfunction. The role of leptin, a hormone made by the fat cell, has been implicated in exercise-induced amenorrhea. Bone loss, particularly in female adolescents, may be an irreversible process (29–31).

- Any over-the-counter and alternative natural medication taken prior to missing menses
- Symptoms of endocrinopathy
    Hypothyroidism: dry skin, lethargy, constipation, intellectual and physical slowness, and menorrhagia may proceed secondary amenorrhea; cold intolerance, decreased appetite, body weight increases, and constipation will be reported
    Hyperthyroidism: anxiety, excessive perspiration, nervousness, restless, sleepiness, emotional instability, palpitations, tremors, excessive sensitivity to heat, daily frequent bowel movement, weight loss, increased appetite
    Cushing syndrome: emotional lability, weakness, and a history of diabetes mellitus may be present.
    Late-onset adrenal hyperplasia: a history of menarche, past and present menstrual pattern (often oligomenorrhea will be reported), and reproductive capacity abnormalities should be explored.
- Brain injury or neurosurgery
- Abdominal or thoracic trauma or surgery

Physical Examination

Results of a general physical examination are usually within normal limits. Height, weight, and vital signs should be recorded (decreasing body fat below 22% or obesity may cause menstrual disturbances, including secondary amenorrhea). In secondary amenorrhea, pregnancy can be determined by the presence of a fetal heart rate with electronic Doppler ultrasonography at about 12 weeks' gestation.

- Hypothyroidism: skin is dry, deep tendon reflexes are prolonged; periorbital puffiness, cramping of muscles
- Hyperthyroidism: skin is silky, moist, and worm; hair is thin and silky; Plummer fingernails observed (separation of fingernails from the nail bed); fine tremors of the tongue and fingers demonstrable; exophthalmos (abnormal protrusion of the eyeball), infrequent blinking, and lid lag.
- Hyperprolactinemia: nipple discharge is present and a hypoestrogenic state may be observed with a negative progesterone/progestin challenge test (estrogen absence disorder)
- Cushing syndrome: skin striae, bruising with ease, buffalo hump (interscapular fat deposition), moon faces (fat deposition in the face), and virilization may be observed.
- Late-onset adrenal hyperplasia: partial defects in adrenal steroid synthesis. Clinical expressions are limited to hirsutism, with minimal virilization, clitoris hypertrophy, and significant acne. It is of clinical importance to distinguish between hirsutism and hypertrichosis (characterized by a male hair pattern distribution and no excess androgen level identified) and hirsutism associated with virilization caused by androgen elevation.

Pelvic Examination

Bimanual examination is essential for ruling out acquired obstruction of lower genital tract outflow and to determine a clinical hypoestrogenic status or hyperandrogenism, such as clitoromegaly [determined by multiplying the length by the width in millimeters; when the result is >40 mm², clitoromegaly is established (7)], hirsutism, acne, oily skin, and voice deepening.

Pregnancy may be determined on pelvic examination when secondary amenorrhea is present; however, today, the early stage of pregnancy is established by measuring the serum human chorionic gonadotropin (hCG) and performing ultrasonography (32). In secondary amenorrhea attributable to pregnancy, the external genitalia and the vagina are bluish and congestive in appearance (Chadwik sign), and the cervix becomes softer (Hegar sign). The uterine enlarges, and its softness is appreciable; in this stage, it is large enough to be palpated abdominally.

Laboratory Tests

Initial laboratory test should include the following:

- A pregnancy test is performed when clinically indicated or needed for documentation of clinical findings.
    A urine pregnancy test may be positive at about 4 weeks from the first day of last menses. Due to the highest concentration of hCG in the morning, the urine specimen should be collected at this time.
    A serum pregnancy test is highly specific and sensitive, is based on the characteristic beta-hCG subunit, and can be obtained in quantitative or qualitative measurement.
- Prolactin levels
- Thyroid-stimulating hormone
- Fasting glucose

If these tests are within normal range and pregnancy was ruled out, the next step is to determine the patient's estrogen status. Such determination can be achieved using the following methods:

- Progesterone challenge test:
    Oral administration of micronized progesterone (Prometrium) at a dosage of 200 mg daily for 5 to 10 days, or
    Intramuscular administration of progesterone at a dose of 150 mg (one injection)
- Progestin challenge test:
    Oral administration of medroxyprogesterone (Provera) at a dosage of 5 to 10 mg daily for 5 to 10 days, or
    Oral administration of norethindrone acetate (Norlutate) at a dosage of 5 mg daily for 5 to 10 days, or
    Oral administration of norethindrone (Norlutin) at a dosage of 5 mg daily for 5 to 10 days
- Plasma estradiol, FSH, and LH determination

If withdrawal bleeding doesn't occur within 2 weeks, the serum FSH level should be determined. It is worthwhile to mention that the progesterone or progestin test is of little value in the diagnosis of premature ovarian failure.

A low serum FSH level (<5 IU/L) and low estradiol level (normal range 20–400 pg/mL or 70–1,500 p*M*) establish a hypogonadotropic hypogonadism state, reflecting either hypothalamic or pituitary dysfunction. On the other hand, an elevated FSH level may indicate premature ovarian failure (hypogonadotropic hypogonadism). To distinguish a hypothalamic disorder from a pituitary disorder, a GnRH challenge test should be performed.

It has been postulated that a low basic metabolic rate, a low free triiodothyronine (T_3) level, a low LH level, and a normal FSH level may confirm the diagnosis of hypogonadic secondary amenorrhea of nutritional origin.

Because ovarian failure can be associated with autoimmune disorders, the following initial tests may be performed:

- Complete blood count and sedimentation rate
- Antinuclear antibody, thyroid antibody, and rheumatoid factor
- Calcium and phosphorous, total protein, and ratio of albumin to globulin
- Morning hormonal study such as cortisol, free thyroxine (T_4), and thyroid-stimulating hormone (TSH)

Low normal levels of serum FSH (normal serum FSH value in adult women is 5–30 IU/L, with the mid-cycle twice as high as the base level) may indicate a uterine abnormality. The confirmatory test for this condition is no withdrawal bleeding in response to the administration of sequential, cyclic estrogen/progestin [oral administration of 0.625 mg conjugated estrogen for 26 consecutive days, adding progestin (10 mg medroxyprogesterone) for last 10 days of the estrogen regimen].

A positive progesterone or progestin challenge test (withdrawal bleeding) indicates an adequate estrogen state. The serum FSH and LH levels should be determined, and a ratio of LH to FSH of 2:1 may support a diagnosis of polycystic ovary syndrome (PCOS). PCOS, hyperthecosis, ovarian tumors, or adrenal gland sources may induce menstrual dysfunction, including secondary amenorrhea, by increasing the secretion of androgens (6,12). To confirm the diagnosis of PCOS, the serum testosterone, dehydroepiandrosterone sulfate (DHEAS), and 17-alpha-hydroxyprogesterone levels should be determined. The last two hormones, DHEAS and 17-alpha-hydroxyprogesterone, essentially are from adrenal sources.

A serum elevation of 17-alpha-hydroxyprogesterone (normal range 100–300 ng/dL or 3–9 n*M*) suggests late-onset congenital adrenal hyperplasia. Cushing syndrome also must be considered because adrenal steroid hormone secretion is increased in this syndrome, which may cause secondary amenorrhea. The free cortisol rate (normal range 10–90 μg/24 h or 28–250 nmol/24 h) is determined via 24-hour urine collection, and the dexamethasone suppression test is performed as needed.

Serum testosterone elevation of over 200 ng/dL, serum DHEAS elevation of over 7 μg/mL, or a decreased sex hormone–binding globulin level is indicative of an *ovarian or adrenal gland androgen-producing tumor*. To identify an adrenal gland tumor, magnetic resonance imaging (MRI) or computed tomography (CT) is helpful. The ovarian origin tumor usually can be detected by ultrasonography; in rare instances, operative inspection of the ovary must be performed (33) .

The serum TSH level will support a diagnosis of either hypothyroidism or hyperthyroidism; secondary amenorrhea is observed in both conditions.

Laboratory data for *hypothyroidism* will characterize primary hypothyroidism (thyroid gland dysfunction) by elevation of TSH (normal range 0.35–6.7 μU/mL or 0.35–6.7 mU/L) and a low level of free T_4 (normal range of free T_4 is 0.8–2.3 ng/L or 10–30 n*M*). Secondary hypothyroidism (pituitary origin dysfunction) is indicated by decreased TSH and a low level of free T_4.

Hyperthyroidism is established when T_4 and T_3 (normal range of free T_3 is 0.13–0.55 ng/dL or 2.0–8.5 p*M*) are elevated and TSH is suppressed or undetectable. It is necessary to rule out a solitary hot nodule within the thyroid gland or multinodular gland; radioactive iodine thyroid uptake and scintigraphic evaluation (radioisotopic scan) will distinguish a hot nodule from a cold nodule.

Isolated TSH hypersecretion causing *hyperthyroidism* is a rare condition, in which elevated levels of TSH, T_4, and T_3 coexist, providing a clue to the diagnosis.

In the presence of *adrenal adenomas*, DHEAS is elevated. Increased levels of DHEAS are also observed in ACTH (corticotropin)-dependent and ACTH-independent hyperandrogenism. To establish ACTH-dependent versus -independent hyperandrogenism, a 24-hour urine free cortisol measurement test is helpful.

An elevation level of prolactin is often associated with compensated hypothyroidism; therefore a high-sensitive TSH level measurement or free T_4 and TSH levels to be determined. *Hyperprolactinemia* (normal range of serum prolactin is 1–20 ng/mL or 44.4–888 p*M*) may be associated with some endocrine gland disorders (polyendocrinopathy), so growth hormone and corticotropin levels should be determined. To rule out pituitary adenoma, CT or MRI should be performed (MRI offers better soft tissue resolution than CT). Macroprolactinoma is characterized by a lesion larger than 10 mm and microprolactinoma by a lesion smaller than 10 mm. It is crucial to perform one of these studies to rule out pseudoprolactinoma, which requires surgical treatment.

In brief, there are three practical steps in the evaluation of hyperprolactinemia:

- To rule out intake of a variety of medications
- To rule out other causes of hyperprolactinemia (head trauma/brain surgery, abdominal or thoracic injury/surgery, pregnancy, and primary hypothyroidism)
- To establish and to verify indication for a treatment and a form of therapy (conservative medical vs. surgical)

In *Asherman syndrome*, an acquired anatomic genital tract obstruction (originally called amenorrhea traumatica atretica by Asherman in 1948), the uterine cavity cannot be visualized or multiple filling defects are detected during radiologic salpingography. It has been documented that hysteroscopic evaluation is superior to hysterosalpingography (34,35). Hysteroscopy is viewed as the safest, least traumatic, and the most accurate diagnostic method (36). Diagnostic and operative hysteroscopic safety can be enhanced under ultrasonographic guidance (37).

Transvaginal ultrasonography has been suggested as a diagnostic tool; however, an independent study showed that less than 63% of intrauterine adhesions can be detected using this method (38). The same study (38) documented that sonohysterography and hysterosalpingography are very useful tools for detecting intrauterine adhesions. Hysteroscopic evaluation for intrauterine adhesions provides additional benefits at the time of the diagnostic procedure:

- Video documentation of adhesions can be made.
- Endometrial biopsy can be performed as indicated.
- Staging of intrauterine adhesions can be established (39):
    Stage I: mild (hysteroscopic score 1–4)
    Stage II: moderate (hysteroscopic score 5–8)
    Stage III: severe (hysteroscopic score 9–12)

The score is established based upon type of adhesions (filmy, score = 1; filmy/dense, 2; dense, 4) and menstrual pattern (normal, score = 0; hypomenorrhea, 2; amenorrhea, 4). Such a classification may provide a uniform method of communication and interpretation between clinicians in reference to the location, extent, and quality of adhesions.

DIFFERENTIAL DIAGNOSIS

- Pregnancy
- Lactation
- Menopause
- Endocrinopathy
- Iatrogenic causes

THERAPY

Specific therapy is aimed at the underlying reversible conditions (endocrine or otherwise) causing secondary amenorrhea. Patients should be informed that the restoration of menstrual cycles most likely would restore reproductive capacity. Therefore, caution should be exercised if preg-

nancy is not desired (7). In broad view, when amenorrhea results from the hypoestrogenic state, it may have a negative impact on the cardiovascular system, lipoprotein profile, bone density, and infertility status. Because the duration of hypoestrogenism is an important factor in the progression of these profiles, it is imperative to commence the appropriate diagnostic algorithm and early therapy.

Conventional Therapy

Hypothalamic secondary amenorrhea may require a multidisciplinary approach:

- A clinician familiar with managing this type of condition
- A psychiatrist or psychologist [psychological stress, lifestyle choices, or psychosomatic disorders may cause menstrual dysfunction and/or or sexual behavior dysfunction (40,41)]
- An exercise physiology specialist [when exercise is inappropriately managed athletic triad may occur: thin body mass, stress fracture, and scoliosis (42)]. It has been shown that bone density correlates with body weight (43) and residual deficit in bone density is an irreversible process with hormonal therapy (44). Therefore, exercise modifications with adequate coordinated therapies should be started early to prevent permanent sequelae of the hypoestrogenic state. Preliminary data indicate that salivary immunoglobulin A holds promise as a useful immunologic marker of the overtrained state. At present, psychological tests including the athlete's mood state are most commonly used for the overtrained state (45).
- A nutritionist [hormonal treatment may be ineffective when an adequate weight is not maintained; hypoleptinemia (low leptin level) is present in secondary amenorrhea (46)]. The hormone leptin is secreted by adipocytes and affects appetite, eating behavior, and energy requirements (47). Serotonin has been implicated in the control of eating behavior (as well as its disturbances) and body weight disorders (48).

Improvement of *nutritional intake* and body composition with a psychological support may reverse hypothalamic amenorrhea (49). Prolonged suboptimal intake of micronutrients leads to impairment of cognitive performance; adequate supplementation will reverse this process, as well as secondary amenorrhea (50).

In idiopathic hypothalamic amenorrhea (low gonadotropin and estrogen levels), if a patient desires pregnancy and pituitary–ovarian functions are preserved, induction of ovulation can be achieved by administration of GnRH or human menopausal gonadotropin.

Administration of *GnRH* stimulates endogenous GnRH secretion and eventually may lead to ovulation, with a cumulative pregnancy rate of 74%. GnRH is administered intravenously via chronic pulsatile (intermittent) injections using a pulse interval/volume-programmable portable pump at a dosage of 5 to 10 µg per pulse. The subcutaneous dose is 10 to 20 µg per pulse, at intervals of 90 minutes. In contrast to hMG therapy, the GnRH modality does not require hCG injection; therefore, ovarian hyperstimulation is avoided. In a well-selected patient, ovulation occurs 10 to 20 days after treatment begins (4,51).

Human menopausal gonadotropin is administered daily regardless of uterine bleeding. At the variable dosage method, 75 to 150 IU is administered intramuscularly (injection is given between 5 and 8 p.m.). On the 4th day of treatment, the serum estradiol level is determined. If follicles response is not observed, the dose of hMG can be increased by 75 to 150 IU per day. The daily hGM maintenance dose should be at the level when estradiol levels begin to increase above 100 pg/mL. At that time, follicle growth and development are evaluated daily by transvaginal ultrasonography. When the dominant follicle diameter is 16 to 20 mm and the optimal serum estradiol level reaches 500 to 2,000 pg/mL, a single dose of 5,000 to 10,000 IU of hCG is injected intramuscularly (24 hours after the last hMG injection). Ovulation is expected within 36 hours from hCG injection. Because hypothalamic hypogonadotropic amenorrhea is associated with hypogonadotropic hypogonadism (hypoestrogenism), hCG supplementation is required at the dose of 2,500 IU and is provided on the 3rd and 6th days after hCG administration.

A patient must be informed about at least two major complications of this mode of therapy: ovarian hyperstimulation syndrome and multiple pregnancies. There are three categories of *ovarian hyperstimulation*:

- Mild type (ovarian size <5 cm, weight gain of <10 pounds, and slight pelvic pain
- Moderate type (ovarian size up to 10 cm, weight gain of ≥10 pounds, and nausea and vomiting
- Severe type (ovarian size >10 cm or any size associated with ascites, hydrothorax, hemoconcentration, or oliguria

If ovarian hyperstimulation is suspected, pelvic and abdominal examinations are avoided, and ultrasonographic studies are chosen instead.

The mild or moderate type of ovarian hyperstimulation requires close clinical observation with daily hematocrit, weight, and abdominal girth measurement. The severe type, a prospectively life-threatening condition, is monitored in a hospital with therapy focused on controlling symptoms such as dyspnea, hypotension, and oliguria. Electrolyte imbalance, coagulopathy, and intraabdominal ovarian hemorrhage should be closely monitored and adequately treated when needed. Ovarian hyperstimulation usually resolves within 7 days; however, when pregnancy occurs it may last for several weeks (4).

In *hypothalamic amenorrhea*, when pregnancy is not desired a therapy can be offered, either in the form of an oral contraceptive (29) or by cyclic hormonal estrogen/progesterone or progestin replacement therapy (HRT) (53). This therapy induces menstrual-like bleeding (menses), and fertility will not be restored. It is a clinical conviction that induced menses four to six times per year is probably sufficient to reduce the risk of endometrial hyperplasia (7).

To induce menstrual-like bleeding, on the first day of each calendar month conjugated estrogen is started at a dose of 0.625 mg and is continued for 25 consecutive days. On the 16th day, progestin is added (medroxyprogesterone acetate 10 mg or norethindrone acetate 5 mg, or norethindrone). Menstrual-like bleeding usually occurs within 3 days after the last dose of progestin.

Micronized progesterone (Prometrium) can be used as a substitute for progestin. It was documented in a double-blind study that withdrawal bleeding was induced in 90% of previously estrogenized patients when oral micronized progesterone was used at the dose of 300 mg for 10 to 14 days per month (48). When bleeding does not occur, increasing the dose of conjugated estrogen to 1.25 mg achieves menstrual-like bleeding.

Without inducing menstrual-like bleeding (for a patient who desires no cyclic bleeding), conjugated estrogen at the dose of 0.625 mg and Provera 2.5 mg should be administered together daily without a break. Prometrium (oral macronized progesterone) 100 mg (54) to 200 mg (55) can be used instead of Provera together with estrogen.

Secondary amenorrhea of idiopathic pituitary origin can be corrected as follows:

- GnRH treatment (see above under hypothalamic amenorrhea)
- Gonadotropin therapy (see above under hypothalamic amenorrhea)
- *Bromocriptine* and cabergoline for hyperprolactinemia. In most instances medical conservative suppression of overproduction of prolactin is highly effective and may:
    Decrease serum prolactin levels
    Resume gonadal function and reproductive capacity
    Reduce adenoma size
    Improve an ophthalmic disorder (peripheral vision) due to macroprolactinoma compression on the optic chiasm

Bromocriptine mesylate is a semisynthetic ergot alkaloid with dopamine receptor agonist activity (4,56). It can be administered orally, vaginally, or intramuscularly. Titration of the dose of bromocriptine is advisable, with an initial oral dose of 1.25 mg daily for 1 week, and can be increased in increments of 1.25 mg weekly until after the customary dose of 2.5 mg twice daily is established. The dose may be increased up to 15 mg daily, but this is rarely indicated, and the dose is appropriately adjusted to sustain the normal range of prolactin (4) .

When nausea, vomiting, orthostatic (postural) hypotension and dizziness, headaches, and nasal congestion occur (4,50), the dose can be reduced or the dose increment can be withheld, and medication can be administered at bed-time or with meals. When these changes fail and general symptoms persist, the oral dose can be reduced to half of a vaginal bromocriptine tablet. This is an effective approach with fewer side effects (57). A long-acting intramuscularly injectable bromocriptine (Parlodel-LAR) at the dose of 50 to 200 mg administered every 28 days is effective and well tolerated (58).

Cabergoline, the newest dopamine agonist, shows high specificity and affinity for the dopamine D2 receptors. It is a potent and very long-acting inhibitor of prolactin secretion. At the dose of 0.5 to 1.0 mg twice weekly, it is more effective than bromocriptine 2.5 to 5.0 mg twice daily (53). Cabergoline is well tolerated [most patients intolerant of other ergot derivatives can tolerate cabergoline (59)], effective, and can be administered orally once or twice weekly (59,60) as well as vaginally at the dose of one 0.5-mg tablet twice weekly (61). At present, due to the teratogenic potential and lack of adequate safety data in pregnancy, cabergoline cannot be recommended as a first-line treatment for infertility (59,62). There are reports of congenital abnormalities in cabergoline-associated pregnancies; however, the pattern of these abnormalities cannot be identified (59). Clinical data show that idiopathic hyperprolactinemia or microprolactinoma requires half the dose of cabergoline as compared with macroadenoma (60). Cabergoline has a proven record as an effective mode of therapy in patients with bromocriptine intolerance or resistance and as a first-line of treatment in all forms of hyperprolactinemia (60,63).

Neurosurgical trans-sphenoidal resection is infrequently indicated for a macroprolactinoma large enough to cause visual impairment by compression of the optic chiasm, when a patient does not tolerate or is resistant to medical therapy (62).

Clomiphene citrate, a nonsteroidal estrogen receptor antagonist, is indicated for the treatment of secondary amenorrhea in a patient with adequate levels of estrogen, FSH, and prolactin. Improper gonadotropin secretion causing an increased ratio of LH to FSH (PCOS) can be treated with clomiphene citrate (4). The initial dosage of 50 mg per day can be administered to induce ovulation in an amenorrheic patient. If the patient is more than 80 kg overweight, the initial dosage is usually increased to 100 mg per day. After commencement of progesterone- or progestin-provoked menstrual bleeding, clomiphene is started on the 3rd to 5th day of bleeding and continued for 5 consecutive days. The dose can be increased in increments of 50 mg if the lower dose does not induce ovulation. Doses of 150 mg or higher are not effective. Clomiphene citrate safety records allow regimens in anovulatory patients for as long as 4 to 6 months without a complete infertility workup (4).

If clomiphene citrate fails to induce ovulation, a 2-month trial of oral contraceptive followed by a repeat course of clomiphene citrate may be tried, which has resulted in a 58% cumulative pregnancy rate (64). However, the overall pregnancy rate with clomiphene citrate therapy is about 40% (4).

A patient with a serum DHEAS level of over 200 μg/dL (normal range 80–320 μg/dL) may benefit from the addition of glucocorticoids (0.5 mg dexamethasone at bedtime) to a clomiphene citrate regimen. Such combined therapy yields significantly higher ovulation and conception rates (65).

Follow-up of clomiphene citrate therapy is clinically indicated to make the following determinations:

- Ovarian enlargement (in the event of residual ovarian enlargement or development of ovarian cysts, clomiphene therapy is postponed)
- Possible pregnancy (contraindication for clomiphene use)

Clinical observations such as a biphasic pattern of basal body temperature and regular menses interval may indicate commencement of the ovulatory cycle. On the 8th day following the last dose of clomiphene citrate, assessment of serum estradiol levels may determine follicle development and maturation. The progesterone level on the 14th day from the last dose of clomiphene citrate may establish the presence of the luteal phase. Ultrasonography may assist in documenting dominant follicle development and collapse at the time of ovulation (4).

In *hypoestrogenic* amenorrhea, osteoporosis and cardiovascular risk constitute indications for assessing bone density and the cardiovascular system. A patient with low bone mineral density and cardiovascular risk should be treated as follows:

- Restoration of circulating estrogen level (when amenorrhea lasts ≥6 months)
- Adequate calcium intake (1,500 mg/day)
- Adequate vitamin D supplementation at the dose of 400 IU per day (7)
- Adequate diet
- Moderate exercise

Asherman syndrome associated with secondary amenorrhea therapy is treated by hysteroscopic synechiolysis (66) (dividing intrauterine adhesions) or hysteroscopic lysis of adhesions, using hysteroscopic scissors, electrocautery, or contact laser. Upon completion of the intrauterine procedure, a no. 8 or 10 pediatric Foley catheter is inserted into the uterine cavity and the catheter bag is filled with 3 mL sterile fluid and left in place for 1 week. In addition, a high stimulatory dose of 2.5 mg conjugated estrogen is given every day, for 25 days. For the last 10 days of estrogen therapy, progestin (Provera 10 mg, Norlutate 5 mg, or Norlutin 5 mg) or micronized progesterone (Prometrium 300 mg) is added. This cyclic mode of therapy is continued for 2 consecutive months.

This method restores menstrual bleeding in secondary amenorrhea in 90.5% of patients, and anatomic distortion is corrected in 86.2%; however, reproductive outcome is about 56% (66). This therapy can be instituted concomitant with laparoscopic treatment (to prevent inadvertent pelvic organ injury that may occur with hysteroscopic uterine perforation). As documented in a randomized prospective study (67), inserting laminaria into the cervical canal preoperatively minimizes potential cervical injury secondary to cervical dilatation (67). Performing this procedure under ultrasonographic guidance has been recommended (37). Blind hysteroscopic division of intrauterine adhesions should be avoided because this risks uterine perforation or could establish a false canal (68). Only in severe cases is abdominal metroplasty performed for intrauterine adhesions (35).

Complementary Therapy

Patient Education

Patient education about secondary amenorrhea is an essential part of the patient's treatment program. It is recognized that stress and environmental factors may lead to secondary amenorrhea. Obesity and malnourishment are well-established causes of this condition. Strenuous, sustained exercise also may induce secondary amenorrhea. Therefore, the physician should speak with the patient on the nature of the condition, nature of medical or surgical management, potential health hazards, benefits from treatment, and current medical conventional-complementary-alternative therapies. Adequate diet; type, intensity, and duration of exercise; and stressful mental and physical factors should be discussed and the patient counseled on how to address these issues. Consequences of secondary amenorrhea such as cardiovascular conditions, osteoporosis, and infertility must be discussed with the patient. More information on this topic is discussed in Chapter 10.

Diet

Nutritional intake for a particular type, intensity, and duration of exercise is essential not only for overall physical performance but also impacts on health in general. The different degrees of extra physical demands require a nutritionally sound diet. However, no scientifically tangible data are available that specify nutritional requirements as they relate to exercise and the treatment of secondary amenorrhea. Many unproven creative dietary approaches have been proposed that do not necessarily accommodate the specific needs of this condition.

In exercise-induced amenorrhea, fats, proteins, and carbohydrates must be well balanced and increased accordingly, and alcohol consumption should be restricted during training or competition. Athletes on low-calorie regimens

should enhance their diets with micronutrients, vitamin B_{12}, and minerals (80).

Secondary amenorrhea caused by nutritional deficiency is best managed with a dietitian specializing in secondary amenorrhea and an exercise physiologist. A diet should be specifically formulated to an individual's needs in order to meet adequate caloric demands to maintain ideal body weight, body fat, and bone mass density, and the diet should be adjusted to compensate for the additional demands of exercise.

Anorexia nervosa and bulimia nervosa require a team approach that includes a psychologist or psychiatrist, an eating disorder counselor, and a physician familiar with hormonal and general therapeutic modalities. Diets usually consist of increased calories, regular, whole foods, increased soy foods, and flax seeds (81).

In patients with secondary amenorrhea due to ovarian failure, diets are composed of plenty of grains, beans (including soy beans), fruits, vegetables (dark leafy greens, nuts, and seeds, especially flax seeds), and fish (salmon, tuna, halibut, sardines) (81).

In patients with chronic anovulation, reduction of carbohydrates and increased protein intake is advised. Increased intake of soy foods, flax seeds, whole grains, fruits, vegetables, beans, nuts, seeds, fish, organic chicken/turkey, low-fat dairy products, and eggs also is recommended (81).

Supplementation

Mineral supplementation for secondary amenorrhea is recommended as follows (81):

- Calcium carbonate, 1,000 to 1,500 mg daily
- Magnesium citrate/malate, 200 to 400 mg daily
- Boron, 3 to 5 mg daily
- Zinc, 15 to 20 mg daily
- Copper, 1.5 to 3.0 mg daily

Vitamin D supplementation at 350 to 400 IU daily also is recommended.

Acupuncture and Electroacupuncture

Clinical studies with a placebo-acupuncture control have documented that acupuncture, particularly auricular acupuncture (ear acupuncture), significantly decreases serum LH concentration levels (69). This finding was confirmed during electroacupuncture investigation. This study also determined that FSH pulsatile frequency significantly increased (70). Another double-blind study discovered that acupuncture applications increase the serum 17-beta-estradiol level (71). Electroacupuncture can influence beta-endorphin mechanisms in the central nervous system and through such interaction may normalize disturbances of the hypothalamic–pituitary–ovarian axis (72). It also has been postulated that electrocautery may influence gene expression on the brain and thereby stabilize hypothalamic GnRH secretion (73). Acupuncture is highly effective in secondary amenorrhea, particularly when the progesterone challenge test result is positive and a normal base hormonal milieu is present (74). Based on these clinical scientific findings, acupuncture may be a viable treatment option for selected patients.

Exercise

Regular exercise in moderation has a positive impact on preventing cardiovascular conditions, decreased bone density, and certain cancers and does not negatively influence menstrual disturbances. However, sustained, strenuous exercise may alter menstrual function in up to 70% of women, depending on the patient's history and prior and current intensity and duration of exercise. Significant weight and body fat reduction through vigorous exercise are the predominant contributory factors to menstrual disorders. An often overlooked problem is the urinary incontinence that is commonly induced by physical stress, even in the young nulliparous population. Therefore, preventive Kegel perineal exercises should be undertaken (75). Long-term consequences of amenorrhea, such as cardiovascular risk, premature osteoporosis, and increased risk of musculoskeletal injury, are potential serious clinical sequelae of strenuous exercise. Diet and exercise program modifications are therefore indicated in exercise-induced secondary amenorrhea. Undertaking simple exercise corrective steps can normalize a menstrual cycle (75–77):

- Modifying the intensity, frequency, and duration of exercise (this approach may require exercise physiologist supervision)
- Temporary suspension of vigorous exercise until a regular menstrual cycle pattern has been established (particularly long-distance running or bodybuilding)
- Reducing or eliminating any type of competition
- Establishing the energy balance (energy intake) to the degree of physical exercise.

Estrogen replacement therapy in exercise-induced secondary amenorrhea significantly increases vertebral and femoral neck bone density (78); therefore it may be a reasonable clinical approach to suggest such therapy when a woman decides not to decrease her sustained strenuous physical activity. Of course, the pros and cons of this treatment must be clearly understood by the patient.

Conversely, amenorrhea associated with obesity requires intensifying physical activity and an exercise program that emphasizes both aerobic and anaerobic metabolism (79). Such approaches are part of the strategies of reducing and maintaining appropriate weight, which in return may normalize a menstrual cycle.

Obesity requires designing a therapeutic form of exercise to overcome or prevent particular medical conditions. It should be well designed to meet a patient's physical and mental abilities and should incorporate recreational activities enjoyed by the specific patient. An overall exercise curriculum should include sustained aerobic or endurance exercise that expands the ability to burn calories (fuel) and to use oxygen (e.g., brisk walking, jogging, bicycle riding, swimming), range-of-motion exercise (e.g., circular movement of a maximally extended arm), and strengthening exercise (e.g., sit-ups, push-ups).

Natural Alternative Therapy

More information on natural alternative therapies is presented in Chapter 10.

Herbal Medicine

The following herbal medicine is recommended for secondary amenorrhea:

- *Black cohosh* (*Cimicifuga racemosa* or *Actaea racemosa*), 40 to 80 mg in standardized extract in the form of caplets or capsules twice daily (82)
- *Chaste tree* (*Vitex agnus-castus* berries), 20-mg capsule twice daily. It has been clinically observed that *Vitex agnus-castus* stimulates multiple follicles to develop in normal cycles, while undergoing unstimulate *in vitro* fertilization. At the same time serum gonadotropin and ovarian hormone measurements were changed (83). However, no independent studies have made appropriate observations in amenorrheic patients.
- *False unicorn root* (*Chamaelirium luteum*), 5 to 10 drops of tincture taken orally four to six times daily or in a decoction drink half a cup twice daily (84,85)

Natural Hormone Replacement

The following natural estrogen/progesterone composition is offered in the therapy of secondary amenorrhea due to ovarian failure or hypoestrogen states:

Estriol 1 mg
Estradiol 0.125 mg
Estrone 0.125 mg

One capsule twice daily is administered for 25 consecutive days per month or on a continuing basis. Micronized progesterone is added from the 16th through 25th days of estrogen therapy at the dose of 100 mg twice daily (81).

Hyperprolactinemia

Hyperprolactinemia may result in various types of menstrual cycle dysfunction, including secondary amenorrhea.

Chaste tree (*Vitex agnus-castus*) extract 40 drops or 175-mg capsule of standardized extract may be taken daily (81).

Results of a randomized placebo-controlled double-blind study demonstrated that chaste tree extract can reduce prolactin after 3 months of therapy (86).

Homeopathic Therapy

A patient may present with personality traits characterized as gentle, mild, yielding, desiring attention, and nervous, with mood swings prevalent and late menses. For such a clinical picture, *Pulsatilla* at a dose of 15 cH (or five granules) twice weekly or 30 cH once or twice monthly (87,88).

A patient also may present personality traits characterized as restless, emotionally indifferent, lacking stamina, and mental exertion. *Calcarea phosphorica* at the dose of 15 cH (or five granules) in the morning three times weekly or 30 cH (5 granules) twice monthly (87).

REFERENCES

1. Association of Professors of Gynecology and Obstetrics. *Medical student educational objectives,* 7th ed. Washington, DC: Association of Professors of Gynecology and Obstetrics, 1997.
2. Council on Resident and Gynecology (CREOG). *Educational objectives core curriculum for residents in obstetrics and gynecology,* 5th ed. Washington, DC: CREOG, 1996.
3. American College of Obstetricians and Gynecologists (ACOG). Technical bulletin No. 134. Washington, DC: ACOG, 1989.
4. American College of Obstetrician and Gynecologists (ACOG). Technical bulletin No. 197. Washington, DC: ACOG, 1994.
5. American College of Obstetrician and Gynecologists (ACOG). Technical bulletin No. 202. Washington, DC: ACOG, 1995.
6. Beckman CRB, Ling WNP, Herbert WP, et al. Obstetrics and gynecology. 3rd ed. Baltimore: Williams & Wilkins, 1998: 430–435, 449–460.
7. McIver B, Romanski S, Nippoldt T. Evaluation and management of amenorrhea. *Mayo Clin Proc* 1977;72:1161–1169.
8. Hallberg L, Hogdahl A, Nilsson L, et al. Menstrual blood loss—a population study. Variation at different ages and attempts to define normality. *Acta Obstet Gynecol Scand* 1966;45:320–351.
9. Skierska E, Leszczynska-Bystrzanowska J, Gajewski AK. Risk analysis of menstrual disorders in young women from urban population. *Przegl Epidemiol* 1996;50:467–474.
10. Hernandez I, Cervera-Aguilar R, Vergara MD, et al. Prevalence and etiology of secondary amenorrhea in a selected Mexican population. *Ginecol Obstet Mex* 1999;67:374–376.
11. Falsetti L, Scalchi S, Villani MT, et al. Premature ovarian failure. *Gynecol Endocrinol* 1999;13:189–195.
12. American College of Obstetricians and Gynecologists (ACOG). Precis—reproductive endocrinology: an update in obstetrics and gynecology. Washington, DC: ACOG, 1998:41–54.
13. Rebar RW, Connolly HV. Clinical features of young women with hypergonadotropic amenorrhea. *Fertil Steril* 1990;53:804–810.
14. Ishizuka B, Kudo Y, Yamada H, et al. Anti-nuclear antibodies in patients with premature ovarian failure. *Hum Reprod* 1999;14: 70–75.
15. Fenichel P, Sosset C, Barbarino-Monnier P, et al. Prevalence, specificity and significance of ovarian antibodies during spontaneous premature ovarian failure. *Hum Reprod* 1997;12:2623–2628.
16. Devi A, Benn PA. X-chromosome abnormalities in women with premature ovarian failure. *J Reprod Med* 1999;44:321–324.
17. Yanai N, Shufaro Y, Or R, et al. Vaginal outflow tract obstruction by graft-versus-host reaction. *Bone Marrow Transplant* 1999;24: 811–812.
18. Speroff L, Galss RH, Kase NG. *Clinical gynecologic endocrinology and infertility,* 5th ed. Baltimore: Williams & Wlikins, 1994: 401–456, 667–687.
19. Klein SM, Garcia CR. Asherman's syndrome: a critique and current review. *Fertil Steril* 1973;24::722–735.
20. Goddijn M, Emanuel MH, Wiers PW, et al. Tuberculosis as an unusual cause of oligomenorrhea and infertility. *Ned Tijdschr Geneeskd* 1997;141:105–107.
21. Keita N, Koulibaly M, Hijazy Y, et al. *Contracept Fertil Sex* 1999; 27:155–161.
22. Bukulmez O, Yarali H, Gurgan T. Total corporeal synechiae due to tuberculosis carry a very poor prognosis following hysteroscopic synechiolysis. *Hum Reprod* 1999;14:1960–1961.
23. Krassas GE, Pontikides N, Kaltsas T, et al. Disturbances of menstruation in hypothyroidism. *Clin Endocrinol* 1999;50:655–659.
24. Ledger GA, Khosala S, Lindor NM, et al. Genetic testing in the diagnosis and management of multiple endocrine neoplasia type II. *Ann Intern Med* 1995;122:118–124.
25. American Psychiatric Association. *Diagnostic and statistical manual of mental disorders,* 4th ed. Washington, DC: American Psychiatric Association, 1994.
26. Pirke KM, Fichter MM, Chloud C, et al. Disturbances of the menstrual cycle in bulimia nervosa. *Clin Endocrin* 1987;27: 245–251.
27. Schweiger U, Pirke KM, Laessle RG, et al. Gonadotropin secretion in bulimia nervosa. *J Clin Endocrin Metab* 1992;74: 1122–1127.
28. Barr SI. Vegetarianism and menstrual cycle disturbances: is there an association? *Am J Clin Nutr* 1999;70(suppl):549–554.
29. Warren MP, Stiehl AL. Exercise and female adolescents: effects on the reproductive and skeletal system. *J Am Womens Assoc* 1999; 54:115–120, 138.
30. Greene JW. Menstruation irregularities associated with athletics exercise. *Compr Ther* 1999;25:209–215.
31. Gidwani GP. Amenorrhea in the athlete. *Adolesc Med* 1999; 10:275–290.
32. Barnhart KT, Simhan H, Kamelle SA. Diagnostic accuracy of ultrasound above and below the beta-hCG discriminatory zone. *Obstet Gynecol* 1999;94:583–587.
33. Dumesic DA. Hormonal evaluation of androgen excess. In: Azziz R, Nestler JE, Dewailly D, eds. *Androgen excess in women.* Philadelphia: Lippincott-Raven, 1997:635–646.
34. Sugimoto O. Diagnostic and therapeutic hysteroscopy for traumatic intrauterine adhesions. *Am J Obstet Gynecol* 1978;131: 539–547.
35. Romer T. Intrauterine adhesions—etiology, diagnosis, therapy and possibilities for prevention. *Zentralbl Gynakol* 1994;116: 311–317.
36. March CM. Intrauterine adhesions. *Obstet Gynecol Clin North Am* 1995;22:491–505.
37. Bellingham FR. Intrauterine adhesions: hysteroscopic lysis and adjunctive methods. *Aust N Z J Obstet Gynecol* 1996;36: 171–174.
38. Salle B, Gaucherand P, de Saint Hilaire P, et al. Transvaginal sonohysterographic evaluation of intrauterine adhesions. *J Clin Ultrasound* 1999;27:131-134.
39. American Fertility Society. Classifications of adnexal adhesions, distal tubal occlusion, tubal occlusion to tubal ligation, tubal pregnancies, müllerian anomalies and intrauterine adhesions. *Fertil Steril* 1988;49:944
40. Neuberg M, Pawlosek W, Jakubowska-Szwed B, et al. Repeated amenorrhea in an adolescent girl in the course of flood disaster in Klodzko Region, July 1997. *Ginecol Pol* 1999;70:378–382.

41. Iglesias EA, Coupey SM. Menstrual cycle abnormalities: diagnosis and management. *Adolesc Med* 1999;10:255–273.

42. Gidwani GP. Amenorrhea in the athlete. *Adolesc Med* 1999;10:275–290, vii.

43. Bachrach LK, Katzman DK, Litt IF, et al. Recovery from osteopenia in adolescent girls with anorexia nervosa. *J Clin Endocrinol Metab* 1991;72:602–606.

44. Jonnavithula S, Warren MP, Fox RP, et al. Bone density is compromised in amenorrheic women despite return of menses: a 2-year study. *Obstet Gynecol* 1993;81:669–674.

45. McKenzie DC. Markers of excessive exercise. *Can J Appl Physiol* 1999;24:66–73.

46. Warren MP, Voussoughian F, Geer EB, et al. Functional hypothalamic amenorrhea: hypoleptinemia and disordered eating. *J Clin Endocrinol Metab* 1999;84:873–877.

47. Miller KK, Parulekar MS, Schoenfield E, et al. Decreased leptin levels in normal weight women with hypothalamic amenorrhea: the effects of body composition and nutritional intake. *J Clin Endocrinol Metab* 1988;83:2309–2312.

48. Leibowitz SF, Alexander JT. *Biol Psychiatry* 1998;44:851–864.

49. Bringer J, Lefebvre P, Renard E. Nutritional hypogonadism. *Rev Prat* 1999;49:1291–1296.

50. Homburg R, Eshel E, Armar NA, et al. One hundred pregnancies after treatment with pulsatile luteinizing hormone releasing hormone to induce ovulation. *BMJ* 1989;296:962–965.

51. Stahelin HB. Malnutrition and mental functions. *Z Gerontol Geriatr* 1999;32(suppl 1):127–130.

52. DeCherney AH, Laufer N. The monitoring of ovulation induction using ultrasound and estrogen. *Clin Obstet Gynecol* 1984;27:993–1002.

53. Gillet JY, Andre G, Faguer B, et al. Induction of amenorrhea during replacement therapy: optimal micronized progesterone dose. A multicenter study. *Maturitas* 1994;19:103–115.

54. Fitzpatrick LA, Good A. Micronized progesterone: clinical indications and comparison with current treatments. *Fertil Steril* 1999;72:389–397.

55. Shangold MM, Tomai TP, Cook JD, et al. Factors associated with withdrawal bleeding after administration of oral micronized progesterone in women with secondary amenorrhea. *Fertil Steril* 1991;56:1040–1047.

56. Parkes D. Bromocriptine. *N Engl J Med* 1979;301:873–878.

57. Kletzky OA, Vermech M. Effectiveness of vaginal bromocriptine in treating women with hyperprolactinemia. *Fertil Steril* 1989;51:266–272.

58. Lengyel AM, Mussio W, Imamura P, et al. Long-acting injectable bromocriptine (Parlodel LAR) in the chronic treatment of prolactin-secreting macroadenomas. *Fertil Steril* 1993;59:980–997.

59. Rains CP, Bryson HM, Fitton A. Cabergoline. A review of its pharmacological properties and therapeutic potential in the treatment of hyperprolactinemia and inhibition of lactation. *Drugs* 1995;49:255–279.

60. Verhelst J, Abs R, Maiter D, et al. Cabergoline in the treatment of hyperprolactinemia: a study in 455 patients. *J Clin Endocrinol Metab* 1999;84:2518–2522.

61. Motta T, deVincentis S, Marchini M, et al. Vaginal cabergoline in the treatment of hyperprolactinemic patients intolerant to oral dopaminergics. *Fertil Steril* 1996;65:440–442.

62. Biller BM. Hyperprolactinemia. *Int J Fertil Womens Med* 1999;44:74–77.

63. Colao A, Di Sarno A, Sarnacchiaro F, et al. Prolactinomas resistant to standard dopamine agonists, respond to chronic cabergoline treatment. *J Clin Endocrinol Metab* 1997;82:876–883.

64. Branigan EF, Estes MA. Treatment of chronic anovulation resistant to clomiphene citrate (CC) by using oral contraceptive ovarian suppression followed by repeat CC treatment. *Fertil Steril* 1999;71:544–546.

65. Daly DC, Qalters CA, Soto-Albors CE, et al. A randomized study of dexamethasone in ovulation induction with clomiphene citrate. *Fertil Steril* 1984;41:844–848.

66. Roge P, D'Ercole, Cravell L, et al. Hysteroscopic management of uterine synechiae: a series of 102 observations. *Eur J Obstet Gynecol Reprod Biol* 1996;65:189–193.

67. Ostrzenski A. Resectoscopic cervical trauma minimized by inserting *Laminaria digitata* preoperatively. *Int J Fertil* 1994;39:111–113.

68. Sadrzadeh S, Wamsteker K, Hummel P, et al. Secondary amenorrhea due to intrauterine adhesions: Asherman's syndrome. *Ned Tijdschr Geneeskd* 1998;142:2329–2332.

69. Kubista E, Boschitsch E, Spona J. Effect of ear-acupuncture on the LH-concentration in serum in patients with secondary amenorrhea. *Wien Med Wochenschr* 1981;131:123–126.

70. Yu J, Zheng HM, Ping SM. Changes in serum FSH, LH and ovarian follicular growth during electroacupuncture for induction of ovulation. *Chung His I Chih* 1989;9:195, 199–202.

71. Zicari N, Ricciotti F, Zicari D. Endocrinology and acupuncture. *Minerva Med* 1983;74:2513–2519.

72. Chen BY, Yu J. Relationship between blood radioimmunoreactive beta-endorphin and hand skin temperature during the electroacupuncture induction of ovulation. *Acupunct Electrother Res* 1991;16:1–5.

73. Chen BY. Acupuncture normalizes dysfunction of hypothalamic-pituitary-ovarian axis. *Acupunct Electrother Res* 1997;22:97–108.

74. Gerhard I, Postneek F. Possibilities of therapy by ear acupuncture in female sterility. *Geburtshilfe Frauenheilkd* 1988;48:165–171.

75. Broso R, Subrizi R. Gynecologic problems in female athletes. *Minerva Ginecol* 1996;48:99–106.

76. Dueck CA, Matt KS, Manore MM, et al. Treatment of athletic amenorrhea with a diet and training intervention program. *Int J Sport Nutr* 1996:24–40.

77. Larsen HM, Hansen IL. Effect of specific training on menstruation and bone strength. *Ugeskr Laeger* 1998;160:4762–4767.

78. Cumming DC. Exercise-associated amenorrhea, low bone density, and estrogen replacement therapy. *Arch Intern Med* 1996;156:2193–2195.

79. Manore MM, Thompson J, Russo M. Diet and exercise strategies of world-class bodybuilder. *Int J Sport Nutr* 1993;3:76–86.

80. Economos CD, Bortz SS, Nelson ME. Nutritional practices of elite athletes. Practical recommendations. *Sports Med* 1993,16:381–399.

81. Hudson T. *Women's encyclopedia of natural medicine. Alternative therapies and integrative medicine.* Lincolnwood, IL: Keats, Division of NTS/Contemporary Publishing Group, 1999:15–27.

82. Lehmann-Willenbrock, Riedel HH. Clinical and endocrinologic studies of the treatment of ovarian insufficiency manifestations following hysterectomy with intact adnexa. *Zentralbl Gynakol* 1988;110:611–618.

83. Cakill DJ, Fox R, Wardle PG, et al. Multiple follicular development associated with herbal medicine. *Hum Reprod* 1994;9:1469–1470.

84. Chopra D, ed. *Alternative medicine. The definitive guide.* Tiburon, CA: Future Medicine Publishing, 1997:936–937.

85. Fetrow CW, Avila JR. The compete guide to herbal medicines. Springhouse, PA: Springhouse Corporation, 1999:126–127, 190.

86. Milewicz A. Gejdel E, Sworen H, et al. Vitex agnus castus extract in the treatment of luteal phase defect due to latent hyperprolactinemia. Results of a randomized placebo-controlled double-blind study. *Arzneimittelforschung* 1993;43:752–756.

87. Holtzscher A, Legros AS. *Pratique homeopathique en gynecologie.* Boiron, France: Centre d'Enseignement et de Developpement de l'Homeopathie, 1994.

10

DYSFUNCTIONAL UTERINE BLEEDING

EDUCATIONAL OBJECTIVES

Medical Students (1) *APGO Objective*	*Residents in Obstetrics/Gynecology (2)* *CREOG Objectives*	*Practitioners (3)* *ACOG Recommendations*
Definition	Pertinent history	Diagnosis
Causes	Physical examination	Differential diagnosis
Pathophysiology	Diagnostic studies	Physical findings
Diagnosis	Diagnosis	Endometrial sampling
Management	Management	Laboratory studies
	Follow-up	Management

DEFINITION

Dysfunctional uterine bleeding (DUB) is characterized by abnormal, irregular endometrial bleeding (excessively heavy, prolonged, or frequent intervals of bleeding) in the absence of an identifiable organic cause or systemic medical illness.

INCIDENCE

The incidence of DUB is unknown; however, a menstrual blood loss of more than 80 mL (menorrhagia) is estimated to occur in 9% to 14% of women (4). In abnormal endometrial bleeding, an identifiable, specific organic cause is diagnosed in less than 5.0%.

CLASSIFICATION

Anovulatory dysfunctional uterine bleeding accounts for 90% of DUB and most commonly takes place at pubertal or perimenopausal ages. Ovulatory dysfunctional uterine bleeding occurs in about 10% of DUB cases and is associated with the luteal phase defect or mid-cycle bleeding.

ETIOLOGY

Dysfunctional uterine bleeding may occur in any medical condition that is associated with a chronic estrus status (constant lack of a cyclic blood level of estrogen). It occurs in medical entities such as obesity, anorexia, polycystic ovar-ian syndrome, adrenal hyperplasia, hypothyroidism, hyperthyroidism, hyperprolactinemia, renal disease, liver disease, and other severe systemic illnesses.

Any disturbance within the hypothalamic–pituitary–ovarian axis or increasing fibrinolytic activity *in utero* may lead to anovulation, or to an inadequate menstrual cycle, even when ovulation occurs. In many instances trivial emotional turbulence such as anxiety, stress, or any psychogenic factor can cause functional breakdown of the hypothalamus. Physical distress associated with substantial weight reduction, anorexia nervosa (malnutrition), obesity, or intense exercise may interfere with pulsatile gonadotropin-releasing hormone (GnRH) secretion from the hypothalamus, even when adequate and timely feedback signals are present. It has been documented that in the anovulatory cycle, pulsatile GnRH secretion is greater due to central opioid tone suppression by the chronic absence of progesterone (5–7). Therefore, LH pulsatile frequency and amplitude are higher when compared with the mid-follicular phase of the regular menstrual cycle (5,8).

A benign anterior pituitary tumor (adenoma) is the principal concern in establishing pituitary dysfunction in DUB. A malignant primary pituitary growth is a remote occurrence (5,9–11); however, it must be borne in mind. A biologically active pituitary adenoma (micro- or macroadenoma) may secrete excessive prolactin and lead to hyperprolactinemia, which causes menstrual disturbances, including, but not limited to, those affecting ovulation.

Uterine fibrinolytic activity is amplified in the DUB due to elevated prostacyclin and an increased ratio of prostaglandin E_2 (PGE_2) to PGF_{2a}. This altered environment enhances vasodilatation, myometrial relaxation, reduced platelet aggregation, and increased endometrial bleeding (12). It has been postulated that angiogenesis [the process of new capillaries developing from preexisting vessels (13)] is an important mechanism in cyclic regeneration of the endometrium, and it appears to be abnormal in DUB (13,14) when compared with an ovulatory cycle (15,16).

In an anovulatory cycle, which is the most common scenario for DUB (17), neuroendocrine [follicle-stimulating hormone (FSH) gonadotropin] secretion can stimulate the follicles and trigger ovarian steroidogenesis; however, the mechanism is insufficient to release the ovum. By this mechanism, ovarian function is limited to producing estrogens, and no progesterone can be synthesized and released by the ovary. Peripherally, the endometrium (the end estrogen target) is constantly under estrogen stimulation and, in return, proliferates, leading to excessive angiogenesis (vascularization) and hyperplasia without parallel stromal build-up to give adequate support. At the same time, the conversion from a proliferative to a secretory type of endometrium will not occur because of a lack of progesterone to oppose the estrogen hormone. In such a scenario, when the level of estrogen is not sufficient to support continuation of endometrial proliferation, breakthrough bleeding develops. Whether gonadotropin secretion is inadequate, follicular response to gonadotropin is encumbered, or both, remains unclear.

Based on this analysis, a question arises: is each anovulatory cycle associated with chronic high plasma estrogen concentration? The answer is no, because chronic low plasma estrogen concentration may produce DUB as well; however, endometrial bleeding is lighter and less frequent than in a high chronic plasma estrogen concentration. Consequently, DUB may precede secondary amenorrhea, because both of these conditions come from chronic anovulation.

In 90% of cases, DUB is associated with an anovulatory cycle and 10% with an ovulatory one. A delicate alternation in the mechanism of ovulation or a physiologic reduction of estrogens in mid-cycle may create endometrial bleeding. An ovulatory cycle does not guarantee an adequate length of the proliferative or secretory phases of the menstrual cycle; therefore, it may result in disturbances in both frequency and duration of the cycle. Such an abnormality may lead to polymenorrhea (a menstrual cycle interval of <21 days) or menorrhagia (excessive menstrual effluent, >80 mL of blood loss per cycle, and prolonged endometrial bleeding for >8 days), or luteal phase deficiency (decreased quantity of progesterone, secreted by the corpus luteum, to support adequately the 13–14 days of luteal phase). Persistent corpus luteum may occur in association with the ovulatory cycle.

Irregular shedding of the endometrium, which is often called uterine lining asynchrony, is another condition in this group (a synchronous or simultaneous desquamation in all parts of the endometrium is expected). These conditions are often self-limiting, and the clinical course is not as dramatic as is encountered in an anovulatory cycle (18).

Systemic hereditary and acquired medical conditions can cause abnormal, excessive endometrial bleeding, such as von Willebrand disease (quantitative and qualitative defects of the von Willebrand factor), including subtypes and acquired forms of this disease, congenital deficiency of factor XI, carriers of hemophilia A or B, idiopathic thrombocytopenic purpura, acquired platelet disorder, acquired autoantibodies against factor VIII, and vitamin K deficiency.

Recently, a hypothesis on the role of subclinical bacteria of the endometrium (bacteria endometrialis) was postulated as a possible cause of DUB.

Other possible causes are microorganisms, possibly those associated with bacterial vaginosis (a noninflammatory condition). These microorganisms may surreptitiously inhibit the endometrium and lead to bleeding (19).

DIAGNOSIS

A diagnosis of DUB is reached via the exclusion of pregnancy and any organic causes of bleeding.

Step I

The menstrual pattern (menstrual interval, duration, and amount of bleeding) will reveal a lack of regular occurrences and the predictability of menses, as well as the absence of premenstrual molimina (abdominal bloating, breast engorgement, peripheral edema, weight gain, uterine cramps, and mood swings). These changes will be noticeable in the ovulatory cycle.

More than 80 mL of menstrual blood loss is considered the cut-off point, and requires a careful patient evaluation and education, because counting sanitary pads or tampons used in clinical assessment is an unreliable method (20) [in a moderately saturated sanitary napkin (perineal pad) or tampon, approximately 10–15 mL of menstrual blood is present]. In the 1990s, a more reliable clinical method was developed to differentiate menorrhagia from expected menstrual blood loss (4,21). A pictorial menstrual blood loss chart is based on diagrams corresponding to lightly, moderately, and heavily soiled sanitary pads or tampons (Fig 10.1). A scoring system requires the comparison of the diagrams with a patient's blood-soiled pads or tampons and multiplying them by 1 when matched with a light diagram, by 5 when matched with a moderate diagram, by 20 for a pad, and by 10 for a tampon when matched with a heavy diagram, respectively. A score of greater than or equal to 100 confirms menorrhagia (21). However, it has been documented that the cut-off point should be individualized (4). Use of the pictorial menstrual blood loss chart method yielded a sensitivity of 86% and a specificity of 89% when the scores were recorded by women, and a sensitivity of 86% and a specificity of 81% when recorded by gynecologists (21). Independent clinical studies verified these data with sensitivity and specificity of 91.0% and 81.9%, respectively (4).

TAMPON	SANITARY NAPKINS	CONSECUTIVE DAYS OF MENSES								MULTIPLICATION FACTOR	
		1	2	3	4	5	6	7	8	Tampon	S. Napkins
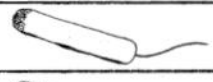	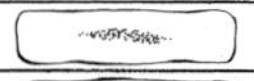									1	1
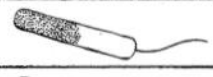	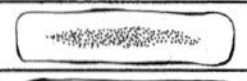									5	5
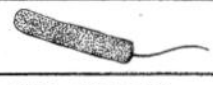	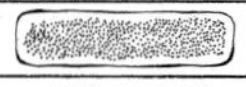									10	10
CLOTS	CLOTS									10	20
									Total Score		

FIGURE 10.1. The pictorial menstrual blood loss chart. (Modifed from Fraser IS, McCarron G, Markham R. Blood and total fluid content of menstrual discharge. *Obstet Gynecol* 1985;65:194–198; with permission.)

The popular clinical conviction that the volume of clots has a predictive capacity has not been verified, so charting the clots to determine blood loss is unnecessary (4).

■ Medication predisposing toward toward endometrial bleeding: gonadal steroids, psychopharmacology agents, autonomic drugs, morphine, reserpine, phenothiazines, monoamine oxidase inhibitors, anticholinergic drugs
■ Natural herbal medicine predisposing toward endometrial bleeding: aloes, *Cascara sagrada,* excessive garlic consumption, ginseng, myrrh (22–29)
■ Methods of contraception [intrauterine devices (IUDs), missed oral contraceptive pills] or low dose of oral contraceptive may cause unexpected endometrial bleeding.

General physical examination is usually within normal limits. Patient's weight should be noted, because being either over or underweight may produce an anovulatory cycle that can result in DUB. Presence of petechiae may indicate thrombocytopenia, and ecchymoses can suggest coagulation disorders.

Pelvic examination will reveal no abnormalities; however, lower genital tract injury must be ruled out. Papanicolaou (Pap) smear and multiple cervical cultures should also be obtained. Endometrial biopsy should be performed in all patients with a history of chronic exposure to unopposed estrogens. In a sexually inactive teenager, a rectal examination is recommended, but no Pap smear or endometrial biopsy is indicated.

Initial laboratory studies should include a complete blood count with a blood smear, which will assist in evaluating blood loss, in order to rule out anemia, and any preexisting hereditary or acquired hematologic conditions. An adequate platelet count excludes thrombocytopenia, and leukocytosis may indicate the possibility of the presence of infection. Blood typing and cross-matching should be performed when indicated.

Clotting studies should include partial thromboplastin time (PTT), prothrombin time (PT), and bleeding time. A serum quantitative beta human chorionic gonadotropin (beta-hCG) test or another pregnancy test is recommended.

Step II

When the pregnancy test result is positive, the following clinical approach is advisable:

■ Determining the existence of an ectopic pregnancy (serial quantitative beta-hCG, ultrasonography, laparoscopy).
■ Determining threatening abortion (serial quantitative beta-hCG, progesterone level, ultrasonography)
■ Determining the presence of a hydatidiform mole (serial quantitative beta-hCG, ultrasonography)

When the pregnancy test result is negative:

■ Initiate an adequate hormonal therapy when profuse bleeding is present
■ Consider the following laboratory studies based on clinical findings: thyroid function tests [triiodothyronine (T_3), thyroxine (T_4) thyroid-stimulating hormone (TSH)], serum prolactin, serum androgens (androstenedione, total and free testosterone), and dehydroepiandrosterone sulfate (DHEAS); and liver function tests, renal function tests, and blood glucose.
■ Further clinical investigation is necessary to exclude an organic cause (Table 10.1). It is crucial to remember that an organic cause for DUB may coexist with chronic anovulation, and both entities should be taken into account in a patient's treatment.

TABLE 10.1. ORGANIC CAUSES OF DYSFUNCTIONAL UTERINE BLEEDING

Vulvar Lesions	Vaginal Lesions	Cervical Lesions	Uterine Lesions	Other Lesions
Infection	Infection	Infection	Infection	Ovarian functional or
Trauma	Trauma	Erosion	Leiomyomata	neoplastic tumor
Benign and malignant	Foreign body	Polyps	Polyps	Polycystic ovary
neoplasm	Pessaries	Benign or malignant	Benign or malignant	Urethral caruncle or
	Benign or malignant	neoplasm	neoplasm	infected diverticulum
	neoplasm		IUD	Gastrointestinal bleeding
			Adenomyosis	Intrauterine device
				Adrenal disorder
				Thyroid disorder
				Liver or renal disease
				Pituitary tumor

The number of procedures are valuable in reaching the diagnosis. *Endometrial biopsy* (EB) is seldom indicated in an adolescent patient, but it is very helpful in a patient with a chronic anovulatory cycle. It is generally acceptable to perform EB on women 35 or older, before initiation of hormone therapy, and on younger patients when a significant risk for endometrial cancer is identified, when bleeding lasts 15 days per month, when the patient is unresponsive to hormonal therapy, when bleeding is severe, or when the patient has frequent or prolonged anemia. Results generated from the EB provide valuable information, not only for premalignancy (cytonuclear atypical changes in endometrial hyperplasia) or malignancy, but also for the proliferative versus secretory endometrium, luteal phase defects, the asynchronous versus synchronous endometrium, acute or chronic endometritis, and chronic focal endometritis. Customarily, EB is performed 2 to 3 days before menses, and no later than 24 hours after commencement of bleeding, including metrorrhagia (irregular occurrence, heavy flow, prolong duration of endometrial bleeding).

It has been documented that a sufficient tissue amount is obtained during endometrial sampling in about 90% of cases, and diagnostic precision for malignancy is about 95%, whereas approximately 90% of endometrial hyperplasias can be diagnosed histologically, and a diagnosis of endometrial polyps can be established in 75% of cases (30–32). It has been recommended that, prior to the initiation of medical therapy, an endometrial biopsy be used to exclude the premalignant or malignant process, depending on the patient's age (33). However, from a practical point of view, the duration of exposure to unopposed estrogens should influence a clinical decision for endometrial biopsy rather than the patient's age. It has been proven that teenagers or young women may present with atypical hyperplasia, carcinoma *in situ,* or invasive endometrial carcinoma (34).

Hysteroscopy is indicated when conservative medical management fails and an intracavitary organic cause for DUB is suspected (30). In today's practice, office hysteroscopy with endometrial sampling, particularly a flexible one, is a useful tool in experienced hands. Women who are unresponsive to initial hormonal therapy or who experience heavy, prolonged, and frequent endometrial bleeding will benefit from this procedure. It will assist in reaching a diagnosis when submucosal leiomyomata, endometrial polyps, or a missing IUD are factors.

Ultrasonography of the pelvis, either with a transabdominal or transvaginal transducer, has a limited role in the diagnosis of endometrial cavity abnormalities. However, sonohysterography (contrast sonography) is considered a very effective method for uterine intracavitary lesions (35). This technique is a superior method of hysterosalpingography (36) and has yielded similar results with less discomfort than an office hysteroscopy (37). Because sonohysterography can be performed independently of the phase of the menstrual cycle, it makes this technique even more attractive (38). A drawback of this method is the inability to obtain a tissue specimen at the same time.

A basal body temperature (BBT) chart may assist in indirectly assuming an anovulatory versus ovulatory cycle, and it may suggest a luteal phase defect. Traditionally, a monophasic cycle is considered to be an indicator of anovulation, but in approximately 75% of cases, when a BBT graph was monophasic, the hormonal assay supported ovulation, thus making BBT an imperfect method (39). However, it is helpful when an unambiguous, biphasic BBT graph is at hand, because it helps to determine the presence of an ovulatory cycle. When a temperature elevation lasts fewer than 10 days for at least two consecutive menstrual cycles, this strongly suggests a defective, overly brief luteal phase (40). For these reasons, some authorities incorporate a BBT chart (recording temperature for 6–8 weeks) into their diagnostic armamentarium for DUB diagnosis (41). However, histologic endometrial dating for luteal phase defects remains the most accepted method of practice. Retrospectively, two separate, consecutive endometrial biopsy results are analyzed. When the results of endometrial dating demonstrate that the endometrium maturation lags more than 2 days behind the time in the cycle, a luteal phase defect is diagnosed.

In an adolescent patient, the clotting mechanism can be impaired in platelet disorders, von Willebrand disease, thalassemia major, leukemia, or Fanconi anemia, and it is quite a common event (30). Therefore, when there is a clinical sign (petechiae or ecchymoses) and laboratory data (platelets, PT, PTT, or bleeding time) indicating possible coagulation disorders, a hematology consultation is advisable.

DIFFERENTIAL DIAGNOSIS

- Pregnancy complications
- Hormonal imbalance
- Pelvic pathology
- Systemic illness
- Coagulopathy

CONVENTIONAL THERAPY

Upon establishing a DUB diagnosis, the primary therapeutic objectives fall into five categories:

- To control an acute episode of endometrial bleeding
- To prevent DUB recurrence
- To minimize the duration and the amount of bleeding
- To establish a rhythm and a predictability of menses
- Iron replacement

With few exceptions, DUB can be managed conservatively, because it is a benign medical entity. However, it is essential to exercise particular caution when conservative management is instituted and atypical endometrial hyperplasia or persistent unresponsive hyperplasia to hormonal therapy is present. DUB is a benign condition, but it may progress to endometrial adenocarcinoma; therefore, precise treatment and follow-up plans should be presented to the patient, including endometrial biopsy after 6 months of therapy. In this particular circumstance, histology results will eventually establish the course of prospective care.

As a general rule, correction of any defined endocrinopathy (e.g., hypothyroidism, hyperthyroidism, hyperprolactinemia, hypercortisonemia, hypocortisonemia), systemic illness (e.g., liver or renal disease), or endometrial infection will yield much better results than hormonally induced menstrual cycles. In the majority of patients, artificial, predictable endometrial bleeding results from estrogen-progesterone therapy; however, this type of management does not induce ovulation in a chronic anovulatory cycle. Ovulation induction can be entertained as a mode of therapy (clomiphene citrate, gonadotropin or other conventional-complementary-alternative medicine methods) when the patient desires pregnancy.

Iron-deficiency anemia (iron-deficient erythropoiesis anemia) is often a sequela of DUB. It has been reported that

60 mL of blood loss per cycle, in a chronic pattern, significantly increases the risk of iron-deficiency anemia (42,43). Clinically, iron-deficiency anemia may present with symptoms such as dizziness, headache, heart palpitations, and fatigue. The following laboratory parameters will assist in making the diagnosis:

- Hemoglobin (Hb) concentration less than 12 g/dL
- Hematocrit less than 37%
- Mean corpuscular volume (MCV) less than 80 g/L,
- Mean corpuscular hemoglobin concentration less than 30%
- Serum iron level less than 50 µg/dL
- Iron saturation less than 30% but more than 10%
- Serum ferritin levels less than 15 µg/L
- Moderately elevated total iron-binding capacity

The therapy is aimed at three goals:

- Treatment of the cause of blood loss
- Oral iron therapy (ferrous sulfate 300- to 325-mg tablets three times daily)
- Parenteral iron therapy is considered when a patient cannot tolerate oral iron intake. For each 1 g/100 mL deficit in hemoglobin concentration, approximately 250 mg of iron dextran (Imferon) is needed. It can be administered intramuscularly (IM) or intravenously (IV). When IV therapy is planned, the total cumulative iron amount required for the therapy should be calculated by the formula:

$$0.3 \times \text{body weight (lbs)} \times [(100 - \text{Hb g/100 mL}) \times 100] = 14.\,8 \text{ total iron, in mg required (1 mL of iron dextran contains 50 mg of iron)}.$$

An anaphylactic reaction is the most serious side effect, but it is not a common event.

Intravenous Therapy and Acute Severe Hemorrhage

Acute, severe genital hemorrhage may lead to hemodynamic and metabolic instability, or to shock. After acute bleeding, resulting in a hematocrit of less than 25%, the first step in treatment is to replete volume with IV crystalloids, colloids, or blood or blood products. At the same time, the cause of bleeding must be eradicated, which can be initiated with IV conjugated estrogen in DUB.

Intravenous conjugated estrogen can be administered in a dose of 20 to 25 mg, every 4 hours, until bleeding stops. It usually takes 12 hours to control hemorrhage (44). When acute, severe bleeding decreases appreciably, and estrogen oral therapy should be instituted in doses corresponding to 1.25 to 3.75 mg of conjugated estrogen per day. If bleeding intensifies during the oral estrogen treatment plan, the dose and interval of estrogen administration may be adjusted (1.25 mg of conjugated estrogen or 2 mg of estradiol every

4 hours). The oral estrogen dose should be continued for 21 consecutive days, followed by a progestational agent for 7 to 10 days (oral medroxyprogesterone acetate 10–20 mg/day, or norethindrone 5–10 mg/day; IM 17-alpha-hydroxyprogesterone 125 mg or progesterone in oil 50–100 mg, monthly). This way, estrogen combined with a progestational agent during the preceding 7 days will create better hormonal support to control withdrawal bleeding.

If bleeding does not stop or considerably subside within 24 hours, dilatation and curettage and reevaluation to determine a possible organic cause of bleeding should be considered.

Intravenous or daily multiple oral doses of estrogen are considered to be a high dose, which raises the possibility of inducing thrombosis, a potentially life-threatening condition. Reviewing the world body of literature, there is no documented case verifying the potential of inducing thrombosis.

In an adolescent patient with heavy, acute endometrial bleeding, using progesterone or progestin will not provide a desirable therapeutic effect because initial endometrial estrogen exposure is required to induce a progesterone effect on the endometrium.

Desmopressin, a synthetic analogue of desamino-8-arginine vasopressin (0.3 μg/kg diluted in 50 mL saline) is given within 30 minutes (45). This medication can release an autologous von Willebrand factor from endothelial cells, correcting factor VIII levels and bleeding time. This mechanism is sufficient to avert bleeding (46). Such clinical management is indicated in a select group of patients with DUB associated with severe coagulation disorders.

Oral Therapy for Dysfunctional Uterine Bleeding

The *oral contraceptive pill*, a monophasic estrogen-progestin with a formulation of 35 μg or less of the estrogen component (the low dose), is administered as one pill, twice a day, and thereafter, continuing for 5 to 7 days, despite bleeding cessation or the significant subsidence of flow within 24 hours. Within 2 to 4 days upon discontinuation of oral contraceptive, heavy endometrial bleeding and cramping recur. Consulting a patient about the expected pattern of heavy bleeding within a short interval (2–4 days) will preclude patient's anxiety associated with thoughts of an incurable condition or the fear of failure of the hormonal therapy. On the 5th day of bleeding, one oral contraceptive pill for the next 21 days is prescribed, with a 7-day break, and this mode is continued for 3 consecutive months. A good prognostic sign is achieved when cramping and the amount of bleeding are decreasing during the course of the 3 months of oral contraceptive therapy.

If the patient requires contraception, oral contraceptives can be offered for both therapeutic and contraceptive purposes. Oral contraceptives must be discontinued when undesirable side effects (headache, nausea, elevated blood pressure, or venous thrombosis) arise. Predictable, timely menses after 3 months of therapy is very reassuring, so the patient should be observed closely. Waiting for spontaneous menses is advised after discontinuing oral contraceptives. If spontaneous menses do not occur on time, an oral progestational agent (Provera, or Norlutate, or Norlutein) is instituted for 10 days, and endometrial bleeding should occur within 2 to 7 days. Starting on the 16th day of an induced menstrual cycle, oral progestin is administered for 10 days.

The effectiveness of oral contraceptives in decreasing DUB is estimated to be 53%, and the treatment is continued until menopause (47) or until the induction of ovulation is considered, when pregnancy is desired. Oral contraceptive pills are usually tolerated well; however, undesirable side effects may not allow continuing treatment (headache, nausea, breast engorgement, mood swing, edema, abdominal bloating, cholelithiasis, thrombotic disease, elevated blood pressure).

Progestin oral therapy is indicated when a proliferative endometrium is documented, and in most instances this mode of therapy will control abnormal endometrial bleeding (47). Such treatment is usually initiated with the following progestational agents:

- Medroxyprogesterone acetate (Provera), 10 to 20 mg daily for 10 to 14 days (5), or from days 19 to 26 of the cycle (47) of each month. This medication will not prevent ovulation; therefore, another form of contraception should be offered to a patient when indicated (a barrier method, tubal sterilization, vasectomy, or IUD).
- Norethindrone acetate (Norlutate), 5 to 10 mg daily for 10 to 14 days (5), or from days 19 to 26 of the cycle (47) each month
- Norethindrone (Norlutin), 5 to 10 mg daily for 10 to 14 days (5), or from days 19 to 26 of the cycle (47) each month
- Megestrol acetate (Megace) 40 mg daily, continuous mode for 3 months

Patient compliance, an adequate dose, and duration of the therapy per cycle are vital to a successful outcome. Unquestionably, progestin, when administered as luteal phase replacement therapy in an anovulatory type of DUB, is a successful modality (47). In a case where all of these parameters are properly addressed and DUB is uncontrollable, reevaluation to establish causation is in order. To prevent DUB from recurring, an intermittent progestin agent or oral contraceptive pills can be used in long-term preventive medical care.

Due to progestin's side effects (e.g., headache, breast tenderness, abdominal bloating, nausea, weight gain, edema, and mood swing) (47,48) and their low clinical effectiveness (20%) in decreasing bleeding during an ovulatory cycle associated with DUB, administrating them as the first line of therapy is not advised (47).

Natural Progesterone Therapy

Micronized progesterone (Prometrium, 100-mg tablet) can be administered orally; however, there is a remarkable variation in the absorption rate between individuals (49). Regardless of these absorption differences, oral macronized progesterone (100 mg/day), when given with estradiol, effectively opposes proliferation in endometrial morphology (50).

It has been documented in randomized clinical trials that administration of transvaginal progesterone gel (Crione 4%, containing 45 g progesterone, or Crione 8%, containing 90 mg or 180 mg progesterone) every other day can transform the proliferative endometrium to a secretory endometrium in each of these doses, despite the low progesterone plasma level. This clinical endometrial response is highly suggestive of local, direct vagina-to-uterus transportation (a direct transit of progesterone into the endometrium).

In order to control and to sustain the release of progesterone, bioadhesives are incorporated into the polycarbophil-based gel (51,52). A vaginal, natural progesterone tablet (effervescent vaginal tablet, 100 mg/day) resulted in adequate progesterone concentrations (53).

Taking all of these parameters into account, natural progesterone can be used in the treatment of DUB; however, there are insufficient clinical studies to determine the safety and efficacy of natural progesterone in oral or local applications.

Danazol, an isoxazole derivative of 17-alpha-ethinyl-testosterone, increases androgenic (hyperandrogenism) levels, while decreasing estrogen levels (hypoestrogenism). This mechanism creates a particular hormonal milieu that is capable of slowing the growth of the endometrium. In randomized studies, danazol (100 mg, twice daily for 60–90 days) yielded a 58.9% reduction of endometrial bleeding (54) and was more statistically significant in its efficacy than progestins or nonsteroidal antiinflammatory drugs (54,55). The drawback to danazol therapy is that it cannot be used for long-term treatment due to its side effects (weight gain, acne, headache/migraine, abdominal bloating, muscle cramps, and premenstrual syndrome). However, in many patients the endometrial bleeding was reduced for up to 4 months after discontinuation of the therapy (47,56).

Intramuscular Injection for Dysfunctional Uterine Bleeding

Progesterone in oil (Lipolutin), 50 to 100 mg, or 17-alpha-hydroxyprogesterone (*Delalutin*), 125 mg, can be administered each month to patients who meet the therapeutic criteria for progestational agents.

Injection of *long-lasting medroxyprogesterone* acetate (150 mg) may indirectly inhibit ovarian function, creating transient hypoestrogenism, which with time will create changes in the endometrium, eventually leading to atrophy. By this mechanism, DUB can be controlled for some time.

Gonadotropin-releasing hormone analogue (injectable Lupron, 375 mg, every 28 days) inhibits the realization of pituitary follicle stimulating (FSH) and luteinizing (LH) hormones, which suppresses ovarian function and eventually leads to secondary amenorrhea (missing at least three previous menstrual cycles, or the absence of menstrual bleeding for 90 days). This medication is highly effective in controlling DUB (52); however, using GnRH for long intervals may inadvertently cause osteoporosis (GnRH increases calcium secretion and causes bone demineralization). When long-term therapy is planned, after 28 days from the initial injection of GnRH analogous, estrogen/progesterone replacement therapy can be instituted (57) (an equivalent of 0.625 mg conjugated estrogen, and 2.5 mg of medroxyprogesterone acetate is added in a continuous daily manner to counteract GnRH agonist side effects (osteoporosis). This modification of GnRH therapy permits treatment to continue for a longer time. GnRH treatment can be helpful after liver transplantation or when DUB is associated with blood dyscrasia or renal failure.

Progestin Intrauterine Device in Therapy for Dysfunctional Uterine Bleeding

A progestin IUD (20 µg of levonorgestrel per day) administered directly to the endometrium appeared to be the most effective therapy for DUB when compared with a prostaglandin synthetase inhibitor (flurbiprogen) and an antifibrinolytic agent (tranexamic acid) (59). This mode of therapy was able to reduce excessive bleeding below 80 mL per menses (80 mL is considered an upper limit for menstrual blood loss). Similarly, satisfactory results were presented with IUD progesterone (60).

Prostaglandin Synthetase Inhibitor in Therapy for Dysfunctional Uterine Bleeding

Prostaglandin synthetase inhibitors demonstrate the ability to reduce DUB bleeding by almost half (61), and when compared with progestational agents, they exhibit less effectiveness than do progestins (62) (Table 10.2).

Prostaglandin synthetase inhibitors are effective when an ovulatory cycle is documented and menorrhagia is present (47). This therapeutic approach should be considered as first-line treatment in this particular condition. This type of management also is effective in diminishing endometrial bleeding secondary to IUDs (63).

Antifibrinolytic Therapy

Upon reaching a diagnosis of DUB, antifibrinolytic medication (primarily epsilon aminocapronic acid or tranex-

TABLE 10.2. SELECTED NONSTEROIDAL ANTIINFLAMMATORY DRUGS FOR DYSFUNCTIONAL UTERINE BLEEDING THERAPY

Generic Name	Trade Name	Loading Dose	Maintenance Dose
Ibuprofen	Motrin	400 mg	400 mg every 4 h
	Rufen	1,200–1,600 mg	600–800 mg every 4 h
	IBU	1,200–1,600 mg	600–800 mg every 4 h
Naproxen	Naprosyn	500 mg	250 mg every 4–6 h
Naproxen sodium	Aflaxen	550 mg	275 mg every 6–8 h
	Anaprox	550 mg	275 mg every 6–8 h
Meclofenamate	Mecolmen	100 mg	50–100 mg every 4–6 h
Mefenamic acid	Ponstil	500 mg	250 mg every 4–6 h

amic acid, given in a single daily dose of 4 g for the first 3–5 days of the menstrual cycle or until the withdrawal of bleeding) (64) will significantly (84%) (47) reduce endometrial bleeding (65,66). Caution should be exercised in patients whose histories are indicative of thrombotic disorders or who are presenting with risk factors for thrombosis. Intracranial thrombosis was directly linked to antifibrinolytic therapy in three cases (47).

Surgical Therapy for Dysfunctional Uterine Bleeding

A surgical approach for the treatment of DUB may be considered for those patients in whom endometrial recurrent bleeding is refractory to conservative medical therapeutic modalities. Today, three surgical procedures are offered for the treatment of DUB:

- Endometrial curettage
- Hysterectomy
- Endometrial ablation

Dilatation and curettage (D & C) used to be the first line of therapy for almost any type of uterine bleeding. Today, by using modern diagnostic tools and methods (sonohysterography, office hysteroscopy, endometrial biopsy, steroid assays, neurohormone assays, and stimulating and inhibiting endocrinologic tests), and by better understanding the physiology of how the endometrium responds to hormones and hormonal therapy, and by implementing adequate conservative medical management, the role of curettage has been greatly reduced. It is still a useful procedure in determining endometrial hyperplasia or cancer; however, it notoriously misses endometrial polyps and focal endometritis submucosus leiomyomata.

When hormonal or nonhormonal conservative managements fails, clinical reevaluation to establish the eventual organic cause of DUB should be initiated, and D & C should be considered if the results of reevaluation are negative.

Hysterectomy for DUB is indicated for only a select group of patients, and it is rarely implemented. As a general recommendation (3), in DUB, the following criteria should be met to qualify the patient for hysterectomy:

- Fertility is no longer desired
- Various schemes of hormonal and iron therapy have failed
- Multiple curettage has failed to control bleeding
- Thorough diagnostic evaluations failed to reveal a specific or correctable pathology
- Atypical endometrial hyperplasia is present

These recommendations were suggested in 1989 by ACOG (3), and they still hold their validity, with one exception: multiple curettage. As stated above, there is little room for D & C in the current practice of medicine. If hysterectomy is ultimately indicated, the patient's care will be enhanced by decreasing numbers of laparotomy and an increasing proportion of vaginal hysterectomy and laparoscopic total abdominal hysterectomy (with suturing and tying intracorporeal and an extracorporeal technique, and the appropriate two-turn flat square knot without a transvaginal surgical approach) (67–69).

Endometrial Ablation

In the 1980s, endometrial ablation was introduced as a method to manage intractable uterine bleeding and to avoid hysterectomy (70). However, a randomized clinical trial has documented that two of every five patients (40%) who was subjected to endometrial ablation require further surgery at the 4-year follow-up evaluation (71). Additionally, the drawbacks to endometrial ablation include intraoperative (or shortly postoperative) hyponatremia and pulmonary edema (72), postsurgical menorrhagia, dysmenorrhea, DUB, pelvic pain, and granulomas of endometrium formation (73).

Regardless of the shortcomings of endometrial ablation, medical treatment is less effective than resection of the endometrium; therefore, early endometrial ablation can be presented for the patient's consideration after the full disclosure of pros and cons of this procedure (74).

The same indications should be applied to endometrial ablation as to the hysterectomy operation for DUB. Endometrial ablation should be performed only for intractable uterine bleeding, and when no other identifiable uterine or endometrial pathology is present. Such pure indications makes this procedure a rare one. Endometrial ablation cannot be considered when atypical endometrial hyperplasia or invasive carcinoma is present, when the patient is not prepared for the potential need of contraceptives (including but not limited to surgical sterilization), when the patient is not aware that menstrual bleeding may occur, and when the long-term effects of endometrial biopsy are unknown (75). Until recently, endometrial ablation was executed on an outpatient basis via a hysteroscope with a contact laser or electrocautery used to ablate the endometrium (65). Today, new, minimally invasive, nonhysteroscopic technologies are emerging to improve outcome and to minimize complications. The following new systems were introduced: thermoregulated, radiofrequency endometrial ablation (76); thermal balloon endometrial ablation (77); photodynamic ablation therapy (78); microwave endometrial ablation (79); and endometrial laser thermoablation, with a diode source (80). The clinical applicability of new technologies has been determined and published; however, documentation of the safety and effectiveness of these technologies is lacking, as are comparison studies among the technologies themselves to establish an eventual superiority.

COMPLEMENTARY THERAPY

Patient Education

One of the forms of DUB is associated with chronic anovulation. Unopposed estrogen levels may result in endometrial hyperplasia, which sometimes characterizes this hormonal milieu; atypical complex hyperplasia may lead to endometrial cancer. The length of hyperestrogenism, and not the age of a patient, determines the choice of this avenue of treatment. Therefore, each patient with a chronic, unopposed estrous status should be educated about such possibilities and how to prevent its precipitation. A patient's basic knowledge about a menstrual cycle is important for clinical communication and can be greatly enhanced using a pictorial menstrual chart. Unquestionably, chronic or severe stress plays a role in creating a hypothalamic type of anovulation; therefore, an effort should be made to familiarize patients with forms of stress control, or to refer them to stress reduction therapy to assist in the management of such cases.

Overweight patients must understand that reducing and maintaining their weight will help in the management of chronic anovulation. When necessary, patients can be referred to a registered, experienced dietitian, a behavioral therapist, and an exercise physiologist.

Nutritional Supplements

Vitamins

Vitamin C (with flavonoids) and vitamin A may help to control menorrhagia. Mixed bioflavonoids (plant compounds that can help maintain the natural state of small blood vessel walls) may decrease endometrial bleeding in mid-cycle or flow between menses therapeutic (83,90).

Acupuncture

Acupuncture can be used to restore hormonal imbalance associated with dysfunctional uterine bleeding, improve patient symptoms, and induce ovulation. Acupuncture is believed to nourish the uterus. Reinforcing and reducing acupuncture applications, liver and kidney function are enhanced. Through these mechanisms, a fine tune-up of the hypothalamus–pituitary–ovarian axis is achieved, and eventually ovulation is reestablished. Acupuncture therapy is applied in 30 separate sessions. Improvement, in various degrees, from this mode of treatment is reported to occur in 82.35% of patients, with marked patient improvement observed in 35.29% (81).

Electroacupuncture treatment is indicated for DUB associated with anovulation. It has been postulated that electroacupuncture induces ovulation through the regulation of hypothalamic–pituitary function. Such therapy establishes FSH and LH secretion within the expected normal range and balances the LH:FSH ratio in induced ovulation. Eliminating a chronic anovulatory cycle cures DUB. In both instances, acupuncture and electroacupuncture therapies present a unique treatment modality for DUB because of the potential for restoring ovulation (82).

Prospectively, these approaches have good potential for reaching long-lasting therapeutic effects by regulating the menstrual cycle, not artificially, but through the induction of ovulation. In contrast, in conventional, conservative medical management, the benefit often lasts only while the patient is on medication.

Exercise

An overweight condition may be the only cause of an anovulatory cycle and the link to DUB. An overweight patient will benefit from a variety of different forms of exercise. A fat-burning exercise program requires slow, continuous activity, which can be achieved with 45 to 60 minutes of brisk walking (83). The effect of life-style activity (walking instead of driving, stairs instead of an elevator or escalator, etc.) may offer similar health benefits to those of structural aerobic activity (84).

Walking is considered to be one of the easiest forms of exercise that burns calories and increases the metabolic rate. The best type of exercise is one that suits the individual's personality and is easy to implement. It is a well-recognized phenomenon that exercise creates a sense of happiness and well-being by increasing endorphins in the central nervous system. Therefore, in stress-related disorders, such as DUB, exercise will provide dual benefits: in weight reduction/maintenance and in coping with stress control. Whether or not weight reduction itself can permanently restore an ovulatory cycle remains an unanswered question. Although weight reduction complements induction of ovulation, weight loss also assists in the clinical management of DUB. An exercise program also helps to enhance the self-discipline that is crucial in developing a pattern of medical compliance.

Vigorous physical exercise or strenuous athletics may cause anovulation that may result in DUB or even in amenorrhea. On the other hand, moderate exercise provides all of the previously mentioned benefits.

Weight Management

In a well-designed weight reduction program for obesity, and the anovulation associated with this entity, weight loss and weight management are essential aspects. Obesity is considered to be a complex, multifactorial (genotype, social, behavioral, cultural, physiologic, and environmental) chronic disease. Guidelines recommend a minimum of 30 minutes of moderate physical activity daily, and reduced calorie consumption (85–87). It also has been established that the consumption of unhydrogenated, monounsaturated, and polyunsaturated fats is beneficial in preventing coronary heart disease in women (86).

Burning calories and decreasing calorie intake without compromising a well-balanced diet are key factors in losing weight and maintaining a reduced weight. Indeed, it is a process that takes time, and not only are the type and amount of food eaten important, but so are behavioral eating habits. Thus, modifications to the latter are also necessary. Any crash diet that includes a period of starvation is more harmful than beneficial in the long run. The daily eating schedule should be established to include breakfast, mid-morning, lunch, mid-afternoon, dinner, and evening. Three of the mealtimes are snacks (mid-morning, mid-afternoon, and evening), and may consist of fruits and vegetables and occasionally seeds or nuts. Eight to ten glasses of water should be consumed daily, six of them preferably 1 hour before each meal. Foods that are low calorie, low fat (preferably unhydrogenated mono- and polyunsaturated fats), balanced in protein quality, and composed of high-fiber carbohydrates should be selected for the remaining three meals.

Aromatherapy

Aromatherapy—using the oil essence of different types of plants, from which molecules travel via the nasal cavity to the limbic system, where a biologic signal raises previous experiences and emotions—may assist indirectly in the clinical management of DUB. There are three ways in which aromas can influence DUB therapy:

- Reducing physical and psychological stress and anxiety, and increasing relaxation (benzoin, basil chamomile, camphor, cedar wood, cypress, geranium, jasmine, juniper, lavender, lemon, lemon grass, mandarin, marjoram, neroli, peppermint, rose, sandalwood)

- Controlling weight (fennel, juniper, black pepper, rosemary, cardamom)
- Providing energy (black spruce, cinnamon, eucalyptus)

Aromatherapy can be instituted via an external application through a bath, massage, cold or hot compresses, or spray, or dispensed through a diffusor or via internal application; however, internal application requires supervision by a properly trained medical practitioner) (83,88).

Meditation

Stress-related hypothalamic disorders leading to an anovulatory cycle are recognized causes of DUB. Therefore, any form of stress reduction/relaxation is a welcome addition to the clinical management of DUB. Meditation (concentrative, mindfulness, transcendental), progressive relaxation (technique relaxing the entire body), and yoga (incorporates posture, breathing exercise, and meditation) are equally beneficial techniques in stress management (83,88).

Hypnotherapy

Hypnosis, particularly in the deep (somnambulistic) state, is proven to be helpful in stress reduction, which often is associated with an anovulatory cycle. DUB, as a sequela of stress-related, chronic anovulation, responds to multilevel relaxation. Hypnosis offers this multilevel relaxation, making the patient receptive to this form of a therapy (83,88).

Manipulative (Chiropractic) Therapy

It is postulated that, in the case of DUB with concomitant low back and lower extremity pain (provided that it exists in the absence of pelvic pain), conservative manipulative treatment is an effective method of treatment. When DUB is suspected to be secondary to a biomechanical or neurologic insult (low back and lower extremity pain), chiropractic, manipulative management should be considered (83,88,89).

Biofeedback Therapy

Biofeedback therapy, alone or in conjunction with other stress-reducing methods, can assist in controlling DUB. As stated above, DUB, as a result of chronic anovulation induced by physical or emotional stress, can be treated by biofeedback as a part of stress-control therapy (83,88).

Imagery

An imagery-relaxation technique is often used as a method of quick stress control, and it can be used in DUB therapy for the same reasons that were explained in each segment above concerning stress and anovulation. A simple, easy-to-learn method makes this an attractive option and is commonly used in today's clinical practice of stress reduction management (83,88).

NATURAL ALTERNATIVE THERAPY

Herbal Medicine

The following phytotherapeutic agents have been recommended:

- *Angelica sinensis* (dong quai): the essential oil and some components increase uterine muscle contractility, and uterine tone in the dose of 12 mL/day of 1:2 fluid extract. Contraindications include a first-trimester pregnancy, a history of spontaneous abortions, and an active viral infection (91,92).
- *Panax notoginseng* (tienchi ginseng), at the dosage of 2 to 9 g/day of the dried root or 4 to 18 mL/day of the 1:2 fluid extract, exhibits antihemorrhagic properties and is contraindicated in pregnancy (92).

The following herbal compositions also have been used (per 5-mL measure):

- *Capsella bursa-pastori* 625 mg
- *Angelica sinensis* 750 mg
- *Paeonia lactiflora* 500 mg
- *Helonias luteum* 625 mg

These remedies are effective in the treatment of menorrhagia, DUB, and breakthrough bleeding in the mid-cycle, but they are contraindicated in the first trimester of pregnancy (93).

- Progesterone-10 skin cream contains 10% or 5,700 mg of *Dioscorea villosa* (wild Mexican yam root) extract, which is considered to be a precursor that is converted to progesterone after transdermal absorption.
- Progesterone-900 skin cream contains 900 mg progesterone and 1,995 mg wild yam extract. These two combinations are structured to deliver progesterone and a precursor of progesterone for the conversion to natural progesterone. To determine the effectiveness, safety, and appropriate dose in potential DUB treatment, further clinical studies are needed.

Homeotherapy

A basis for the selection of a homeopathic therapeutic regimen rests on the amount of bleeding and the appearance of the menstrual effluent. Particular attention is directed to the color of the blood and its general appearance. When endometrial bleeding is bright red and glassy, a different type of medication is selected than when bleeding is heavy with dark blood.

- *Achillea millefolium* (yarrow) is prescribed in a dilution of 5 cH, five granules, three to four times daily, when blood is red and glassy (94). This regimen is contraindicated in pregnancy (95) or in a documented allergic reaction (96).
- Witchhazel leaves (*Hamamelis virginiana*) is prescribed in a dilution of 5 to 9 cH, five granules, two to three times daily, when the appearance of the blood is deep/dark red (94). Toxic cardiac effects have been observed, so possible side effects such as increased potassium loss, heart palpitations, and increased blood pressure should be taken into account (95,96).
- Phosphorus has been recommended in a dilution of 15 to 30 cH, once a day, when coagulopathy is present (94).

REFERENCES

1. Association of Professors of Gynecology and Obstetrics. *Medical student educational objectives,* 7th ed. Washington, DC: Association of Professors of Gynecology and Obstetrics, 1997.
2. Council on Resident and Gynecology (CREOG). *Educational objectives core curriculum for residents in obstetrics and gynecology,* 5th ed. Washington, DC: CREOG, 1996.
3. American College of Obstetrician and Gynecologists (ACOG). Technical Bulletin No. 134. Washington, DC: ACOG, 1989.
4. Janssen CAH, Scholten P, Heintz PM. A simple visual assessment technique to discriminate between menorrhagia and normal menstrual blood loss. *Obstet Gynecol* 1995;85:977–982.
5. Speroff L, Galss RH, Kase NG. *Clinical gynecologic endocrinology and infertility,* 5th ed. Baltimore: Williams & Wilkins, 1994: 457–482, 860–861.
6. Barnes RB, Lobo RA. Central opioid activity in polycystic ovary syndrome with and without dopaminergic modulation. *J Clin Endocrinol Metab* 1985;61:779–786.
7. Siiteri PK, MacDonald PC. Role of extraglandular estrogen in human endocrinology. In: Geyer SR, Astwood EB, Greep RO, eds. *Handbook of physiology.* Washington, DC: American Physiology Society, 1973:615–629.
8. Burger CW, Korsen T, van Kessel H, et al. Pulsatile luteinizing hormone patterns in the follicular phase of the menstrual cycle, polycystic ovarian disease (PCOD) and non-PCOD secondary amenorrhea. *J Clin Endocrinol Metab* 1985;61:1126–1131.
9. Walker JD, Grossman A, Anderson JV, et al. Malignant prolactinoma with extracranial metastases: a report of three cases. *Clin Endocrinol* 1993;38:411–415.
10. Mountcastle RB, Roof BS, Mayfield RK, et al. Case report: pituitary adenocarcinoma in an acromegalic patient. Response to bromocriptine and pituitary testing: a review of the literature on 36 cases of pituitary carcinoma. *Am J Med Sci* 1989;298: 109–112.
11. Schelthauer BW, Randall RV, Laws ER Jr, et al. Prolactin cell carcinoma of the pituitary. *Cancer* 1985;55:985–988.
12. American College of Obstetricians and Gynecologists. Precis V. An update in obstetrics and gynecology. Washington, DC: ACOG, 1994:398.
13. Abulafia O, Sherer DM. Angiogenesis of the endometrium. *Obstet Gynecol* 1999:94:148–153.
14. Kooy J, Taylor NH, Healy DL, et al. Endothelial cell proliferation in the endometrium of women with menorrhagia and in women following endometrial ablation. *Hum Reprod* 1996;11: 1067–1072.
15. Rogers PA, Abberton KM, Susil B. Endothelial cell migratory signal produced by human endometrium during the menstrual cycle. *Hum Reprod* 1992;7:1061–1066.
16. Au CL, Rogers PA. Immunohistochemical staining of von Willebrand factor in human endometrium during normal menstrual cycle. *Hum Reprod* 1993;8:17–23.
17. Claessons EA, Cowell CL. Acute adolescent menorrhagia. *Am J Obstet Gynecol* 1981;139:377–381.

18. Mattox JH. In: Seltzer V, Pearse WH, eds. *Women's primary health care. Office practice and procedures.* New York: McGraw-Hill, 1995:149–163.
19. Viniker DA. Hypothesis on the role of sub-clinical bacteria of the endometrium (bacterial endometrialis) in gynecological and obstetric enigmas. *Hum Reprod Update* 1999;5:373–385.
20. Fraser IS, McCarron G, Markham R. Blood and total fluid content of menstrual discharge. *Obstet Gynecol* 1985;65:194–198.
21. Higham JM, O'Brien PMS, Shaw RW. Assessment of menstrual blood loss using a pictorial chart. *Br J Obstet Gynaecol* 1990:97:734–739.
22. Sherman JA. *The complete botanical prescriber,* 2nd ed. Portland, OR: National College of Naturopathic Medicine, 1979.
23. Brinker F. *The toxicology of botanical medicines,* 2nd ed. Sandy, OR: Electronic Medical Publishers, 1996.
24. Harper-Shove F. *Prescriber and clinical repertory of medicinal herbs.* Rustington, UK: Health Science Press, 1952.
25. Brinker F. Botanical medicine research summaries. In: *Eclectic dispensatory of botanical therapeutics.* Vol. II. Sandy, OR: Eclectic Medical Publishers, 1995.
26. Rose KD, Parliament CF, Levin MB. Spontaneous spinal epidural hematoma with associated platelet dysfunction from excessive garlic ingestion. A case report. *Neurosurgery* 1990;26:880–882.
27. Hopkins MP, Andronff L, Benninghoff AS. Ginseng face cream and unexplained vaginal bleeding. *Am J Obstet Gynecol* 1988;159:1121–1123.
28. Hammond TG, Whitworth JA. Adverse reactions to ginseng. *Med J Aust* 1981;1:492–494.
29. McGuffin M, Hobbs C, Upton R, et al., eds. *Botanical safety handbook.* Boca Raton, FL: CRC Press, 1997.
30. Laufer MR, Goldstin DP. Pediatric and adolescent gynecology. In: Ryan KJ, Berkowitz RS, Barbieri RL, eds. *Kistner's gynecology. Principles and practice.* St. Louis: Mosby-Year Book 1995:571–632.
31. Goldchmit R, Katz Z, Blickstein I, et al. The accuracy of endometrial sampling with and without sonographic measurement of endometrial thickness. *Obstet Gynecol* 1993;82:727–730.
32. Claessons EA, Cowell CA. Acute adolescent menorrhagia. *Am J Obstet Gynecol* 1981;193:377–380.
33. American College of Obstetrician and Gynecologists (ACOG). Technical bulletin No. 191. Washington, DC: ACOG, 1994.
34. Farhi B, Nosanchuk J, Silverberg S. Endometrial adenocarcinoma in women under 25 years of age. *Obstet Gynecol* 1991;68:741–744.
35. Cleveger-Hoeft M, Syrop CH, Stovall DW, et al. Sonohysterography in premenopausal women with and without abnormal bleeding. *Obstet Gynecol* 1999;94:516–520.
36. Gaucherand P, Piacenza JM, Salle B, et al. Sonohysterography of the uterine cavity: preliminary investigations. *J Clin Ultrasound* 1995;23:339–348.
37. Widrich T, Bradley LD, Mitchinson AR, et al. Comparison of saline infusion sonography with office hysteroscopy for the evaluation of the endometrium. *Am J Obstet Gynecol* 1996;174:1327–1334.
38. Parsons AK, Lense JJ. Sonohysterography for endometrial abnormalities: preliminary results. *J Clin Ultrasound* 1993;21:87–95.
39. Bauman JE. Basal body temperature: unreliable method of ovulation dedaction. *Fertil Steril* 1981;36:729–732.
40. Dowans KA, Gibson M. Basal body temperature graph and the luteal phase defect. *Fertil Steril* 1983;40:466–469.
41. Beckman CRB, Ling WNP, Herbert WP, et al. *Obstetrics and gynecology,* 3rd ed. Baltimore: Williams & Wilkins, 1998:430–435.
42. Hallberg L, Hogdahl AM, Nilsson L, et al. Menstrual blood loss—a population study. Variation at different ages and attempts to define normality. *Acta Obstet Gynecol Scand* 1966;45:320–351.
43. Hallberg L, Hogdahl AM, Nilsson L, et al. Menstrual blood loss and iron deficiency. *Acta Med Scand* 1966;180:639–650.
44. DeVore GR, Owens O, Kase N. Use of intravenous premarin in the treatment of dysfunctional uterine bleeding—a double blind randomized control study. *Obstet Gynecol* 1982;59:285–290.
45. Kubrinsky NL, Tulloch H. Treatment of refractory thrombocytopenic bleeding with desamino-8-D-arginine vasopressin (desmopressin). *J Pediatr* 1988;112:993–998.
46. Castaman G, Rodeghiero F. Current management of von Willebrand's disease. *Drugs* 1995;50:602–614.
47. Shaw RW. Assessment of medical treatments for menorrhagia. *Br J Obstet Gynaecology* 1994;101(suppl 11):15–18.
48. Stabinsky SA, Einstein M, Breen L. Modern treatments of menorrhagia attributable to dysfunctional uterine bleeding. *Obstet Gynecol Surv* 1998;54:61–72.
49. Bolaji II, Tallon DF, O'Dwyer E, et al. Assessment of bioavailability of oral micronized progesterone using a salivary progesterone enzyme immunoassay. *Gynecol Endocrinol* 1993;7:101–110.
50. Gillet JY, Faguer B, Andre G, et al. A "no-bleeding" substitute hormone treatment with an oral microdose progesterone. A prospective multicenter study. *J Gynecol Obstet Biol Reprod (Paris)* 1994;23:407–412.
51. Fanchin R, Ziegler D, Bergeron C, et al. Transvaginal administration of progesterone. *Obstet Gynecol* 1997;90:396–401.
52. Warren MP, Shantha S. Use of progesterone in clinical practice. *Int J Fertil Womens Med* 1999;44:96–103.
53. Levy T, Gurevitch S, Bar-Hava I, et al. Pharmacokinetics of natural progesterone administered in the form of a vaginal tablet. *Hum Reprod* 1999;14:606–610.
54. Dockeray CJ, Sheppard BL, Bonner J. Comparison between mefenamic acid and danazol in the treatment of established menorrhagia. *Br J Obstet Gynaecol* 1989;96:840–844.
55. Higham JM, Shaw RW. A comparative study of danazol, a regimen of decreasing doses of danazol, and norethindrone in the treatment of objectively prover unexplained menorrhagia. *Am J Obstet Gynecol* 1993;169:1134–1139.
56. Chimbira TH, Anderson AB, Naish C, et al. Reduction of menstrual blood loss by danazol in unexplained menorrhagia: lack of effect of placebo. *Br J Obstet Gynaecol* 1980;87:1152–1158.
57. Shaw A. Treatment of menorrhagia. *Br J Obstet Gynaecol* 1984;91:913–916.
58. Thomas EJ, Okuda KJ, Thomas NM. The combination of depot gonadotropin releasing hormone agonist and cyclical hormone replacement therapy for dysfunctional uterine bleeding. *Br J Obstet Gynaecol* 1991;98:1155–1159.
59. Milsom I, Anderson K, Andersch B, et al. A comparison of flurbiprogen, tranexamic acid, and levonorgestrel-releasing intrauterine contraceptive device in the treatment of idiopathic menorrhagia. *Am J Obstet Gynecol* 1991;164:879–882.
60. Bergqvist A, Rybo G. Treatment of menorrhagia with intrauterine release of progesterone. *Br J Obstet Gynecol* 1983;90:255–258.
61. Hall P, Maclachlan N, Thorn N, et al. Control of menorrhagia by the cyto-oxygenase inhibitors naproxen sodium and mefenamic acid. *Br J Obstet Gynecol* 1987;94:554–559.
62. Cameron IT, Haining R, Lumsden MA, et al. The effects of mefenamic acid and norethistrone on measured menstrual blood loss. *Obstet Gynecol* 1990;76:85–88.
63. Ylikorkala O, Pekonen F. Naproxen reduces idiopathic but not fibromyomata-induced menorrhagia. *Obstet Gynecol* 1986;68:10–12.
64. Ong YL, Hull DR, Mayne EE. Menorrhagia in von Willebrand disease successfully treated with single daily dose tranexamic acid. *Haemophilia* 1998;4:63–65.

65. Dockeray CJ, Shappard BL, Daly L, et al. The fibrinolytic enzyme system in normal menstruation and excessive uterine bleeding and the effect of tranexamic acid. *Eur J Obstet Gynecol Reprod Biol* 1987;24:309–318.

66. Edlund M, Andersson K, Rybo G, et al. Reduction of menstrual blood loss in women suffering from idiopathic menorrhagia with a noval antifibrinolytic drug (Kabi 2161). *Br J Obstet Gynaecol* 1995;102:913–917.

67. Ostrzenski A. Laparoscopic total abdominal hysterectomy by suturing technique, with no transvaginal surgical approach: a review of 276 cases. *Int J Gynecol Obstet* 1996;55:247–257.

68. Ostrzenski A. New retroperitoneal culdoplasty at the time of laparoscopic total abdominal hysterectomy (L-TAH). *Acta Obstet Gynecol Scand* 1998;77:1017–1021.

69. Ostrzenski A. A systematic arrangement of laparoscopic total hysterectomy: a new technique. *J Natl Med Assoc* 1999;911:404–409.

70. DeCherney AH, Diamond MP, Lavy G, et al. Endometrial ablation for intractable uterine bleeding: hysteroscopic resection. *Obstet Gynecol* 1987;70:668–670.

71. Aberdeen Endometrial Ablation Trials Group. A randomized trial of endometrial ablation versus hysterectomy for the treatment of dysfunctional uterine bleeding: outcome at four years. *Br J Obstet Gynecol* 1999;106:360–366.

72. Klinzing S, Schlensog M, Klein U. Hyponatremia and lung edema in endometrium ablation with rollerball ablation. *Zentralbl Gynakol* 1999;121:98–100.

73. Silvernagel SW, Harshbarger KE, Shevlin DW. Postoperative granulomas of the endometrium: histological features after endometrial ablation. *Ann Diagn Pathol* 1997;1:82–90.

74. Cooper KG, Parkin DE, Garrat AM, et al. A randomized comparison of medical and hysteroscopic management in women consulting a gynaecologist for treatment of heavy menstrual loss. *Br J Obstet Gynecol* 1997;104:1360–1366.

75. American College of Obstetrician and Gynaecologists (ACOG). Criteria Set No. 1, 1994.

76. Desquesne JH, Gallinat A, Garza-Leal JG, et al. Thermoregulated radiofrequency endometrial ablation. *Int J Fertil Med* 1997;42:311–318.

77. Buckshee K, Banerjee K, Bhatla H. Uterine balloon therapy to treat menorrhagia. *Int J Gynaecol Obstet* 1998;63:139–143.

78. Tadir Y, Hornung R, Pham TH, et al. Intrauterine light probe for photodynamic ablation therapy. *Obstet Gynecol* 1999;93:299–303.

79. Hodgson DA, Feldberg IB, Sharp N, et al. Microwave endometrial ablation: development, clinical trials and outcomes at three years. *Br J Obstet Gynaecol* 1999;111106:684–694.

80. Donnez J, Polet R, Squifflet J, et al. Endometrial laser intrauterine thermo-therapy (ELITT): a revolutionary new approach to the elimination of menorrhagia. *Curr Opin Obstet Gynecol* 1999;11:363–370.

81. Mo X, Li D, Pu Y, et al. Clinical studies on the mechanism for acupuncture stimulation of ovulation. *J Trad Chin Med* 1993;13:115–119.

82. Yu J, Zheng HM, Ping SM. Changes in serum FSH, LH and ovarian follicular growth during electroacupuncture for induction of ovulation. *Chung His I Chieh Ho Tsa Chih* 1989;9:199–202.

83. Burton Goldberg Group. Alternative medicine. The definitive guide. Tiburon, CA: Future Medicine Publishing, 1997:53–72, 769.

84. Andersen R, Wadden TA, Bartlett SJ, et al. Effect of lifestyle activity vs structured aerobic exercise in obese women. *JAMA* 1999;281:335–340.

85. Ness AR, Powles JW. Fruit and vegetables, and cardiovascular disease: a review. *Int J Epidemiol* 1997;26:1–13.

86. Hu FB, Stampfer MJ, Manson JE, et al. Dietary fat intake and the risk of coronary heart disease in women. *N Engl J Med* 1997;337:1491–1499.

87. Eliopoulos C. Integrating conventional and alternative therapies. Holistic care for chronic conditions. St. Louis: CV Mosby, 1999:83–85, 121, 122.

88. van Dale D, Saris WH. Repetitive weight loss and weight regain: effect on weight reduction , resting metabolic rate, and lipolytic activity before and after exercise and/or diet treatment. *Am J Clin Nutr* 1998:49:409–416.

89. Stude DE. Dysfunctional uterine bleeding with concomitant low back and lower extremity pain. *J Manipulative Physiol Ther* 1991;14:472–477.

90. Cohen JD, Rubin HW. Functional menorrhagia: treatment with bioflavonoids and vitamin C. *Curr Ther Res* 1960;2:539–542.

91. Chang HM, But PP. Pharmocology and applications of Chinese Materia Medica. Vol. 2. Singapore: World Scientific, 1987.

92. Bone K. *Clinical applications of ayurvedic and Chinese herbs. Monographs for the Western herbal practitioner.* Queensland, Australia: Phytotherapy Press, 1997:3–7, 43–45.

93. Bone K, Burgess N, McLeod D. *Phytosynergistic prescribing. A professional prescriber reference guide to herbal formulas.* Portland, OR: Professional Complementary Health Formulas, 1994:63–64.

94. Holtzscherr A, Legros AS. *Pratique homeopathique en gynecologie.* Boiron, France: Centre d'Enseignement et de Developpement de l'Homeopathie. 1994.

95. Brinker F. The toxicology of botanical medicine, 2nd ed. Sandy, OR: Eclectic Medical Publishers, 1996.

96. Wichtel M. Herbal drugs and phytopharmaceuticals. Boca Raton, FL: CRC Press, 1994.

11

INFERTILITY

EDUCATIONAL OBJECTIVES

Medical Students (1) *APGO Objective No.52*	*Residents in Obstetrics/Gynecology (2)* *CREOG Objectives*	*Practitioners (3–5)* *ACOG Recommendations*

Definition of primary and
    secondary infertility
Causes of male and
    female infertility
Evaluation and management
Psychological issues
    associated with infertility
	Pertinent history: failure to conceive
	    Sexual practices
	    Gynecologic disorders
	    Male factors
	    Menstrual history
	Physical examination
	Diagnostic studies
	Diagnosis
	Management
	Follow-up
	Reproductive technologies
		Initial assessment
		Basic workup
		The male factor
		The pelvic factor
		Ovulatory factor
		Cervical factor
		Unexplained infertility

DEFINITION

Infertility is defined, in general, as failure to conceive after 1 year of regular, unprotected coitus in women of reproductive age (15–44 years) (4). The European Society for Human Reproduction and Embryology defines infertility as failure to conceive after 2 years of regular unprotected coitus in women of reproductive age (5).

Infertility is a reduced capacity to conceive when compared with the mean capacity of the general population. *Fecundability* is the statistically determined physiologic autonomy of conception during any given menstrual cycle and is predicted to be 20% to 25% per healthy cycle (6).

Fecundity is the ability to conceive and achieve a live birth within one menstrual cycle (6).

Cumulative fertility is the statistical probability of conceiving within 12 months (6). *Sterility* is the inability to reproduce.

OCCURRENCE

The prevalence of infertility is estimated at 10% to 15%. When both the U.S. and European definitions are applied, the infertility rate in North America and Europe is estimated to be 5% to 6% (4,5).

CLASSIFICATION

Infertility is classified into two categories:

- Primary infertility is clinically considered when the couple has never conceived.
- Secondary infertility is considered when the couple achieved conception once or more and thereafter became infertile.

PHYSIOLOGY OF CONCEPTION

Preconceptional maturation of the oocyte and spermatozoa must reach morphologic and functional capacity compatible with fertilization. More detailed information on the menstrual function is presented in Chapter 3. The oocyte resumes meiosis and reaches metaphase II, which is characterized by expulsion of the first polar body. The matured spermatozoa must express the capacity to activate motility and the acrosomal cap must come off (acrosomal reaction). Upon completion of this process, a spermatozoa can release proteolitic enzymes essential for the attachment of spermatozoa to the vitelline (the oocyte membrane) and penetration of the zona pellucida of the oocyte. Upon entering the oocyte, the haploid spermatozoon chromosomal arrangement triggers the second oocyte meiotic division, which reduces chromosomes from diploid to haploid; at the same time, the ejection of the second polar body takes place. Fusion of the pronuclei of the spermatozoon and oocyte completes the process of fertilization, which occurs in the ampulla of the fallopian tube. The first cleavage division of the embryo occurs 24 hours after fertilization.

Spermatozoa are produced in the testes. There are several structures in which the synchronized process of sperm production and maturation takes place:

- Sertoli cells hold spermatogonia and line the seminiferous tubules, in which the maturation process from spermatids (spermatogonia) to spermatozoa takes place.
- Leydig cells are located in interstitial testicular tissue and are responsible for androgen synthesis.
- The epididymis is a pool, in which sperm are deposited at the time of sperm maturation. A spermatozoon upon arriving to the epididymis is functionally immature and usually takes approximately 12 days to reach motility.
- The vas deferens is a connector between the epididymis and the ejaculatory ducts. Lateral head movements and fast tail movements are necessary to achieve forward, progressive, rapid motility, and this transformation occurs in the epididymis.
- The seminal fluid is produced and secreted by the seminal vesicles, prostate (contains proteolitic enzymes) gland, and the Cowper gland (the bulbourethral gland).

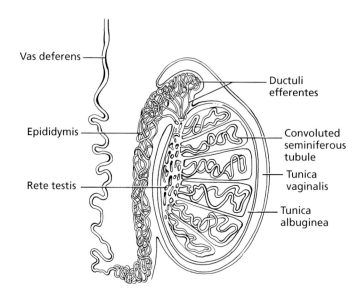

FIGURE 11.2. Paratesticular and testicular structures.

Schematic illustrations of these structures along with the spermatozoa are presented in Figs. 11.1 to 11.3.

The sperm generation time is about 73 to 74 days, during which spermatogonia are transformed to spermatozoa in excess of total sperm count per ejaculation (more than 40×10^6 spermatozoa).

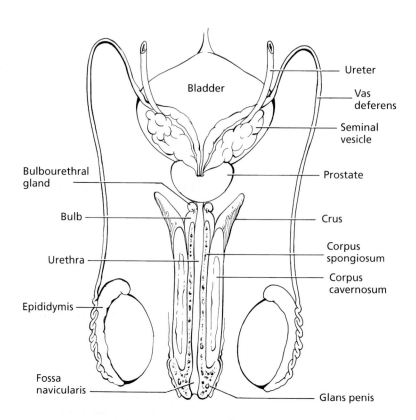

FIGURE 11.1. Male uroreproductive system.

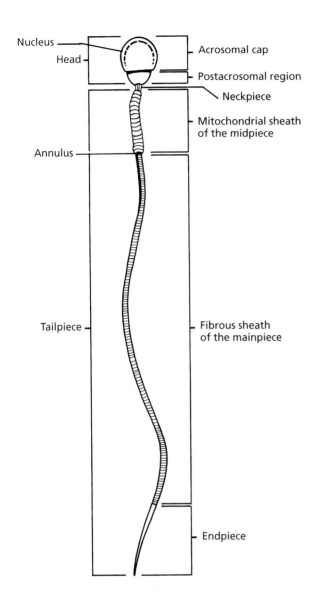

Nucleus
Head
Acrosomal cap
Postacrosomal region
Neckpiece
Mitochondrial sheath of the midpiece
Annulus
Tailpiece
Fibrous sheath of the mainpiece
Endpiece

FIGURE 11.3. Matured spermatozoa.

The following phases of sperm formation and maturation have been identified (7):

- Spermatocytogenesis is the process whereby spermatogonia type A is transformed by mitotic division to spermatogonia type B and through subsequent division produces primary spermatocytes.
- Meiosis is the process of reduction of chromosomal number in half, furnishing each gamete with a haploid chromosomal number.
- Spermiogenesis is the process of recruiting, developing, and transforming a germ cell to a flagellum that is changed from a spermatid to a matured form of spermatozoon.

In contrast to the pulsatile pattern of luteinizing hormone (LH) secretion in women, LH secretion in men exhibits a tonic pattern. In response to LH stimulation, Leydig cells produce testosterone and the germinal epithelium initiates spermatogenesis. In response to follicle-stimulating hormone (FSH) stimulation, Sertoli cells secrete inhibin. The sperm ejaculation process is initiated in the distal vas deferens, which triggers the release of prostate fluid and, shortly after, seminal vesicle fluid. In the ejaculation phase, semen coagulates to a gel, a state in which spermatozoa is incapable of fertilization. Within 20 to 30 minutes, the ejaculate liquefies in the presence of prostatic proteolitic enzymes. The process of capacitation occurs in cervical mucus and is a necessary step for conception. The final preparation of a spermatozoon for fertilization is the acrosomal reaction, which is the process leading to collapse of the sperm plasma membranes, combining them with the external acrosomal membrane, and accumulating proteolitic enzymes within the acrosome, needed for sperm to penetrate the ovum (the cumulus cell mass, corona radiata, and zona pellucida). Upon successful sperm penetration, the oocyte commences the cortical reaction (distribution of the secretory granules just below the vitelline membrane). This process prepares the oocyte to be impenetrable by other spermatozoa.

Other factors play a role in successful conception, and abnormality in any one of them will affect fecundity. The following aspects of sexual intercourse are essential in achieving successful conception:

- Delivering adequate volume, morphology, and functional sperm to the posterior fornix of the vagina
- Optimal timing of 1 to 2 days before ovulation (spermatozoa remain fertility capacity for approximately 48 hours in the female reproductive tract)
- Effective frequency of coitus every other day or often
- Accumulating ejaculate in the posterior fornix of the vagina, when the uterus is in an anteroverted position; occasionally, ejaculate should remain in the anterior vaginal fornix in a case of acute uterine retroversion

Cervical mucus should be considered a tissue and not a fluid (8). This tissue creates a netlike matrix made from mucoprotein. The netlike appearance of cervical mucus fluctuates in response to estrogens levels. The peak of cervical production by endocervical glands or peak of cervical mucus receptivity coincides with the mid-cycle estradiol peak level. The peak of cervical mucus receptivity dissipates within 2 to 3 days after progesterone/estrogen-opposed action occurs. The cervical mucus netlike function is to act as a filter, allowing sperm with adequate motility to pass through.

The ovum uptake and its transport depends on the healthy tubal fimbriae, ciliary endotubal mucosa, preserved tubal patency, and absence of adnexal adhesion.

The endometrial quality, its full secretory transformation from the proliferative status, its receptivity for blactocyst nidation, and its decidualization are the crucial elements in preservation of fertility integrity. Because it is a process in time, endometrial histology from one point in this process will not provide clinically valuable information in this respect.

ETIOLOGY

Etiologic factors of infertile couples are divided into four major categories: the female factor, the male factor, combined factors, and unexplained infertility.

Female factors (approximately 35%) can be related to an ovulatory dysfunction, which account for about 25% of all fertility failure (8) and are suspected when any abnormality of the menstrual cycle is reported, included delayed menarche. The clinical manifestation of anovulation is oligomenorrhea or amenorrhea. The conception rate in patients with oligomenorrhea is lower than in patients with amenorrhea on appropriate therapy, and essentially depends on the diagnostic precision. Advancing age also influences fecundability in terms of decreasing oocyte quality, which may result in decreasing endometrial capacity for implantation, without affecting ovulation and fertilization potential (8). Hyperprolactinemia, polycystic ovary syndrome (PCOS), thyroid, adrenal dysfunction and other causes of anovulation are discussed in other chapters.

Luteal phase defect (also called inadequate luteal phase) is most likely a result of insufficient progesterone secretion or its expression on the target tissue (endometrium). An inadequate luteal phase is a relatively uncommon cause of infertility (3%–4%). It can be identified by histologic endometrial dating and is considered (a) when the endometrium secretory maturity lags behind or is out of phase for more than 2 days of the menstrual cycle (9,10) (the discrepancy between the actual dates of the menstrual cycle and endometrial dating must be documented in more than one consecutive cycle), (b) when a single serum progesterone level in the mid-luteal phase (approximately on day 22 or within 1 week prior to onset of menses) is less than 10 ng/mL (31.8 nM), or (c) when the sum of three serum progesterone levels is less than 30 ng/mL (10). The diagnostic accuracy of endometrial biopsy and its clinical usefulness has been called into question (11,12). The controversy surrounds endometrial out-of-phase dating and using it as a criterion for the diagnosis of luteal phase defect. Luteal phase defects are thought to occur in the fertile cycle at a rate of approximately 20% to 30%, and they occur in about 5% of consecutive cycles (13). Nevertheless, it has been shown that the sensitivity and specificity of the test appears to be marginally acceptable (10).

Initial data suggest that *antiendometrial antibodies*, detected by enzyme-linked immunosorbent assay, are associated with infertility, mainly ovulatory dysfunction and tubal occlusion (14).

Another factor that may play a role in conception and early pregnancy support is immunomodulatory protein, known as *the progesterone induced blocking factor*. This factor has been found to positively correlate with early pregnancy beta-human chorionic gonadotropin (beta-hCG) levels (15).

Tubal and peritoneal factors are usually secondary to pelvic inflammatory disease (PID), abdominopelvic surgery, endometriosis, and tuberculosis, among other conditions.

Functional damage to the tubal mucosa and to fimbriae is critical. Microsurgical correction, either by fimbrioplasty (the opening of the distal tubal end) or tubal reconstruction, to reestablish the patency of the fallopian tubes, does not usually involve any technical difficulties. However, the resulting pregnancy rates, particularly with distal tube occlusion with hydrosalpinx or proximal tubal occlusion due to salpingitis isthmica nodosa, are low. All types of adhesions (e.g., filmy, fibrotic, dense) on intraabdominal reproductive organs (fallopian tubes and ovaries) may cause infertility. Regardless, the visual assessment of adhesions (mild, moderate, severe, extensive) (16) will not provide appropriate information in terms of extent of irreversible functional damage, fibrosis, or occlusion of the tubal mucosa. Bilateral tubal obstruction caused by a disease process (not tubal ligation) treated surgically may result in a pregnancy rate of approximately 10%, with an ectopic pregnancy rate as high as 5% (8).

Other causes of infertility include endometriosis (5%), cervical mucus defects or cervical mucus hostility (3%), uterine anatomic abnormalities and leiomyomata (low percentage as a true cause of infertility), systemic illness (rare), and reproductive organ tuberculosis (rare in Western countries) (8).

Coexisting factors affecting fertility should be explored as a possible cause, which in some instances may be difficult to rectify:

- Age as a contributory factor to infertility begins progressively affecting women after 30 years of age. A significant decrease is observed between 35 and 38 years of age, and a sharp decline after 40 years of age. The age factor not only influences fecundability but also increases the risk for spontaneous abortion. An aging ovary with a declining number of follicles and declining functional capacity is the recognizable phenomenon. Rising basal serum FSH in a young woman with the decreased ovarian reserve is a poor prognostic factor for successful natural or assisted conception (17). Serum basal estradiol levels in combination with basal FSH and chronologic age are suggested as useful predictive values for cumulative pregnancy rate. When the estradiol level is less than or equal to 80 pg/mL, the basal FSU is greater than or equal to 13 mIU/mL, and chronologic age is at least 42 years, the chances for conception decrease (18).

- Duration of infertility among untreated infertile couples in combination with the female partner's age, pregnancy history, tubal disease, endometriosis, and male factor is an effective predictive method in the untreated couple (19). Unattended infertility diminishes fecundity, particularly when the cause of infertility is not established (8,19,20).

- Previous pregnancy (and its clinical history and outcome) is one of the predictive factors for conception (19,20).
- Body mass index (BMI), when it indicates either obesity or low body weight, is a factor in infertility because it may interfere with menstrual function and ovulation.
- Cigarette smoking and use of other tobacco products may directly affect oocytes, resulting in decreased fertility and impaired nidation. Smoking presents significant detrimental effects on conception (21) and contributes to the risk for miscarriage (22). Fecundity decreases in about 20% of smoking women. In women who smoke and who qualify for *in vitro* fertilization (IVF), decreased fecundity is even more pronounced, approximately 40% (23). The negative effect of smoking on infertility has been demonstrated even with a low number of cigarettes, ranging from one to nine cigarettes daily (24). It also has been documented that natural conception returns to the expected fecundity level and the rate of spontaneous abortion decreases after cessation of smoking (23). For men, cigarette smoking lowers sperm density, but its effect on the conception rate is probably far less significant (25,26).

The male factor (approximately 30%) usually refers to semen quality (total volume of ejaculate, number of spermatozoa, motility, and morphology), but also includes sperm defects and impaired function. *Oligozoospermia* (decreased number of sperm) and *azoospermia* [failure to produce (spermatogenesis) or eject spermatozoa] occur in about 1% to 2% of men. *Anizoospermia* or *asthenozoospermia* (decreased sperm motility) may occur in association with varicocele (1%–2%) and seminal sperm antibodies (5%) (8).

Combined factors (approximately 20%) include either infrequent sexual intercourse for conception or coital failure. Both partners' coital history and any dysfunctions should be documented.

Unexplained infertility accounts for approximately 15% of cases.

DIAGNOSIS

Initial Infertility Evaluation

An initial diagnostic process of infertility should include evaluation of both partners.

Female Partner Pertinent Medical History

Pertinent medical history should cover the following areas:

- Ovulatory disorders can be suspected when late menarche, abnormal frequency, duration, increased or decreased menstrual flow, intermenstrual bleeding or spotting, premenstrual symptoms, hot flushes or flushes

(premature ovary failure), and excessive weight changes are reported.

- Iatrogenic causes such as hormones, antiestrogen agents, or gonadotropin-releasing hormone (GnRH) agonists may cause transient infertility. Transient induced infertility also is observed with neuroleptic, antidepressant, and hypotensive medications, as well as any medication that increases prolactin levels. It has been suggested that recreational drugs such as marijuana and cocaine may negatively influence fertility. Permanently induced infertility is expected from cytostatic agents, radiation therapy, and surgery (bilateral oophorectomy).
- Systemic illnesses such as adrenal, thyroid, or liver disease, renal dysfunction, hyperprolactinemia, pituitary conditions, and diabetes mellitus may have an adverse influence on infertility.
- A vaginal factor is suspected with recurrent infections, the underdeveloped vagina, or the inadequately canalized vagina.
- A cervical factor is related to infections and cervical surgery performed, such as cervical conization.
- A pelvic factor represents pelvic organs (the uterus, ovaries, fallopian tubes, and neighboring organs) that may influence negatively fertility. A uterine factor manifested by hypomenorrhea or amenorrhea shortly after intrauterine manipulation may indicate endometrial adhesions obliterating the uterine cavity (Asherman syndrome). Abnormal, heavy, or prolonged endometrial bleeding with or without associated pelvic pain or pressure may suggest endometrial polyps, chronic endometritis, missing intrauterine devices (IUDs), or uterine leiomyomata. Secondary dysmenorrhea, cyclic abdominopelvic pain, hypermenorrhea, and dyspareunia strongly suggest endometriosis. Fallopian tube infections (salpingitis) as a part of PID, pelvic tuberculosis, ruptured appendix, septic abortion, ectopic surgery, adnexal surgery, or exposure to diethylstilbestrol (DES) should be explored.
- Previous pregnancy and its outcome, such as artificial abortion, spontaneous abortion, molar pregnancy, and ectopic pregnancy, should be noted.

Female Partner Physical Examination

The physical examination should focus on the following areas:

- Determining BMI (body mass index)
- General physical examination, with particular attention to cardiopulmonary systems and gastrointestinal tract
- Phenotype characteristics and stature should be determined. Type of hair distribution (female vs. male), skin androgenization signs (oily skin, acne, hirsutism), and nipple discharge (spontaneous vs. induced) should be determined.

- Pelvic examination should concentrate on external genitalia inspection (type of hair distribution, pigmentation, clitoromegaly), the vagina [length, discharge, fornices, with special attention to the posterior fornix's shape, depth, and any nodularity in the posterior cul-de-sac (e.g., possible endometriosis)], the cervix, (cervical external os and mucus appearance), and uterine enlargement, symmetry, shape, consistency, irregularity, mobility, tenderness, and retroflexion, if present, and to what degree. Adnexa pathology should be identified.

Male Partner Pertinent Medical History

Medical history should focus on the following areas:

- Coital history, decreased libido, ejaculate volume reduction
- General health, presence of asthenia, use of marijuana, cigarette smoking, and alcohol consumption
- Genital anatomic abnormalities such as hypospadias or retrograde ejaculation
- Postpubertal mumps or other genitourinary infection (including sexually transmitted infections)
- Drug history
- Testicular surgery, genital radiation, chemotherapy, or genital trauma
- Testicular exposure to heat (sitting for long periods, tight underwear, use of hot tubs and saunas)
- Sexual history

Male Partner Physical Examination

Physical examination should include a general examination, with special emphasis on the following areas:

- Habitus (male phenotype vs. eunuchoid)
- Presence or absence of gynecomastia
- Decreased beard growth, sparse or absent body hair
- Visual genital inspection
- Penile abnormality (particularly the location of and integrity of the urethral meatus), urethral discharge, and skin lesions
- Testicular evaluation: testicular descent (cryptorchidism), size (average 4.5×2.8 cm), shape (elliptical), consistency, tenderness, and presence or absence of varicocele are assessed (with patient standing, a Valsalva maneuver is executed by the patient, and a reflux impulse is appreciated by a patient; several invasive and noninvasive methods are available, the most commonly used being a Doppler stethoscope). Testicular volume (at least 20 cm^2 or >15 mL) is assessed by scrotal palpation, and testes are measured using an orchidometer (known ellipsoid volumes are used in the calculations). A testicular volume of less than 15 mL may imply dysfunction of the seminiferous tubules [spermatozoa production] (27).

- Epididymis evaluation commences with determination of location (the posterolateral area of testes) and indurations (may indicate occlusion).
- Vas deferens consistency should be determined.
- Rectal examination of the prostate and the area just above is performed to rule out dysfunction of the ejaculatory duct (dilated seminal vesicles).

Evaluation of Ovulatory Function

The use of basal body temperature (BBT) in the evaluation of female infertility is controversial. However, its pragmatic application in the clinical setting has gained global clinical interest.

The reliability, acceptability, and application of the BBT graph have been called into question. It has been determined that BBT is not an optimal parameter for infertility assessment (28,29). However, it appears that BBT can provide useful information, as long as its interpretation and limitations are well defined. Temperature reading and recording on a chart should be properly executed. Each morning, upon awakening and before any activity, oral temperature is taken with a specially designed infertility thermometer or a disposable thermocrystal thermometer. This routine is commenced on the first day of menses, which corresponds to day 1 of the menstrual cycle. It is important to establish a systematic approach for the clinical use of BBT.

Limitations of Basal Body Temperature

- BBT graph analysis represents a retrospective identification of parameters and does not reflect an upcoming menstrual cycle.
- The BBT graph can be adversely influenced by reading temperature fluctuation from any cause and by cycle length variability itself.
- The BBT does not establish the precise day of ovulation; however, it is a relatively accurate guide for retrospective identification of the preovulatory period (30).
- The monophasic BBT graph does not establish an anovulatory menstrual cycle (up to 75% of a monophasic BBT graph can present hormonal evidence of ovulation) (29).
- BBT elevation of greater than 98°F does not match an LH surge, which occurs approximately 48 hours later (following the nadir of the BBT graph) (31).
- The protracted elevation of BBT is not indicative of abnormal function of the menstrual cycle.

Interpretation of Basal Body Temperature

- In the proliferative phase of the menstrual cycle, the temperature reading is approximately 97°F in a healthy woman.

- The monophasic BBT graph is the absence of temperature elevation above 98°F throughout a menstrual cycle.
- The biphasic BBT graph is an increase in temperature greater than 98°F in the luteal phase for 13 to 14 days and is indicative of a presumptive normal ovulatory cycle in about 90%.
- The biphasic BBT graph with a luteal phase fewer than 10 days duration is suggestive of a short luteal phase
- The biphasic BBT graph with a temperature elevation for longer than 16 days is highly suggestive of pregnancy.
- The biphasic BBT graph shows a decreasing the temperature 14 to 36 hours after commencing menses.

Basal body temperature graphs are an instrumental guidance tool for patients in conjunction with diagnostic procedures such as hysterosalpingography (HSG), diagnostic hysteroscopy, ultrasonography, hysterography, ultrasonographic follicular assessment, and hormonal assays.

Indicial Laboratory Diagnostic Tests

Indicial laboratory diagnostic tests universally ordered for infertility include those for general screening, ovulation confirmation, ovulation prediction, postcoital testing, tubal patency, and semen analysis.

General Screening
Among general screening tests, the following are most commonly indicated:

- General health
- Female rubella serology
- Hepatitis serology (both partners)
- Human immunodeficiency virus (HIV) serology, when indicated (both partners)
- Cervical cytology
- Cervical bacteriologic screening is recommended for common infections, gram-positive and gram-negative bacteria, *Chlamydia trachomatis* [serology test for specific immunoglobulin G (IgG) and IgA antibody to *Chlamydia trachomatis* can be useful because all cases of salpingitis demonstrate IgA specific for *Chlamydia,* regardless of cervical culture results (32)] *Neisseria gonorrhoeae, Ureoplasma urealyticum,* and *Mycoplasma hominis.* Screening is indicated when pelvic pain is present or vaginal discharge is identified.

Ovulation Confirmation
At mid-luteal phase a progesterone assay is recommended as the best test for confirming ovulation. A plasma progesterone concentration of greater than 5.6 ng/mL (>5.6 n*M*) on at least two occasions in a mid-luteal phase in two to six cycles confirms ovulation (33). The test is usually performed when a patient's medical history suggests a menstrual cycle dysfunctional pattern and when such a pattern is documented on BBT graphs (for at least 3 months) (3).

Ovulation Prediction
Daily measurement of preovulatory LH to establish the LH surge (a twofold elevation of serum LH from the baseline) is the best single assay, because ovulation usually occurs 34 to 36 hours later (34,35). Ovulation prediction is most accurate when both the serum LH surge and serum preovulatory estradiol levels are established.

Postcoital Testing
The postcoital test or Sims-Huhner test is usually performed after a vaginal/cervical infection has been ruled out and optimal timing of coitus in relation to the preovulatory/ovulatory cycle has been established. The test is performed *in vivo* and determines the presence or absence of cervical mucus hostility toward spermatozoa. A period of sexual abstinence is observed for 48 hours, beginning 24 to 48 hours before expected ovulation (established with some degrees of certainty, either by urinary LH home test kits or by analyzing current and previous BBT graphs). The cervical mucus is evaluated within 2 to 8 hours after sexual intercourse, and the woman is advised to stay in bed in the prescribed position for at least 45 minutes after coitus to prevent sperm from coming out. The following parameters may identify the absence of a so-called cervical factor of infertility:

- Adequate quantity and clarity of mucus
- A spinnbarkeit of greater than 8 cm
- Clear, acellular mucus with 5 to 10 progressively motile spermatozoa present per microscopic high-power (×400) field

Abnormal cervical mucus–sperm interaction can be determined only when a good quantity and quality of the cervical mucus is present. Both normal or abnormal postcoital test results have poor predictive and validity values (36,37). When quantity and quality of cervical mucus is good (cervical score >10), the postcoital test result is abnormal, and spermiogram results are normal, cervical mucus antisperm antibody determination is warranted.

Tubal Patency
Tubal patency assessment is performed when ovulation is confirmed, no abnormality is found on a postcoital test, and no conception occurs within 6 to 12 months.

Essentially, tubal patency can be determined by hysterosalpingography (HSG), which is usually performed between menstrual cycle days 5 and 10 (to avoid potential radiation exposure of a product of conception or inadvertently dislodging a fragment of the endometrium that could develop into an endometriosis implant). The procedure is best performed under fluoroscopy visualization; however, when fluoroscopy is not available, radiographs can be obtained sequentially using water-soluble contrast material [oil contrast may cause lipid granulomas and lipid embolization, and injury, and death have been reported (38,39) due to intravasations].

Intravasation can be identified at the beginning of the procedure by streaklike contrast opacities traversing from the uterine cavity toward the pelvic side walls; such an event warrants termination of the procedure. Nevertheless, when oil contrast media was compared with water-soluble contrast, oil contrast expressed a better therapeutic effect on pregnancy rate [13% with water-soluble vs. 29% with oil contrast media (40)] when injected at volumes of 3, 5, 8, and 10 mL. Radiographs should be taken under fluoroscopic guidance when the uterine cavity is filled with contrast, and at the interstitial and proximal parts of the fallopian tubes, because the rate of proximal, cornual, or interstitial tubal obstruction can be as high as 50% among infertile patients. Tubal obstruction can be caused by salpingitis isthmica nodosa, which is frequently associated with chronic inflammation (41). When contrast reaches the ampullae of the fallopian tubes, the next radiograph is obtained. Distal tube occlusion is established by the absence of peritoneal spillage. Periadnexal adhesions are suspected when irregular, loculated aggregations of contrast are trapped around the distal tube. Both false-positive and false-negative findings have been reported with HSG. More accurate assessment of fimbriae, the endosalpinx mucosa, and ciliary action can be achieved endoscopically (falloposcopy is performed by means of tubal catheterization via laparoscopy or hysteroscopy). HSG can be used to identify the following abnormalities:

- Uterine filling defects
- Müllerian anomalies
- Periadnexal adhesions
- Occlusion of one or both fallopian tubes

When an HSG study reveals tubal patency, laparoscopic chromotubation with methylene blue dye (usually performed at days 20 to 24 of the menstrual cycle) can be postponed [the rate of tubal occlusion after patency documented by HSG is very low (42)]. HSG should not be performed, if pregnancy has not been ruled out, if the patient has a history of acute PID (41), or if a severe male factor has established that an assisted reproductive technique (ART) is indicated [e.g., IVF with embryo transfer (IVF-ET) or intracytoplasmic sperm injection (ICSI)]. Antibiotic prophylaxis with doxycycline at the dosage of 100 mg daily for 3 days is widely recommended for all patients undergoing HSG. Hysterosalpingography with selective salpingography has not only diagnostic value but also therapeutic potential for some infertile women when tubal disease is present (43,44).

Semen Analysis

A semen analysis is an inseparable, integral part of infertility evaluation (Tables 11.1 and 11.2). Findings on semen analysis can be defined as follows (33):

- Normospermia: spermiogram within the expected normal range
- Oligozoospermia: sperm concentration of less than 20×10^6/mL
- Asthenozoospermia: less than 50% of spermatozoa demonstrate forward progression
- Teratozoospermia: less than 30% of spermatozoa have normal morphology
- Oligoasthenoteratozoospermia: abnormalities in all three parameters
- Aspermia: no ejaculation
- Azoospermia: no spermatozoa in the analyzed ejaculate
- Necrospermia: no live spermatozoa present

Semen should be collected by masturbation or during coitus, using a silicone semen collection pouch. Before semen is collected, the partners should abstain from coitus for 2 to 3 days and the collected ejaculate should be delivered to a laboratory within 1 hour.

A semen analysis holds predictive value when no abnormality is identified or when aspermia or azoospermia is present. However, with substandard semen quality, the predictive value is greatly limited. Once the initial semen analysis is determined to be within the normal range, there is no need to repeat the test, unless a clinical condition could have influenced the results. If clinical pathology is derived

TABLE 11.1. NORMAL RANGE OF SEMEN ANALYSIS

Volume	>2 mL
PH	7.2–80
Sperm concentration	$>20 \times 10^6$ spermatozoa/mL
Total sperm count	$>40 \times 10^6$ spermatozoa/ejaculate
Motility	>50% with forward progression or >25% with rapid progression within 60 min of ejaculation
Morphology	>30% normal forms
Vitality	>75% live
White blood cells	$<1 \times 10^6$/mL
Immunobead test	<20% spermatozoa with adherent particles
Mixed agglutination reaction test	<10% spermatozoa with adherent particles

Reprinted from the World Health Organization. *WHO manual for the standardized investigation and diagnosis of the infertile couple.* Cambridge, UK: Cambridge University Press, 1993; with permission.

TABLE 11.2. OPTIONAL SEMEN TESTS

Alpha-glucosidase (neutra)	>20 mU/ejaculate
Zinc (total)	>2.4 µmol/ejaculate
Citric acid	>52 µmol/ejaculate
Acid phosphatase (total)	>200 U/ejaculate
Fructose (total)	>13 µmol/ejaculate

Reprinted from the World Health Organization. *WHO manual for the standardized investigation and diagnosis of the infertile couple.* Cambridge, UK: Cambridge University Press, 1993; with permission.

from the semen analysis, the test should be repeated after at least 6 to 12 hours have elapsed. A computer-assisted semen analysis is not diagnostically superior to the traditional method (5).

Specific Infertility Evaluation

Initial infertility evaluation results usually indicate functional impairment of a specific organ or of the endocrine system. Evaluation also may specifically indicate a female factor, a male factor, or factors relating to both partners as potential causes of infertility.

Female-specific infertility evaluation is directed toward the most probable cause that surfaces during the initial infertility evaluation.

Oligomenorrhea or *secondary amenorrhea* requires a pregnancy test, followed by a progesterone challenge test to determine estrogens levels in a sufficient concentration to induce endometrial growth. Direct measurement of estradiol levels, FSH, LH, and prolactin should be determined in the follicular phase of the menstrual cycle.

When oligomenorrhea or amenorrhea is associated with a clinical picture of androgen excess (hirsutism, oily skin, acne, etc.), the serum testosterone, dehydroepiandrosterone sulfate, androstenedione, and 17-hydroxyprogesterone levels should be determined:

- If 17-hydroxyprogesterone is elevated, 21-hydroxylase deficiencies are possible and an adrenocorticotropic hormone stimulation test or a dexamethasone test should be performed.
- If the LH:FSH ratio is greater than 2:1, and increased androgen levels, obesity (BMI > 25), and hirsutism are present, PCOS is suspected. Some clinicians recommend transvaginal ultrasonography for documentation of ovarian polycysts; however, there is no unanimous clinical approval of this approach. More detailed information on this subject is presented in Chapter 8.
- Elevated FSH levels call for establishing estrogen levels (1 month apart), particularly when a women is under 40 years of age. Premature ovarian failure is possible, so additional clinical investigations such as karyotype, anti–ovarian-specific antibody, polyglandular endocrinopathy, other autoimmune disorders, and pelvic ultrasonography should be used to reach the diagnosis.

Elevated prolactin levels can be associated with not only pituitary adenoma or functional hypersecretion of prolactin but also with primary hypothyroidism or the uses of medications; therefore, those conditions must be excluded. More information on this topic is presented in Chapters 8, 9, and 10.

To rule out pituitary micro- or macroadenoma, as well as suprasellar organic pathology, magnetic resonance imaging (or x-ray computerized tomography) should be ordered.

Tubal occlusion diagnosed by HSG requires further laparoscopic evaluation with tubal chromotubation (tubal lavage) and assessment of potential pelvic pathology, particularly periadnexal adhesions. In approximately 57.67% of patients, HSG findings agree with the laparoscopic diagnosis. Laparoscopic evaluation in cases of unexplained infertility revealed existing pelvic pathology in 57.14% of patients (45). In about 73% of patients whose HSG showed proximal tubal occlusion, laparoscopic tubal dye perfusion under general anesthesia did not confirm this diagnosis owing to a cornual spasm (46). Diagnostic laparoscopy is an irreplaceable tool for visualization or biopsy, and operative laparoscopy is instrumental as a treatment modality for endometriosis, pelvic adhesions, periadnexal adhesions, phimotic fimbriae, hydrosalpinx, and tubal occlusion.

Falloposcopy or *salpingoscopy* is an endoscopic procedure that allows visualization of the ciliated tubal epithelium that is essential for oocyte retrieval and (after conception) embryo transport. Salpingoscopy can assist in identifying endosalpinx polyps, intratubal adhesions, and mucosal plugs. Performed from a transfimbrial or a transcervical approach, falloposcopy is a technically demanding procedure. Nevertheless, falloposcopic evaluation is a superior diagnostic technique compared with HSG, laparoscopy with dye perfusion, and transvaginal ultrasonographic salpingography (47,48).

Uterine abnormalities related to infertility are either of the congenital or acquired type. A congenital uterine anomaly such as uterine hypoplasia or uterine agenesia is an obvious cause of infertility. On the other hand, uterine didelphis or uterine septa is more often associated with early fetal wastage or mid-trimester pregnancy loss.

Acquired uterine abnormalities include endometrial polyps, intrauterine synechiae (Asherman syndrome), submucosal or large intramural leiomyomata, and abnormalities resulting from *in utero* exposure to diethylstilbestrol (postulated as an etiologic factor in infertility not as it relates to uterine and uterine cavity contour changes, but also to the increased risk of tubal or cervical factors and increased incidence of endometriosis). The uterine factor in infertility is not definitively linked to infertility and is more associated with recurrent pregnancy losses. The diagnosis is based on exclusion of other causes of infertility. Although uterine leiomyomata are frequently considered as the cause of infertility, supporting clinical scientific data are lacking. It is presumed that myomata interfere with sperm transport and implantation. The anatomic location of myomata (submucosal) is clinically a more important prognostic factor in infertility than the size of myomata.

Hysterosalpingography is a good screening method, and hysteroscopy is the best technique for evaluating the uterine cavity and for confirming the initial HSG diagnosis and determining the extent of intrauterine abnormality.

Transabdominal, transvaginal, or contrast ultrasonography is also considered a reliable method for identifying uterine abnormalities.

Chromosomal aberrations may be expected in long-term infertility, and primary or secondary amenorrhea is associated with highly elevated serum FSH levels. In such cases, chromosomal karyotyping is necessary to reach the diagnosis.

In most cases of *endometriosis*, ovulation is present and the fallopian tubal mucosa is healthy, but this condition may still cause infertility in the following ways (8):

- Interference with the ovum released
- Blockage of oocyte access to the tubal fimbriae
- Restriction of tubal function with adhesions
- Functional impairments of the granulosa cells and oocyte
- Release of local peritoneal prostaglandin which causes abnormality in the oocyte passage and pick-up, and also interferes with spermatozoa function (48)

The diagnosis of endometriosis is established through direct visualization via laparoscopy with or without biopsy for histologic verification. When the ovary is unilaterally or bilaterally affected by adhesions (intense, local, or fibrotic) or cystic formations (endometrioma), the prognosis for successful pregnancy is poor. More detailed information on endometriosis and its classification is presented in Chapters 5, 6, and 9.

Male-specific infertility evaluation is necessary when volume, density, function, or morphology of sperm is called into question. A semen analysis alone cannot determine the fertilizing ability of spermatozoa. The function of sperm can be categorized as follows:

- Ability to penetrate cervical mucus
- Ability to migrate and reach the distal part of the fallopian tubes
- Ability to penetrate and fertilize the oocyte (several tests are available to determine spermatozoa's ability to fertilize oocytes in *in vitro* tests) (49)

The sperm penetration assay is a commonly accepted tool. However, this test does not determine the sperm's ability to penetrate the zona pellucida. The assay is based on the sperm-penetrating ability of zona-free hamster ova. A sperm penetration rate of less than 10% is indicative of male infertility (50).

Hormonal evaluation is undertaken to determine the following serum concentrations:

- FSH elevation in view of normal LH and testosterone levels, decreased testicular volume to less than 10 to 12 mL, with normal ejaculate volume of greater than 2 mL imply *spermatogenesis dysfunction* (51).
- Low FSH, LH, and testosterone levels are indicative of hypogonadic hypogonadism. Functioning or nonfunctioning pituitary adenoma should be excluded.

Immunologic evaluation should be considered with asthenozoospermic or oligoasthenozoospermic patients after infection had been ruled out. Specific antibodies to spermatozoa are responsible for male infertility in about 3% to 7% of patients. Antibodies can be identified from a patient's serum blood or ejaculate, or from a partner's cervical mucus (52).

Bacteriologic examination is indicated when asymptomatic leukocytospermia is present or physical examination suggests infection. Semen cultures for gram-positive and gram-negative bacteria, *Chlamydia trachomatis, Neisseria gonorrhoeae, Ureoplasma urealyticum,* and *Mycoplasma hominis* should be performed.

Testicular biopsy is indicated for the following:

- Diagnosis of spermatogenesis dysfunction in patients with azoospermia, serum FSH levels in the normal range, and normal testicular volume, implying occlusion
- Treatment of male infertility caused by obstruction, in which spermatozoa are retrieved from testes and used for ICSI (53)
- Karyotyping is indicated in male infertility associated with azoospermia and severe oligozoospermia with serum FSH elevation and testicular volume of less than 10 to 12 mL.
- Vasography is offered to a patient with obstructive azoospermia or severe oligospermia. Before vasography is performed, completion of endocrinology assays such as FSH, LH, prolactin, and thyroid-stimulating hormone, as well as those for immunologic or infectious factors, are performed.

CONVENTIONAL THERAPY
Female Partner
Induction of Ovulation

Pelvic ultrasonography should precede induction of ovulation to rule out the presence of an adnexal mass or uterine pathology. Patients on clomiphene citrate should be checked monthly for ovarian cysts, preferably via transvaginal ultrasonography. It is not necessary to determine follicular maturation when a GnRH agonist or antiestrogen agent is used for ovulation induction. To avoid ovarian hyperstimulation, close monitoring of follicular maturation is advised using an ultrasonographic transvaginal transducer every other day, with parallel determination of serum estradiol levels. When ovulation induction is attempted with human menopausal gonadotropin (hMG) and hCG (or FSH and hCG), close monitoring is mandatory. If ultrasonography and estradiol elevations indicate possible ovarian hyperstimulation, induction of ovulation should be aborted. Induction of ovulation is discussed at length in Chapter 10.

Irregular or chronic ovulation is a recognizable cause of infertility. When a hormonal abnormality is identified, the cause of infertility can be attributed either to the absolute hormone level of secretions or to an inappropriately balanced ratio between hormones. Based on these two components, the following categories of anovulation, as a cause of female infertility, can be identified and a specific therapy can be instituted.

In eugonadotropic anovulation, the LH:FSH ratio is elevated due to the increased serum LH levels. Such an imbalance among gonadotropins is observed in PCOS, and this condition is discussed in more detail in Chapter 8. The treatment is provided with antiestrogen agents such as clomiphene citrate or occasionally tamoxifen. Weight reduction is recommended when a patient's BMI is over 25. There is no clinical evidence that administration of either human chorionic gonadotropin or sequential estrogen will provide additional benefits in ovulation induction.

GnRH agonists or recombinant FSH may be used when patient is resistant or unresponsive to antiestrogen agents. It has been suggested that insulin-sensitizing agents can improve the outcome in PCOS; however, validation of this therapy is needed. Surgical ovarian wedge resection either through laparotomy or laparoscopy in patients with PCOS that is resistant to conservative medical therapies is an acceptable approach.

Hypogonadotropic anovulation can be related to the following types of dysfunction:

- Primary pituitary gland dysfunction leading to anovulation: induction of ovulation can be achieved with gonadotropin treatment.
- Secondary pituitary gland dysfunction leading to hypothalamic disorder: ovulation can be induced with pulsatile GnRH therapy.

Hypergonadotropic anovulation is associated with premature ovary failure and FSH levels of over 40 mIU/L. No effective therapy is available. The potential solutions include ovum donation and adoption. In the early stages of premature ovary failure, when FSH levels are not yet at the menopausal range (e.g., 15-25 mIU/L), remaining oocytes can be harvested under controlled ovarian hyperstimulation, and IVF or oocyte cryopreservation can be offered for later ART.

Hyperprolactinemic anovulation correction can be achieved with bromocriptine therapy in functional hyperprolactinemia or hyperprolactinemia associated with microadenoma or macroadenoma (prolactinoma). When prolactinoma is unresponsive to conservative medical management, trans-sphenoidal adenectomy is indicated (53).

Conditions such as *systemic illnesses, endocrinopathy* of other endocrine systems, endometriosis, and underweightedness (BMI of <19) can negatively affect ovulation. An appropriate therapy for the underlying cause may restore ovulation.

A more detailed description of therapeutic modalities for ovulation induction in different causes is presented in Chapter 10.

The role of the luteal phase defect and its therapy in infertility have been called into question. Most of practitioners take this condition into account in infertility management. It has been postulated that a luteal phase shorter than 8 days may affect the implantation process. Clomiphene citrate appears to be effective in normalizing luteal phase defects in the ovulatory cycle, or natural progesterone supplementation may be used.

Surgical Therapy for Female Infertility

Surgical correction of reproductive organs can be categorized as follows:

- Reconstructive microtubal surgery
- Ovarian surgery
- Uterine reconstructive or restorative surgery
- Endometriosis therapy
- Cervical factor

Reconstructive Microtubal Surgery

The outcome of *tubal ligation reversal* must be balanced against the outcome that ART can offer. In properly selected patients, tubal ligation reversal using laparotomy and magnifying loupes may yield pregnancy and delivery rates of up to 75% (56). There are several prognostic factors, such as method of surgical sterilization, fimbrial function preservation, surgical technique, and surgeon microsurgery skill. Most influential on the pregnancy rate is the patient's age and the tubal length after anastomosis. Age at tubal reversal of over 35 years and tubal length postanastomosis of less than 4 cm are significant factors for a successful outcome (tubal length postanastomosis of >7 cm is associated with the best outcome rate) (57,58). Pregnancy and the overall live birth rate in this group is about 14.3%, with the spontaneous abortion rate approximately 23.8% and the ectopic pregnancy rate 2.4% (59). A cumulative analysis of one-tube versus two-tube reconstruction demonstrated the same fecundity rate (60). The most successful tubal reversal pregnancy outcomes are reconstruction following Falope ring placement (about 83%); the worst outcome is observed in fimbriectomy. The highest success is noted when isthmic–isthmic or cornual–isthmic anastomosis is performed with 81% and 67% term live delivery rates, respectively (61,62).

The advances in laparoscopic surgical skill and technology allow execution of tubal reconstruction (isthmic–isthmic, cornual–isthmic, isthmic–ampullary, and ampullary–ampullary anastomosis) with resulting pregnancy rates compatible with those achieved via classic laparotomy (59,61,62).

Tubal reconstruction outcomes for occluded fallopian tubes are varied and depend on the cause of tubal obstruction (PID, endometriosis, previous pelvic surgery, ruptured appendix, etc.). Poor results of surgery can be expected when distal tubuocclusion is present with hydrosalpinx. Microsurgical techniques are applicable in the same way as for tubal ligation reversal.

Ovarian Surgery
Ovarian surgery for infertility is performed for endometrioma excision, lysis of periovarian adhesions, ovarian wedge resection, or ovarian drilling for PCOS resistant to medical management. The procedures can be executed via laparotomy or laparoscopy with the similar outcome (63).

Uterine Reconstructive or Restorative Surgery
Myomectomy for uterine leiomyomata (myomata) is infrequently performed for infertility. Submucosal, large intramural or penetrating uterine myomata warrant myomectomy to restore fertility. The indication and verification for surgical treatment for infertility are reached by exclusion of other causes of infertility. The size of myomata is less important than the anatomic location. Clinical findings show that postmyomectomy pelvic adhesions may lead to a mechanical type of infertility, particularly when the myomectomy incision is on the posterior wall of the uterus (64). Myomectomy can be executed either via laparotomy or a laparoscopic approach, with compression of the uterine isthmic vessels, repair of endometrial defects, and reconstruction of the myometrium in three layers (65). Submucosal uterine fibroids are usually resected using a hysteroscopic approach. This technique avoids creation of intraabdominal adhesions, but may lead to intrauterine adhesions, which may be prevented with estrogen supplementation at the oral dose of 2.5 conjugated estrogen daily for 30 days, adding either 200 mg micronized natural progesterone or 10 mg medroxyprogesterone daily for the last 10 days of estrogen supplementation. Upon completion of submucosal myomata resection, an IUD or pediatric Foley catheter may be inserted; however, the clinical scientific data are lacking to support this empiric approach. A prophylactic broad-spectrum antibiotic is administered concomitantly (66). Operative hysteroscopy is best performed in the early proliferative phase of the menstrual cycle. To reduce uterine medium distention, intravasation, and intraoperative bleeding, 20 U of diluted vasopressin in 50 mL of sterile saline can be injected into the cervical stroma (the vasoconstrictive effect of vasopressin occurs after about 30 minutes).

Metroplasty for the intrauterine septum using the classic transabdominal approach (either the Jones or Tampkins technique) has been replaced by hysteroscopic resection. Uterine septum hysteroscopic resection is indicated either for infertility or recurrent pregnancy losses. The septum can be excised using the semirigid hysteroscopic scissors or a resectoscopic loop electrode. Bleeding is minimal during the resection process; intensification of bleeding indicates the nearness of the myometrium. Upon entering the myometrium stratum, the procedure is completed. Uterine septum resection is advocated for its simplicity and minimal risk and sequelae, and it significantly improves reproductive outcome. This procedure is among the safest and most effective means for conception, in clinical practice (67–69). Prevention of postoperative intrauterine adhesions is similar to that presented in the preceding paragraphs on myomectomy.

Adhesiolysis of the uterine cavity associated with Asherman syndrome is performed using the hysteroscopic approach, with good surgical outcome. The live birth rates range from 81.3% in patients with mild disease to 31.9% in patients with severe disease (70).

Endometrial polypectomy is thought to have little consequence on infertility. Hysteroscopic enucleation of polyps or curettage for multiple polyps can be applied. Pedunculated polyps and polyps protruding from the external os of the cervical canal can be removed in the office.

Endometriosis Therapy
Medical conservative management is usually chosen for patients infertile due to endometriosis. Ovulation suppression is induced with GnRH agonists (nasal spray or an injectable form), danazol, medroxyprogesterone acetate (oral or an injectable form), or oral contraceptives. The success rate of endometriosis therapies, when compared with the placebo, were for medroxyprogesterone acetate 41%, oral contraceptive 40%, GnRH agonists 36%, danazol 35%, and placebo 41% (71). Medical conservative approach is offered for women classified with the minimal to mild stage endometriosis [staging classification was adopted from the American Fertility Society (72)]. More advanced stages of endometriosis are surgically treated or, when endometriosis meets criteria, ART is planned.

Detailed information on endometriosis is presented in Chapters 9 and 10.

Cervical Factor
Cervical factor, such as mucus hostility and inflammation, can be treated with artificial insemination, as can some other causes of infertility. Upon determining the type of cervical infection and sensitivity with bacteriologic culture, parenteral antibiotic therapy and local intravaginal treatment may restore fertility. There are several forms by which artificial insemination can be executed.

Artificial insemination with the husband's semen (AIH) is one of the oldest forms of infertility treatment. It involves semen placement into the cervical canal [intracervical insemination (ICI)]. This type of insemination is indicated when male anatomic impairment (such as hypospadias) is present. However, a randomized controlled prospective study documented no improvement with AIH, regardless of semen analysis results or the presence or absence of sperm antibodies (the cumulative pregnancy rate was 3.8% in the AIH group and 3.9% in the untreated group) (73).

Artificial insemination with donor semen (AID) is indicated when a severe, irreversible form of male factor infertility is diagnosed. The fecundity success rate for artificial insemination with fresh donor sperm is higher than with cryopreserved (frozen) donor sperm (74). Nevertheless, the U.S. Food and Drug Administration, the American Fertility Society, and the Centers for Disease Control and Prevention recommend insemination with cryopreserved donor sperm over fresh specimen to prevent HIV infection (semen from an HIV-negative donor is accepted for use only when the report on HIV is still negative after 60–180 days).

Intrauterine insemination (IUI) is insertion of 0.3 mL of washed or prepared semen into the uterine cavity through a catheter after ovulation. Based on the meta-analysis of prospective randomized studies comparing IUI and ICI, IUI provides significantly higher fecundity rates than ICI with cryopreserved specimens (75). IUI conception can be expected when 1 to 2×10^6 motile spermatozoa are used with a controlled multiovulation cycle. If no conception occurs with the first three consecutive cycle attempts, gamete intrafallopian transfer (GIFT), zygote intrafallopian transfer (ZIFT), or IVF should be considered (71).

Fallopian tube sperm perfusion (FSP) is intratubal insemination with 4 mL of processed semen through catheter and superovulation induced with gonadotropins (76) [a pediatric Foley catheter can be used, which prevents the reflux of sperm suspension (77)]. This form of artificial insemination with washed and resuspended spermatozoa is successful in about 40% in couples with unexplained infertility and is a less invasive procedure than GIFT, ZIFT, and IVF, and does not require culturing of human oocytes and embryos (76). Invalidated clinical data indicate that FSP is more successful than IUI (78).

Direct intraperitoneal insemination (DIPI) or *in vivo* transperitoneal fertilization (IVTPF) is offered to a couple with either unexplained infertility or with a male subinfertility factor. Processed and resuspended sperm is injected using a 19-gauge needle on the peritoneal surface of the posterior cul-de-sac (the pouch of Douglas) with controlled ovulation. In an observational study, the pregnancy rate was higher than reported from IUI studies (79).

Male Partner Therapy

When treatment of the male partner is indicated, careful reevaluation of all parameters should be considered before offering any specific therapy. Male factor therapeutic effectiveness is notoriously low, and the prognosis for live birth among untreated infertile couples at 12 months is approximately 14.3% (80,81). Therefore, when a female partner is relatively young (<30 years), infertility has been present for only a short period (<3 years), and a male partner is diagnosed with oligozoospermia or asthenozoospermia, or a combination of both, expectant management should be recommended.

Male infertility has many causes. Infection in male infertility with a full clinical picture of active stage is not difficult to identify or to treat. The diagnostic challenge comes into play when an asymptomatic subclinical male genital tract infection is present. Transurethrally obtained swab culture, following digital prostatic massage, is the best way to identify the type of infection and to establish the degree of sensitivity to antibiotics. Appropriate antibiotics are administered to both partners. Difficulty arises when the male partner's ethnic background or culture disapproves of the concept of male infertility and believes that only a woman can be blamed for reproduction failure. The clinician must decide whether to treat both partners empirically with broad-spectrum antibiotics or to obtain a cervical culture from the female partner. The cervical culture, performed as a part of the female routine fertility workup, adequately identifies *Chlamydia trachomatis* (the most common sexually transmitted infection), *Ureoplasma urealyticum* (the prevalence varies in human semen from 10% to 40%), or *Mycoplasma hominis*. *Enterobacteria* is found in both partners in about 94% of cases and is the most common cause of subclinical infection (82,83). Clinical research is underway analyzing the detection of viruses in semen and their potential role in infertility (83). The specific therapy is determined by the sensitivity of the microorganism to antibiotics. If the sensitivity is unknown, tetracycline oral therapy for 10 days to 2 weeks, followed by repeat cervical culture is recommended.

Varicocele is present in about 20% to 40% of males undergoing infertility evaluation (varicocele is unilaterally or bilaterally present in approximately 15% of the general population) (84). Most authorities suggest varicocelectomy (high ligation of the internal spermatic vein above the internal inguinal ring) as treatment, improving sperm count, motility, and morphology (85–88). It has been postulated that even a small palpable right varicocele can have a detrimental effect on bilateral testis function, and the presence of bilateral varicoceles requires bilateral varicocelectomy (88). It is not uniformly accepted among clinicians that varicocele ligation improves fecundity (89).

The American Fertility Society suggests the following criteria when considering varicocelectomy:

- Documented infertility
- Potential fertility documented in a female partner
- Palpable varicocele
- The male partner has one or more semen parameter abnormalities.

It has been shown that spermatogenic failure can be associated with varicoceles and that varicocelectomy can result in reversal of azoospermia. A selected group of men with spermatogenic failure and varicoceles may be good candidates for varicocele ligation before testicular biopsy for sperm extraction in preparation for ICSI (90).

Ejaculation disorders may be identified in any of the physiologic events that occur in the process of ejaculation. The following synchronized actions take place in ejaculation:

- A phase accumulation of semen components in the prostatic part of urethra
- Sperm emission (a phase of expulsion) with accessory gland fluids into the urethra (controlled by a thoracolumbar symptomatic reflex with supraspinal modulation and mediated by the alpha-adrenergic system)
- Closure of the bladder neck
- Forceful semen ejaculation via the urethra (controlled by a sacrospinal reflex mediated by the pudendal nerve)

An asynchronic event in the process of ejaculation may result in ejaculation dysfunction.

The orgasmic phase of sexual function disturbances can be clinically categorized as either premature ejaculation or retrograde ejaculation.

Premature ejaculation is divided into primary and secondary types (organic etiology such as vein leakage or arterial insufficiency or other causes). Primary premature ejaculation therapy is addressed by sexual therapeutic behavioral training and, if necessary, prescription of diazepam or chlorodizepoxid (91). Secondary premature ejaculation treatment is directed to an underlying organic cause.

Retrograde ejaculation (unphysiologic passage of seminal fluids from the posterior urethra into the bladder) should be suspected in any case of azoospermia and can be determined by microscopic demonstration of sperm in postejaculation urine. Retrograde ejaculation can be congenital, acquired (bladder neck lesion, nephropathic disorders, diabetes), iatrogenic, or idiopathic in origin. To convert retrograde ejaculation to antegrade ejaculation, intact anatomy and innervations of the bladder neck are necessary prerequisites.

Therapy for retrograde ejaculation includes the following:

- Pharmacologic therapy can be effective, such as imipramine hydrochloride (tricyclic antidepressant) 25 to 50 mg daily 7 days before the planned ejaculation or expected ovulation of a female partner. Conservative medical therapy is ineffective when anorgasmia is present (91).
- Intrauterine insemination with retreated spermatozoa from male partner urine (92,93). To ensure the best possible survival of spermatozoa, the pH (7.2–8.2) and osmolarity (300–380 mosmol/kg) of urine can be adjusted by administering bicarbonate and water to a patient a few hours before ejaculation (94).
- Electroejaculation and electrovibration stimulation are discussed later in the section on Complementary Therapy.
- Surgical bladder neck reconstruction is recommended if all other methods fail. Bladder neck reconstruction is

performed to convert retrograde ejaculation to physiologic antegrade ejaculation (95).

Idiopathic anejaculation in male infertility usually responds to psychotherapy, or sexual, marital, or behavioral therapy. Electroejaculation also is a useful treatment method in this condition. However, the average sperm motility may decrease with electrostimulation (96).

Secondary anejaculation is caused by spinal cord injury [infertility is due to ejaculatory dysfunction, impaired spermatogenesis, and poor semen quality (97)] or retroperitoneal lymphadenectomy. Electroejaculation with sperm retrieval and female partner stimulation for superovulated cycles appears to improve the pregnancy rate in both of these conditions (98). Even though technologic advances have been made in the management of ejaculation dysfunction, the sperm quality (density motility, and function) remains poor (93,97–99).

Diabetes also may cause secondary anejaculation. Appropriate control of diabetes with electroejaculation may assist in overcoming this condition (99).

Secondary anejaculation of psychogenic origin is treated by psychotherapy with a sexual therapist. If necessary, diazepam or chlorodizepoxid can be added (91). Psychogenic anejaculation also may be treated by electroejaculation, but sperm quality is poor (100,101).

Many treatment modalities are available for *obstructive azoospermia*:

- Vasectomy reversal (vasovasostomy) is a microsurgical procedure that restores the patency of the vas deferens. The success rate of vasovasostomy to reach patency is about 86%, and the associated pregnancy rate is approximately 28% (102). The fertility rate decreases with the more time elapsed since vasectomy (103).
- Vaseopididymostomy is microsurgical restoration of patency between the vas deferens and the epididymis. For other obstructive azoospermic conditions, patency is restored in about 45% of men; the associated pregnancy rate is approximately 18% (104).
- Microsurgical sperm aspiration from the epididymis is used as an ART when congenital absence of the vas is documented or reconstructive microsurgery has failed (105).

Hypogonadotropic hypogonadism is the result of either hypothalamic or hypophyseous dysfunction. In hypothalamic dysfunction, pulsatile GnRH therapy (25–600 ng/kg/120 min) is a quite successful method of attaining quality semen. When the diagnosis of pituitary disorder is established, combination therapy with hMG and hCG provides satisfactory results.

Oligospermia can be improved with the split ejaculation technique, which concentrates sperm in a small volume, so that even with a severe form of oligospermia, conception may occur. Sperm density increases significantly with split ejaculation; although, sperm motility improvement is variable. When mild oligospermia is present (10–40 × 10^6 of whole semen) and high semen volume is documented (>5 mL), improvement in both semen density and motility is observed (106).

Therapies such as androgens, clomiphene citrate, bromocriptine, and kallicreine are considered anecdotal therapeutic modalities because none of these medications has demonstrated efficacy in randomized, double-blind, controlled clinical trials (107).

Antisperm antibodies can be effectively treated by IVF. Other methods such as condom use, IUI, sperm processing, or glucocorticoid therapy have proved to be ineffective in the treatment of this entity.

Necrospermia (immotile spermatozoa) prevalence is reported to occur in approximately 0.2% to 0.48% of men. The diagnosis of necrospermia is reached by analysis of at least three semen samples. Infection may cause up to 40% of immotile spermatozoa. In about 20% the epididymis is abnormal. The remaining etiologic factors have not been established and are considered to be an idiopathic form. Therapy is recommended for the underlying etiology. If the etiology is unknown, there is no specific treatment (108,109).

Karyotyping is indicated when azoospermia, low normal or low serum testosterone levels, and elevated serum gonadotropins are present, and testicular biopsy disclosed no spermatogenesis (110,111).

Assisted Reproductive Techniques

A detailed description of ART is beyond the scope of this chapter. However, a brief appraisal of these techniques is offered.

Intrauterine insemination is a simple method of insertion of previously selected spermatozoa into the uterine cavity via catheterization. The placement of spermatozoa should be synchronized with the female partner's ovulation. IUI is indicated when the male factor in not severe, ovulation is either spontaneous or induced, and no tubal factor is present. Combined superovulation and IUI yeilds pregnancy rates of about 10% to 25% per cycle, an average of approximately 15% per cycle (8).

Intracytoplasmic sperm injection is the placement of a single spermatozoon into the oocyte cytoplasm. This technique is particularly beneficial in severe male factor infertility, including azoospermia. The oocyte cytoplasm is injected after microsurgical sperm aspiration from the epididymis, after testicular sperm aspiration with a needle, or after open biopsy testicular sperm extraction.

In vitro fertilization and embryo transfer is undertaken after the induction of multiple follicles; the harvesting of oocytes is accomplished under transvaginal ultrasonographic guidance. Retrieved oocytes are incubated for 3 to 6 hours followed by *in vitro* insemination. The embryo cleaves within 2 days after insemination. Upon grading,

two or three embryos are selected and inserted into the uterine cavity. IVF-ET is indicated in instances of either female or male factor infertility. The overall pregnancy rate is approximately 25% per controlled ovulation cycle (8).

Zygote intrafallopian transfer is a combination of IVF and ZIFT. After IVF, the zygote is transferred to the fallopian tube under general anesthesia and through a laparoscopic approach.

Gamete intrafallopian transfer is performed under general anesthesia and under direct laparoscopic visualization, sperm and oocytes are introduced into the ampullary part of the fallopian tube, where IVF occurs. A prerequisite for GIFT fertilization is the presence of intact fallopian tubes. The pregnancy rate is about 35% for each cycle (8).

Gamete micromanipulation incorporates several different methods:

- ICSI
- Partial zona dissection, designed to assist sperm in the penetration process
- Subzonal sperm injection or microinsemination sperm transferred (MIST) facilitates fertilization.

Partial zona dissection and MIST have a low live birth rate, ranging from 1% to 5% (112); the pregnancy rate for ICSI is 31% (113).

Endometriosis and Assisted Reproductive Techniques

Endometriosis and its influence on infertility are well documented. A therapeutic approach for endometriosis associated with infertility is based mainly on retrospective observational studies and small randomized clinical trials. The following clinical management has been suggested (114):

- Minimal to mild endometriosis may favorably respond to controlled ovarian hyperstimulation.
- Data on the treatment of severe stages of endometriosis have not been generated by randomized controlled studies. The therapy offered is often based on a practitioner's personal conviction. Overall birth life success with ART in treatment for all stages of endometriosis appears to be valuable.
- Ovarian endometriomas and their influence on fecundity, apart from the stage of endometriosis, have not been clearly established. A surgical conservative treatment is indicated in any management plan.
- GnRH agonist therapy seems to be beneficial not only for pelvic pain associated with endometriosis but also presumptively has a positive effect on infertility, but no data from randomized controlled studies support this notion.
- Surgical conservative treatment for endometriosis has long been used, although evidence-based high-ranking clinical trials have not specifically advocated this modality.

Karyotyping is indicated when primary amenorrhea or hypergonadotropic hypogonadism (serum FSH elevation) manifested by secondary amenorrhea is identified. Long-standing unexplained infertility or habitual abortion, particularly in the first trimester, also has been documented.

Turner syndrome is one of the clinical entities that presents a challenge for the practitioner. In this syndrome, only 5% to 10% of patients will undergo spontaneous puberty; the rest will require hormonal replacement therapy not only to develop secondary sex characteristics, but also to provide protection from cardiovascular disease and osteoporosis. Spontaneous pregnancy may occur in about 2% to 5%. Consequently, sexually active patients with Turner syndrome require contraceptive counseling, and oral contraceptive pills will protect against unwanted pregnancy. In fertility counseling the following options can be presented to a patient with Turner syndrome (115):

- Ovarian tissue with oocytes present can be obtained from young girls with Turner syndrome via ovarian full-thickness laparoscopic biopsy (116) and preserved using a cryotechnology technique. The optimal time for ovarian full-thickness biopsy has not been determined.
- Oocyte donation with embryo transfer yields a pregnancy rate of approximately 46%.

Upon completion of sequential diagnostic steps, treatment choices should be presented according to the best expected outcome for the particular cause or causes of the couple's infertility. Table 11.3 illustrates the effectiveness of different ART methods.

Unexplained Infertility Therapy

The negative results of both partners' infertility evaluations are defined as a form of unexplained infertility (normal but infertile), found in about 10% of cases. The natural cumulative conception rate decreases with the increasing duration of unexplained infertility, with the cut-off point at 3 years. When unexplained infertility is shorter than 3 years duration, greater than 30% of conceptions occur from expectant management (80). However, this rule cannot be applied across the entire population with unexplained infertility, and when the female patient is over 30 years of age, other methods of ART should be offered. IUI combined with clomiphene citrate is suggested as the first line of therapeutic approach; if this therapy fails, hMG plus hCG and IUI should be tried before IVF is offered to the couple (118,119).

When clomiphene citrate or hMG and IUI are not successful, IVF combined with superovulation appears to be en effective therapeutic modality (120).

Age and reproductive capacity are well-established interrelationship phenomena. Oocyte quantity and quality decline with progressing age. Ovarian responsiveness to gonadotropin stimulation weakens, and the endometrium's preimplantation and postimplantation ability to maintain the early stage of pregnancy is progressively diminished.

Also with aging, the chances of acquiring reproductive organ dysfunction or systemic disease may influence reproductive capacity (121,122). Fetal genetic abnormalities such as Down syndrome also increase in women over 35 years of age (120).

Ovarian cancer, infertility, and induction of ovulation have been linked for some time. Despite numerous publications, a definitive connection between infertility and induction of ovulation and epithelial ovarian cancer has not been established (123,124).

Adoption is an alternative approach when the success of a live birth cannot be secured. Through a formal legal process, couples can start a new family and a physician should be a part of the decision-making process.

TABLE 11.3. PREGNANCY RATE OF DIFFERENT ART METHODS

Method	Effectiveness
Tubal/pelvis surgery	50% after 2 years (8)
Tubal/pelvic surgery for severe infective damage	≤10% after 2 years (8)
Intracervical donor insemination	5%–10%(8)
IUI with combined superovulation	15% per cycle (8)
IUI alone	5%–10% per cycle (8)
IVF-ET	26% deliveries per retrieval (117)
GIFT	29% deliveries per retrieval (117)
ZIFT	30.9% deliveries per retrieval (117)
ICSI	31% per cycle (113)
PZD and MIST	1% to 5% live birth (112)
Cryopreserved ET from donated oocytes	20.8% deliveries per transfer (117)
ET using a host uterus	31.3% deliveries per emergency room (117)

IUI, intrauterine implantation; IVF-ET, *in vitro* fertilization with embryo transfer; GIFT, gamete intrafallopian transfer; ZIFT, zygote intrafallopian transfer; ICSI, intracytoplasmic sperm injection; PZD, partial zona dissection; MIST, microinsemination sperm transfer.

COMPLEMENTARY THERAPY

Both Partners

Education

A couple in search of infertility treatment is best served when a detailed explanation for both partners about infertility is provided. A diagnostic process, its steps, and potential therapeutic options should be presented. Potentially harmful environmental, occupational, and life-style factors can compromise fertility capacity and should be identified. Systemic illness negatively influencing fecundability should be discussed. Evaluation does not always yield a definitive diagnosis, and unexplained infertility is difficult to treat and is associated with a low rate of conception. Expectant management in selective cases is successful. Therefore, avoiding alcohol consumption, smoking tobacco, drugs, caffeine, self-administered medication, vigorous exercise, and changing life-style may assist in conception.

Diet

A balanced diet with intake of whole foods, high protein, high fiber, and vegetables is optimal. A vegetarian diet has a more beneficial effect than other diets for infertility (150). A very low-fat and high-fiber diet will not affect ovulation; although, it will positively influence general health (151). Therefore, a diet that incorporates soy, almonds and other nuts, cold water fish (salmon, mackerel, herring), carrots, kale, cabbage family vegetables, brussels spouts, onions, garlic, and leeks, with reduced red meat and sugar consumption, will benefit patients with infertility.

Female Partner

Female Partner Supplementation

Minerals

- Selenium, 200 to 400 µg per day (deficiency may lead to subinfertility)
- Magnesium, 600 mg per day (improves outcome of conception in unexplained infertility within 4 months of therapy; if conception does not occur, adding selenium at the dose of 200 mg daily may enhance fecundity (152)
- Zinc, 80 mg per day (improves function of the reproductive organs)
- Manganese, 10 mg per day (enhances gonadal hormone production)

Vitamins

- Vitamin C, 2,000 to 6000 mg per day in divided doses (a key component in gonadal function) (153)

- Vitamin E, 400 to 1,000 IU daily (starting dose of 200 mg daily, gradually increasing)
- Vitamin A, 15,000 IU daily (improves gonadal function)
- Vitamin B complex, 50 mg (improves gonadal function)

Acupuncture

Acupuncture is particularly suggested for oligomenorrheic/amenorrheic patients or those with luteal phase defects. It has been postulated that approximately 44% of women respond to this mode of therapy (125). Electroacupuncture is recommended in normalizing hypothalamic–pituitary–ovarian axis dysfunction (126). Acupuncture and acupressure are recommended for therapeutic application in infertility, mostly based on observational studies (127), and more randomized controlled clinical trials are needed to substantiate these clinical claims. Additional information on acupuncture applications for ovulation induction is discussed in Chapters 8, 9, and 10.

Exercise

Regular exercise as a part of life-style changes, particularly for weight control and as part of a stress reduction program, is very helpful. The emotional aspect of infertility is accentuated more by both partners than in the general population. Hence, regular, moderate daily exercise should be incorporated into infertility management. More information is presented in Chapters 8, 9, and 10.

On the other hand, excessive exercise may lead to several clinical reproductive dysfunction manifestations (delayed menarche, luteal phase deficiency, and anovulation). The diagnosis is reached by exclusion, and exercise modification with nutritional support is recommended for this condition. Such a therapeutic approach is often effective (128).

Life-Style

Life-style factors such as cigarette smoking, alcohol and caffeine consumption, physical exercise, BMI, and drug use may negatively influence reproductive capacity, particularly in the female partner. Primary tubal infertility risk factors include use of IUDs, particularly the Dalkon Shield type, and cigarette smoking. Obesity is identified as the risk factor for ovulatory dysfunction. Drugs such as cocaine, marijuana, alcohol, and caffeine may contribute to various subtypes of primary infertility (129,130).

Hypnosis

The clinical application of hypnotherapy in recent years has increased and has captured public attention. Improvement in research methodology in this field has enhanced its clinical use and availability (131). Hypnosis may mediate intimate mind–body communications in terms of the central nervous system, autonomic nervous system, neuropeptides, neurohormones, and hormones. Although the effects of hypnosis may be subjective, physiologic changes can be measured (132). Information in the scientific literature in reference to the role of hypnosis in the treatment of functional infertility is limited. However, case reports suggest that hypnotherapy may provide a beneficial effect through modification of attitude, optimism, anxiety, and body–mind interaction (133,134). It also has been reported, based on meta-analysis studies, that the beneficial effect of hypnosis increases substantially over time (135).

Behavioral Therapy

Behavioral modification therapy may increase fecundity by reducing the emotional aspects of infertility (significant decrease in anxiety, depression, and fatigue). Behavioral treatment also increases enthusiasm and energy. Within 6 months following the behavioral modification program, 34% women conceived. Such an improvement in fecundability suggests that the emotional component of infertility plays a significant role in the conception rate. Based on these findings, behavioral treatment should be recommended for an infertile couple before or in conjunction with other infertility treatments (136). Although this management suggestion sounds promising, it remains untested at present.

Male Partner

Male Partners Supplementation

Minerals

- Selenium, 200 to 400 mg daily (may improve sperm count and motility). Supplementing selenium with vitamin E significantly increases sperm count, motility, and percentage of live spermatozoa (154).
- Zinc, 80 mg daily (zinc and folate are participants in the DNA and RNA synthesis (155). Zinc is considered a necessary element for spermatozoa maturation and function (156). Excessive high zinc concentration may cause defective sperm motility. Physiologic zinc seminal plasma concentration is necessary for normal sperm function (157).

Vitamins

- Vitamin C in high doses is considered an antioxidative treatment and anecdotally has been offered to improve sperm quality (158). However, a randomized, placebo-controlled, double-blind study revealed no improvement in conventional semen parameters, even when high-dose vitamin C and E were administered (159).

- Vitamin B_{12} is suggested for improvement of sperm quality (158). However, there is not sufficient scientific data to support this notion.

Other Therapies

- Glutathione at the dose 600 mg daily for 2 months may improve sperm mobility, as has been presented in observational studies (160).
- Carnitine supplementation, 3 g daily for 3 to 4 months, may increase sperm density and rapid linear progressive motility in patients with idiopathic asthenozoospermia. Only observational clinical studies are available (161,162).
- Folinic acid, 15 mg per day for 3 months, is beneficial in increasing sperm number and motility in male infertility. Significant variation in improvements was noted after treatment in an observational clinical trial (163).

Acupuncture

A prospective controlled study documented that acupuncture therapy may improve sperm quality (viability, density, mobility, and the integrity of axonema). Improvement has been noticed in male patients with oligozoospermias, oligoasthenozoospermia, and azoospermia. Men with very poor sperm density associated with postgenital infections were the best candidates for this approach (137). It usually required a total of 10 treatment sessions over 3 weeks to observe statistically significant improvement in sperm quality (140,141). However, ejaculate volume is insignificantly improved with acupuncture treatment (140).

Electroejaculation

Electroejaculation is a useful therapeutic modality in the treatment of ejaculation dysfunction, particularly retrograde ejaculation. Vibroejaculation (electrovibration stimulation) can be applied in retrograde ejaculation or other forms of ejaculation disorders (93).

Exercise

Moderate exercise positively influences men in maintaining homeostasis due to an improved integrated endocrine response to changes in homeostatic balance (137). There are conflicting data in reference to endurance or resistant athletic training. The data suggest significant changes in gonadal hormonal ambience (total and free testosterone) and sperm quality (oligospermia) (142–144). Sperm density, motility, and morphology also may be significantly altered in endurance-trained runners (145). Other studies contradict this notion (146,147).

Life-Style

It is postulated, based on the results of a questionnaire study on life-style and sperm quality, that no association exists between the two. There is no relationship between sperm quality and moderate tobacco smoking, coffee drinking, alcohol intake, exposure to heat generated from a sauna, hot bath, type of underwear, or sedentary activities. The average ejaculation frequency significantly increases sperm progressive motility and the number of abnormal sperm morphology, and decreases semen volume. Life-style has little, if any, impact on semen quality (148). In contrast, other studies implicate numerous unfavorable influences on reproduction from alcohol consumption, cigarette smoking, and coffee drinking. Additional studies are needed to validate these preliminary findings (149).

NATURAL ALTERNATIVE THERAPY

Herbal Medicine

Female Partner

Herbal therapies have been used for many years; however, scientific clinical data is scarce. But, evaluation of the safety and efficacy of these remedies is available. Herbalists offer the following recommendations in the treatment of infertility.

Damiana (also called rosemary, old woman's broom, Mexican damiana, or herba de la pastora) is distributed in the form of tincture (orally 2.5 mL three times daily) and powdered herb (18 g in 500 mL, taken as tea three times daily). Side effects include hallucination, urethral irritation, and, in higher doses, liver toxicity. It is contraindicated during pregnancy and lactation, when operating a car or other equipment, or performing hazardous activities (164).

Dong quai (Chinese angelica, dry-kuei, tang-kuei, women's ginseng) is available in 0.5-mg tablets or the raw root (4.5 to 30 mg) is soaked or boiled in wine (1 g of the root). Side effects include skin sensitivity to sunlight, fever, diarrhea, or bleeding. It is contraindicated during pregnancy and lactation (164).

Hachimijiogan, 7.5 g daily, is recommended for infertile women associated with hyperprolactinemia with no pituitary adenoma present. This herbal remedy reduces prolactin and restores ovulation. In a clinical observational study, no side effects were observed; however, a randomized, controlled study has not been conducted (165).

Chaste tree (*Vitex agnus-castus*, agneau chaste, chastberry, gatillier, hemp tree, keuschbaum or monk's pepper) is indicated for oligomenorrhea/amenorrhea, scanty, irregular menstrual cycles, or luteal phase insufficiency. The remedy is particularly effective when latent hyperprolactinemia is present. It has been recommended at a dose of one 20-mg capsule once or twice daily (166). Ovarian hyperstimulation may by induced by Chaste tree (168). Side effects include a cramping type of abdominal pain, hypermenorrhea, headaches, diarrhea, skin rush, and itching (164).

Ginseng (American ginseng, Asiatic ginseng, Chinese ginseng, Japanese ginseng, Korean ginseng, Oriental ginseng, Western ginseng, five-fingers, jintsam, schinsent, seng and sang, tartar root) is recommended at a dose of 200 to 600 mg in one or two doses (available in 100-, 250-, and 500-mg capsules; root extract 2 ounces in alcohol base; root powder 1 or 4 ounces). Side effects such as breast or chest pain, headaches, gastrointestinal symptoms, elevated blood pressure, rapid pulse, skin symptoms, insomnia, and vaginal bleeding have been reported. There is no specific indication, only a general indication for the treatment of infertility (164).

Licorice (Chinese licorice, Persian licorice, Russian licorice, Spanish licorice, licorice root, sweet root) is available in 100- to 520-mg capsules and 7-mg tablets, and a dose of 200 to 600 mg is recommended. Often reported side effects are headaches, muscle weakness, and water retention. Serious complications may occur with overdose, such as heart failure, high blood pressure, and rhabdomyolysis (a muscle disorder). It is contraindicated during pregnancy and lactation (164).

Most of these remedies' therapeutic benefits are based on anecdotal clinical observation. Well-designed randomized controlled clinical trials are needed to substantiate such approaches.

Male Partner

Chinese herbal medicine supposedly is quite beneficial in improving sperm quantity and quality. Clinical data are established predominantly on observational clinical trials. Selected Chinese herbal remedies that may play role in improving sperm quality are described below.

Guizhi-Fuling-Wan, 7.5 g per day for at least 3 months, is recommended for oligoasthenozoospermia associated with varicocele. It has been reported that varicoceles totally vanish in about 80%, with improvement of sperm concentration and motility of approximately 71.4% and 62.1%, respectively (169).

The Shengjing pill significantly improves sperm quantity and quality and reduces antisperm antibody. It has been reported to result in live births in 53.4% (170).

Ju Jing powder is of assistance for improving sperm density and motility in approximately 85.4% when compared with pretreatment sperm quality (171).

Hachimijiogan, 7.5 mg three times daily for 4 months, is helpful in the treatment of oligozoospermia or asthenozoospermia, or a combination of both. Sperm density is improved in 21% and sperm motility in about 50% (172). Another clinical observational study supports these interesting findings (17).

Ninjinotoh, 5.1 g three times per day, is indicated for oligozoospermia or asthenozoospermia, or a combination of both. Sperm counts increase in about 31% and sperm motility improves in approximately 45% (172).

Hochu-Ekki-To is administered orally for mild oligospermia (sperm density $20–40 \times 10^6$) and is beneficial in about 51.1% with the pregnancy rate about 20% (174).

Homeopathy

Homeopathy and its application for infertility are not represented in the literature. Nevertheless, some data are available that may be used indirectly, such as other reproductive organ illnesses influencing conception. Homeopathic remedies are further described in Chapters 3, 8, and 10.

REFERENCES

1. Association of Professors of Gynecology and Obstetrics. *Medical student educational objectives,* 7th ed. Washington, DC: Association of Professors of Gynecology and Obstetrics, 1997.
2. Council on Resident and Gynecology (CREOG). *Educational objectives core curriculum for residents in obstetrics and gynecology,* 5th ed. Washington, DC: CREOG, 1996.
3. American College of Obstetrician and Gynecologists (ACOG). Technical bulletin No.125. Washington, DC: ACOG, 1989.
4. Mosher WD. Reproductive impairment in the United States, 1965–1982, *Demography* 1985;22:415–430.
5. Crosignani PG, Rubin B. The ESHRE Capri Workshop. Guidelines to the prevalence, diagnosis and management of infertility. *Hum Reprod* 1996;11:1775–1807.
6. Cramer DW, Walker AN, Schiff I. Statistical methods in evaluating the outcome of infertility therapy. *Fertil Steril* 1979;32:80–86.
7. Adelman MM, Cahill EM. *Atlas of sperm morphology.* Chicago, IL: American Society of Clinical Pathology, 1989.
8. Hull MGR, Cahill DJ. Female infertility. *Endocrinol Metab Clin North Am* 1998;27:851–876.
9. Klentzeris LD, Li TC, Dockery P, Cooke ID. The endometrial biopsy as a predictive factor of pregnancy rate in women with unexplained infertility. *Eur J Obstet Gynecol Reprod Biol* 1992;45:119–124.
10. Jordon J, Craig K, Clifton DK, et al. Luteal phase defect: the sensitivity and specificity of diagnostic methods in common clinical use. *Fertil Steril* 1994;62:54–62.
11. Balasch J, Fabregues F, Creus M, et al. The usefulness of endometrial biopsy for luteal phase evaluation in infertility. *Hum Reprod* 1992;7:973–977.
12. Peters AJ, Lloyd RP, Coulam CB. Prevalence of out-of-phase endometrial biopsy specimens. *Am J Obstet Gynecol* 1992;166:1738–1745.
13. Batista MC, Cartledge TP, Merino MJ, et al. Midluteal phase endometrial biopsy does not accurately predict luteal function. *Fertil Steril* 1993;59:294–300.
14. Palacio JR, Iborra A, Gris JM, et al. Anti-endometrial autoantibodies in women with a diagnosis of infertility. *Am J Reprod Immunol* 1997;38:100–105.
15. Check JH, Ostrzenski A, Klimek R. Expression of an immunomodulatory protein known as progesterone induced blocking factor (PIBF) does not correlate with first trimester spontaneous abortions in progesterone supplemented women. *Am J Reprod Immunol* 1997;37:330–334.
16. Wu CH, Gocial B. A pelvic scoring system for infertility surgery. *Int J Fertil* 1988;33:341–346.
17. Scot RT, Opsahl MS, Leonardi MR, et al. Life table analysis of pregnancy rate in a general infertility population relative to ovarian reserve and patient age. *Hum Reprod* 1995;10:1706–1710.
18. Buyalos RP, Daneshmand S, Brzechffa PR. Basal estradiol level and follicle-stimulating hormone predict fecundity in women of advanced reproductive age undergoing ovulation induction therapy. *Fertil Steril* 1997;68:272–277.
19. Collins JA, Burrows EA, Wilan AR. The prognosis for live birth among untreated infertile couples. *Fertil Steril* 1995;64:22–28.
20. Snick HK, Snick TS, Evers JL, et al. The spontaneous pregnancy prognosis in untreated subfertile couples: the Walcheren primary care study. *Hum Reprod* 1997;12:1582–1588.
21. Augood C, Duckitt K, Templeton AA. Smoking and female infertility: a systemic review and metaanalysis. *Hum Reprod* 1998;13:1532–1539.
22. Suonio S, Saarikoski S, Kauhanen O, et al. Smoking does affect fecundity. *Eur J Obstet Gynecol Reprod Biol* 1990;34;89–95.
23. Hughs EG, Brennan BG. Does cigarette smoking impair natural or assisted fecundity? *Fertil Steril* 1996;66:679–689.
24. Alderete E, Eskenazi B, Sholtz R. Effect of cigarette smoking and coffee drinking on time to conception. *Epidemiology* 1995;6:403–408.
25. Vine MF, Margolin BH, Morrison HI, et al. Cigarette smoking and sperm density: a meta-analysis. *Fertil Steril* 1994;61:35–43.
26. Bolumar F, Olsen J, Boldsen J. Smoking reduces fecundity: a European multicenter study on infertility and subinfertility. The European Study Group on Infertility and Subfecundity. *Am J Epidemiol* 1996;143:578–587.
27. Steeno OP. Clinical and physical evaluation of the infertile male: testicular measurement or orchidometry. *Andrologia* 1989;21:103–112.
28. Lenton EA, Weston GA, Cook ID. Problems in using basal body temperature recordings in an infertility clinic. *BMJ* 1977;1:803–805.
29. Bauman JE. Basal body temperature: unreliable method of ovulation detection. *Fertil Steril* 1981;36:729–733.
30. Martinez AR, van Hoof MH, Schoute E, et al. The reliability, acceptability and applications of basal body temperature (BBT) records in the diagnosis and treatment of infertility. *Eur J Obstet Gynecol Reprod Biol* 1992;47:121–127.
31. Morris N, Underwood L, Easterling W Jr. Temporal relationship between basal body temperature nadir and luteinizing hormone surge in normal women. *Fertil Steril* 1976;27:780–783.
32. Osborne NG, Hecht Y, Winkelman J, et al. Detection of specific IgG and IgA antibodies to *Chlamydia trachomatis* in women with salpingitis confirmed by laparoscopy. *J Natl Med Assoc* 1989;81:541–543.
33. World Health Organization. WHO manual for the standardized investigation and diagnosis of the infertile couple. Cambridge, UK: Cambridge University Press, 1993.
34. Hoff JD, Quigly ME, Yen SS. Hormonal dynamics at midcycle: a reevaluation. *J Clin Endocrinol Metab* 1983;57:792–796.
35. Hull MGR. Managed care of infertility. *Curr Opin Obstet Gynecol* 1996;8:305–316.
36. Griffith CS, Grines DA. The validity of the postcoital test. *Am J Obstet Gynecol* 1990;162:615–620.
37. Oei SG, Helmerhorst FM, Keirse MJ. When is the post-coital test normal? A critical appraisal. *Hum Reprod* 1995;10:1711–1714.
38. Siegler AM. *Hysterosalpingography.* New York: Medcon Press, 1974.
39. Bateman BG, Nuley WC JR, Kitchin JD. Intravasation during hysterosalpingography using oil base contrast media. *Fertil Steril* 1980;34:439–443.
40. DeCherney AH, Kort H, Barney JB, et al. Increased pregnancy rate with oil soluble hysterosalpingography dye. *Fertil Steril* 1980;33:407–410.
41. Rice JP, London SN, Olive DL. Reevaluation of hysterosalpingography in infertility investigation. *Obstet Gynecol* 1986;67:718–721.
42. Mol BW, Collins JA, Burrows EA, et al. Comparison of hysterosalpingography and laparoscopy in predicting fertility outcome. *Hum Reprod* 1999;14:1237.

43. Gazzera C, Gallo T, Faissola B, et al. Tubal catheterization and selective salpingography. *Rays* 1998;23:735–741.
44. Kamiyama S, Miyagi H, Kanazawa K. Therapeutic value of selective salpingography for infertile women with patent fallopian tubes: the impact on pregnancy rate. *Gynecol Obstet Invest* 2000;49:36–40.
45. El-Minawi MF, Abdel-Hadi M, Ibrahim AA, et al. Comparative evaluation of laparoscopy and hysterosalpingography in infertile patients. *Obstet Gynecol* 1978;51:29–32.
46. Hutchins CJ. Laparoscopy and hysterosalpingography in the assessment of tubal patency. *Obstet Gynecol* 1977;49:325–327.
47. Sueoka K, Asada H, Tsuchiya S, et al. Falloposcopic tuboplasty for bilateral tubal occlusion. A novel infertility treatment as an alternative for in-vitro fertilization? *Hum Reprod* 1998;13:71–74.
48. Lundberg S, Rasmussen C, Berg AA, et al. Falloposcopy in conjunction with laparoscopy: possibilities and limitations. *Hum Reprod* 1998;1490–1492.
49. Martinez-Roman S, Balasch J, Creus M, et al. Immunological factors in endometriosis-associated reproductive failure: studies in fertile and infertile women with and without endometriosis. *Hum Reprod* 1997;12:1794–1799.
50. Krausz C, Bonaccorsi L, Maggio P, et al. Two functional assays of sperm responsiveness to progesterone and their predictive values in in-vitro fertilization. *Hum Reprod* 1996;11:1661–1667.
51. Rogers BJ. The sperm penetration assay: its usefulness reevaluation. *Fertil Steril* 1985;43:821–840.
52. Bergmann M, Behre HM, Nieschlag E. Serum FSH testicular morphology in male infertility. *Clin Endocrinol (Oxf)* 1994;40:133–136.
53. Haas GG. How should sperm antibody tests be used clinically? *Am J Reprod Immunol Microbiol* 1987;15:106–111.
54. Friedler S, Raziel A, Strassburger D, et al. Testicular sperm retrieval by percutaneous fine needle sperm aspiration compared with testicular sperm extraction by open biopsy in men with non-obstructive azoospermia. *Hum Reprod* 1997;12:1488–1493.
55. Wilson CB. Surgical management of pituitary tumors. *J Clin Endocrinol Metab* 1997;82:2381–2385.
56. Hulka JF, Halme J. Sterilization reversal: results of 101 attempts. *Am J Obstet Gynecol* 1988;159:767–774.
57. Boeckx W, Gordts S, Buysse K, et al. Reversibility after female sterilization. *Br J Obstet Gynecol* 1986;93:839–842.
58. Rouzi AA, Mackinnon M, McComb PF. Predictors of success of reversal of sterilization. *Fertil Steril* 1995;64:29–36.
59. Glock JL, Kim AH, Hulka JF, et al. Reproductive outcome after tubal reversal in women 40 years of age or older. *Fertil Steril* 1996;65:863–865.
60. Isaacs JD Jr, Young RA, Cowan BD. Cumulative pregnancy analysis of one tube versus two-tube tubal anastomosis. *Fertil Steril* 1997;68:217–219.
61. Henderson SR. The reversibility of female sterilization with the use of microsurgery: a report on 102 patients with more than one year of follow-up. *Am J Obstet Gynecol* 1984;149:57–65.
62. Barjot PJ, Marie G, Von Theobald P. Laparoscopic tubal anastomosis and reversal of sterilization. *Hum Reprod* 1999;14:1222–1225.
63. Ostrzenski A. Endoscopic carbon dioxide laser ovarian wedge resection in resistant polycystic ovarian disease. *Int J Fertil* 1992;37:295–299.
64. Tulandi T, Murray C, Guralnick M. Adhesions formation and reproductive outcome after myomectomy and second-look laparoscopy. *Obstet Gynecol* 1993;82:213–215.
65. Ostrzenski A. A new laparoscopic myomectomy technique for intramural fibroids penetrating the uterine cavity. *Eur J Obstet Gynecol Reprod Biol* 1997;74:189–193.
66. March CM, Israel R. Hysteroscopic management of recurrent abortion cause by septate uterus. *Am J Obstet Gynecol* 1987;156:834–842.
67. Szamotowicz J, Tomaszewska I, Szamotowicz M. The effectiveness of hysteroscopic intrauterine septum resection in terms of reproductive outcome. *Ginecol Pol* 1998;69:757–760.
68. Poreu G, Cravello L, D'Ercole C, et al. Hysteroscopic metroplasty for septate uterus and repetitive abortions: reproductive outcome. *Eur J Obstet Gynecol Reprod Biol* 2000;88:81–84.
69. Homer HA, Li TC, Cooke ID. The septate uterus: a review of management and reproductive outcome. *Fertil Steril* 2000;73:1–14.
70. Valle RF, Sciarra JJ. Intrauterine adhesions: hysteroscopic diagnosis, classification, treatment, and reproductive outcome. *Am J Obstet Gynecol* 1988;158:1459–1470.
71. Crosignani PG, Rubin B. The ESHRE Capri Workshop. Guidelines to the prevalence, diagnosis, treatment and management of infertility. *Hum Reprod* 1996;11:1775–1807.
72. The American Fertility Society. Revised American Fertility Society classification of endometriosis. *Fertil Steril* 1985;43:351.
73. Glazener CM, Coulson C, Lambert PA, et al. The value of artificial insemination with husband's semen in infertility due to failure of postcoital sperm-mucus penetration—controlled trial of treatment. *Br J Obstet Gynecol* 1867;94:774–778.
74. Subak LL, Adamson GD, Boltz NL. Therapeutic donor insemination: a prospective randomized trial of fresh versus frozen sperm. *Am J Obstet Gynecol* 1992;166:1597–1604.
75. Goldberg JM, Mascha E, Falcone T, et al. Comparison of intrauterine and intracervical insemination with frozen donor sperm: a meta-analysis. *Fertil Steril* 1999;72:792–795.
76. Kahn JA, Sunde A, von During V, et al. Treatment of unexplained infertility. Fallopian tube sperm perfusion (FSP). *Acta Obstet Gynecol Scand* 1993;72:193–199.
77. Nuojua-Huttunen S, Tuomivaara L, Juntunen K, et al. Comparison of fallopian tube sperm perfusion with intrauterine insemination in the treatment of infertility. *Fertil Steril* 1997;67:939–942.
78. Kuhan JA, Sunde A, Koskemies A, et al. Fallopian tube sperm perfusion (IUI) in the treatment of unexplained infertility: a prospective randomized study. *Hum Reprod* 1993;8:890–894.
79. Lesec G, Manhes H, Hardy RI, et al. In-vivo transperitoneal fertilization. *Hum Reprod* 1989;4521:526.
80. Collins JA, Burrows EA, Wiln AR. The prognosis for live birth among birth among untreated infertile couples. *Fertil Steril* 1995;64:22–28.
81. Snick HK, Snick TS, Evers JL, et al. The spontaneous pregnancy prognosis in untreated subfertile couples: The Walcheren primary care study. *Hum Reprod* 1997;12:1582–1588.
82. Trum JW, Pannekoek Y, Spanjaard L, et al. Accurate detection of male subclinical genital tract infection via cervical culture and DNA hybridization assay of the female partner. *Int J Androl* 2000;23:43–45.
83. Keck C, Gerber-Schafer C, Clad A, et al. Seminal tract infection: impact on male fertility and treatment options. *Hum Reprod Update* 1998;4:891–903.
84. American College of Obstetrician and Gynecologists (ACOG). Technical bulletin No.142. Washington, DC: ACOG, 1990.
85. Krause W. Effects of varicocele therapy on spermatozoan function. *Urologie* 1998;37:254–257.
86. Schatte EC, Hirshberg SJ, Fallick ML, et al. Varicocelectomy improves sperm strict morphology and motility. *J Urol* 1998;160:1338–1340.
87. Ismail MT, Sedor J, Hirsch IH. Are sperm motion parameters influenced by varicocele ligation? *Fertil Steril* 1999;71:886–890.

88. Scherr D, Goldstein M. Comparison of bilateral versus unilateral varicocelectomy in men with palpable bilateral varicoceles. *J Urol* 1999;162:85–88.

89. Lund L, Larsen SB. A follow-up study of semen quality and infertility in men with varicocele testis and in control subjects. *Br J Urol* 1998;82:682–686.

90. Kim ED, Leibman BB, Grinblat DM, et al. Varicocele repair improves semen parameters in azoospermic men with spermatogenic failure. *J Urol* 1999;162:737–740.

91. Ochsenkuhn R, Kamischke A, Neischlag E. Imipramine for successful treatment of retrograde ejaculation caused by retroperitoneal surgery. *Int J Androl* 1999;22:173–177.

92. Glander HJ. Disorders of ejaculation. *Fortschr Med* 1998;116:26–28.

93. Kamischke A, Nieschlag E. Treatment of retrograde ejaculation and anejaculation. *Hum Reprod Update* 1999;5:448–474.

94. Dirken JJ, Cleine JH. Retrograde ejaculation: a treatable fertility problem. *Ned Tijdschr Geneeskd* 1997;141:1149–1151.

95. Middleton RG, Urry RL. The Young-Dees operation for the correction of retrograde ejaculation. *J Urol* 1986;136:1208–1209.

96. Stewart DE, Ohl DA. Idiopathic anejaculation treated by electroejaculation. *Int J Psychiatry Med* 1989;19:263–268.

97. Monga M, Bernie J, Rajasekaran M. Male infertility and erectile dysfunction in spinal cord injury: a review. *Arch Phys Med Rehabil* 1999;80:1331–1339.

98. Chung PH, Verkauf BS, Eichberg RD, et al. Electroejaculation and assisted reproductive techniques for anejaculatory infertility. *Obstet Gynecol* 1996;87:22–26.

99. Lucas MG, Hargreave TB, Edmond P, et al. Sperm retrieval by eletro-ejaculation: preliminary experience in patients with secondary anejaculation. *Br J Urol* 1991;67:191–194.

100. Ohl DA. Electroejaculation. *Urol Clin North Am* 1993;20:181–188.

101. Hovav Y, Shotland Y, Yaffe H, et al. Electroejaculation and assisted fertility in men with psychogenic anejaculation. *Fertil Steril* 1996;66:620–623.

102. Casell R, Luscher U, Gasser TC, et al. Results of microsurgical reconstruction after vasectomy. *Schweiz Rundsch Med Prax* 1997;86:933–936.

103. Fox M. Vasectomy reversal—microsurgery for best results. *Br J Urol* 1994;449–453.

104. Engelmann UH, Schramek P, Tomamichel G, et al. Vasectomy reversal in central Europe: results of questionnaire of urologists in Austria, Germany and Switzerland. *J Urol* 1990;143:64–67.

105. Marmar JL, Corson SL, Batzer FR, et al. Microsurgical aspiration of sperm from the epididymis: a mobile program. *J Urol* 1993;149:1368–1373.

106. Marmar JL, Praiss DE, Debenedictis TJ. Statistical comparison of the parameters of semen analysis of whole semen versus the fractions of the split ejaculation. *Fertil Steril* 1978;30:439–443.

107. Nieschlag E. Care for the infertile male. *Clin Endocrinol (Oxf)* 1993;38:123–133.

108. Nduwayo L, Barthelemy C, Lansac J, et al. Management of necrospermia. *Contracept Fertil Sex* 1995;23:682–685.

109. Jewett MA, Greenspan MB, Shier RM, et al. Necrospermia or immotile cilia syndrome as a cause of male infertility. *J Urol* 1980;124:292–293.

110. Nishino Y, Fujihiro S, Hatano K, et al. A case of 46XX male. *Hinyokika Kiyo* 1993;39:93–95.

111. Terada H, Yamaguchi Y, Ushiyama T, et al. A case of male infertility with chromosomal abnormality of 45, x146, x+mar. *Nippon Hinyokika Gakkai Zasshi* 1995;86:1294–1297.

112. Fishel S, Symonds M. *Gamete and embryo micromanipulation in human reproduction.* Boston: Little, Brown, 1993.

113. Schlegel PN, Girardi S. In vitro fertilization for male factor infertility. *J Clin Endocrinol Metab* 1997;82:709–716.

114. Dokras A, Olive DL. Endometriosis and assisted reproductive technologies. *Clin Obstet Gynecol* 1999;42:687–698.

115. Hovatta O. Pregnancies in women with Turner's syndrome. *Ann Med* 1999;31:106–110.

116. Ostrzenski A. A new, laparoscopic full-thickness slice ovarian biopsy (from antimesenteric to mesenteric margin). *J Gynecol Surg* 1995;11:109–112.

117. American Society for Reproductive Medicine, Society for Assisted Reproductive Technology Registry. Assisted reproductive technology in the United States: 1996 results generated from the American Society for Reproductive Medicine/Society for Assisted Reproductive Technology Registry. *Fertil Steril* 1999;71:789–907.

118. Guzick DS, Sullivan MW, Adamson GD, et al. Efficacy of treatment for unexplained infertility. *Fertil Steril* 1998;70:207–213.

119. Belaish-Allart J, Mayenga JM, Plachot M. Intra-uterine insemination. *Contracept Fertil Sex* 1999;27:614–619.

120. Crosignani PG, Walters DE, Soliani A. The ESHRE multicenter trial on the treatment of unexplained infertility: a preliminary report. *Hum Reprod* 1991;6:953–958.

121. Fitzgerald C, Zimon AE, Jones EE. Aging and reproductive potential in women. *Yale J Biol Med* 1998;71:367–381.

122. Masseri A, Grifo JA. Genetics, age, and infertility. *Maturitas* 1998;30:189–192.

123. Goshen R, Weissman A, Shoham Z. Epithelial ovarian cancer, infertility and induction of ovulation: possible pathogenesis and update concepts. *Baillieres Clin Obstet Gynecol* 1998;12:581–591.

124. Burmeister L, Healy DL. Ovarian cancer in infertility patients. *Ann Med* 1998;30:525–528.

125. Gerhard I, Postneek F. Auricular acupuncture in the treatment of female infertility. *Gynecol Endocrinol* 1992;6:171–181.

126. Beal MW. Acupuncture and acupressure. Applications to women's reproductive health care. *J Nurse Midwifery* 1999;44:217–230.

127. Chen BY. Acupuncture normalizes dysfunction of hypothalamic-pituitary ovarian axis. *Acupunct Electrother Res* 1997;22:97–108.

128. Chen EC, Brzyski RG. Exercise and reproductive dysfunction. *Fertil Steril* 1999;71:1–6

129. Buck GM, Sever LE, Batt RE, et al. Life-style factors and female infertility. *Epidemiology* 1997;8:435–441.

130. Silva PD, Cool JL, Olson KL. Impact of lifestyle on female infertility. *J Reprod Med* 1999;44:288–296.

131. Manusov EG. Clinical applications of hypnotherapy. *J Fam Pract* 1990;31:180–184.

132. Gansalkorale WM. The use of hypnosis in medicine: the possible pathways involved. *Eur J Gastroenterol Hepatol* 1996;8:520–524.

133. Gravitz MA, Hypnosis in the treatment of functional infertility. *Am J Clin Hypn* 1995;38:22–26.

134. Smith WH. Hypnosis in the treatment of anxiety. *Bull Menninger Clin* 1990;54:209–216.

135. Kirsh I. Hypnotic enhancement of cognitive-behavioral weight loss treatments—another meta-reanalysis. *J Consult Clin Psychol* 1996;64:517–519.

136. The mind/body program for infertility: a new behavioral treatment approach for women with infertility. *Fertil Steril* 1990;53:264–249.

137. Siterman S, Eltes F, Wolfson V, et al. Does acupuncture treatment affect sperm density in males with very low sperm count? A pilot study. *Andrologia* 2000;32:31–39.

138. Fischel F, Riegler R, Biegluayer C, et al. Modification of sperm quality by acupuncture in subfertile males. *Gesburtshilfe Frauenheilkd* 1984;44:510–512.

139. Siterman S, Eltes F, Wolfson V, et al. Effect of acupuncture on

sperm parameters of males suffering from subfertility related to low sperm quality. *Arch Androl* 1997;39:155–161.

140. Riegler R, Fishl F, Bunzel B, et al. Correlation of psychological changes and spermiogram improvements following acupuncture. *Urologie* 1984;23:329–333.

141. De Souza MJ, Miller BE. The effect of endurance training on reproductive function in male runners. A "volume threshold" hypothesis. *Sports Med* 1997;23:357–374.

142. Hackney AC. The male reproductive system and endurance exercise. *Med Sci Sports Exerc* 1996;28:180–189.

143. Jensen CE, Wiswedel K, McLoughlin J, et al. Prospective study of hormonal and semen profiles in marathon runners. *Fertil Steril* 1995;64:1189–1196.

144. Arce JC, DeSouza MJ, Pescatello LS, et al. Subclinical alternations in hormone and semen profile in athletes. *Fertil Steril* 1993;59:398–404.

145. Cumming DC, Wheeler GD, McColl EM. The effect of exercise on reproductive function in men. *Sports Med* 1989;7:1–17.

146. Struder HK, Hollmann W, Platen P, et al. Hypothalamic-pituitary-adrenal and gonadal axis function after exercise in sedentary and endurance trained elderly males. *Eur J Appl Physiol* 1998;77:285–288.

147. Arce JC, De Souza MJ. Exercise and male factor infertility. *Sports Med* 1993;15:146–169.

148. Oldereid NB, Rui H, Purvis K. Lifestyle of men in barren couples and their relationship to sperm quality. *Eur J Obstet Gynecol Reprod Biol* 1992;43:51–57.

149. Gerhard I, Runnebaum B. Harmful substances and infertility. Substances of abuse. *Gesburtshilfe Frauenheilkd* 1992;52:509–515.

150. Ritter MM, Richter WO. Effects of a vegetarian life style on health. *Fortschr Med* 1995;113:239–242.

151. Bagga D, Ashley JM, Geffrey SP, et al. Effects of a very low fat, high fiber on serum hormones and menstrual function. Implication for breast cancer prevention. *Cancer* 1995;76: 2491–2496.

152. Howard JM, Davis S, Hunnisett A. Red cell magnesium and glutathione peroxidase in infertile women—effects of oral supplementation with magnesium and selenium. *Magnes Res* 1994; 7:49–57.

153. Luck MR, Jeyaseelan I, Scholes RA. Ascorbi acid and fertility. *Biol Reprod* 1995;52:262–266.

154. Vezina D, Mauffette F, Roberts KD, et al. Selenium-vitamin E supplementation in infertile men. Effects on semen parameters and micronutrient levels and distribution. *Biol Trace Elem Res* 1996;53:65–83.

155. Fuse H, Kazama T, Ohta S, et al. Relationship between zinc concentrations in seminal plasma and various sperm parameters. *Int Urol Nephrol* 1999;31:401–408.

156. Henkel R, Bittner J, Weber R, et al. Relevance of zink in human sperm flagella and its relation to motility. *Fertil Steril* 1999; 71:1138–1143.

157. Wong WY, Thomas CM, Merkus JM, et al. Male factor subinfertility: possible causes and the impact of nutritional factors. *Fertil Steril* 2000;73:435–442.

158. Sinclair S. Male infertility: Nutritional and environmental considerations. *Altern Med Rev* 2000;5:28–38.

159. Rolf C, Cooper TG, Yeung CH, et al. Antioxidant treatment of patients with asthenozoospermia or moderate oligoasthenozoospermia with high-dose vitamin C and vitamin E: a randomized, placebo-controlled, double-blind study. *Hum Reprod* 1999;14:1028–1033.

160. Lenzi A, Lombardo F, Gandini L, et al. Glutathione therapy for male infertility. *Arch Androl* 1992;29:65–68.

161. Costa M, Canale D, Filicori M, et al. L-carnitine in idiopathic asthenozoospermia: a multicenter study. Italian Study Group on Carnitine and Male Infertility. *Andrologia* 1994;26:155–159.

162. Vitali G, Parente R, Melotti C. Carnitine supplementation in human idiopathic asthenospermia: clinical results. *Drugs Exp Clin Res* 1995;21:157–159.

163. Bentivoglio G, Melica F, Cristoforoni P. Folinic acid in the treatment of human male infertility. *Fertil Steril* 1993;60:698–701.

164. Fetrow CW, Avila JR. *The complete guide to herbal medicines.* Springhouse, PA: Springhouse Corporation, 1999.

165. Usuki S, Kubota S, Usuki Y. Treatment with hachimijiogan, a non-ergot Chinese herbal medicine, in two hyperprolactinemic infertile women. *Acta Obstet Gynecol Scand* 1989;68:475-478.

166. Veal L. Complementary therapy and infertility: an Icelandic perspective. *Complement Ther Nurs Midwifery* 1998;4:3–6.

167. Milewicz A, Gejdel E, Sworen H, et al. *Vitex agnus* extract in the treatment of luteal phase defects due to latent hyperprolactinemia. Results of randomized placebo-controlled double-blind study. *Arzneimittelforschung* 1993;43:752–756.

168. Cahill DJ, Fox R, Wrdle PG, et al. Multiple follicular development associated with herbal medicine. *Hum Reprod* 1994;9: 1469–1470.

169. Ishikawa H, Ohashi M, Hayakawa K, et al. Effect of guizhi-fuling-wan on male infertility with varicocele. *Am J Chin Med* 1996;24:327–331.

170. Chen RA, Wen H. Clinical study on treatment of male infertility with shengjing pill. *Chung Kuo Chung His I Chieh Ho Tsa Chih* 1995;15:205–208.

171. Zhai Y, Xu L, Xu F, et al. TCM treatment of male infertility due to seminal abnormality—a clinical observation of 82 cases. *J Tradit Chin Med* 1990;10:26–29.

172. Okuyama A, Namiki M, Sonoda T, et al. Effects of hachimijiogan and ninjintoh on fertility in males with sterility. *Hinyokika Kiyo* 1984;30:409–413.

173. Usuki S. Hachimijiogan changes serum hormonal circumstance and improves spermatogenesis in oligozoospermic men. *Am J Clin Med* 1986;14:37–45.

174. Yoshida H, Tanifuji T, Sakurai H, et al. Clinical effects of Chinese herbal medicine (hochu-ekki-to) on infertile men. *Hinyokika Kiyo* 1986;32:297–302

12

MENOPAUSE AND OSTEOPOROSIS

EDUCATIONAL OBJECTIVES

Medical Students (1)
APGO Objective No. 51

Physiologic changes in the
   hypothalamic–
   pituitary–ovarian axis
Symptoms and physical
   findings associated with
   hypoestrogenism
Long-term changes associated
   with hypoestrogenism
Management:
   hormonal therapy, nutrition
   and exercise, and nonhormonal
   therapeutic options
Risks and benefits of hormonal
   replacement therapy

Residents in Obstetrics/Gynecology (2)
CREOG Objectives

Pertinent history
Physical examination
Diagnostic studies
Diagnosis of perimenopause
Management
Factors influencing
   decisions regarding intervention,
   potential complications of
   intervention, and potential
   complications of nonintervention
Follow-up
Problems of menopause,
   osteoporosis, hyperlipidemia,
   cardiovascular disease, diagnosis
Management
Follow-up

Practitioners (3–5)
ACOG Recommendations

Hormonal replacement therapy:
   indications, risk factors,
   therapeutic options, and
   strategies to improve
   compliance
Hormonal replacement therapy
   in women with previously
   treated breast cancer
Estrogen replacement therapy
   and endometrial cancer

DEFINITION

Menopause can be natural, physiologic, or induced [either by surgical (oophorectomy), iatrogenic (chemotherapy), or radiation treatment] as a result of the termination of ovarian follicular function. This biologic event is expected to occur between the ages of 44 and 55 years (average in the United States, 50–52 years; median, 51.5 years) (6).

Postmenopause is clinically defined as the absence of menses for 12 months following the onset of menopause (7). Perimenopause (the menopause transition) is defined as the 2 to 8 years preceding the final menstrual bleeding (menopause) (7,8).

OCCURRENCE

Within the next decade, over 36 million women will go into a menopause period in the United States (3).

CLASSIFICATION

- Natural biological menopause
- Induced menopause [by surgical castration or iatrogenic ablation of ovarian function (chemotherapy, radiation treatment), with transient menopause induced by gonadotropin-releasing hormone (GnRH) agonists] (9)
- Premature ovarian failure (spontaneous cessation of ovarian function before age 40) (8)

PHYSIOLOGY

Climacterium encompasses three distinct biological events:

- Perimenopause
- Menopause
- Postmenopause

Perimenopause, or the menopause transition (which lasts 2–8 years) (7), is a gradual process, in which ovarian function decreases. A natural biologic evolution occurs from premenopause through perimenopause to menopause, then finally to a postmenopause period. The mechanisms of this bodily process are not clearly understood, and clear clinical symptoms have not been well defined. The interpretation of this period as a biologic phase of female reproductive changes can be analyzed in three stages.

The early menopausal transition period (*perimenopause*) is characterized by a progressively loosening cyclic regulatory capacity of hypothalamic–pituitary neurohormone secretion with no influence on the length of the menstrual cycle.

The middle menopausal transition period is typified by overt changes in the frequency and duration of the menstrual cycle (often with a longer interval between menses, and an irregular and shorter cycle) (10). Such an alteration of the menstrual cycle is most likely related to an erratic maturation process of the remaining ovarian follicles (some of the cycles are ovulatory, whereas others are anovulatory) (11). Clinically, this stage can be characterized by erratic menstrual cycles with menorrhagia (endometrial hyperplasia may be identified as a result of unopposed estrogen stimulation), breast tenderness or enlargement, and the occurrence of postmenopausal symptoms (12). This symptomatology correlates with elevated follicle-stimulating hormone (FSH) levels (>25 mIU/mL) and decreased estrogen concentrations, in the early follicular phase of the menstrual cycle (13).

The late menopausal transition is characterized by extended time lapses between menses, decreased estrogen levels that correspond to postmenopausal concentrations (<20 pg/mL), and an absence of ovulation due to the presence of gonadotropins (14).

The transition affects not only the menstrual cycle but also other organs and systems, such as the skin, genitourinary system, and neuroendocrine secretion (7–9,14).

In the menopause transition period, neurohormones and estrogen concentrations fluctuate. FSH may reach postmenopausal levels and may return to a perimenopausal serum concentration during the same or subsequent menstrual cycles; therefore, using a high FSH concentration (>40 mIU/mL) to make the diagnosis of menopause in menstruating women appears to be an inappropriate diagnostic approach. Such fluctuations of neurohormone concentrations may lead to a classic picture of postmenopausal symptoms. Perimenopause will eventually show the way to the next stage, which is menopause.

Menopause, or the final natural menses, normally occurs between the ages of 48 and 52 years and indicates the cessation of ovarian follicular function (15). Predisposing factors for the occurrence of menopause at an earlier age include chemotherapy involving cyclophosphamide, methotrexate, or fluorouracil (16); cigarette smoking (1–2 years younger at menopause than nonsmokers), and surgical procedures that compromise ovarian circulation (no well-documented events). The occurrence of menopause at

a later age may be due to oral contraceptive use (controversial, because an earlier menarche may lead to a later age of menopause) (14).

The postmenopause phase, whose beginning is not clearly defined, is considered as commencing either immediately or 12 months after the final menses regardless of the reason (whether natural or induced) for menopause (9,14).

There are several types of postmenopausal symptoms.

Vasomotor symptoms, such as hot flashes, night sweats, and heart palpitations, are considered to be indirectly related to changing estrogen levels, causing the increase of gonadotropin. This process may result in dysregulation of the hypothalamic temperature control center (thermoregulatory instability) or a decreased hypothalamic opioid tone (14). Classic hot flashes (the perception of a wave of high temperature within or on the body) are considered the hallmark symptom of menopause. The intensity of symptoms varies and ranges from a minor nuisance to an unbearable state, in which hot flashes may occur more than 100 times per day. These symptoms may interfere with daily activities, work performance, concentration, sex life, and a woman's comfort in general. They usually occur approximately 2 years before menopause (in approximately 40%–58% of women) and eventually subside spontaneously (10). About 80% of women report this symptom in Western countries, whereas as little as 10% of women report it in East Asian countries (7,14). These women have central flushing on the face, neck, and upper torso, and they are usually afflicted with sweating followed by a cold feeling, when the core body temperature drops. Night sweats may cause sleep disturbances and lead to general fatigue. Hot flashes usually occur at night, in a warm atmosphere, after alcohol or caffeine consumption, and under stressful circumstances. The frequency of hot flashes varies from less than once a day to several times per hour, and the duration may be anywhere from seconds to an hour. Hot flashes may persist for a few years or for decades (17,18).

Estrogen-dependent target tissue symptoms (of the urogenital tract), such as dryness of the vagina and vulva, and increased frequency and urgency of urination (atrophy of the urethra and trigone of the bladder mucosa), are common in the postmenopausal phase due to the large number of estrogen receptors in these organs (9). Vaginal subepithelial and epithelial transformation leads to a pale, fragile, thin, smooth, and narrowed vagina. Loss of vaginal transverse rugae is observed, and sometimes a blood-stained discharge. Clinical documentation of vaginal epithelium changes during the postmenopausal period can be assessed on the vaginal cytology maturation index (a biologic assay of estrogen's influence on the vaginal epithelium), which reflects the shift in proportion of matured squamous superficial cells to less mature parabasal (intermediate cells) and basal cells. Clinically, the maturation index does not reflect vaginal symptoms associated with the postmenopausal phase (19). These symptoms may include dryness, itching, burning, increased vaginal discharge (frequently blood stained), painful sexual intercourse (dyspareunia), and offensive odor. In addition, vaginal atrophy depletes the natural bacterial flora of *Lactobacillus acidophilus,* which change the acidic vaginal environment to one with an alkaline pH (9).

It has been documented that the prevalence of sexual activity declines with aging [to 70% among women 45–54 years of age (20) and to 60% among women 55–64 years of age (21)]. Additionally, postmenopausal vaginal symptomatology decreases sexual arousal in women (22).

Urinary tract symptoms, such as incontinence, infection (urethritis and/or cystitis frequently without the presence of microflora), and increased frequency and urgency of urination, occur more frequently in postmenopausal women (23).

Emotional symptoms are another recognizable part of the postmenopausal event. These symptoms are either directly or indirectly related to vasomotor symptomatology. Nightly hot flashes and sweating may result in chronic sleep deprivation (24) (early waking, insomnia), which may lead to irritability and fatigue. However, the onset of natural menopause is not associated with an increased risk for depression, and if it does occur, it is transitory (25). The most common emotional instability associated with climacterium manifests as anxiety, irritability, mood depression, mood swings, nervousness, tension, crying easily, and apathy (26).

Among *general symptoms*, skin changes may occur as collagen synthesis and maturation correspond to changing estrogen levels (27). Clinical manifestations of decreased estrogen levels are dry skin and the increased appearance of wrinkles. Muscle pain, joint pain, paresthesia, dryness of the eyes, mouth, and nose, oily skin, acne, hirsutism, and male-pattern alopecia are also often present (9,25).

In the *late postmenopausal phase*, pubic hair loss and breast atrophy (decreased breast size) are also noticeable (28).

ETIOLOGY

Premature Ovarian Failure

The causes of premature ovarian failure (POF; spontaneous menopause before the age of 40 years), which is a multifactorial form of premature depletion of oocytes, may have the following causes.

Genetic disorders (karyotypic aberrations) may cause menopause to occur in a young woman (under 30 years); infertility is also usually reported (14). It has been documented, using a DNA hybridization technique, that the deletion of the interstitial portion of the distal long arm of the X chromosome may be such a cause. However, these findings also have established that a combination of cytogenetic and DNA hybridization analysis is necessary to substantiate a diagnosis (29). Such an approach provides a specific cause of

POF (29–31). Other genetic causes, such as hereditary reduction of the number of germ cells, germ cell migration failure, increased atresia of primordial follicles, or chromosomal abnormalities (gonadal dysgenesis, the X-chromosome trisomy with or without chromosomal mosaicism), also may be responsible for the occurrence of POF.

Recently, genes located on the X chromosome were coded for their involvement in follicular atresia; GDF9 and connexin 37 are implicated in the process of ovarian follicle maturation (32).

Autoimmune disorders also may cause POF and are considered when a woman of reproductive age with a normal karyotype spontaneously enters premature menopause. Ovarian failure, with the presence of serum antiovarian antibodies, may exist as an isolated medical entity; however, the specificity of ovarian antibodies as a marker for autoimmune POF is questionable (33,34). In addition, POF may result from polyendocrine autoimmune disorders such as hypothyroidism, hypoparathyroidism, adrenal insufficiency (Addison's disease), diabetes mellitus, myasthenia gravis, vitiligo, and pernicious anemia (8,35).

Autoimmune oophoritis usually presents in the form of cystic ovarian enlargement (36–38), which contrasts with classic POF in which small ovaries are present. Such cystic ovarian enlargement is usually treated by oophorectomy, which can actually be avoided (this enlargement is most likely an ovarian response to increased gonadotropin secretion) (36).

Ovarian infection as a result of the mumps virus (mumps oophoritis) is also a probable cause of premature ovarian failure (39–41). Mumps oophoritis is a rare medical condition but may affect the ovaries as it affects other organs.

Induced premature ovarian failure is associated with a premature loss of ovarian function by one of the following:

■ Physical cause (radiation therapy in the pelvis area for malignant neoplasia)
■ Chemotherapy (for cancer with cyclophosphamide, methotrexate, or fluorouracil) (16)
■ Surgical removal of the ovaries (oophorectomy or surgical castration)

Galactosemia, which results from a congenital deficiency of the enzyme galactose-1-phosphate uridyl transferase, may cause premature ovarian failure (42–44). Homozygotic women, specifically, are at a high risk for developing ovarian failure (42).

The following factors also influence premature menopause:

■ Low body weight may predispose women to experience menopause at a younger age, and the menopause symptomatology may be more accentuated and more difficult to treat.
■ Smoking cigarettes may cause menopause to take place 3 to 5 years ahead of the expected age.

■ Hysterectomy accelerates the onset of menopause, causing it to occur 3 to 5 years before the anticipated time.

DIAGNOSIS

Pertinent Medical and Surgical History

A patient's initial medical history should include the age, parity, menstrual pattern, surgical and gynecologic history, sexual history, and current sexual activity (pregnancy symptomatology should be explored in women with an oligomenorrheic or amenorrheic state). A history of heart disease, hypertension, headaches, deep-vein thrombosis or pulmonary embolism should be addressed. It is necessary to obtain a history of genital tract infection, particularly of mumps virus infection, when a patient is suspected of having premature menopause. A family history of heart disease, breast cancer, or other gynecologic cancer should be obtained.

When ascertaining classic climacteric symptoms, the focus is on the following conditions:

■ Estrogen deficiency may interrupt the balance between norepinephrine and dopamine neurotransmitters; this imbalance leads to vasomotor instability (25). Clinically, it manifests as hot flashes, night sweats, heart palpitations, emotional lability (mood swing, irritability, tension, nervousness, anxiety, depression), sleep disorder (insomnia or early waking), dryness of the skin, eyes, or vagina, dyspareunia, or vaginitis.
■ Urethritis, cystitis (abacterial or bacterial), urinary frequency, urgency, and stress incontinence
■ Progesterone deficiency, which is suspected when irregular, heavy endometrial bleeding with or without clots is present
■ Androgen-related deficiency, which may reduce libido, decrease sexual arousal, and interfere with orgasm

A review of systemic and social history provides valuable information regarding current and past prescription and nonprescription medications, alternative remedies, supplements, vitamins or complementary therapy, or off-the-shelf phytohormones or other hormonal remedies. In addition, information on dietary habits, alcohol consumption, cigarette smoking (>10 cigarettes per day), and type of exercise performed may enlighten the diagnostic process. It is a generally accepted clinical practice not to perform any specific laboratory test when the absence of menses occurs in the presence of an intact uterus and characteristic climacteric symptomatology at the expected menopausal age.

Physical Examination

Upon general examination, vital signs, height, and weight should be recorded. Skin turgor and elasticity may be decreased, along with an oily complexion, acne, hirsutism, and alopecia; the skin and mucosal tissue also may exhibit dryness. Breast atrophy and pallor of the areola may occur. The thyroid gland and cardiovascular system also should be examined.

Pelvic examination of women experiencing menopause shows pallor and thin external genitalia upon visual inspection. The vagina appears pale, thin, smooth, and fragile with petechiae, with no transverse rugae present; a blood-stained vaginal discharge may be seen. A vaginal atrophic state may be observed with or without symptoms suggesting atrophic vaginitis, which is not clearly defined and may incorporate symptoms and signs (or symptoms only or signs only). A cervix without a mucosal plug and atrophic changes may be noted. An ecto-endo-cervical/vaginal smear should be obtained to screen for cytology (Papanicolaou test). An atrophic uterus and bilaterally impalpable ovaries may be encountered.

Laboratory Studies

Serum elevation of FSH levels (> 30 mIU/mL), serum reduction of 17-beta-estradiol concentration (E_2 < 20–40 pg/mL), patient age appropriate for menopause confirm and document the postmenopausal phase of climacterium. These tests, however, are indicated only for a hysterectomized woman with at least one ovary intact. A simple, practical approach (once pregnancy has been ruled out) in assessing an estrogenic state is the use of a progesterone challenge test. This test is composed of a progesterone withdrawal test using either (a) progesterone in oil (Lipolutin) 50 to 100 mg or 17-alpha-hydroxyprogesterone (Delalutin) 125 mg intramuscularly (IM); or (b) oral progesterone [micronized progesterone (Prometrium, 100 mg twice daily), medroxyprogesterone (Provera, 10 mg), norethindrone acetate (Norlutate, 5 mg), or norethindrone (Norlutin, 5 mg) one tablet a day for 7 to 10 days]. A negative test (no bleeding) implies hypoestrogenism and a lack of endometrial proliferation or occlusion in the uterine outflow.

Premature ovarian failure can be substantiated by laboratory tests, such as a negative pregnancy test (of which serum quantitative beta-human chorionic gonadotropin is the most reliable test), a negative progesterone challenge test result, and an indication of serum elevation of FSH (>30 mIU/mL).

Clinically, possible POF in an older woman (which may manifest as an absence of puberty) can be confirmed by a significant increase of baseline and poststimulation plasma gonadotropins (although congenital galactosemia should also be considered as a cause of POF) (43).

A presumed diagnosis of ovarian autoimmunity is based on the presence of serum ovarian-specific autoantigens, and despite recent progress in molecular characterization of target ovarian autoantigens, the diagnosis still remains elusive for POF (34). The definitive diagnosis of POF is established by histopathologic verification (37,38) through either classic ovarian laparotomy or laparoscopic biopsy (45).

A genetic study may be useful in older girls to rule out chromosomal or genetic aberrations.

A diagnosis of viral mumps–related oophoritis can be established by isolating the virus from cervicovaginal secretions; a serologic test of mumps-specific immunoglobulin M antibodies also may provide evidence confirming the diagnosis of this condition (41).

DIFFERENTIAL DIAGNOSIS

- Gonadotropin-resistant ovary syndrome (Savage syndrome or receptor or postreceptor defects)
- Turner syndrome
- Congenital thymic aplasia
- Gonadotropin secretion aberration (producing and secreting a biologically imperfect and inactive alpha or beta chain)

THERAPY

Conventional Therapy

Although climacteric symptomatology merely reflects a natural biologic physiologic occurrence in a woman's life, it is important to consider the preventive aspects of hormonal replacement therapy (HRT, estrogen/progesterone therapy) or estrogen replacement therapy (ERT) as indicated. A practitioner should develop a step-by-step, individual, systematic, clinical system for preventive long-term therapy. The physician and patient should collaborate to make a decision about appropriate medical management. One such systematic clinical approach can be achieved as follows (46):

- Establishing the type (natural or premature, or induced) and phase of climacterium
- Defining objectives of HRT or ERT, or alternative therapies:
    - To control vasomotor symptoms and their potential sequelae
    - To prevent potential illness associated with hormonal changes that accompany climacterium (osteoporosis, coronary heart disease, urinary stress incontinence, vaginal atrophy, urinary infections, sexual dysfunction, and other less common chronic disease such as arthritis, periodontal disease, skin atrophy, cataract formation, ovarian or colon cancer, etc.) (7)
- Establishing risk factors, in which HRT may present a negative clinical effect on a preexisting medical condition

The clinical scenario precludes temporary or permanent contraindications to implementing HRT. Absolute contraindications are as follows (47):

- Pregnancy
- Undiagnosed abnormal genital bleeding
- Estrogen-dependent malignancy, such as breast or endometrial cancer, constitutes a contraindication for HRT. However, it is not a generally accepted approach, and controversy exists as to whether or not to use HRT or ERT in breast cancer. Some incorporate ERT in the management of short-term treatment (<5 years) (4); it is implemented when severe menopausal symptoms are present and alternative management is ineffective (8). After adequate therapy for endometrial cancer, HRT may be implemented (5,48) based on prognostic indicators (the differentiation of cell type and the depth of invasion). Well-differentiated endometrial cell types with superficial invasion present a risk for persistent disease of approximately 5%; moderately differentiated endometrial cancer with one-half myometrial invasion constitutes a risk for persistent disease of 10% to 15%. When nonendometrioid-type cells or serous papillary-type cells are present, the risk for persistent disease is as high as 50%. Poorly differentiated tumors, regardless of cell type, with over one-half myometrial invasion present a risk for persistent disease that is estimated at 40% to 50% (5).
- Recent vascular thrombosis
- Informed patient's refusal
- Active liver disease can be exacerbated by oral estrogen administration because estrogen inactivation takes place in the hepatic first pass. To avoid exacerbation, the hepatic first-pass transdermal estrogen patch (Estraderm, 0.05 mg) may provide estrogen replacement that is safer than the oral route in this clinical situation (7).
- Anaphylaxis-like reaction (anaphylactoid attack) is a potentially life-threatening medical entity, related either to progesterone sensitivity or hypersensitivity to some metabolic substance in menstrual fluid.

Relative contraindications are as follows (47):

- Malignant melanoma may constitute a relative contraindication. However, there is no persuasive evidence to support this view (49); the conclusion thus far has been based on clinical progression of malignant melanoma in oral contraceptive users and pregnant women.
- History of thromboembolic disease
- Family history of breast cancer
- Hypertriglyceridemia: when the triglyceride level is higher than 300 mg/dL, oral estrogen can be administered with very close monitoring for the first 2 to 3 months of therapy with yearly follow-ups, because patients are at risk for developing pancreatitis (8).
- Gallbladder disease
- Migraine headaches (an interruption of estrogen for a few days may exacerbate migraine headaches, and the frequency of migraines may increase with the accentuated estrogen fluctuation of the menopause transition (28).

- Uterine leiomyomata
- Seizure disorder

Hypertension is not considered a contraindication for HRT or ERT (3,50). Contrary to the clinical conviction, HRT or ERT can be used safely in symptomatic post-menopausal women, although appropriate clinical supervision should be exercised (50). In addition, cigarette smoking does not constitute a contraindication, nor is there a higher incidence of stroke [no clinical association has been established between HRT users and stroke (50)] with HRT (3).

Patient education about the pros and cons of HRT must be undertaken. Particular attention should be directed to elucidating the relationship between HRT and cancer and addressing the fear of cancer associated with this mode of treatment, namely reassuring the patient that the risk for endometrial cancer does not increase when progesterone or a progestin agent is administered (51). Endometrial cancer is usually diagnosed at an early stage. It has been observed that the relative risk for breast cancer increases after 10 years of HRT and ERT, but neither therapy is associated with increased mortality at any cancer site (51). Possible vaginal bleeding is a side effect of HRT, but it is usually a transient event and frequently self-limited.

The long-term compliance with HRT or ERT is poor, and it is estimated that only 20% of postmenopausal women will continue therapy (52). Women with a high level of education and who consume a high-fiber diet and exercise regularly are found to observe good compliance (53). In contrast, those women who had high parity, who were young during their first complete pregnancy, and who have not undergone gynecologic surgery (hysterectomy or oophorectomy) refused HRT or stayed on HRT in the short-term with poor compliance (53).

The relative risk for deep-vein thrombosis increases with HRT, even though the absolute risk remains small. In temporal immobilization (trauma or surgery), HRT should be withheld.

A patient–physician collaborative decision about HRT falls into several categories. Regarding short-term versus long-term administration of medication, poor compliance may result in endometrial bleeding when medication is not properly administered on a daily basis.

The nature of menopausal symptoms and their influence on a woman's general well-being, along with the nature of preventive treatment and potential management of side effects, should be discussed with the patient (54). It has been well established that in women with moderate to severe postmenopausal symptoms, HRT is an obvious choice of treatment. However, when HRT is entertained only as a preventive treatment, the decision is not straight-forward, and it is necessary to address potential health benefits as well as safety concerns to reach a proper decision. From a clinical pragmatic point of view, most symptomatic women who request HRT or ERT as preventive treatments and who meet the risk-benefit criteria of inclusion should not be deprived of such treatment (55).

The selection of an appropriate regimen, its route of administration, the duration of therapy, as well as an established follow-up schedule, are the final steps in determining a management plan. An adequate estrogen dose should be selected to eliminate climacteric symptoms and at the same time provide preventive benefits. A continuous vs. cyclic method with progesterone (a continuous progesterone or progestin therapeutic manner prevents withdrawal endometrial bleeding) is advised. ERT should be recommended for hysterectomized women.

The initial follow-up should be scheduled after 3 months of HRT or ERT, and during that period it is advisable to keep a contemporaneous record of symptoms on a daily basis. Upon establishing an adequate estrogen dose and mode of administration, a patient should have an annual routine health check-up with cervical cytology, and a mammography should be obtained as indicated.

Clinical Management of Postmenopausal Symptoms

Estrogens

Vasomotor symptoms (hot flashes, night sweats, and heart palpitation), in a majority of cases, are not so severe as to be disruptive, and they eventually resolve spontaneously. In addition, postmenopausal symptoms themselves do not lead to any adverse health consequences.

The most effective medical therapy in reducing vasomotor symptoms (severity and frequency) is HRT. Young climacteric women, women with induced menopause, or women with POF who exhibit severe and frequent symptoms may require a higher dose of estrogen (at least double the starting dose), 1.25 mg daily to suppress symptoms, than the standard daily dose (0.625 mg conjugated estrogen daily is considered the standard dose to control vasomotor symptoms and to prevent bone density diminishment and coronary artery disease). However, higher doses of estrogen should be reduced whenever a clinical condition warrants it to minimize potential long-term risks (although the lessened dose should not be lower than standard starting doses) (7,9). Patients in whom such an estrogen dose causes related adverse side effects (mastalgia, fluid retention, etc.) may receive a lower equivalent conjugated estrogen dose of 0.3 mg. This dose may control postmenopausal symptoms, but any preventive aspects, particularly of bone density, are lost and other drugs can be added to prevent bone density disease. Alendronate sodium, (Fosamax) 10 mg orally daily in the morning on an empty stomach in an upright position (56), can be used and has been approved by the U.S. Food and Drug Administration (FDA) for prevention of osteoporosis (9).

Intranasal calcitonin spray can be prescribed when alendronate cannot be used (in cases of esophageal or peptic problems, or renal insufficiency).

The FDA has approved the following common estrogen equivalents at the lowest estrogen doses that prevent bone loss and coronary artery disease and that may control vasomotor symptoms:

Oral

- Conjugated equine estrogens (Premarin, 0.625 mg daily)
- Estropipate, Ogen or Ortho-Est (0.625 mg daily)
- Esterified estrogens (Estratab or Menest, 0.625 mg daily)
- Micronized estradiol [Estrace, 0.5 mg twice a day (due to short half-life) or 1 mg daily)
- Micronized estradiol (Climaval, 2 mg daily)

Transdermal

- Transdermal estradiol (Estraderm, 0.05) avoids first-pass enterohepatic metabolism and does not affect hepatic coagulation proteins. A transdermal patch is sometimes indicated because (7,9,28):

    Oral estrogen may cause side effects such as nausea or estrogen-induced hypertension (an uncommon event)

    Hepatic dysfunction can occur

    High triglycerides may be noted

    Patient prefers this method

- Percutaneous estradiol gel patches (Oestrogel, Divigel, or Sandrena, 1 mg applied topically daily) deliver the medication through a metered dose measurement system.
- Estradiol subcutaneous implants (Riselle, 25 mg, replaced every 6 months) are placed into the abdominal wall or buttock. Once the pellet is inserted, it is difficult to remove.

Vaginal

- Conjugated equine estrogens (Premarin vaginal cream, 0.625 mg)
- Dinestrol vaginal cream, 0.01%
- Estradiol vaginal cream (Estrace 0.01%) is applied at a dosage of 2 g daily for 2 weeks, then 1 g one to three times each week). This treatment is usually added to oral estrogen therapy for women with residual genitourinary atrophy. Systemic absorption of estradiol from the vagina is negligible (9).
- Estropipate vaginal cream (Ogen, 1.5 mg)
- Estriol vaginal cream (Ovestine, Synopause, 1 mg/g, 0.5 mg twice a week)
- Estradiol vaginal tablet (Vagifem, one tablet twice a week)
- The estriol vaginal ring (Estring) is replaced every 90 days. Estring is usually added to oral estrogen for women with residual genitourinary atrophy or for women who

declined HRT or ERT with symptoms and signs of atrophy, and systemic absorption or endometrial stimulation is not significant (9). However, it has been documented and reported that Estring expresses a clinical capacity to preserve bone density; therefore, peripheral blood concentration measurement does not always reflect therapeutic-preventive capabilities (58).

Follow-ups are based on the clinical suppression of vasomotor symptoms. The first visit is usually scheduled 3 months after the commencement of HRT or ERT and is then scheduled on a yearly basis. In selected cases, however, it may be advisable to schedule more follow-ups to determine serum estradiol levels (in order to maintain 60 pg/mL concentration) (7,59).

A patient should be informed about common side effects of estrogen:

- Bloating, fluid retention, weight gain
- Breakthrough bleeding
- Breast tenderness
- Headaches
- Increased cervical mucous secretion
- Gastrointestinal symptoms (nausea)

Progestin also may cause bloating, breast tenderness, headaches and gastrointestinal symptoms.

Estrogen alone (unopposed), as a mode of oral treatment for postmenopausal symptoms and for preventive benefits, is indicated in the form of conjugated estrogen 0.625 to 1.25 mg daily in a hysterectomized woman. Other routes of estrogen administration also can be used in the same dosage.

Usually, unopposed ERT (either low dose or standard dose) is not recommended for women with an intact uterus, due to the fivefold increased risk for endometrial cancer (60).

Estrogen/Progesterone (or Progestin) Regimens

Unopposed estrogens therapy will eventually cause endometrial hyperplasia that may predispose women with an intact uterus to develop endometrial cancer; adding progesterone or progestin should prevent this undesirable endometrial stimulation. The following progesterone/progestin regimens are usually incorporated into HRT:

Oral Administration

- Micronized natural progesterone (Prometrium or Uterogestan) is given at a cyclic daily dose of 200 mg for 12 days each month (61) or at a 100-mg dose daily for continuous administration (7,28,61). A high metabolic rate during the first hepatic pass (>90%) greatly compromises the efficacy of once-daily administration, and due to this metabolic process, unphysiologic accumulation of progesterone metabolites may lead to side effects such as dizziness and drowsiness (62). It has also been clinically documented that micronized progesterone can induce antiproliferative changes in the endometrium at lower doses than those required for transformation of the endometrium to a secretory state (63). Natural micronized progesterone does not decrease estrogen-increased high-density lipoprotein (HDL) levels (7).

■ Medroxyprogesterone acetate (C-21 progesterone derivatives, including Provera, Cycrin, Amen, and Curretab) are given at a cyclic dose of 5 to 10 mg for 12 days each month or at 2.5 to 5 mg daily for continuous treatment. It exhibits weak androgenic predisposition even though it displays no effect on lipid profiles (7,28,61).

■ Dydrogesterone (C-21 progesterone derivatives, including Duphaston and Teroulut) at the cyclic daily dose of 10 to 20 mg for 12 days each month has no androgenic activities and no effect on beneficial estrogen-increased HDL levels (7).

■ Norethisterone (C-19 nortestosterone derivatives, including Micronor, NorQD, Primolut, and Nor) is given at a cyclic daily dose of 0.7 to 1.0 mg for 12 days each month or at 0.35 to 0.5 mg daily for continuous treatment. It has an androgenic effect, and this group of progestins displays antagonistic effects on estrogen-increased HDL levels (7).

Transdermal Administration

■ Norethindrone acetate (62)
■ Transdermal micronized progesterone administration in a sequential mode with continuous transdermal estrogen is insufficient to induce endometrial transformation from a proliferative to a secretory state (64).

Vaginal Administration

Progesterone vaginal gel, administered at a dose of 45, 90, or 180 mg, induces secretory transformation of the endometrium despite low plasma levels (65). Such endometrial transformation suggests a local and direct vagina-to-uterus method of transport (62,65). Transvaginal gel therapy may offer fewer side effects) (62).

In a clinical observational study, natural progesterone vaginal effervescent tablets (100 mg daily in a continuous mode) sufficiently produced antiproliferative endometrial stimulation, with only a 6% occurrence of side effects (mild vaginal irritation) (66). It is premature to suggest a vaginal tablet as a course of treatment because of the lack of satisfactory clinical trials. This vaginal route of progesterone administration avoids the hepatic first-pass of progesterone metabolism and does not influence lipid profiles (65).

Intranasal Administration

A nasal spray of progesterone at the dosage of 11.2 mg three times daily for 10 days appears to transform the endometrium from a proliferative to a secretory state (67).

This observational study requires well-designed controlled clinical trials before such administration can be recommended.

Intrauterine Administration

Levonorgestrel-releasing intrauterine devices display the ability to protect endometrial hyperstimulation, and no endometrial hyperplasia has been observed within 3 years (68) and 5 years of treatment (69). However, an initial report indicates that it does cause negative effects similar to those of norethisterone on beneficial estrogen-increased HDL levels (70).

Progestin may cause the following side effects, and a patient should be notified of this before HRT is started:

■ Acne or oily skin
■ Alopecia or growth of excess hair
■ Bloating
■ Breast tenderness
■ Changes in libido
■ Depression or premenstrual dysphoric disorder-like symptoms
■ Gastrointestinal symptoms
■ Headaches
■ Insomnia
■ Skin itching or rashes

Estrogen also may produce bloating, breast tenderness, gastrointestinal symptoms, and headaches.

Androgenic effects are directly related to the androgenicity and dose of a progestin agent. Natural micronized progesterone (Prometrium or Uterogestan) has the weakest androgenic potency, whereas ethindrone (Aygestin, Micronor, Nor, Nor QD, or Primolut) has the strongest androgenic capacity, and medroxyprogesterone (Amen, Curretab, Cycrin, or Provera) falls between these two androgenicities (28,61). The androgenic predilection of progestins minimizes the preventive effects of estrogen on lipoproteins, particularly on the HDL cholesterol profile (71); therefore, prescribing natural micronized progesterone seems logical.

Progesterone, or progestin itself, can both prevent and reverse endometrial hyperplasia and, in combination with estrogen, will reduce endometrial hyperstimulation. Progesterone or progestin can be administered in combination with estrogen in the following manner:

■ Daily: a continuous mode of estrogen-progesterone or progestin therapy is currently the most commonly accepted method by both patients and physicians, because endometrial hyperplasia is encountered at a rate of less than or equal to 1% and menstrual-like bleeding is absent (7,72).
■ Monthly: a cyclic method is suggested, in which a patient takes progestin for the last 10 to 12 days instead of estrogen [the longer the duration of progestin treat-

ment, the lower the risk for endometrial cancer (73)], and the patient is usually advised to administer progestin on calendar days 1 through 12 of each month (7).

- Quarterly: although progestins can be used, this method is not often prescribed due to an unacceptably high occurrence of endometrial hyperplasia (7).

Progestin alone can be used when estrogen therapy is contraindicated. Usually, oral medroxyprogesterone acetate (10–20 mg daily) or depo-medroxyprogesterone acetate (150 mg IM for 1–3 months) is administered. Megestrol acetate (oral daily dose of 40 mg) also may be suggested as an option (8).

Estrogen-progesterone (or progestin) combined therapy is recommended in any case when a woman with an intact uterus chooses estrogen as a form of postmenopausal management. There are several clinical options in the administration of combined regimens for HRT to treat vasomotor symptoms and to prevent chronic diseases associated with a hypoestrogenic state:

- Cyclic (sequential) HRT can be administered in the form of an estrogen component (0.625 mg conjugated estrogen, 0.625 mg estrone sulfate, or 1.0 mg micronized estradiol) for 25 days monthly. Progesterone component (micronized natural progesterone 200 mg daily) or progestin component (medroxyprogesterone acetate 5–10 mg, dydrogesterone 10–20 mg, or norethindrone 0.7–1.0 mg) is added for the last 10 to 12 days of the estrogen regimen. Expected withdrawal bleeding (on average, bleeding will show after the 9th day of progestin treatment) will occur monthly in 70% to 90% of women, but an absence of monthly withdrawal bleeding should not be a clinical concern (7). Pragmatically, it is advisable to start an estrogen regimen on the 1st day of each calendar month and to add progestin from the 14th to the 25th days. A downside of this method is that a patient may experience vasomotor symptoms during the HRT lapse.
- Combined cyclic method: estrogen is prescribed for 21 days, as in the cyclic method presented above, with a concomitant continuous progesterone or progestin regimen for 21 days (micronized progesterone at the dose of 100 mg, medroxyprogesterone at the dose of 2.5–5 mg, or norethisterone at the dose of 0.35–0.5 mg). Regular menstrual-like bleeding occurs during the 7-day medication-free period.
- Continuous estrogen with sequential progesterone or with the progestin regimen is designed to provide estrogen replacement on a continuous basis (dosages as described for cyclic HRT). Such a clinical approach eliminates the 7-day medication-free period, in which a patient may experience postmenopausal symptoms. A progesterone or progestin regimen should be prescribed for the first or last 12 days of each calendar month (dosages as described for cyclic HRT). Withdrawal men-

strual-like bleeding may occur. A combination of 0.625 mg of conjugated equine estrogen and 5 mg of medroxyprogesterone in one tablet is the suggested dose to be taken for 14 days (Premphase).

- Continuous combined method: administer estrogen and progesterone or progestin regimens for the duration of therapy (dosages are for the combined cyclic method). Erratic mild endometrial bleeding or spotting may occur within the first 12 months. Regimens are available that contain estrogen and progestin in one tablet or one transdermal patch. An oral combination of conjugated equine estrogen (0.625 and 2.5 mg) with medroxyprogesterone acetate is available in one tablet, 28 pills total in a package. Because this mode of therapy is designed for continuous use, 28 tablets in one package is not enough for an average monthly supply. Therefore, a patient is forced to obtain 13 instead of 12 packages per year).
- Transdermal estradiol (Combipatch) at the dose of 0.05 mg estrogen and norethindrone acetate at the daily dose of 0.14 mg or 0.25 mg can be used.
- Continuous estrogen (unopposed) method: indicated only for a hysterectomized woman (dosages as for cyclic HRT). A low dose (equivalent of 0.3 mg conjugated estrogen) may provide relief of vasomotor symptoms, but it will not provide preventive benefits.

The menopause transition clinically manifests with vasomotor symptoms (14) such as cyclic mastalgia and irregular uterine bleeding, which result from serum-unopposed elevated estrogen levels (74). These symptoms can be controlled with micronized natural progesterone (Prometrium or Uterogestan) at the daily dose of 100 to 200 mg for the duration of any menstrual-like bleeding. When vasomotor symptoms cannot be controlled, estrogen-progesterone or progestin regimens may be prescribed (8). In the menopausal transition, ovulation occurs in about 37% of women (74), and low-dose oral contraceptives can be used to provide protection against unwanted pregnancy (8). During the menopausal transition period or in the postmenopausal phase, women who are on unopposed ERT and who experience unexpected prolonged endometrial bleeding may have endometrial hyperplasia (75).

Follow-up

A clinical follow-up is initially scheduled after 3 months of HRT to assess relief of symptoms, endometrial withdrawal bleeding or erratic bleeding, degree of medication compliance, possible adverse side effects and their management, and dosage adjustment. After the initial follow-up visit, an annual schedule of follow-ups is recommended (47). The endometrial bleeding pattern is the best indicator of endometrial response to HRT stimulation, and any departure from an expected individual pattern (in frequency, duration, and intensity) warrants endometrial assessment.

Expected menstrual-like flow begins after the 6th day of the progestin regimen. If bleeding occurs before the 6th day or is abnormally heavy (>80 mL per cycle) or prolonged (>8 days), endometrial assessment should be performed (76). The integrity of the endometrium may be evaluated in the following ways.

- Office hysteroscopic uterine cavity investigation with a biopsy is now a preferable and more accurate mode of endometrial cavity assessment.
- Office endometrial biopsy is an accurate method of endometrial investigation if the disease affects the entire endometrium. When a focal abnormality is present, an endometrial biopsy is insufficient, and a hysteroscopic study should be performed.
- Dilatation and curettage (fractional) has limited value today, because hysteroscopic evaluation is widely accessible; however, dilatation and curettage has a therapeutic significance as well as diagnostic importance when it is indicated.
- Transvaginal ultrasonographic measurement of endometrial double-layer thickness has been considered a noninvasive method of monitoring the endometrium in postmenopausal women on HRT with a 5-mm cut-off point of endometrial thickness (77). The negative predictive value in ERT is 100%; however, 5-mm endometrial thickness in postmenopausal women on ERT or HRT is very low (60,78). Ultrasonographic endometrial surveillance shows that 23% to 53% of women have an endometrial thickness greater than or equal to 5 mm while on HRT, and only 4% of them will actually have endometrial pathology (79). Therefore, endometrial ultrasonography may lead inadvertently to an invasive form of endometrial assessment.

When a continuous combined method of HRT is selected, it is expected that up to 75% of women may experience endometrial bleeding within the first 12 months of therapy [bleeding ceases in about 90% of women during this period (7)], and 10% to 15% may continue to experience erratic endometrial bleeding (80,81). Initiating the continuous combined method of HRT in older women may result in fewer cases of endometrial bleeding than in younger patients (7).

The American College of Obstetricians and Gynecologists (ACOG) recommends endometrial evaluation after 6 months of endometrial bleeding (82). If spotting occurs, increasing the dose of progesterone or progestin may prevent the endometrium from bleeding.

During each annual visit, particular attention should be directed to the patient's medical history, blood pressure, and breast and pelvic examination. Cervical cytology must be obtained as indicated for an individual woman, and a screening mammography should be scheduled. Other aspects of postmenopausal prevention and sexual function should be addressed (47).

Androgen Replacement Therapy

Sex steroid hormones gradually decline during climacterium. The ovaries are responsible for about 50% of androgen production during the premenopausal period (about 25% of total daily testosterone synthesis and 25% of peripheral conversion from weak androgens). In the adrenal gland, dehydroepiandrosterone (DHEA) and dehydroepiandrosterone sulfate (DHEAS) decrease slowly and gradually from the age of 25 years, and significant serum concentration reduction occurs between the ages of 50 and 60 years. Consequently, oophorectomy in reproductive age abruptly decreases 50% of the circulating testosterone. Testosterone, androstenedione, and DHEA are not exceptions, and significant decreases in serum concentration have been observed in the late menopausal transition and within the first 2 years of the postmenopausal period (83–86). Androgen deficiency symptomatology in postmenopausal women has not yet been established definitively (87); still, it is a clinical conviction that androgens may influence several health functions (7,8,28,84,87).

Sexual function such as *libido* (the desire phase of sexual function) depends on many factors, among which emotional, environmental, and hormonal milieu play a considerable role, and it has been postulated that serum testosterone concentration influences the frequency of sexual intercourse (88). *Orgasmic* function is not androgen-dependent (8). As a result of this link, androgens are added to ERT to increase libido in postmenopausal women (89). This claim has been challenged by other authorities (90,91). In view of these conflicting data establishing efficacy in sexual function, low-dose androgens are being prescribed. Low-dose androgens are attractive because virilization is low, with methyltestosterone at the dose of 1.25 mg. However, at least one virilization symptom usually develops at the end of 2 years of therapy (92) (acne, alopecia, hirsutism, clitoromegaly, deepening of the voice, etc.), and it is self-limited upon discontinuation of treatment. Hepatotoxicity has not been reported. This treatment does not mitigate the beneficial effects of standard dose of estrogen on lipid profiles (93).

The idea that combined therapy of estrogen/androgen regimens is superior to estrogen therapy alone is inconclusive in light of conflicting data from different randomized controlled clinical studies (87,89,92,94). Therefore, adding androgen to the estrogen therapy offers little, if any, benefit to postmenopausal women.

Preliminary data from a randomized, placebo-controlled, double-blind clinical trial with *DHEA* administration at the dose of 50 mg daily in postmenopausal women showed improvement in physical (fatigue, insomnia, and heart palpitation) and psychological well being (95).

Recently, attention has focused on an estrogen/androgen regimen replacement therapy and its influence on mood and well-being, and the initial results have been encouraging (96).

Bone density in postmenopausal women treated with estrogen/androgen implants (estradiol 50 mg and testosterone 50 mg) demonstrated increased bone density by dual-energy x-ray absorptiometry (97). A similar effect was noted using markers of bone formation (osteocalcin, bone-specific alkaline phosphatase, and C-terminal procollagen peptide) with oral regimens (esterified estrogens at 1.25 mg combined with 2.5 mg of methyltestosterone) (92,96). *Anabolic steroids* (Nandrolone decanoate) present another option for increased bone mineral density (BMD) (98). In addition, conflicting clinical data are present in reference to the increase of bone density with DHEA at the oral dose of 100 mg daily or daily application of a 10% cream on the skin (99,100).

The combination of estrogen and androgen in one oral tablet is available in two different dose compositions:

■ Esterified estrogens of 0.625 mg and methyltestosterone of 1.25 mg (Estratest HS)
■ Esterified estrogens of 1.25 mg and methyltestosterone of 2.5 mg (Estratest)

The customary dose of Estratest is one tablet daily for short-term use. Because this combination of estrogen and androgen does not contain a progesterone or progestin component, very close clinical endometrial monitoring should be carried out or a progesterone regimen should be added (84).

There are other routes of androgen administration, such as micronized testosterone in vegetable oil capsules (2.5–5 mg of testosterone), transdermal 17-beta-testosterone skin patches, subcutaneous pellets (50 mg), and IM injectable testosterone (87).

Cardiovascular disease sharply increases shortly after menopause (101) and is attributed to two factors:

■ Lipoprotein changes [increased total cholesterol and low-density lipoprotein (LDL) with decreased HDL (102)]
■ Inefficient function of the vascular endothelium, predominantly due to advancing atherosclerosis (103)

An evaluation of the overall negative effect of androgen on the cardiovascular system must be carefully balanced, if this regimen is considered. The cardiovascular mortality rate did not show signs of increase when postmenopausal women received the androgen therapy for 2 years (87,104).

Surgically induced menopause (bilateral oophorectomy) raises questions about the appropriate time to initiate HRT and the best hormones to use. The acute onset of menopause immediately following oophorectomy warrants initiation of ERT as soon as possible after the procedure. It has been postulated that this therapy should be commenced in the recovery room; an estrogen/androgen regimen will provide not only relief of vasomotor symptoms but also an androgenic anabolic effect, which enhances the postopera-

tive healing process and assists in later sexual function (increase libido, sexual arousal) in this relatively young patient population. Such combination replacement therapy is continued for 6 months. At the 6-month point, an evaluation is conducted, and a decision is made whether or not to continue estrogen/androgen therapy, to modify to ERT only, or to change to another form of management (105).

Conventional Nonhormonal Treatment for Menopausal Symptoms

The following agents can be used to cope with post-menopausal vasomotor symptomatology:

■ Bellergal-Retard at the dose of one tablet twice a day
■ Clonidine oral administration at the dose of 0.1 to 0.2 mg twice daily
■ Methyldopa at the dose of 250 to 500 mg once daily

Local vaginal dryness can be relieved using the following intravaginal lubricant regimens:

■ Astroglide (vaginal application, as needed)
■ Lubrin (vaginal application, as needed)
■ Replens (one vaginal application daily)
■ Vegetable oil (vaginal application, as needed)

POSTMENOPAUSAL PREVENTION AND THERAPY

Osteoporosis

Definition

Osteoporosis is a disease characterized by low bone mass and microarchitectural deterioration of bone tissue leading to increased bone fragility and risk for fracture (106).

Incidence

Over 20 million individuals are currently affected by osteoporosis in the United States (107), and this number will probably increase with the growing aging population. Osteoporosis may develop despite adequate prevention with ERT or HRT. A growing number of handicapped women who reach postmenopausal age are predisposed to osteoporosis (108). Prevention of osteoporosis with HRT is limited by poor compliance, particularly in older patients.

Etiology

Through a remodeling procedure, the old bone structure is removed (resorption) and the bone deficit is repaired. The delicate balance between resorption (osteoclasts) and repair (new bone is formed by osteoblasts) is maintained in harmony until the end of the third decade of life (at which point women reach peak bone mass or maximal bone density); after that point, this balance slowly and gradually becomes unstable, and resorption outweighs repair. This imbalance is more accentuated in the menopausal transition and continues into old age. Bone loss may affect either the cortical (shafts of long bones) or trabecular (flat bone such as vertebrae, pelvis, and ends of long bones) bone structure. Several factors affect the bone architectural structure and BMD, such as race (black population has greater bone density than white or Asian population), genetics [accountable for up to 70% of maximal bone density and familial predisposition to osteoporosis (109)], gender, time of puberty, frequency and intensity of exercise, calcium intake (important during bone growth and consolidation period), and vitamin D concentration. It has been estimated that postmenopausal women may lose about 1% of trabecular bone yearly (110).

There are two recognizable forms of osteoporosis. *Type I* osteoporosis is excessive, accelerated, disproportional, menopause-related predominantly trabecular bone loss [up to 5% yearly (111)]. The postmenopausal accelerated phase of trabecular bone loss predisposes women to common side fractures, such as vertebrae (43%), the hip (17%), and the distal part of the forearm (13%). Approximately 40% of women carry the lifetime risk for fracture of any side (112).

Type II osteoporosis is the loss of both trabecular and cortical bone structures, and it affects women in their seventies or older. This type is characterized by skeletal deformity such as dorsal kyphosis (dowager's hump), multiple wedge-type vertebral fractures, as well as fractures of the hip, pelvis, humerus (proximal part), and tibia (112).

In order to maintain a remodeling bone process at its most dynamic, calcium, renal calcium reabsorption, intestinal calcium absorption, and the biologically active vitamin D metabolite (1,25-dihydroxyvitamin D) are necessary (112–115). It is a well-established phenomenon that postmenopausal women require higher doses of calcium than premenopausal women to maintain calcium balance (116). Postmenopausal hypoestrogenism predisposes women to decreasing intestinal and renal tubular calcium absorption, which may lead to a negative calcium balance (112, 117–119).

Classifications

Osteoporosis is classified as either the primary or secondary type (120). Secondary osteoporosis is associated with the following medical conditions (120,121):

- Anticonvulsant therapy
- Chronic neurologic disease
- Chronic obstructive lung disease
- Connective tissue disease
- Heparin therapy
- Hypogonadism
- Hypercortisolism

- Hyperthyroidism
- Malabsorption syndrome
- Primary hyperparathyroidism
- Rheumatoid arthritis

Diagnosis

Diagnosis of primary osteoporosis is reached by exclusion; this medical entity develops gradually and insidiously. Pertinent medical history may not be adequate to diagnose primary osteoporosis; however, if a practitioner suspects osteoporosis, the following symptoms may assist in confirming a diagnosis:

- Acute pain associated with bone fracture that is disproportional to trauma or non–weight-bearing activities
- Chronic back pain
- Hypoestrogenism and its symptomatology (discussed elsewhere in this section)

Physical examination is usually negative among younger women, whereas skeletal deformity may be identified in older women.

Bone Density Measurement

Bone mineral density accounts for 75% to 85% of all bone strength (121). Therefore, clinically assessing this bone parameter efficiently predicts the risk for bone fracture (122). All methods used for bone mass measurement have a radiation exposure comparable with the dose received from chest x-ray or computed tomography of the abdomen (123).

Currently, there are several techniques available to measure bone mass (121):

- Single-photon absorptiometry (SPA) or single-energy x-ray absorptiometry (SXA) can be used to assess the radius and os calcis.
- Dual-photon absorptiometry (DPA) or dual-photon X-ray absorptiometry (DXA) can be used to determine BMD in the spine, proximal femur, and other locations.
- Quantitative computed tomography (QCT) provides similar information to DXA.
- Standard radiography is inferior to any of the above-presented techniques with an accuracy of 30% to 50% in measuring bone mass.
- Radiographic densitometry can be used to measure bone density at a peripheral side (preferably the hand) with accuracy comparable with that of SPA and SXA.
- Ultrasonographic measurement also may provide information regarding bone quality.

The World Health Organization (106) and the National Osteoporosis Foundation (124) recommend the following indications for bone density assessment:

- Hypoestrogenic (estrogen-deficient) state in women is documented.

- Osteoporosis is clinically suspected (radiographically documented vertebral bone loss or deformities present).
- Primary hyperparathyroidism is diagnosed.
- Hypercortisolism is established due either to medical or iatrogenic condition.
- Prolonged heparin therapy
- Follow-up of osteoporosis therapy should be performed within 2 years of initial therapy.

Based on BMD and standard deviation (SD) of mean reference for young adult women, the World Health Organization established the following diagnostic criteria for osteoporosis (106):

- Low bone mass (osteopenia) is diagnosed when BMD is lower, with SD between −1.0 and −2.5.
- Osteoporosis is confirmed when BMD is lower, with SD of −2.5.
- Severe osteoporosis is diagnosed by BMD measurement and at least one fragility fracture.

The diagnosis of secondary osteoporosis is established by a properly underlined medical condition evaluation utilizing the techniques and technology used in the primary osteoporosis diagnostic process.

Cardiovascular Disease Prevention

Primary coronary heart disease increases remarkably after menopause, and taking estrogen significantly decreases the mortality rate associated with postmenopausal coronary heart disease (125). Presently, it is a clinical conviction that the risk for primary coronary artery disease can be reduced in about 35% to 55% of women by administering postmenopausal estrogen (9,28,125).

Estrogen's role in the prevention of secondary coronary heart disease was scrutinized in a randomized controlled clinical trial, and the conclusion was that postmenopausal women with preexisting coronary heart disease should not be taking HRT (126).

Prevention of Cognitive Function Disorder and Dementia

It has been suggested that estrogen may lower the risk for cognitive (memory) function disorder and prevent dementia, including Alzheimer disease, in women (127,128). At present, due to the lack of randomized, controlled clinical studies, HRT as a preventive therapy for memory function disorder and dementia should not be recommended (129).

Prevention of Cerebrovascular Disease

Currently, the hypothesis that estrogen increases or decreases the risk for stroke has not yet been proved or disproved conclusively (125).

Conventional Prevention and Therapy

Osteoporosis

Prevention is unquestionably the best method of management of osteoporosis, and the FDA has approved ERT and HRT as a part of preventive treatment (28).

Estrogen effectiveness in the prevention of osteoporosis has been documented. It has been established that the presence of estrogen receptors in bones helps inhibit the osteoclastic activity responsible for bone resorption. Such estrogen activity increases the mean bone density by more than 5%, and this increase in bone density reduces the vertebral fracture rate by 50% and the hip fracture rate by 25%. Upon discontinuation of estrogen therapy, the beneficial estrogen effect stops, and the bone loss process quickens, reaching baseline after 10 years.

It has been established that the optimal, preventive, effective minimal dose of conjugated estrogen is 0.625 mg (7–9,28,112). The type of hormones, dosage, and route of administration are presented elsewhere in this chapter.

Calcium is an important factor in the prevention of osteoporosis (calcium may reduce age-related bone loss). However, it cannot be considered as a substitute for estrogen-related bone loss. Optimal daily calcium intake has been established by the National Institutes of Health Consensus Development Conference on calcium (130):

- During childhood: 800 to 1,000 mg
- Between 12 and 24 years of age: 1,200 to 1,500 mg
- Between 25 and the time of menopause, or 65 years of age: if estrogen is depleted, 1,000 mg
- After the age of 65 or after menopause: if estrogen is depleted, 1,500 mg

Vitamin D forms in the skin with exposure (15 minutes daily) to sunlight (in the range of 230- to 313-mm wavelengths) from precursors produced by the liver. The recommended dietary allowance of vitamin D is 200 IU daily, but up to 800 IU daily is safe. Daily intake of vitamin D_3 (cholecalciferol) should be in the range of 200 to 800 IU, with an average of 400 IU daily (112). Vitamin D itself or in combination with calcium supplementation may reduce the risk for common-site fracture (131,132). However, vitamin D in excess is toxic. Most foods do not contain vitamin D, but there are a few exceptions, such as milk, corn flakes, eggs, margarine, and salmon with bones. People who have decreased intestinal absorption and who are elderly or housebound have compromised vitamin D levels.

Bisphosphonates are an effective nonhormonal inhibitor of bone resorption. Alendronate at a dose of 10 mg daily has been approved by the FDA for osteoporosis management and should be administered with water on an empty stomach. It should be given at least 30 minutes before or after any other medication, and the patient should remain in an upright position for some time after ingesting it.

Fosamax 5 mg daily has been approved for women who are diagnosed with osteopenia and who cannot be on ERT or HRT (9,112).

The FDA has approved *calcitonin* for the treatment of osteoporosis, and it can be administered through either nasal spray or subcutaneous injection. However, intranasal spray is less effective than subcutaneous injection, HRT, or alendronate (112,133).

Selective estrogen receptor modulators are a new modality [with a mixed estrogen agonist/antagonist effect (134)] for the prevention and treatment of osteoporosis and have demonstrated a favorable, significant effect on the spine, hips, and overall peripheral skeleton in postmenopausal women. Preliminary, multicenter clinical studies of raloxifene hydrochloride (*Evista*) have shown not only a significant increase of BMD but also a significant decrease of serum cholesterol and LDL cholesterol, with little effect on serum HDL cholesterol and triglycerides (135). Evista has been approved for the prevention (increased bone mass, nontraumatic vertebral fractures, improved lipid profile) and treatment of osteoporosis in postmenopausal women and is recommended at the dose of 60 mg daily (can be taken any time of day regardless of meals). In addition, raloxifene clinically expresses a beneficial effect on the cardiovascular system and breasts without stimulation of the endometrium or breast tissues, or an increased risk for phlebitis. Therefore, it can be used alone or in combination with calcium, vitamin D, bisphosphonates, and calcitonin in women with an identifiable risk for breast or endometrial cancer (134–136). Hot flashes are the most frequently observed undesirable side effect, but they are of low intensity and generally occur during the first month of treatment only (135). Existing data suggest that ERT in clinical trials has greater positive effects on BMD than does raloxifene (137).

Other therapeutic agents, such as *sodium fluoride*, a bone formation–stimulating drug (at the dose of 75 mg), produce conflicting results by increasing bone mass but not significantly decreasing the risk for vertebral fractures. However, when these agents are used at the daily dose of 50 mg for over 4 years, the risk for vertebral fracture decreases (112). Therefore, clinical application of sodium fluoride remains to be determined. Other regimens, such as *parathyroid hormone* and strontium, are still under clinical investigation.

In primary *cardiovascular disease*, ERT is recommended in the standard dose. This method of approach is based on observational clinical study and therefore should not be considered definitive. In secondary cardiovascular disease, ERT is not recommended.

Prevention of cognitive function disorder and dementia with ERT has not yet been proven, so ERT or HRT should be administered only as part of regular postmenopausal management.

Uterine leiomyomata do not constitute a contraindication for prescribing HRT in standard doses (0.625–1.25 mg conjugated equine estrogen) for postmenopausal asymptomatic women (138). Symptomatic uterine leiomyomata and HRT present a clinical dilemma, and surgical therapy is usually offered before an estrogen therapy is instituted. This mode of therapy is practiced today, even though such an approach is based on a clinical tradition rather than on scientific clinical data. An alternative to surgery is to postpone HRT for 6 months to 1 year (it is a clinical conviction, based on anecdotal data, that uterine leiomyomata will undergo spontaneous involution). During this period, alternative treatment for postmenopausal symptomatology and prevention for osteoporosis should be used.

Complementary Therapy

Patient Education

Patient education in pre- and postmenopausal management is essential, particularly in improving compliance . It is a well-known phenomenon that compliance with conventional and natural ERT is poor. One third of postmenopausal women discontinue the treatment due mainly to side effects, fear of cancer, and the advice of practitioners (146). It should be recognized that a natural approach, such as taking soybeans or soy foods, practicing relaxation and stress reduction techniques, and exercising regularly, may relieve vasomotor postmenopausal symptoms to some degree, but such methods may not provide sufficient prevention of coronary heart disease, osteoporosis, or dryness of the mucosa or skin or both. The following areas of postmenopausal management should be well-understood by both a physician and a patient in order to make collaborative management decisions:

- Consideration should be given to either natural or conventional ERT or HRT as a process, in which women must learn about the pros and cons of existing conventional-complementary-natural therapeutic paradigms. With time, a woman's symptoms and concerns fluctuate, so a practitioner should maintain a dialogue with a patient throughout the climacterium period and afterward. It is worthwhile to emphasize that therapeutic and preventive effects of ERT will disappear upon discontinuation.

- A physician's knowledge of this ever-changing field should be updated to keep up with new proven clinical progress.

- There should be a balance between medical evidence and facts against myths, particularly in view of a fatality rate from coronary heart disease that is almost 10 times higher than that of breast cancer in postmenopausal women.

- Side effects occur on an individual basis, and particular attention should be directed to the fact that estrogen may exacerbate preexisting medical conditions, such as coronary artery disease (estrogen is very useful in the prevention of primary coronary artery disease but should not be prescribed in secondary coronary heart disease), liver function disorder, gallbladder disease, coagulation disorders, migraine headaches, and unexplained endometrial bleeding.

■ It is important to address a patient's fears of cancer. The risk for breast cancer may increase on HRT; those patients with recent breast cancer (within the past 5 years) or a family history of two or more first-degree relatives (mother or sisters) should avoid ERT. The risk for endometrial cancer can be reduced to the expected prevalence level of nonestrogen users when an adequate dose and duration of natural progesterone or progestin are prescribed with estrogen.

■ Adequate prevention of heart disease, bone mass loss, vaginal dryness, urinary incontinence, urinary infections, and potential cognitive function disorders should be discussed. The significance of life-style, including smoking habits, alcohol consumption, diet, and exercise, should be stressed, as should the importance of compliance with prescribed regimens.

Diet

Nutritional support during the climacteric period is usually addressed in terms of either general dietary recommendations or specific diet. General nutritional recommendations for climacteric women include consuming unprocessed, natural foods such as fruits, vegetables, whole grains, beans, seeds, nuts, and healthy oil, and foods that are low in animal fat (147).

■ Nutrition to ease vasomotor symptoms is provided with foods containing phytoestrogens, which usually contain a nonsteroidal estrogen substance that demonstrates an affinity to bind estrogen receptors (known as an estrogen receptor alpha). These foods may demonstrate an antiestrogen effect (prevention of breast and endometrial cancer) and at the same time act as a weak estrogen (estrogen-like activity on lipoprotein profiles and bone mass). As a result of this dual affinity (estrogen-agonist and estrogen-antagonist), such foods can be considered selective estrogen receptor modulators (148). The primary sources of phytoestrogens are phenolic phytoestrogens (isoflavones: genistein, daidzein, and glycitein), lignanes (such as enterodion and enterolactone), and coumestans. Isoflavones and lignanes make up the major component of dietary phytoestrogens (148).

■ Isoflavones are found in soybeans (a vegetable protein with no cholesterol and low in saturated fat that contains vitamin B, iron, calcium, zinc, and fiber). It has been clinically established that by taking at least 75 mg of total isoflavones (isoflavone concentrations per gram of soy protein vary among different products) (149). Isoflavones in a concentrated form (one 55-mg tablet contains mostly isoflavone genistein) are not an equivalent substitute for soy protein (which also contains daidzein, genistein, and glycitein isoflavones) (128).

■ It is essential to furnish a patient with the pertinent clinical information regarding soy protein. Hot flashes can be reduced by approximately 45% with soybeans (standard doses of ERT or HRT reduce hot flashes in 80%–90% of women) (150).

■ Soy protein consumption of 47 g daily (20 g of soy protein contains approximately 34 mg of phytoestrogens) decreases LDL cholesterol levels by 12.9% and triglyceride levels by 10.5%, but it does not significantly elevate HDL cholesterol levels (these data were established by meta-analysis) (15). However, recent randomized, double-blind, placebo-controlled clinical trials using 55 mg of isoflavones (predominantly genistein) did not support the claim that phytoestrogens can improve serum lipoprotein profiles (152). This controversy may have resulted from using one isoflavone, such as genistein, in a tablet form versus soybean-based isoflavones, such as daidzein, genistein, and glycitein.

The following foods contain phytoestrogens:

■ Soy protein: cooked soybeans, half a cup contains 150 mg of isoflavones; roasted soy nuts, half a cup contains 60 mg of isoflavones; texture soy protein granules, half a cup contains 62 mg of isoflavones; tofu (regular or low fat), half a cup contains 35 mg of isoflavones; tempeh, half a cup contains 35 mg of isoflavones; regular soy milk, 1 cup contains 30 mg of isoflavones; low-fat soy milk, 1 cup contains 20 mg of isoflavones; soy beverage powders, one to two scoops contain 25 to 75 mg of isoflavones.
■ Flax seed flour or flax seed meal
■ Seaweeds
■ Whole grains (corn, oats, wheat)
■ Legumes (beans, peas, peanuts)

Soy protein may cause gastrointestinal side effects, such as bloating, constipation, and nausea (150).

Nutritional prevention of heart disease is part of the lifestyle category, which includes eating habits and a specific diet. Changes in eating behavior involve decreasing calorie intake, reducing consumption of high-cholesterol foods, as well as foods high in saturated fats (such as beef, butter, cheese, coconut oil, palm oil, and pork), and limiting total fat intake to less than 30% of total calorie intake. The most influential postmenopausal diet for preventing coronary artery disease would minimize consumption of animal and other fats, dairy products, sugar and salt, refined grains, flours, and alcohol (147). It would also maximize consumption of cold-water fish (such as halibut, herring, mackerel, salmon, and tuna), which prevents clots and inflammation in vessel walls, and promotes vasodilatation as well as regular heart rhythm (147). Apples and raw carrots decrease cholesterol more effectively than oats

(153,154), and a high intake of fruits and vegetables, whole grains, and legumes decreases the risk for coronary artery disease (147). The FDA approved the notion that soy protein reduces coronary heart disease and authorized food labels making this claim.

Nutrition plays an essential role in the prevention of bone loss and in the maintenance of bone mass. Dietary prevention of bone loss incorporates large amounts of green leafy vegetables (such as kale, collard greens, romaine lettuce, and spinach) (147). Several dietary factors are important for proper bone remodeling. Among them is adequate calcium intake, which can be found in the following natural sources:

- Cow's milk, goat's milk, cheese, buttermilk, yogurt, and other dairy products
- Fish, such as salmon with bones, sardines, and other seafood
- Green leafy vegetables, such as asparagus, cabbage, broccoli, and dandelion greens
- Nuts, such as almonds or sesame seeds
- Other food sources, such as brewer's yeast, oats, prunes, figs, kale, and soy protein
- Herbs, such as alfalfa, burdock root, chamomile, chickweed, chicory, dandelion, eyebright, fennel seed, horsetail, kelp, lemon grass, mullein, nettle, oat straw, paprika, parsley, peppermint, plantain, raspberry leaves, red clover, rose hips, shepherd's purse, violet leaves, yarrow, and yellow dock

Vitamin D is required for intestinal absorption and utilization of calcium and phosphorous. Vitamin D from food or supplements must undergo conversion in the liver and then the kidneys before reaching its full activity potential. The following sources of vitamin D are available:

- The skin has the ability to synthesize a vitamin D precursor from cholesterol in the presence of ultraviolet rays (exposing the face and arms to sunlight for 15 minutes three times a week provides an adequate amount of vitamin D).
- Foods that contain vitamin D include fish, such as halibut, sardines, salmon, tuna and fish oil (liver oil, cod liver oil); milk; egg yolks; butter; oatmeal; liver; sweet potatoes; dandelion greens; and vegetable oils.
- Herbs rich in vitamin D are parsley, nettle, horsetail, and alfalfa.

There should be a balanced intake of calcium and phosphorous (low calcium and high phosphorus, for example, may predispose a patient to osteoporosis). Nutritional elements that may interfere with calcium levels include refined sugar, salt, grains, and flours.

Acupuncture

The effects of standardized acupuncture treatment for postmenopausal symptoms, blood pressure, and serum lipoprotein profile have been evaluated in randomized, placebo-controlled clinical trials, and it has been documented that acupuncture transitionally (over a period of 2 months) reduces postmenopausal symptoms. Additionally, no influence on blood pressure or serum lipid profiles has been observed (139). Therefore, acupuncture cannot offer either long-term relief of postmenopausal vasomotor symptoms or prevent cardiovascular disease.

Chiropractic

There is no clinical data that spinal manipulation (chiropractic) techniques are effective in alleviating climacteric symptoms.

Exercise

Exercise is one of the components of life-style that positively influences postmenopausal symptomatology, coronary artery disease (systolic blood pressure, lipoprotein profile, and the vascular endothelial function), and bone mass (stabilized and increased bone mineral component and density). Postmenopausal hormonal ambience changes are more closely related to decreased bone density levels than to life-style factors. Thus, exercise has a more profound effect when combined with estrogen (140). Physical exercise increases levels of muscle strength and bone density; however, the amount of improvement depends on age, race, estrogen use, and commitment to life-style changes (141). It has been observed that only 38% of women over age 19 exercise regularly and that those who initiate exercise have a low compliance rate (142). Therefore, a general lack of interest in exercise may compromise the effect of this form of postmenopausal management. Existing literature supports the overall moderately supportive effect of aerobic exercise (the most natural way to stimulate new bone growth) as a nonpharmacologic approach to increase bone density of the hips in postmenopausal women (143).

Endermologic Therapy

Endermologic therapy is a motorized rhythmic folding-unfolding and suction technique of the panniculus adiposus (the subcutaneous fat) in a 40-minute therapeutic session. It is an emerging complementary approach for premenopausal and postmenopausal women. Preliminary data suggest some benefit, as of yet unspecified, in postmenopausal management (144).

Behavioral Therapy

A paced respiration behavioral treatment for hot flashes in randomized clinical trials has been documented to decrease hot flashes significantly in postmenopausal women. Based on this study, paced respiration training is recommended as a complementary treatment for the reduction of hot flashes in women who cannot take supplemental estrogen (145).

Biofeedback

There is no medical evidence that biofeedback therapy has been used specifically for climacteric symptoms. However, this technique is beneficial for common symptoms such as headaches, hypertension, anxiety, and urinary stress incontinence. Biofeedback may relieve these symptoms in selected patients.

Stress Management

Stress management is an essential part of life-style changes and should be recommended for climacteric women. It is common knowledge that some forms of stress may suppress the immune system and increase blood pressure, epinephrine levels, serum cholesterol levels, platelet aggregation, and vulnerability to disease. Additionally, emotional liability during climacterium makes a postmenopausal woman more susceptible to the negative effects of stress. Through any form of relaxation and meditation, stress, anxiety, heart rate, blood pressure, respiration rate, muscle tone, and even pain can be reduced.

Yoga itself reduces stress through meditation, breathing exercises, and specific posture. Such an approach uses mind-spirit-body balance that in turn decreases blood pressure and heart rate, improves physical conditioning, and reduces overall stress. Yoga usually complements ayurvedic medicine that offers balance through diet, massage, meditation, purging, vomiting, and enemas. With stress reduction, postmenopausal vasomotor symptoms may improve; however, this notion is speculative due to the lack of supporting clinical scientific data.

Medical Massage

Medical massage plays a positive role in relaxation and thus can be used as a form of stress management. It has not been documented that the use of medical massage is beneficial for climacteric symptoms.

T'ai Chi

T'ai chi is a combination of meditation, exercise, improvement of balance , and strength training; it may be helpful in reducing stress, lowering heart rate, lowering blood pressure, and improving body balance (which may reduce falls in the elderly). There are no data to support the use of T'ai chi for climacteric symptoms.

Nutritional Supplements (Nutraceuticals)

Bioflavonoids administered with vitamin C reportedly control vasomotor symptoms (155). A combination of isoflavones and *vitamin C* is recommended in the following formula:

- Hesperidin 900 mg
- Hesperidin methyl chalcone 300 mg
- Vitamin C 1,200 mg

Such a combination may alleviate hot flashes in about 53% of women and decrease their occurrence in about 34% of women. Another simple formula is to administer 1,000 mg of bioflavones and 1,000 to 1,500 mg of vitamin C (147).

Vitamin B6 (pyridoxine) at the daily dose of 50 to 200 mg may reduce insomnia and irritability. However, vitamin B6 at 50 mg daily can be toxic when taken for several months (147).

Vitamin E at the daily dose of 400 to 800 IU has been used for a long time in the nonhormonal management of vasomotor symptoms. Randomized, placebo- controlled, cross-over clinical trials documented that vitamin E significantly reduced hot flashes during the initial stage of the study; however, by the end of the trial, patients did not favor vitamin E over the placebo (155).

Magnesium intake of 600 mg daily is recommended to maintain an adequate ratio of calcium to magnesium (2:1) and to maintain an appropriate magnesium reserve in the bones (magnesium deficiency may decrease trabecular bone). Comprehensive bone-building formulas that incorporate calcium, magnesium, vitamin D, and other minerals and vitamins can be recommended.

Evening primrose oil at the daily dose of 1,500 to 3,000 mg is recommended. Gamma linolenic acid from evening primrose oil has been clinically tested, but the outcome of this study does not support the clinical concept that evening primrose oil is effective in the management of hot flashes (156).

Gamm-oryzanol contains the active substance ferulic acid, which can be found in rice, wheat, barley, oats, tomatoes, asparagus, olives, berries, peas, citrus fruits, and other foods. Results of observational studies involving gamm-oryzanol suggest that 53% to 85% of climacteric symptoms may be reduced with a dose of 300 mg daily (100 mg three times a day) (147).

Natural Alternative Therapy
Herbal Medicine

Herbal phytoestrogens are derivatives of medicinal plants. Edible plants and medicinal plants have a component of phytoestrogens that displays estrogen receptor affinity (antiestrogens) and weak estrogen agonist activity (the strength of phytoestrogens is estimated to be 1/100 to 1/1,000 that of estrogens). It has been postulated that phytoestrogens present antiproliferative effects on the breast and positive effects on serum lipoprotein profile, bone density, and climacteric symptoms (157).

Among the most commonly used herbal phytoestrogens is *red clover (Trifolium praetense)*, which has one of the highest levels of isoflavones (daidzein, genistein, and quercetin glycosides) in its flower head. Red clover is recommended at the standardized extract dose of 40 mg total isoflavones, one tablet daily, or as a dry herb capsule of 500 mg, one capsule daily (147). Red clover is available in tablets (100 mg), capsules (200, 354, 375, and 430 mg), and liquid form (1 or 2 ounces). Red clover is contraindicated for women with estrogen-responsive tumors, and during periods of pregnancy and lactation. There is a known interaction between red clover and aspirin, Coumadin (Du Pont, Wilmington, DE), and oral contraceptives. Red clover is also known as beebread, cow clover, meadow clover, Missouri milk vetch, purple clover, trefoil, and wild clover (158).

Estrogenic activity is associated with fukinolic acid, which is found in *black cohosh* (*Cimicifuga racemosa*) (159). The safety and efficacy of *Cimicifuga racemosa* for climacteric symptoms and vaginal atrophy have been studied, and preliminary data indicate that black cohosh is safe and effective as a therapeutic agent (160–162). Black cohosh effectively relieves climacteric symptoms; however, it does not demonstrate any preventive capacity for diseases associated with hypoestrogenism (coronary artery disease or osteoporosis, etc.) (147). Black cohosh is recommended as a standardized extract in 40-mg caplets, one to two caplets twice a day, or in standardized liquid extract, half to 1 tablespoon twice a day for postmenopausal therapy. It is available in caplets (40, 400, or 420 mg) and capsules (25 or 525 mg). Side effects include gastrointestinal symptoms (nausea or vomiting), lowered blood pressure (causing dizziness), increased uterine contraction (which may lead to miscarriage), and interaction with antihypertensive medications. Black cohosh is also known as black snakeroot, bugbane, bugwort, cimicifuga, rattleroot, rattleweed, and squawroot (158).

Dong quai used alone neither relieves climacteric symptoms significantly nor produces an estrogen-like response in target tissue (the endometrium or the vagina) (163). Still, it has been clinically recommended in combination with other herbs (147) as a phytosynergistic agent in the following formula (164):

Dong quai 750 mg
Capsella bursa-pastoris 625 mg
Paeonia lactiflora 500 mg
Helonias luteum 625 mg

Side effects of dong quai include dizziness or faintness and lowered blood pressure. It may interact with Coumadin (158).

Dong quai is also known as angelica, angelique, angelica root, garden angelica, wild angelica, engelwurzel, the root of holy ghost, tang-quai, and heiligenwurzel.

Ginkgo (*Ginkgo biloba*) is used at the standardized extract capsule dose of 40 to 80 mg, three times a day, or tinctured doses of half to 1 tablespoon, three times a day, to improve perimenopausal/postmenopausal symptoms. *Ginkgo biloba* increases blood circulation to the brain (may improve memory), hands, and feet, and may improve sexual function. No clinical study is available to support these benefits in climacteric women (147). Side effects of ginkgo include gastrointestinal function abnormalities (nausea, vomiting, diarrhea, flatus), headaches, seizures, skin irritation, and bruising. It may interact with aspirin and Coumadin (158). Ginkgo is also known as ginkogink, rokan, sophium, tanakan, tebofortan, and tebonin.

Hyperizine-A (shuaangyiping), like Ginkgo, is recommended for improving memory and concentration during the menopause transition and general symptoms during postmenopause. It is administered in 50-mg tablets or capsules at the dosage of 200 mg twice a day. Preliminary data indicate that this remedy may improve memory and behavioral function more than the placebo, but the available data are inconclusive (165).

Ginseng (*Panax ginseng*) assists in the management of physical and emotional stress, and because of this ability is quite often used in the treatment of postmenopausal symptoms. As of yet, there are not enough scientific clinical data to support its usefulness in reducing postmenopausal symptoms. Ginseng is recommended at the standardized daily dose of 200 mg (147) and is available in capsules (100, 250, and 500 mg), tea bags (containing 1,500 mg ginseng root), root extract (2 ounces in alcohol base), root powder (1 and 4 ounces), oil, and unprocessed root (offered in bulk by the pound). Side effects of ginseng include breast pain, chest pain, headaches, nausea, vomiting, diarrhea, tachycardia, elevated blood pressure, nosebleeds, vaginal bleeding, insomnia, nervousness, skin rash, itching, and impotence. It may interact with antidepressant drugs [monoamine oxidase (MAO) inhibitors such as Marplan and Nordil] and drugs that lower blood sugar (insulin, Amaryl, Diabeta, Diabinese, Glucophage, Glucotrol, Precose, and Rezulin). Because of the possible adverse reactions to ginseng and the lack of clinical scientific evidence, it can only be used for a short time. Ginseng is also known as American ginseng, Chinese ginseng, Asiatic ginseng, Japanese ginseng, Korean ginseng, Oriental ginseng, Western ginseng, schinsent five fingers, g115, jintsam, seng and sang, and tartar root (158).

St. John's wort (*Hypericum perforatum*) has been extensively tested in clinical randomized, placebo-controlled trials, and its antidepressant, antianxiety, and sleep-promoting therapeutic effectiveness have been well established (166). For these particular abilities, it is prescribed for postmenopausal symptoms as a standardized extract at a dosage of 300 mg of 3% hypericin, three times a day (147). Possible side effects include allergic reaction, sensitivity to sunlight, restlessness, insomnia, dizziness, dry mouth, and constipation. It may interact with antidepressants, such as MAO inhibitors (Nordil and Parnate), selective serotonin reuptake inhibitors (Paxil and Prozac), tricyclic antidepressants, and Desyrel . St. John's wort is also known as amber, amber touch and heal, chassediable, weed mellepertuis, rosin rose, and witches' herb (158).

Valerian, with its pharmacologic activity as a sedative and sleeping aid, while not being addictive, is often used in the treatment of irritability, anxiety, epilepsy, and insomnia. Although there are no credible data in existing literature to indicate that valerian is an effective therapeutic regimen for climacteric symptoms, it has been used to help alleviate the anxiety, stress, and sleep dysfunction associated with menopause.

Kava is recommended for the treatment of emotional symptoms associated with climacterium, and anecdotal data suggest that beneficial effects include a feeling of peacefulness and well-being, and a reduction of pain and anxiety. Taking the 60- to 100-mg standardized daily dose is significantly effective in improving vasomotor instability and in decreasing anxiety and stress (167). Fresh kava beverage doses should be between 400 and 900 grams a week, and it is available in the form of tablets, capsules, or extracts. Side effects include visual disturbances, poor judgment, and reduced muscle control. Kava may interact with Xanax, Mebutol, L-dopa, or benzodiazepines, and it should not be used in children under the age of 12, or in women who are pregnant or breast-feeding. Long-term use may cause significant side effects. Kava is also known as ava, awa, kava-kava, kew, sakau, tonga, and yagona (158).

Chamomile has traditionally been used for relaxation. Chamomile acts on certain brain receptors through its active component of apigenin, which causes sedation, and it is usually used as part of a multiherbal composition for the treatment of postmenopausal symptoms (168).

It is available in the form of capsules (354 and 360 mg), liquid, and tea (1 tablespoon of the flower heads in hot water for 10 to 15 minutes, four times a day). Side effects include conjunctivitis, skin irritation, chest tightness, wheezing, hives, itching, rash, and vomiting. This regimen may interact with Coumadin and should be avoided during pregnancy and lactation, and by patients with asthma and allergic dermatitis. It is also known as English, German, Hungarian, and Roman chamomile, as well as sweet false chamomile, true chamomile, and wild chamomile (158).

Damiana (rosemary) is considered to have aphrodisiacal properties, and it has been suggested that this remedy may act as testosterone. For this reason, it is recommended for postmenopausal women as a way to increase libido. However, no clinical evidence supports this potential benefit.

Yohimbine (yohimbe) is also suggested for the management of decreased libido in postmenopausal women. Clinical scientific data to support this claim are available only from studies conducted on men. Yohimbine is available in 3-mg and 5.4-mg tablets, which should be taken twice a day. Side effects with a dose of 20 to 30 mg a day include tachycardia and elevated blood pressure.

Yohimbe may interact with antidepressants (Prozac, Norpramin, or Tofranil), stimulant products (caffeine), or medication containing phenylephedrine or phenylpropanolamine (158).

Herbal combinations containing phytoestrogens can be offered to a symptomatic postmenopausal patient at an identifiably low risk for coronary artery disease and osteoporosis.

Natural progesterone cream ($^1/_4$ to $^1/_2$ tablespoon twice a day, 3 weeks on and 1 week off) also can be given (147). There are no published scientific data to substantiate such an anecdotal clinical approach.

Natural Hormone Replacement Therapy

There is a natural hormone derived from plants that matches the original human hormone in both molecular structure and biologic activity. Natural hormone replacement (NHR) therapy is based on the same clinical concept as conventional HRT, but it offers natural hormones instead of synthetic substances.

Natural hormone replacement therapy is offered in three different formulas. The single-estrogen formulation of oral micronized natural estradiol is given at a daily dose of 1–2 mg (unopposed by progesterone) when indicated (for hysterectomized women) or in combination with micronized natural progesterone (at a daily dose of 100 mg continuously), if endometrial bleeding is not desired by a patient. The cyclic mode consists of 200 mg micronized natural progesterone once a day for 12 days a month (147). This mode of therapy appeared to improve not only climacteric symptoms but also lipoprotein profiles with minimal side effects and the presence of amenorrhea without endometrial proliferation or hyperplasia (169). In addition, the bone density improvement with this mode of therapy is comparable to that of conjugated equine estrogens and medroxyprogesterone combinations (170,171).

The bi-estrogen formulation is one of the most common prescribed forms of postmenopausal NHR therapy. It is made up of the following combination of natural estrogens and natural progesterone:

Estriol 1 mg
Estradiol 0.250 mg
Micronized natural progesterone 40 mg

These compound natural hormones are administered orally, one capsule twice a day (147).

The tri-estrogen formulation is a compound prescription:

Estriol 1 mg
Estradiol 0.125 mg
Estrone 0.125 mg
Micronized natural progesterone 40 mg

Because estrone may exhibit possible negative effects on breast tissue and estrone metabolites may produce undesirable side effects, this formulation is less desirable than single or bi-estrogen formulations. All these formulations are made up of a standard dose of conjugated equivalent estrogen and 2.5 mg of medroxyprogesterone (Provera) (147).

Natural Progesterone Therapy

Micronized natural progesterone alone is effective in opposing estrogen (prevents endometrial hyperplasia) and has a positive influence on serum lipoprotein profiles (61,172), but it is ineffective in the prevention of bone loss (173).

Natural progesterone cream (approximately 400 mg per ounce) is usually applied to the inner arms, palms, chest, inner thighs, or under the breast; doses vary (147):

- In the menopause transition from days 8 to 21 of a menstrual cycle, ¼ tablespoon twice a day, or from days 22 to 28 of a menstrual cycle, ½ tablespoon twice a day. Progesterone cream should not be used during menses.
- In the postmenopausal period, from day 8 to the end of each month at the dosage of ¼ tablespoon once or twice a day (147).

Recently, a randomized clinical study revealed significant improvement in vasomotor symptoms in patients using transdermal progesterone cream; however, no protective effect on bone density was established (174).

Oral and transvaginal progesterone administration and doses were discussed earlier in this chapter.

Natural Androgens

Natural androgens are prescribed for improving sexual function or enhancing NHR therapy in postmenopausal women. *Nonmethylated testosterone* is incorporated into NHR therapy in the form of 0.5-mg to 1-mg capsules taken twice a day. Oral natural testosterone can be combined with estrogen/progesterone formulations or taken separately. *Testosterone cream* 0.5%, 1%, or 2% can be applied to the vulva twice a day.

Dehydroepiandrosterone is indicated for symptoms such as sexual dysfunction, fatigue, or loss of a general sense of well-being (associated with low serum DHEA levels). The usual recommended daily dose of DHEA is 5 to 25 mg (147).

There is a lack of sufficient scientific clinical data on the safety and efficacy of natural androgens for the treatment of climacteric symptoms and their preventive effects.

Homeopathy

Homeopathic therapy is based on specific symptoms in a patient's detailed history and on personal characteristics. A homeopathic practitioner may recommend different diluted remedies to match both the symptoms associated with climacterium and those of personality. The prescribing medicine philosophy ("*similia similibus curantur*," which means "like cures like," called the Law of Similar) differs between a homeopathic and allopathic practitioner in that a remedy matches individual characteristics and symptoms in the former while the latter uses a remedy that opposes a patient's symptoms. It is a homeopathic conviction that high concentrations of a substance may induce symptoms of the disease, whereas the same substance in a highly diluted solution may treat the disease. Still, the precise mechanism must be elucidated.

The following remedies are recommended for the given diseases(175):

- Hot flashes
  Lachesis (surucucu, bushmaster) is prepared from the venom of a *Lachesis muta* snake, and is administered in dilution from 9 to 30 mL once a day. It is recommended for the postmenopausal symptom of hot flashes accompanied by cold extremities.
  Sepia is made from the pigment fluid of the cuttlefish and is offered in the diluted dose of 15 to 30 mL with one to three times a week. Usually it is prescribed for vasomotor symptoms causing lowered body temperature during the day, increased body temperature at night, or night sweats accompanied by chills that may lead to sleep disorders.
  Sulphur is administered in daily alternation with Lachesis in a diluted dose of 15 mL, each in the form of granules. Sulphur is used for the sensation of warmth that may lead to excessive perspiration.
  Sanguinaria (blood root) is prepared from the fresh root of *Sanguinaria canadenis,* and it is given in combination with lachesis and sulphur in a diluted dose of 15 mL, up to five granules daily. Usually, it is prescribed for vasomotor instability and headaches.
  Glonoinum is made from nitroglycerine and is taken in 5 to 9 cH one to two times a day.
  Folliculinum in a diluted dose of 5 or 9 mL once a day may decrease the secretion of FSH.
  Phosphorous is prepared from bone ash, and it is recommended at a daily diluted dose of 15 to 30 mL. It is indicated for vasomotor symptoms, such as heart palpitation, dizziness, and anxiety.
- Headaches
  Sanguinaria at the dose presented above
  Cyclamen in a diluted dose of 30 mL once a day or as seldom as once a week
  Melilotus in a diluted dose of 5 mL once to twice a day
- Heart palpitation
  Aurum metallicum in a diluted dose of 5 or 9 mL once to twice a day
  Strontium carbonicum in a diluted dose of 9 mL twice a day
- Bone joint pain
  Kalium carbonicum in a diluted dose of 5 to 30 mL, three granules one to three time a day

Natrium sulfuricum in a diluted dose of 15 or 30 mL, five granules daily or every 8 days as needed

■ Vaginal dryness

Lycopodium in a diluted dose of 15 mL, five granules every other night

Natrium muriaticum in a diluted dose of 15 mL, five granules every other night

Folliculinum in a diluted dose of 7 mL, five granules every other night

Bryonia alba is prepared from either the *Bryonia alba* or the *Bryonia diocia* plant and is taken in a diluted dose of 15 mL once or twice a day

■ Emotional symptoms

Pulsatilla (wind flower) is prepared from the entire fresh plant of *Pulsatilla nigricans* and is administered in a daily diluted dose of 15 mL, five granules. This remedy is offered for vasomotor symptoms associated with stress and anxiety.

Lachesis in a daily diluted dose of 15 or 30 mL

Sepia in a daily diluted dose of 15 or 30 mL

Lilium tigritum in a daily diluted dose of 15 or 30 mL

It is recommended that each homeopathic remedy be taken 30 minutes to 1 hour before any food or drink consumption, and that nothing be ingested for 1 hour afterward. The therapy is discontinued upon reaching a symptom-free state. Relief from symptoms is expected within a few days, and treatment may last up to 8 weeks. If expected results are not achieved, an experienced homeopathic practitioner should reevaluate the case.

Feminon N is a multihomeopathic formula for postmenopausal symptoms that reduces FSH significantly (this formula is used in Europe) (176).

There are no credible scientific clinical data to support these traditional approaches in the management of climacterium. Nevertheless, a meta-analysis of placebo-controlled clinical trials documented that homeopathy in general is an effective form of therapy when compared with a placebo; however, there is insufficient evidence that homeopathy is clearly efficacious for any single clinical condition. In addition, methodologic shortcomings and inconsistencies of analyzed clinical studies have resulted in a lack of convincing evidence (177,178).

REFERENCES

1. Association of Professors of Gynecology and Obstetrics. *Medical student educational objectives,* 7th ed. Washington, DC: Association of Professors of Gynecology and Obstetrics, 1997.
2. Council on Resident and Gynecology (CREOG). *Educational objectives core curriculum for residents in obstetrics and gynecology,* 4th ed. Washington, DC: CREOG, 1992.
3. American College of Obstetricians and Gynecologists (ACOG). Technical bulletin No. 247. Washington, DC: ACOG, 1998.
4. American College of Obstetricians and Gynecologists (ACOG). Committee opinion No. 226. Washington, DC: ACOG, 1999.
5. American College of Obstetricians and Gynecologists (ACOG). Committee opinion No. 126. Washington, DC: ACOG, 1993.
6. Beckman CRB, Ling WNP, Herbert WP, et al. *Obstetrics and gynecology,* 3rd ed. Baltimore: Williams & Wilkins, 1998: 430–435, 449–460.
7. Greendale GA, Lee NP, Arriola ER. The menopause. *Lancet* 1999;353:571–580.
8. Johnson SR. Menopause and hormone replacement therapy. *Med Clin North Am* 1998;82:297–320.
9. Kothari S, Thacker HL. Risk assessment of the menopause patient. *Med Clin North Am* 1999;83:1489–1502.
10. McKinlay SM, Brambilla PJ, Posner JG. The normal menopause transition. *Maturitas* 1992;14:103–115.
11. Treloar AE, Bonton RE, Behn BG, et al. Variation of the human menstrual cycle through reproductive life. *Int J Fertil* 1967; 12:77–126.
12. Sherman BM, West JM, Korenman SC. The menstrual transition: analysis of LH, FSH, estradiol and progesterone concentration during menstrual cycles of older women. *J Clin Endocrinol Metab* 1976;42:629–636.
13. Burger HG. Diagnostic role of follicle stimulating hormone (FSH) measurements during the menopause transition—an analysis of FSH, oestradiol and inhibin. *Eur J Endocrinol* 1994;130:38–42.
14. Greendale GA, Sowers MF. The menopause transition. *Endocrinol Metab Clin North Am* 1997;26:261–277.
15. MacMahon B, Worcester J. Age at menopause: United States 1960–1962. *US Vital Statistics II* 1966;19:1–19.
16. Richards MA, O'Reilly SM, Howell A, et al. Adjuvant cyclophosphamide, methotrexate, and fluorouracil in patients with axillary node–positive breast cancer: an update of the Guy's/Manchester trial. *J Clin Oncol* 1990;12:2032–2039.
17. Voda AM, Climacteric hot flashes. *Maturitas* 1981;3:73–90.
18. Tulandi T, Samarthji L. Menopausal hot flush. *Obstet Gynecol Surv* 1985;40:553–563.
19. Stone SC, Mickal A, Rye PH. Postmenopausal symptomatology, maturation index, and plasma estrogen levels. *Obstet Gynecol* 1975;45:625–627.
20. Fantel JA, Cardozo L, McClish DK. Estrogen therapy in the management of urinary incontinence in postmenopausal women: a meta-analysis. *Obstet Gynecol* 1994;83:12–18.
21. Greendale GA, Hogen P, Shumaker S. Sexual function in postmenopausal women: the postmenopausal estrogen/progestin interventions trial. *J Womens Health* 1996;5:445–458.
22. Osborn M, Hawton K, Gath D. Sexual dysfunction among middle age women in community. *BMJ* 1988;296:259–256.
23. Rekers H, Drogendijk AC, Valkenburg HA, et al. The menopause, urinary incontinence and other symptoms of the genitourinary tract. *Maturitas* 1992;15:101–111.
24. Stone AB, Pearlstein TB. Evaluation and treatment of changes in mood, sleep, and sexual functioning associated with menopause. *Obstet Gynecol Clin North Am* 1994;21:391–403.
25. Avis NE, Bambilla D, McKinlay SM, et al. A longitudinal analysis of the association between menopause and depression: results from Massachusetts Women's Health Study. *Ann Epidemiol* 1994;4:214–220.
26. Moore AA, Noonan MD. A nurse's guide to hormone replacement therapy. *J Obstet Gynecol Neonatal Nurs* 1996;25:24–31.
27. Kao KY, Hitt WE, McGavack TH. Effect of estradiol benzoate upon collagen synthesis by sponge biopsy connective tissue. *Proc Soc Exp Biol Med* 1965;119:364–369.
28. McNagny SE. Prescribing hormone replacement therapy for menopausal symptoms. *Ann Intern Med* 1999;131:605–616.
29. Krauss CM, Turksoy RN, Atkins L, et al. Familial premature

ovarian failure due to an interstitial deletion of the long arm of the X chromosome. *N Engl J Med* 1987;317:125–131.

30. Veneman TF, Beverstock GC, Exalto N, et al. Premature menopause because of inherited deletion in the long arm of the X-chromosome. *Fertil Steril* 1991;55:631–633.

31. Davison RM, Quilter CR, Webb J, et al. A familial case of X-chromosome deletion ascertained by cytogenetic screening of women with premature ovarian failure. *Hum Reprod* 1998;13; 3039–3041.

32. Christin-Maitre S, Bouchard P. Genes and ovarian insufficiency. *Ann Endocrinol (Paris)* 1999;60:118–122.

33. Wheatcroft NJ, Salt C, Milford-Ward A, et al. Identification of ovarian antibodies by immunofluorescence, enzyme-linked immunosorbent assay or immunoblotting in premature ovarian failure. *Hum Reprod* 1997;12:2617–2622.

34. Weetman AP. Autoimmunity and endocrinology. *Exp Clin Endocrinol Diabetes* 1999;107(suppl 3):63–66.

35. Kasperlik-Zaluska AA, Czarnocka B, Czech W, et al. Secondary adrenal insufficiency associated with autoimmune disorders: a report of twenty-five cases. *Clin Endocrinol (Oxf)* 1998;49: 779–783.

36. Biscotti CV, Hart WR, Lucas JG. Cystic ovarian enlargement resulting from autoimmune oophoritis. *Obstet Gynecol* 1989; 74;492–495.

37. Lonsdale RN, Roberts PF, Trowell JE. Autoimmune oophoritis associated with polycystic ovaries. *Histopathology* 1991;19:77–81.

38. Kalantaridou SN, Braddock DT, Patronas NJ, et al. Treatment of autoimmune premature ovarian failure. *Hum Reprod* 1999; 14:1777–1782.

39. Morrison JC, Givens JR, Wiser WL, et al. Mumps oophoritis: a cause of premature menopause. *Fertil Steril* 1975;26:655–659.

40. Cramer DW, Welch WR, Cassells S, et al. Mumps, menarche, menopause, and ovarian cancer. *Am J Obstet Gynecol* 1983;147: 1–6.

41. Taparelli F, Squadrini F, De Rienzo B, et al. Isolation of mumps virus from vaginal secretion in association with oophoritis. *J Infect* 1988;17:255–258.

42. Saardharwalla IB, Wraith JE. Galactosaemia. *Nutr Health* 1987; 5:175–188.

43. Beauvais P, Guilhaume A. Ovarian insufficiency in congenital galactosemia. *Presse Med* 1984;13:2685–2687.

44. Kaufman FR, Donnell GN, Roe TF, et al. Gonadal function in patients with galactosemia. *J Inherit Metab Dis* 1986;9: 140–146.

45. Ostrzenski A. A new, laparoscopic full-thickness slice ovarian biopsy (from antimesenteric to mesenteric margin). *J Gynecol Surg* 1995;11:109–112.

46. Johnson SR. The clinical decision regarding hormone replacement therapy. *Endocrinol Metab Clin North Am* 1997;26: 413–435.

47. American College of Obstetricians and Gynecologists (ACOG). Criteria Set, Committee on Quality Assessment, No. 23, Washington, DC, 1997.

48. Creasman WT. Recommendations regarding estrogen replacement therapy after treatment of endometrial cancer. *Oncology* 1992;6:23–26.

49. Franceshi S, Baron AE, La Vecchia C. The influence of female hormones on malignant melanoma. *Tumori* 1990;76:439–449.

50. Lip GY, Beevers M, Churchill D, et al. Hormonal replacement therapy and blood pressure in hypertensive women. *J Hum Hypertens* 1994;8:491–494.

51. Paganini-Hill A. Estrogen replacement therapy and stroke. *Prog Cardiovasc Dis* 1995;38:223–242.

52. Persson I, Yuen J, Bergkvist L, et al. Cancer incidence and mortality in women receiving estrogen and estrogen-progestin ther-

apy—long term follow-up of a Swedish cohort. *Int J Cancer* 1996;67:327–332.

53. Brett KM, Madans JH. Use of postmenopausal hormone replacement therapy: estimates from a nationally representative cohort study. *Am J Epidemiol* 1997;145:536–545.

54. Persson I, Bergkvist L, Lindgren C, et al. Hormone replacement therapy and major risk factors for reproductive cancer, osteoporosis, and cardiovascular diseases: evidence of confounding by exposure characteristics. *J Clin Epidemiol* 1997;50:611–618.

55. Greendale GA, Judd HL. The menopause: health implications and clinical management. *J Am Geriatr Soc* 1993;41: 426–436.

56. Daly E, Vessey MP, Barlow D. Hormone replacement therapy in a risk-benefit perspective. *Maturitas* 1996;23:247–259.

57. Cummings SR, Black DM, Thompson DE. Effect of alendronate on risk of fracture in women with low bone density but without vertebral fractures. *JAMA* 1998;280:2077–2082.

58. Naessen T, Bergund L, Ulsten U. Bone loss in elderly women prevented by ultralow doses of parenteral 17-beta-estradiol. *Am J Obstet Gynecol* 1997;177:115–119.

59. Thacker HL. Women's hormonal health issues: menopause, hormone replacement therapy, and hormonal contraceptive. In: Stoller, Ahmad, Longworth, eds. *The Cleveland Clinic intensive review of internal medicine.* Baltimore: Williams & Wilkins, 1998:13–26.

60. Cushing KL, Weiss NS, Voigt LF, et al. Risk of endometrial cancer in relation to use of low-dose, unopposed estrogens. *Obstet Gynecol* 1998;91:35–39.

61. Effects of estrogen or estrogen/progestin regimens on heart diseases risk factors in postmenopausal women. The postmenopausal estrogen/progestin interventions (PEPI) Trial. The Writing Group for the PEPI Trial. *JAMA* 1995;273:199–208.

62. Wrren MP, Shantha S. Uses of progesterone in clinical practice. *Int J Fertil Womens Med* 1999;44:96–103.

63. Kim S, Korhonen M, Wilborn W, et al. Anti-proliferative effects of low-dose micronized progesterone. *Fertil Steril* 1996; 65:323–331.

64. Waren BG, McFarland K, Edwards L. Micronized transdermal progesterone and endometrial response. *Lancet* 1999;354: 1447–1448.

65. Fanchin R, De Ziegler D, Bergeron C, et al. Transvaginal administration of progesterone. *Obstet Gynecol* 1997;90:396–401.

66. Levy T, Gurevitch S, Bar-Hava I, et al. Pharmocokinetics of natural progesterone administered in the form of a vaginal tablet. *Hum Reprod* 1999;14:606–610.

67. Cicinelli E, Cignarelli M, Resta L, et al. Effect of the repetitive administration of progesterone by nasal spray in postmenopausal women. *Fertil Steril* 1993;60:1020–1024.

68. Suhonen S, Holmstrom T, Lahteenmaki P. Three-year follow-up of the use of a levonorgestrel-releasing intrauterine system in hormone replacement therapy. *Acta Obstet Gynecol Scand* 1997; 76:145–150.

69. Suvato-Luukkonen E, Kauppiala A. The levonorgestrel-releasing intrauterine system in menopausal hormone replacement therapy: five-year experience. *Fertil Steril* 1999;72:161–163.

70. Raudaskoski TJ, Lahti EI, Kauppiala AJ, et al. Transdermal estrogen with a levonorgestrel-releasing intrauterine device for climacteric compliance. Clinical and endometrial responses. *Am J Obstet Gynecol* 1995;172:114–119.

71. Speroff L, Rowan J, Sympsons J, et al. The comparative effect on bone density, endometrium, and lipids of continuous hormones as replacement therapy (CHART study). A randomised controlled trial. *JAMA* 1996;276:1397–1403.

72. Woodruff JD, Picker JH. Incidence endometrial hyperplasia in postmenopausal women taking conjugated estrogens (Pre-

marin) with medroxyprogesterone acetate. *Am J Obstet Gynecol* 1994;170:1213–1223.

73. Ross D, Cooper AJ, Pryse-Davise J, et al. Randomized, double-blind, dose-ranging study of the endometrial effects of a vaginal progesterone gel in estrogen-treated postmenopausal women. *Am J Obstet Gynecol* 1997;177:937–941.

74. Wypych K, Spiewankiewich B, Sawicki W. Evaluation of endometrial changes in women with cyclical mastalgia. *Ginecol Pol* 1995;66:451–456.

75. Pickar JH, Archer DF. Is bleeding a predictor of endometrial hyperplasia in postmenopausal women receiving hormone replacement therapy? Menopause Study Group (United States, Italy, Netherlands, Switzerland, Belgium, Germany, and Finland). *Am J Obstet Gynecol* 1997;177:1178–1183.

76. Spencer CP, Cooper AJ, Whitehead MI. Management of abnormal bleeding in women receiving hormone replacement therapy. *BMJ* 1997;315:37–42.

77. Holbert TR. Transvaginal ultrasonographic measurement of endometrial thickness in postmenopausal women receiving estrogen replacement therapy. *Am J Obstet Gynecol* 1997;176:1334–1338.

78. Ballester MJ, Serra V, Raga F, et al. The effect of hormone replacement therapy on uterine arterial blood flow in postmenopausal women. *J Ultrasound Med* 1995;14:497–501.

79. Langer RD, Pierce JJ, O'Hanlan KA. Transvaginal ultrasonography compared with endometrial biopsy for detection of endometrial disease. *N Engl J Med* 1997;337:1792–1798.

80. Gillet JY, Andre G, Faguer B, et al. Induction of amenorrhea during hormone therapy: optimal micronized progesterone dose. *Maturitas* 1994;19:103–115.

81. Nand SL, Webster MA, Baber R, et al. Bleeding pattern and endometrial changes during continuous combined hormone replacement therapy. The Ogen/Provera Study Group. *Obstet Gynecol* 1998;91(part 1):678–684.

82. American College of Obstetrician and Gynecologists (ACOG). Technical Bulletin No. 166. Washington, DC: ACOG, 1992.

83. Labrie F, Belanger A, Cusan L, et al. Marked declined in serum concentrations of adrenal C19 sex steroid precursors and conjugated androgen metabolites during aging. *J Clin Endocrinol Metab* 1997;82:2396–2402.

84. Devaprabu A, Carpenter P. Issues concerning androgen replacement therapy in postmenopausal women. *Mayo Clin Proc* 1997;72:1051–1055.

85. Judd HL, Lucas WE, Yen SS. Effect of oophorectomy on circulating testosterone and androstenedione levels in patients with endometrial cancer. *Am J Obstet Gynecol* 1974;118:793–798.

86. Zumoff B, Strain GW, Miller LK, et al. Twenty-four-hour, mean plasma testosterone concentration declines with age in normal postmenopausal women. *J Clin Endocrinol Metab* 1995;80:1429–1430.

87. Hoeger KM, Guzick DS. The use of androgens in menopause. *Clin Obstet Gynecol* 1999;42:883–894.

88. McCoy NL, Davidson JM. A longitudinal study of the effects of menopausal on sexuality. *Maturitas* 1985;7:203–210.

89. Sherwin BB, Gelfand MM. The role of androgen in the maintenance of sexual functioning in oophorectomied women. *Psychosomatic Med* 1987;49:397–409.

90. Myers LS, Dixon J, Morrissette D, et al. Effects of estrogen, androgen, and progestin on sexual psychophysiology and behavior in postmenopausal women. *J Clin Endocrinol Metab* 1990;70:1124–1131.

91. Dennerstein L, Dudley EC, Hopper JL, et al. Sexuality, hormones, and the menopause transition. *Maturitas* 1997;26:833–893.

92. Watts NB, Morris N, Timmons MC, et al. Comparison of oral estrogens plus androgen on bone mineral density, menopausal

symptoms, and lipid-lipoprotein profiles in surgical menopause. *Obstet Gynecol* 1995;85:529–537.

93. Hicckok LR, Toomey C, Spiroff L. A comparison of esterified estrogens with and without methyltestosterone: effects on endometrial histology and serum lipoproteins in postmenopausal women. *Obstet Gynecol* 1993;82:919–924.

94. Simon JA, Kaiber E, Witta B, et al. Double-blind comparison of estrogen-androgen combination and estrogen therapy in menopausal women. Effects on symptoms and neuroendocrine parameters. *Fertil Steril* 1996;66(suppl):71.

95. Morales AJ, Nolan JJ, Nelson JC, et al. Effects of replacement dose of dehydroepiandrosterone in men and women of advancing age. *J Clin Endocrinol Metab* 1994;78:1360–1367.

96. Raisz LG, Witta B, Arttis A, et al. Comparison of the effects of estrogen alone and estrogen plus androgen on biochemical markers of bone formation and resorption in postmenopausal women. *J Clin Endocrinol Metab* 1996;81:37–43.

97. Davis SR, McCloud P, Strauss BJG, et al. Testosterone enhances estradiol's effects on postmenopausal bone density and sexuality. *Maturitas* 1995;21:227–236.

98. Erdtsieck RJ, Pols HAB, Van Kuijk C, et al. Course of bone mass during and after hormonal replacement therapy with and without addition of nandrolone decanoate. *J Bone Miner Res* 1994;9:277–283.

99. Morales AJ, Haubrich RH, Hwang JY, et al. The effect of 6-months treatment with a 100 mg daily dose of DHEA on circulating sex steroids, body composition, and muscle strength in age-advanced men and women. *Clin Endocrinol* 1998;49:421–432.

100. Labrie F, Dimond P, Cusan L, et al. Effect of 12 months Dehydroepiandrosterone replacement therapy on bone, vagina, and endometrium in postmenopausal women. *Clin Endocrinol Metab* 1997;82:3498–3505.

101. Kuhn FE, Rackley CE. Coronary artery disease in women. Risk factors, evaluation, treatment, and prevention. *Arch Intern Med* 1993;153:2626–2636.

102. Ginsberg HN. Lipoprotein metabolism and its relationship to atherosclerosis. *Med Clin North Am* 1994;78:1–20.

103. O'Brien KD, Chait A. The biology of the artery wall in atherosclerosis. *Med Clin North Am* 1994;78:41–67.

104. Barret-Connor E, Timmons C, Young R, et al., and the Estratest Working Group. Interim safety analysis of a 2-year study comparing oral estrogen-androgen and conjugated estrogens in surgically menopausal women. *J Women Health* 1996;5:593–602.

105. Gelfand MM. Role of androgens in surgical menopause. *Am J Obstet Gynecol* 1999;180:325–327.

106. World Health Organization. Assessment of fracture risk and its application to screening for postmenopausal osteoporosis. *World Health Organ Tech Rep Ser* 1994;843:1–129.

107. Dempster DW, Lindsay R. Pathogenesis of osteoporosis. *Lancet* 1993;341:797–801.

108. Ziegler R. Osteoporosis will never be a disease of the past. *Osteoporosis Int* 1994;4(suppl):3–4.

109. Slemenda CW, Turner CH, Peacock M, et al. The genetics of proximal femur geometry, distribution of bone mass and bone mineral density. *Osteoporosis Int* 1996;6:178–182.

110. Ravn P, Hetland ML, Overgaard K, et al. Premenopausal and postmenopausal changes in bone mineral density of the proximal femur measured by dual-energy X-ray absorptiometry. *J Bone Miner Res* 1994;9:1975–1980.

111. Riggs BL, Melton LJ III. Involutional osteoporosis. *N Engl J Med* 1986;314:1676–1686.

112. Hurley DL, Khosla S. Subspecialty clinics: endocrinology, metabolism, and nutrition. Update on primary osteoporosis. *Mayo Clin Proc* 1997;72:943–949.

113. Ledger GA, Burritt MF, Kao PC, et al. Role of parathyroid hor-

mone in mediating nocturnal and age related increases in bone resorption. *J Clin Endocrinol Metab* 1995;80:3304–3310.

114. Epstein S, Bryce G, Hinman JW, et al. The influence of age on bone mineral regulating hormones. *Bone* 1986;7:421–426.

115. Eastell R, Yergey AL, Vieira NE, et al. Interrelationship among vitamin D metabolism, true calcium absorption, parathyroid function, and age in women: evidence of an age-related intestinal resistance to 1,25-dihydroxyvitamin D action. *J Bone Miner Res* 1991;6:125–132.

116. Heaney RP, Recker RR, Saville PD. Menopausal changes in calcium balance performance. *J Lab Clin Med* 1978;92:953–963.

117. MacKane WR, Khosla S, Risteli J, et al. Role of estrogen deficiency in pathogenesis of secondary hyperparathyroidism and increased bone resorption in elderly women. *Proc Assoc Am Physicians* 1997;109:174–180.

118. MacKane WR, Khosla S, Burritt MF, et al. Mechanism of renal calcium conservation with estrogen replacement therapy in women in early postmenopause—a clinical research center study. *J Clin Endocrinol Metab* 1995;80:3458–3464.

119. Gennari C, Agnusdei D, Nardi P, et al. Estrogen preserves a normal intestinal responsiveness to 1,25-hydroxyvitamin D in oophorectomized women. *J Clin Endocrinol Metab* 1990;71:1288–1293.

120. Khosla S, Riggs BL, Melton LJ III. Clinical spectrum. In: Riggs BL, Melton LJ III, eds. *Osteoporosis: etiology, diagnosis, and management,* 2nd ed. Philadelphia: Lippincott-Raven, 1995:205–223.

121. Pejovic T, Olive DL. Contemporary use of bone densitometry. *Clin Obstet Gynecol* 1999;42:876–882.

122. Cummings SR, Black DM, Nevitt MC. Bone density at various sites for prediction of hip fracture. *Lancet* 1993;341:72–75.

123. Boshong SC. *Radiologic science for technologists: physics, biology and protection,* 4th ed. St. Louis: CV Mosby, 1988.

124. Johnston CC Jr, Melton LJ III, Lindsay R, et al. Clinical indications for bone mass measurement. *J Bone Miner Res* 1989;4(suppl 2):1–28.

125. Grady D, Rubin SM, Petitti DB, et al. Hormone therapy to prevent disease and prolong life in postmenopausal women. *Ann Intern Med* 1992;117:1016–1037.

126. Hulley S, Grady D, Bush T, et al. Randomized trial of estrogen plus progestin for secondary prevention of coronary heart disease in postmenopausal women. Heart and Estrogen/Progestin Replacement Study (HERS) Research Group. *JAMA* 1998;280:605–613.

127. Yaffe K, Sawaya G, Lieberburg I, et al. Estrogen therapy in postmenopausal women: effect on cognitive function and dementia. *JAMA* 1998;279:688–695.

128. Tang MX, Jacobs D, Stern Y, et al. Effect of oestrogen during menopause on risk and age at onset of Alzheimer's disease. *Lancet* 1996;348:429–432.

129. Sherwin BB. Hormones, mood, and cognitive functioning in postmenopausal women. *Obstet Gynecol* 1996;87(suppl):20–26.

130. Optimal calcium intake (consensus conference). *JAMA* 1994;272:1942–1948.

131. Matkovic V, Jellic T, Wardlaw GM, et al. Timing of peak bone mass in caucasian females and its implication for the prevention of osteoporosis. *J Clin Invest* 1994;93:799–808.

132. Chapuy MC, Arlot ME, Duboeuf F, et al. Vit D₃ and calcium to prevent hip fractures in elderly women. *N Engl J Med* 1992;327:1637–1642.

133. National Osteoporosis Foundation. *Physician guide to prevention and treatment of osteoporosis.* Washington, DC: National Osteoporosis Foundation, 1998.

134. Roe B, Chiu KM, Arnaud CD. Selective estrogen receptor modulators and postmenopausal health. *Adv Intern Med* 2000;45:259–278.

135. Agnusdei D, Liu-Leage S, Augendre-Ferrante B. Results of international clinical trials with raloxifene. *Ann Endocrinol (Paris)* 1999;60:242–246.

136. Burckhardt P. Selective estrogen receptor modulators (SERM): new substances for hormone replacement therapy. *Schweiz Med Wochenschr* 1999;129:1926–1930.

137. Umland EM, Rinaldi C, Parks SM, et al. The impact of estrogen replacement therapy and raloxifene on osteoporosis, cardiovascular disease, and gynaecologic cancer. *Ann Pharmacother* 1999;33:1315–1328.

138. American College of Obstetricians and Gynecologists (ACOG). Technical Bulletin No. 192. Washington, DC: ACOG, 1994.

139. Kraft K, Coulon S. Effect of a standardized acupuncture treatment on complaints, blood pressure and serum lipids of hypertensive, postmenopausal women. A randomised, controlled clinical study. *Forsch Komlementarmed* 1999;6:74–79.

140. Landin-Wilhelmsen K, Wilhelmsen L, Bengtsson BA. Postmenopausal osteoporosis is more related to hormonal aberrations than to lifestyle factors. *Prev Med* 1998;27:789–807.

141. Chumalea WC, Guo SS. Body mass and bone mineral quality. *Curr Opin Rheumatol* 1999;11:307–311.

142. Burghardt M. Exercise at menopause: critical differences. *Medscape Womens Health* 1999;4:1.

143. Kelly GA. Aerobic exercise and bone density at hip in postmenopausal women: a meta-analysis. *Prev Med* 1998;27:798–807.

144. Benelli L, Berta JL, Cannistra C, et al. Endermologie: humoral repercussions and estrogen interaction. *Aesthetic Plast Surg* 1999;23:312–315.

145. Freedman RR, Woodward S. Behavioral treatment of menopausal hot flashes: evaluation by ambulatory monitoring. *Am J Obstet Gynecol* 1992;167:436–439.

146. Vihtamaki T, Savilahti R, Tuimala R. Why do postmenopausal women discontinue hormone replacement therapy? *Maturitas* 1999;33:99–105.

147. Hudson T. Women's encyclopedia of natural medicine. Los Angeles: Keats Publishing, 1999:135–216.

148. Murkies A, Wilcox G, Davis S. Phytoestrogens. *J Clin Endocrinol Metab* 1998;83:297–303.

149. Knight DC, Eden JA. A review of the clinical effects of phytoestrogens. *Obstet Gynecol* 1996;87:897–904.

150. Albertazzi P, Pansini F, Bonaccorsi G, et al. The effect of dietary supplementation on hot flashes. *Obstet Gynecol* 1998;91:6–11.

151. Anderson JW, Johnstone BM, Cook-Newell ME. Meta-analysis of the effects of soy protein on serum lipids. *N Engl J Med* 1995;333:276–282.

152. Hodgson JM, Puddey IB, Beilin LJ, et al. Supplementation with isoflavonoid phytoestrogens does not alter serum lipid concentration: a randomised controlled trial in humans. *J Nutr* 1998;128:728–732.

153. Kris-Etherton P, Krummel D. Role of nutrition in the prevention and treatment of coronary artery disease in women. *J Am Diet Assoc* 1993;93:987–993.

154. Robertson J, Brydon W, Tadesse K. The effect of raw carrot on serum lipids and colon function. *Am J Clin Nutr* 1979;32:1889–1892.

155. Barton DL, Loprinzi CL, Quella SK, et al. Prospective evaluation of vitamin E for hot flashes in breast cancer survivors. *J Clin Oncol* 1998;16:495–500.

156. Chenoy R, Hussain S, Tayob Y, et al. Effect of oral gamma linolenic acid from evening primrose oil on menopausal flushing. *BMJ* 1994;308:503–506.

157. Brzezinski A, Debi A. Phytoestrogens: the "natural" selective estrogen receptor modulators? *Eur J Obstet Gynecol Reprod Biol* 1999;85:47–51.

158. Fetrow JR, Avila CW. *The complete guide to herbal medicines.* Springhouse, PA: Springhouse Corporation, 1999:61, 176–177, 212–215, 411–412.

159. Kruse SO, Lonhning A, Pauli GF, et al. Fukiic and piscidic acid esters from the rhizome of *Cimicifuga racemosa* and the *in vitro* estrogenic activity of fukinolic acid. *Planta Med* 1999;65:763-764.

160. Stoll W. Phytopharmacon influences atrophic vaginal epithelium. Double-blind study—Cimicifuga av estrogenic substances. *Therapeuticum* 1987;1:23–31.

161. Lieberman S. A review of the effectiveness of *Cimicifuga racemosa* (black cohosh) for the symptoms of menopause. *Womens Health* 1998;7:525–529.

162. Liske E. Therapeutic efficacy and safety of *Cimicifuga racemosa* for gynaecologic disorders. *Adv Ther* 1998;15:45–53.

163. Hirata JD, Swiersz LM, Zell B, et al. Does dong quai have estrogenic effects in postmenopausal women? A double-blind, placebo-controlled trial. *Fertil Steril* 1997;68:981–986.

164. Bone K, Burgess N, McLeod D. *Phytosynergistic prescribing.* Portland, OR: Health Formulas, 1994:63–54.

165. Xu SS, Cai ZY, Qu ZW, et al. Huperzine-A in capsules and tablets for treating patients with Alzheimer disease. *Chung Kuo Yao Li Hsueh Pao* 1999;20:486–490.

166. Morazzoni P, Bombardelli E. *Hypericum perforatum. Fitoterapia* 1995;66:43–68.

167. Warmecke G. Neurovegetative dystonia in the female climacteric: studies on the clinical efficacy and tolerance of kava extract WS 1490. *Fortschr Med* 1991;109:120–122.

168. Mills S. *Essential book of herbal medicine.* Arkana, NY: Penguin, 1991.

169. Hargrove JT, Maxson WS, Wentz AC, et al. Menopausal hormone replacement therapy with continuous daily oral micronized estradiol and progesterone. *Obstet Gynecol* 1989;73:606–612.

170. Souza M, Prestwood K, et al. A comparison of the effect of synthetic and micronized hormone replacement therapy on bone mineral density and biochemical markers of bone metabolism. *Menopause* 1996;3:140–148.

171. Ettinger B, Gennent H, Steiger P, et al. Low-dosage micronized 17-beta estradiol prevents bone loss in postmenopausal women. *Am J Obstet Gynecol* 1992;166:479–488.

172. Kim S, Korhonen M, Wilborn W, et al. Antiproliferative effects of low-dose micronized progesterone. *Fertil Steril* 1996;65:323–331.

173. Ikram Z, Dulipsingh L, Prestwood KM. Lack of effect of short-term micronized progesterone on bone turnover in postmenopausal women. *J Womens Health Gend Based Med* 1999;8:973–978.

174. Leonetti HB, Longo S, Aasti JN. Transdermal progesterone cream for vasomotor symptoms and postmenopausal bone loss. *Obstet Gynecol* 1999;94:225–228.

175. Holtzsherer A, Legros MS. *Pratique homeopathique en gynecologie.* Boiron, France: CEHD, 1994.

176. Warenik-Szymankiewich A, Meczekalski B, Obrebowska A. Feminon N in the treatment of menopausal symptoms. *Ginekol Pol* 1997;68:89–93.

177. Lende K, Clausius N, Ramirez G, et al. Are the clinical effects of homeopathy placebo effects? A meta-analysis of placebo-controlled trials. *Lancet* 1997;350:834–843.

178. Linde K, Melchart D. Randomised controlled trials of individualized homeopathy: a state-of-art review. *J Altern Complement Med* 1998;4:371–388.

13

BENIGN VULVAR DISORDERS

EDUCATIONAL OBJECTIVES

Medical Students (1)
APGO Objectives Nos. 38 and 55

Evaluation and management:
dermatologic conditions, –
    Bartholin gland disease,
    vulvodynia, trauma
Vulvar neoplasia: risk factors,
    methods of diagnosis,
    diagnosis and management

Residents in Obstetrics/Gynecology (2)
CREOG Objectives

Vulvar infections
Vulvar dystrophies and dermatoses
Vulvar malignancies: preinvasive
    vulvar lesions, invasive vulvar
    carcinoma

Practitioners (3,4)
ACOG Recommendations

Vulvar non-neoplastic epithelial
    disorders: lichen sclerosus,
    lichen simplex chronicus,
    lichen planus, squamous
    cell hyperplasia, vulvar
    vestibulitis, vestibular
    papillomatosis, idiopathic
    vulvodynia
Vulvar cancer: squamous cell
    carcinoma, melanoma,
    Bartholin gland carcinoma,
    Paget disease of the vulva,
    verrucous carcinoma

VULVAR ANATOMY

The vulva is a female reproductive organ that encompasses several external genital structures. The mons pubis or the mons veneris lies over the anterior-superior part of the symphysis pubis and is composed of skin, hair, and subcutaneous fat. During puberty, crispy, curly, coarse pubic hair distribution develops. Characteristically, female hair distribution is in a triangular shape and is not expected to extend upward toward the umbilical area, but normal racial and familial variations can occur (Fig.13.1).

The labia majora are two symmetrical folds of skin in a U shape. The longitudinal arm of the skin folds includes the clitoris, labia minora, and fossa navicularis. The upper parts of the U-shaped arms insert laterally into the clitoris, creating bilateral fat pads, where the clitoris is situated. The fusion part connecting the U-shaped arms is located caudally and is termed the posterior commissure. The labia majora extend from the mons anteriorly to the posterior fourchette and are homologous to the male scrotum. The interior structures of fat pats present as small lobules separated from each other by connective and elastic tissues, creating a saclike structure. The sac opens anteriorly to the inguinal canal; through this open-

ing, the round ligaments (corresponding structure in males is the gubernaculum) insert into these connective-elastic tissues. The skin covers the fat pads, and the skin in this area is reached in both apocrine (sebaceous glands) and eccrine (sweat glands). Postpubertally, hair follicles grow on the labia majora skin (Fig. 13.1).

Blood supply and blood return to the labia majora primarily come from:

■ Posterior branch of the internal pudendal artery and veins
■ Small branches of the obturator artery and veins
■ The vein's drainage connects with the inferior hemorrhoidal veins and the vesicovaginal plexus.

Nerve distribution is provided by:

■ Pudendal nerve (derived from S2–4), from which the posterior labia nerve begins as the branch of the perineal branch. The posterior labia nerve innervates the labia majora and the lateral aspect of the urethral triangle.
■ Ilioinguinal nerve
■ Internal branch of the genitocrural nerve
■ Genital nerve, which is a branch of the posterior femoral cutaneous, or lesser sciatic, nerve (Fig. 13.2)

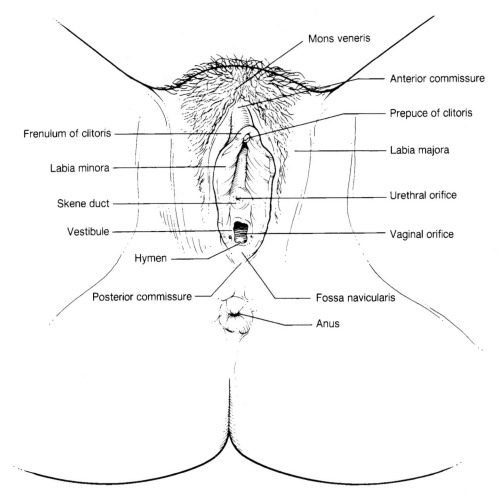

FIGURE 13.1. Anatomy of the external genitalia.

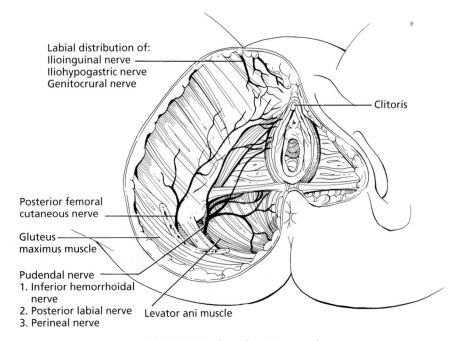

FIGURE 13.2. The vulva nerve supply.

The labia minora refer to the skin, not the mucosa. Two thin, firm, pigmented skin folds create these symmetrical structures bilaterally, with anteriorly located free margins. These structures extend between the vaginal openings and the labia majora. The cephalic part of labia minora fuses from each site and embraces the clitoris. Such fusion creates the prepuce of the clitoris superiorly and the frenulum of the clitoris inferiorly (homologous male structures are the penile urethra and the skin of the penis). The size of the labia minora varies, and the labia majora can cover them or the labia minora can project beyond the labia majora. The labia minora have abundant blood vessel distribution. The skin of the labia minora is not covered with hair and contains very few eccrine glands. On the other hand, the apocrine glands are densely distributed, particularly on the lateral aspects. Stimulation during foreplay and sexual intercourse induces the sebaceous glands and vestibular glands to secrete lubrication. Additional functions include protecting the distal clitoris and preventing urine from spraying, as happens in vulvectomized women.

Blood supply and return, the labial vessels, and the dorsal vessels of the clitoris (terminal branches of the pudendal vessels) create the blood circulation system for the labia minora.

Nerve distribution to the labia minora comes from the same sources that innervate the labia majora (Figs. 13.1 and 13.2).

The fossa navicularis is a curved depression in the vulvar area. The borders are delineated anteriorly by the hymenal ring and posteriorly by the fourchette. The blood circulatory system and innervation come from the labia minora.

The clitoris is a cylindrical, erectile organ located at the anterior lower border of the symphysis pubis and almost hidden by the anterior portion of the labia majora (no corpus spongiosum and not as much erectile tissue are present, as in the penis). The clitoris is homogenous to the glans of the penis and serves as the sexual nerve center (the most erotically sensitive organ).

The glans of the clitoris is the most distal and visible part of the clitoral body. Two folds of the labia minora create the prepuce and frenulum of the clitoris, which surround the glans.

The body of the clitoris is the result of fusion of the two roots or crura of the clitoris in one structure, reaching 2.5 to 3.0 cm in length and 1 cm in width.

The crura or roots of the clitoris contain erectile tissues. In the flaccid clitoral state they are approximately 3 to 4 cm long, and in the erectile state they are 4.5 to 5.0 cm. They run closely to the ischiopubic rami. The ischiocavernous muscle covers the clitoral crura and body.

The function of the clitoris is said to be responsible for orgasm, because female orgasm can be reached by clitoral stimulation. To support this view, circumcised women have been examined, and results have documented that this group of patients had difficulty reaching orgasm. The clitoris is removed as a part of total vulvectomy for malignancy; in contrast, patients so treated can reach orgasm. Such events show that the clitoris is not the sine qua non organ for orgasmic gratification.

Blood supply and return are provided by the clitoris artery and accompanying clitoral vein. The dorsal clitoris vein also connects clitoral blood return with the pelvis vein directly.

The dorsal clitoral nerve (the branch of the pudendal nerve) provides innervation for the clitoris.

The vestibulum is the space between the labia minora extending from the frenulum anteriorly to the posterior fourchette. Upon separating the labia minora, the following anatomic structures are found within this space:

- The hymen is usually a thin, well-vascularized membrane, although varying thickness is often observed. The membrane separates the vagina from the fossa navicularis and partially occludes the vaginal orifice. The shapes of the natural openings of the hymen are referred to as the anular hymen, septate hymen, cribriform hymen, and parous introitus. After vaginal delivery, the hymenal remnants are called carunculae hymenales or carunculae multiformes (Fig. 13.3).
- The vaginal orifice
- The opening of the Bartholin ducts (about 1 cm in length) is the conduit between the Bartholin glands and the vestibulum. The Bartholin glands (homologous to the bulbourethral glands or Cowper glands in the male) produce colorless mucus, particularly during the excitement state of sexual stimulation and vaginal intercourse. The openings of the Bartholin glands are situated at the

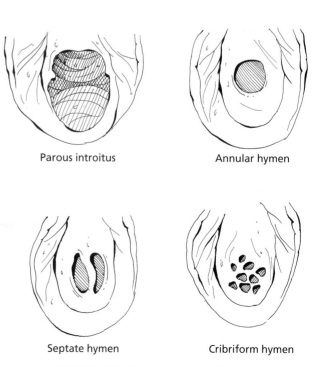

Parous introitus   Annular hymen

Septate hymen   Cribriform hymen

FIGURE 13.3. The shapes of the hymen.

5 and 7 o'clock positions between the hymen and labia minora. Growth is accentuated during the puberty, and atrophy occurs in the postmenopausal period.

- The urethral meatus is a papilla-like structure that slightly protrudes from the surface of the vestibulum and is usually 2 cm below the clitoris. It is the most distal part of the urethra and is the highest anatomic structure within the vestibulum.
- The Skene gland ducts (approximately 1 cm in length) run parallel to the urethra and are located lateral and posterior to the urethral meatus. The Skene glands or paraurethral glands are homologous to the prostate gland in the male.
- The minor vestibular glands release mucus to the vestibulum.
- The vestibular bulbs are an accumulation of erectile tissue that extends from the crura of the clitoris to the vaginal orifice, where they open bilaterally. They are located superiorly to the inferior fascia of the pelvic diaphragm and below the bulbocavernous muscles. Anteriorly, Bartholin glands become thinner and narrow to match and to fuse with the opposing bulb. Posteriorly, the ends of the vestibular bulbs and Bartholin glands remain in contact. Vestibular bulbs are homologous to the corpus spongiosum or bulb of the penis.

VULVAR EPITHELIAL DISORDERS

Vulvar non-neoplastic epithelial disorders include the following conditions.

Lichen Sclerosus

Definition

A lichen sclerosus is a hypopigmented, atrophic, wrinkled vulvar lesion affecting women of all ages and is associated with labial agglutination and vaginal orifice stenosis.

Incidence

The incidence or prevalence of lichen sclerosus is unknown. it has been estimated that among women with vulvar symptomatology, lichen sclerosus occurs in about 10% (3).

Etiology

The etiology of lichen sclerosus is unknown. Several hypotheses have developed:

- Sexual abuse (evidence is inconclusive) (5)
- Hormonal causes (6)
- Autoimmune diseases (strong association with lichen sclerosus in all ages) (7)
- Genetics (8)
- Trauma to the vulvar area (9)

Diagnosis

Pertinent medical history usually discloses the following symptoms:

- Vulvar symptoms
  Irritation
  Pruritis
  Soreness
  Superficial dyspareunia
- Periurethral symptoms
  Voiding difficulties
  Dysuria
- Perianal symptoms
  Constipation
  Dyschezia
  Anal stenosis

Physical examination of the vulva in the presence of lichen sclerosus shows the following (10):

- The skin appears to be atrophic or wrinkled.
- The area is affected symmetrically and is hypopigmented.
- Epithelial excoriation, ecchymosis, superficial ulcers, scarring, and subepithelial hemorrhage with hematoma formation in small vessels may be present.
- Agglutination of the labia minora or prepuce or frenulum of the clitoris can occur.
- Perianal area has a classic figure-of-eight appearance [extragenital lesions of lichen sclerosus occur in about 6% (11)].
- It is not typical that lichen sclerosus will extent to the labia majora.

The definitive diagnosis is reached from histologic examination of the material obtained by direct lesion biopsy.

Differential Diagnosis

- Pemphigoid and pemphigus
- Lichen planus
- Scleroderma
- Morphea
- Lupus erythematosus
- Radiation fibrosis

Conventional Therapy for Lichen Sclerosus

Conventional therapy for lichen sclerosus depends on the severity of symptoms. Asymptomatic women with lichen sclerosus need no treatment. Vulvar, perineal, and perianal hygiene is the only recommendation.

A mild form usually responds to the following treatment:

- A combination of vitamin A and vitamin D ointment and hygiene are initially recommended.

- Topical corticosteroids can be administered when local treatment with vitamins fails. Potent local steroids in cream for topical application such as clobetasol propionate 0.05% or betamethasone dipropionate 0.05% twice daily are suggested for a period of 2 to 12 weeks (12,13). This is decreased to once-daily application at bedtime, finally tapering to one to three times per week. Such an approach is safe for long-term treatment with high-potency corticosteroid cream (14).
- Topical progesterone and topical testosterone can be used. However, the results are not superior to corticosteroids, and this treatment can induce oily skin, acne, and excessive hair growth (15).
- Topical estrogens are not effective in lichen sclerosus therapy (3).

Surgery is occasionally indicated in the form of a reconstructive procedure to free the clitoris from the hood (results from agglutination of the labia minora) or restoration of an adequate size of the stenotic vaginal introitus.

The long-term risk of vulvar squamous cell carcinoma associated with lichen sclerosus ranges from 3.5% to 10% (11,16); therefore, any suspicious changes within lichen sclerosus, such as an ulceration or nodule, should be subjected to direct biopsy or local excision (3).

Complementary Therapy

Hypnosis
A wide spectrum of dermatologic conditions can be improved or even cured by hypnosis. There is no explicit information in reference to lichen sclerosus treatment with hypnosis; however, pruritis is one of the primary symptoms in lichen sclerosus and can be improved with hypnosis (17).

Alternative Therapy

Herbal Remedy
No herbal remedy recommendation for lichen sclerosus is offered; nevertheless, an antipruritogenic effect may be successful.

Kochiae fructus or *Hocia scoparia* fruit in the form of 70% ethanol extract, 200 to 500 mg/kg orally, inhibits skin itching and scratching (18). No study is available to validate the safety and effectiveness of this approach.

Triticum aesstivum or wheat is used in folk medicine for itching and inflammatory dermatoses. Externally is applied in a form of a bran bath (19).

Squamous Cell Hyperplasia

Definition
Vulvar squamous cell hyperplasia is a chronic, focal, nonspecific epithelial thickening of the skin.

Incidence
The incidence of squamous cell hyperplasia is unknown.

Etiology
The cause of this condition is a chronic reactive response to nonspecific agents without atypia and inflammation. Squamous cell hyperplasia is most commonly observed in women 30 to 60 years of age, and there is no racial predilection.

Diagnosis
Pertinent medical history is significant for vulvar itching (pruritis). Physical examination reveals the following symptoms:

- Affected vulvar skin color is white to gray and is distributed asymmetrically (contrary to the symmetric appearance of lichen sclerosus) and usually is confined to the focal area.
- Scratch marks are present on the affected and adjacent vulvar area.
- Excoriation and fissures can be visualized.

The diagnosis is reached by exclusion of other pruritic conditions affecting the vulva.

Differential Diagnosis
The characteristic microscopic findings of *lichen simplex chronicus* incorporate fibrosis, collagenization, and chronic inflammatory cells on the superficial dermis (20). Such histologic changes are not observed in squamous cell hyperplasia.

Lichen planus is histologically distinguished by the presence of inflammatory infiltration below the epithelium and surroundings. It is often found on the vaginal walls or oral mucosa (20).

Psoriasis is often considered in the differential diagnosis, even though the clinical picture does not resemble squamous cell hyperplasia. Characteristically, vulvar lesions are red and white (the range of color is white to gray in squamous cell hyperplasia). Histologic examination shows inflammation and acanthosis in the dermis and epithelium (20).

Seborrhea and *chronic fungal infection* are often associated with squamous cell hyperplasia. Microscopic examination of a specimen with 10% KOH assists in the diagnosis of fungal infection. A culture will identify not only the presence of the fungal microorganism but also will allow isolation of a specific mycotic type.

Condylomata acuminata, particularly occurring in the flat form of human papillomavirus (HPV) infection, is often a perplexing condition (subclinical HPV infection presents with more burning than itching). A clinical feature of condylomata acuminata is occurrence in multiple locations. Histologically, condylomata acuminata is distinguished from squamous cell hyperplasia by the presence of koliocytosis, cellular links, an accentuated granular layer, and parabasal cell hyperplasia (20).

Vulvar intraepithelial neoplasia (VIN) is clinically distinguishable by the characteristic presence of white, red, or pigmented maculopapular lesions and multifocal location. A microscopic study establishes not only the presence of VIN but also the severity of atypia (21).

Conventional Therapy

Conventional therapy is very successful when the underlying provocative cause of squamous cell hyperplasia can be established. Because the cause of squamous cell hyperplasia is often nonspecific, a nonspecific treatment is offered. Clinically, topical corticosteroid creams are considered curative.

The following management is recommended:

- General personal hygiene is essential, especially keeping the vulva dry.
- Guarding the vulvar area from contact with irritants is helpful.
- Triamcinolone acetonide 0.1% (medium-strength corticosteroid) cream is applied twice daily until symptoms subside, at which point application can be decreased to once daily at bedtime. The treatment is typically continued for 2 to 6 weeks (22–24).
- Antipruritogenic agents can assist in interrupting the itching/scratching sequence.

Complementary Therapy

No specific therapy is available for squamous cell hyperplasia; nevertheless, pruritis can be treated as presented in the section on lichen sclerosus.

Alternative Therapy

Alternative therapies can be applied for vulvar itching as described earlier for lichen sclerosus. No specific alternative therapy has been designed for treatment of squamous cell carcinoma.

OTHER VULVAR DERMATOSES

Lichen Simplex Chronicus

Lichen simplex chronicus is considered a form of squamous cell hyperplasia and has the same clinical picture, the same differential diagnosis, and the same therapies (20). However, some histologic features distinguish this condition from squamous cell hyperplasia.

Lichen Planus of the Vulva

Definition

Lichen planus is an inflammatory skin disease.

Incidence

The incidence of lichen planus is unknown; although, it is estimated to affect approximately 5% of women with vulvar disorders (3).

Etiology

The etiology of lichen planus has not been established; a psychogenic cause has been suggested.

Diagnosis

Pertinent medical history discloses either an asymptomatic or symptomatic status. The following symptoms may be present:

- Vulvar pruritis
- Vulvar burning
- Vulvar pain

Occasionally, vulvar, vaginal, and gingival symptoms associated with erosions can coincide, suggesting the presence of a vulvo-vaginal-gingival syndrome (25).

Physical examination can establish the following vulvar findings:

- Erythematous, friable vestibule with adherent exudates may be observed.
- Variable appearance of vulvar lesions, particularly occurring in the vestibulum and on the vaginal walls, and ranging from delicate papules to erosions, as well as scarring and stenosis of the vaginal introitus may be identified.
- Marked resorption and agglutination of the labia minora, clitoral prepuce, and frenulum may be present in the advanced stage of the disorder. The process also affects the labia minora by thinning and hypopigmentation. In the advanced stage, lichen planus is clinically difficult to distinguish from lichen sclerosus.

A direct biopsy with a histologic examination will establish the definitive diagnosis (20).

Differential Diagnosis

- Lichen sclerosus does not involve the vaginal wall or gingival mucosa, and histopathologic characteristics help to differentiate these two conditions (20).
- Cicatricial pemphigoid exhibits subepithelial blisters, and typically an immunofluorescence study shows linear

immunoglobulin A deposits, which are absent in lichen planus (20).

- Morphea (scleroderma) clinically is present in a location other than the vulva, particularly on the back. Microscopic features can assist in making the diagnosis (20).
- Psoriasis
- Kaposi sarcoma is observed in immunocompromised patients (HIV infection, transplant recipient, or drug induced).
- VIN

Conventional Therapy

The early diagnosis and therapy of lichen planus is essential because it is a progressive vulvar skin condition leading to adhesion formation, labia minora agglutination, scarification, and shrinkage of the vulva and vagina. There is no cure for lichen planus; nevertheless, continuous, indefinite treatment can manage symptoms and prevent the sequelae of an uncontrolled disease process (26).

In view of the fact that the vulva and vagina are usually involved in this clinical process, the following management is recommended:

- Vulvar treatment
    Betamethasone valerate 0.1% cream is applied twice daily until acute symptoms abate. After the initial period of treatment, cream application should be reduced to once daily at bedtime. Eventually the dose will be reduced to three times per week, and such vulvar application may continue indefinitely.
    Topical estrogens in a hypoestrogenic state may be of assistance. However, estrogen creams containing alcohol should be avoided because they increase irritation.
- Vaginal synchronized therapy with vulvar treatment
    Vaginal foaming cortisone enema is recommended for an acute state, or betamethasone valerate 0.1% cream may be applied once daily for 2 weeks.
    Hydrocortisone vaginal suppositories are administered at the daily dose of 25 mg after the acute stage subsides.
    Estrogen vaginal cream in a hypoestrogenic state is recommended (see Chapter 12).
- Retin-A and topical corticosteroids may control symptoms and diminish vulvar skin lesions.

Complementary Therapy

No clinical suggestion is available for a lichen planus treatment.

Alternative Therapy

No specific remedy is proposed for lichen planus.

Psoriasis

Definition

Psoriasis is an inflammatory skin disorder that may affect the vulva.

Incidence

Psoriasis is estimated to affect 2% of the population in the United States; about 5 million women are affected by this condition (28). No incidence data are available for vulvar psoriasis disorder.

Etiology

Psoriasis is an autosomal-dominant trait with incomplete penetrance. The vulva is not the most common site. The scalp, nails, muscle extender surfaces of the elbows, knees, and sacrum skin area are more commonly affected. New lesions and superimposed infections are typically associated with scratching.

Diagnosis

Pertinent medical history shows periods of exacerbation and remission of skin lesion and itching.

Physical inspection of the vulva determines the presence of well-marginated plaque and silver-topped erythematous papules that are symmetrically distributed. Scratch marks, the Auspitz sign (multiple punctuated blood-oozing sources are observed, upon removing loose silvery scales), and the Koebner phenomenon (occurring within 7–30 days of new psoriatic lesions on the skin microtraumatic area often result from scratching) may be present. Medical history and physical examination is diagnostic; direct skin lesion biopsy verifies the clinical diagnosis.

Differential Diagnosis

- Paget disease
- Fungal infection
- Reactive dermatitis
- VIN
- Lymphoma

Conventional Therapy

Conventional therapy includes the following approaches:

- Topical 2% to 10% salicylic acid ointment is applied.
- Topical short-term fluorinated corticosteroids used long-term can maximize local skin atrophy and fibrosis.
- Methotrexate

Complementary Therapy

Complementary therapy for psoriasis includes the following options:

- Ultraviolet light (either sunlight or artificial light)
- Hypnotherapy (17)
- Other forms such as acupuncture, magnetic field therapy, biofeedback therapy, and meditation are suggested. Nevertheless, no sufficient clinical studies are available to support their effectiveness.

Diet

A diet that includes 50% raw foods for a patient affected by psoriasis should be considered. Consumption of the following nutritional products are recommended:

- Seafood high in omega-3 fatty acids (herring, mackerel, salmon, sardines)
- Rotating olive, flax seed, and canola oils, 1 tablespoon daily
- Freshly squeezed juice of garlic, apple, carrot, grape, cucumber, and beet
- Avoidance of alcohol, nuts (except almonds), aromatic spices (e.g., curry, mustard, pepper), citrus foods or juice

Supplemental Therapy

Supplemental therapy recommendations are based on anecdotal evidence.

Vitamins

- Vitamin A, 75,000 IU daily for the first 2 weeks; 50,000 IU daily for the next 3 months; 25,000 IU per day thereafter
- Vitamin B complex, 50 mg three times daily
- Vitamin B_1, 50 mg three times daily
- Vitamin B_5, 100 mg three times daily
- Vitamin B_6, 50 mg three times daily
- Vitamin B_{12}, sublingually 2,000 µg daily
- Vitamin C, 2,000 to 10,000 mg daily
- Vitamin D, as directed by label or vitamin D analogue (calcipotril) topically
- Vitamin E, 400 to 1,200 IU daily
- Folic acid, 400 µg daily

Minerals

- Zinc, 50 to 100 mg daily
- Calcium, 1,500 mg daily
- Magnesium, 750 mg daily
- Selenium, 200 µg daily

Other Supplement

- Kelp 1,000 to 1,500 mg daily (balanced minerals)
- Shark cartilage 1 g/15 pounds body weight divided into three doses daily

Alternative Therapy

Herbal Therapy

Herbal therapy for psoriasis is based on folk medicine tradition, and there are not sufficient scientific data to support its use. Among many herbal remedies, the following are commonly suggested:

- Black nightshade or *Salane nigrum* is applied externally in the form of a compress or rinse.
- Burdock or *Arctium loppa* is used topically for psoriasis in the form of burdock oil.
- Red clover or *Trifolium pratense* is externally applied as a liquid extract 1:1 in 25% ethanol alcohol three times daily.
- Sunflower or *Helianthus annuus* oil dressing is applied to psoriatic lesions.
- Coal tar or fototar cream is applied to affected skin area one to four times daily for relief of itching, irritation, and skin flaking associated with psoriasis.

Homeopathic Therapy

- Black nightshade homeopathic is administered in a parenteral dose of five drops of extract every hour until the acute stage subsides, one to three times daily thereafter.
- Mountain laurel is administered in a dose of five drops of extract every hour until the acute stage subsides, one to three times daily thereafter.
- *Arsenicum album* is given in a diluted dose of 15 cH, five granules three times daily.
- Sulfur is administered in a diluted dose of 15 cH, five granules daily

Seborrheic Dermatitis or Atopic Dermatis

Seborrheic dermatitis or atopic dermatis is not a disease of the sebaceous glands. It is a skin disorder characterized by vulvar itching, scaling, and dryness. The diagnosis is clinical, and histology is nonspecific. The differential diagnosis includes fungal infection, psoriasis, Paget disease, and reactive dermatitis. There is no cure for this condition, and treatment should include personal hygiene and application of Burow solution and topical corticosteroids.

Herbal medicine treatment, such as burdock or coal tar cream, has been suggested for external use.

Allergic Dermatitis or Contact Dermatis

Allergic dermatitis or contact dermatis is the vulvar skin's response to allergen or irritant exposure. An individual can react to her body products, such as sweat or urine. Semen also can induce contact dermatitis, but it is a rare occurrence.

Symptoms include burning, itching, pain, and tenderness. Occasionally, dysuria and urinary retention are observed. On inspection, edema, erythema, and vesicles are present.

The diagnosis is based on medical history and physical examination. If any diagnostic questions remain, vulvar culture and biopsy should be performed.

The differential diagnosis includes vulvar infections or other skin itching conditions affecting the vulva.

Conventional therapy includes eliminating the allergens or irritants from contact with the vulvar skin. Water and soap are the most common cause of contact dermatitis; therefore, using filtrated or boiled water and natural soap with no perfume can be very helpful. Avoiding tight clothing, bubble bath, and washing detergents is advised.

A low-potency corticosteroid such as fluocinolone acetonide 0.01% cream, desonide (Desowen) 0.05% cream, or hydrocortisone acetate 1.0% cream is sufficient therapy for symptoms associated with contact dermatitis. Infrequently, a medium-potency corticosteroid such as triamcinolone acetonide 0.1% is topically applied. Corticosteroids are usually applied two or three times daily depending on the severity of the contact dermatis.

Alternative Therapy

The following alternative herbal remedies are suggested for the symptoms of allergic dermatitis:

- Marigold or *Calendula officinalis* in the form of 4% ointment is applied twice daily on the affected skin areas (19).
- Chamomile or *Matricaria recutita* exhibits antiinflammatory, antispasmodic, and sedative properties. Externally, chamomile extract or cream is applied to skin lesions. Clinical effectiveness has not been established for vulvar contact dermatitis (29).

Pigmented Lesions of the Vulva

Nevi

Nevi are pigmented, benign skin lesions. Acquired nevi typically occur during adolescence; congenital nevi usually are recognized before adolescence. The vulva is not affected as often as skin exposed to sunlight.

Junctional nevi involve only the epidermis and present as tan to black lesions (uniform color) that are smooth, and have well-demarcated margins. They are small (2–3 mm), predominantly flat lesions, but can be slightly elevated. Inspection of the vulva, in most instances, establishes the clinical diagnosis. A direct biopsy is occasionally recommended, when clinical diagnosis is uncertain. Follow-up every 6 to 12 months is advisable, and a patient should be instructed to observe the lesion. If any change occurs, such as size, configuration, symmetry, color, or margins, excisional biopsy and histologic examination are indicated.

Compound or intradermal nevi can grow *de novo* or can arise from junctional nevi. In contrast to junctional nevi, compound nevi penetrate both the epidermis and dermis and are larger (4–10 mm) and of uniform color, and have regular well-demarcated margins. Diagnosis is made by inspection and palpation. When symptomatic (irritation or bleeding present), excisional biopsy is usually the recommended diagnostic and therapeutic procedure. Hyperpigmented polypoid or popular nevi should be excised to avoid the potential for malignant transformation.

Acanthosis Nigricans

Acanthosis nigricans is a symmetric, diffused, velvetlike brown to gray-black vulvar skin lesion. This hyperpigmented lesion is usually located in inguinal folds, the labia majora, lateral labia minora, and pubis (the axilla, neck, and back also can be affected). In adults, acanthosis nigricans can be associated with abdominal viscera disorders, particularly the stomach. In adolescence, this entity is frequently observed in association with endocrine disorders. When hyperandrogenism, insulin resistance, and acanthosis nigricans coexist, it is called the HAIR-AN syndrome. In adults, the presence of the HAIR-AN syndrome warrants clinical investigation of endocrine dysfunction (diabetes, hyperandrogenism) and malignant neoplasia (gastric adenocarcinoma). In adolescence, endocrine evaluation also should be considered. Obesity and autoimmune endocrinopathy or lipodystrophy can produce pseudoacanthosis nigricans. Upon ruling out potentially associated conditions, symptomatic therapy is begun, mostly addressing vulvar itching associated with sudden onset. Management consists of a symptomatic antipruritic treatment, weight reduction, and reassurance.

Vitiligo

Vitiligo is a disorder, in which the previously normally pigmented vulvar skin becomes depigmented. Etiology is unknown, and familiar occurrence is about 10%. Autoantibodies are elevated. There is a noticeable absence of the basilar melanocytes and melanin granules. Vulvar vitiligo lesions are characterized by the presence of white patches. The lesions are sharply demarcated, with irregular border areas frequently present in different locations (e.g., trunk, extremities, or face). Symmetry usually is a feature of vitiligo lesion distribution. It is an asymptomatic condition, and no cure is available (20).

VULVAR VESTIBULITIS

Definition

Vulvar vestibulitis or vulvar vestibular syndrome is a chronic inflammatory process manifested by tenderness of the vulvar vestibule to pressure, superficial (introital) dyspareunia, and vestibular erythema.

Incidence

The prevalence of vulvar vestibulitis has been reported at rates of 12% to 26% among adult women.

Etiology

The etiology of this entity is unknown. Nevertheless, several hypothesis have been proposed: excessive used of topical corticosteroids, exposure to irritants [5-fluorouracil (5-FU), trichloroacetic acid (TCA), podophyline, topical antibiotics, gentian violet, perfumes, deodorants, irritant soaps], infections, allergic reaction, hormonal imbalance, pelvic floor dysfunction, urinary oxalates, sexual trauma, sexual abuse, and vulvar laser therapy (3,30).

Classification

Primary vestibulitis (persistent dyspareunia from the onset of sexual life) is more refractory to a therapy than secondary vestibulitis. Secondary vestibulitis is painless sexual intercourse preceding dyspareunia.

Diagnosis

Pertinent medical history provides the following information related to vulvar vestibulitis:

- Varied degrees of discomfort of the vaginal introitus or vestibulum associated with insertion, touch, or tampons are present. In most advanced cases, women avoid coitus due to excessive pain.
- Vulvar vestibule burning and itching are reported.
- Increased urinary frequency can be associated with vestibular syndrome.

Physical examination reveals the following:

- Vulvar vestibule inflammation is visualized particularly around the openings of the periurethral glands and can extend to minor and major vestibular duct openings.
- Cotton swab pressure evokes pinpoint tenderness.

A patient's medical history and physical findings usually are sufficient for establishing the diagnosis of vulvar vestibulitis. A direct vestibular biopsy is not a conclusive diagnostic tool, and a histologic examination demonstrates periductal inflammation without vestibular gland involvement. However, a differential diagnosis can be reached based on histologic information.

Differential Diagnosis

- Pudendal neuralgia clinically manifests with the presence of vulvar burning exacerbated by coitus.
- Vulvodynia

- Vaginismus (31)
- Psychogenic aspect (32)
- Fungal, bacterial, and viral infections can be associated with vulvar vestibulitis. However, infection per se cannot be considered as a cause of vulvar vestibulitis.

Conventional Therapy

Identifying associated diseases constitutes a specific therapy. Because the cause of vulvar vestibulitis is unknown, symptomatic management is recommended.

Several modalities for vulvar vestibulitis treatment are available. Among conservative medical options, the following topical agents may be used:

- Corticosteroid cream or ointment (medium-potency triamcinolone acetonide 0.1% cream or high-potency betamethasone valerate 0.1% ointment) is recommended once or twice daily, tapering to once or twice a week (33).
- Estrogen cream in a hypoestrogenic state, 1 g daily, is recommended.
- Lidocaine gel (2%–5%) is applied in a small amount to the vaginal introitus prior to vaginal penetration. Capsaicin, a natural topical analgesic cream, also is recommended (see section on Alternative Therapy).

Oral medication is aimed toward an associated disease process, particularly chronic fungal infection [fluconazole, 150 mg weekly for 3 months is recommended (34); although, clinical validation of this approach is lacking]. An antidepressant, amitriptyline hydrochloride, 10 mg at bedtime, can be increased in 10-mg increments every 2 weeks until therapeutic response is achieved. The daily dose should not exceed 75 mg per day (35). Supportive clinical data for this therapy are not available. Calcium citrate and a low-oxidate diet (see section on Alternative Therapy) also are suggested.

Intralesional interferon (intravestibular) injection is administered using a 30-gauge needle and a 1-mL syringe. Recombinant alpha-interferon injection is recommended (1×10^6 per injection; 1 mL contains 3×10^6 IU) (3). Twelve total sites are injected within 4 weeks. Interferon therapy is indicated when an HPV-associated condition is histologically documented (36). The success rates for this approach vary from 49% to 88% (30).

Systemic interferon therapy can be used, with intramuscular injection of beta-interferon at a total dose of 45×10^6 over 20 days (37).

Surgical therapy is indicated when coitus becomes unbearable and either the condition is refractory to conservative therapy or a patient does not wish to continue it. It is a general clinical consensus that laser vaporization therapy is not recommended for vulvar vestibulitis (3,36).

Several surgical approaches are offered for vulvar vestibulitis:

- Vestibuloplasty
- Partial vestibulectomy with vaginal advancement
- Total vestibulectomy with vaginal advancement

With a properly established indication for surgical treatment, improvement is achieved at a rate of 60% to 90% (30).

Complementary Therapy

Complementary therapy for vulvar vestibulitis embraces the following:

- Warm sitz baths are advocated based on anecdotal clinical experience, but no clinical scientific data is available to validate this approach (3).
- Biofeedback treatment of vulvar vestibulitis with electromyographic stimulation of the pelvic floor muscles yields approximately 83% improvement in patients with moderate to severe disease. Such therapy demonstrates satisfactory effects on an average of 16 weeks of biofeedback exercise. Short-term (6-month) follow-up has established persistent beneficial effects of this modality (3,38). Unfortunately, this observational descriptive study has yet not been clinically validated.
- Vaginal dilatation with graduated vaginal dilators and analgesic cream can be useful in selective cases (3).

Diet

A well-balanced nutritional diet with low-oxalate components is recommended for vulvar vestibulitis management (39). The benefits of the diet have not been clinically evaluated.

Minerals

Calcium citrate tablets (200 mg calcium and 950 mg citrate) at the daily dose of six tablets can induce significant improvement of vulvar vestibulitis (39). Reproducing these clinical results failed in a general population of patients with vulvar vestibulitis. Nevertheless, treatment with calcium citrate yielded improvement in 24% of selected patients with vulvar vestibulitis and urinary oxalate spikes of greater than 1 mg/40 mL (30).

Alternative Therapy

Herbal Therapy

Capsaicin is a natural ingredient of the pepper plant, and its ability to temporarily relieve pain has been used in vulvar vestibulitis. Capsaicin cream (Doublecap, contains 0.05% capsaicin cream) at the concentration of 0.025% (half of the commercial dose) is clinically recommended. Severe vestibular burning has been reported with capsaicin cream treatment (30).

OTHER VULVAR DISORDERS

Vulvodynia

Vulvodynia is an enigmatic condition characterized by the presence of vulvar pruritis, pain, and tenderness. The spe-

cific cause of this condition is unknown, but organic, mental-physical-sexual abuse, as well as psycho-social-sexual-economical background have been postulated (40). The diagnosis is reached by exclusion, and consultation with dermatologists, psychologists, sexologists, and medical neurologists is encouraged. *Conventional management* includes a multidisciplinary approach to the cluster of symptoms, personal vulvar hygiene, antipruritic treatment, local anesthetic, and aggressive therapy for any vulvar infection.

Complementary therapy is suggested with acupuncture, biofeedback, hypnosis (17), and nutritional therapy as presented above. *Alternative therapy*, generally for pruritis, includes herbal medical treatment with jasmine, wheat, wild thyme, houseleek, speedwell, sweet gale, or vervain (19). The clinical effectiveness of either complementary or alternative therapy has not yet been documented.

Vestibular Papillomatosis

Vestibular papillomatosis is a vulvar skin condition associated with pruritis and characterized by the appearance of small papillar lesions (2–3 mm in length and 1 mm in diameter) that are clustered (can reach several centimeters in diameters) on the medial surface of the labia minora close to the hymenal ring. The lesions are predominantly asymptomatic, but vulvar itching can be present (41).

Conventional therapy is to promote vulvo-perineal-perianal hygiene, to avoid contact with irritating substances, and to remove lesions.

Complementary and alternative therapies can be applied for pruritis as presented above.

Vulvar Manifestation of Systemic Disease

Vulvar manifestation of systemic disease encompasses a variety of conditions. *Crohn disease* or regional enteritis is a chronic noncaseating granulomatous condition primarily affecting the gastrointestinal tract. However, the vulva can be involved as early as childhood (42). The vulvar manifestation of Crohn disease most commonly consists of edema, erythema followed by ulcer formation (cutlike, deep, multiple with or without secondary infections). The labia majora and minora can be enlarged, and vulvar polyps, a vulvar mass, and pyoderma gangrenosum can be present (43). Vulvar signs and symptoms can be present with or without general symptoms of gastrointestinal dysfunction.

The diagnosis frequently presents a challenge, and a direct lesion biopsy is indicated. The differential diagnosis includes Behçet syndrome, condylomata acuminata, condylomata lata, herpetic/ulcerative conditions, hidradenitis suppurativa, granuloma inguinale, lymphogranuloma venereum (LGV), sarcoidosis, and tuberculosis.

Conventional therapy is directed toward the underlying disease with steroids and antibiotics. A surgical approach is not contemplated until the healing process advances. Surgical treatment unaccompanied by medical therapy is ineffective.

Behçet Syndrome

Behçet syndrome is an infrequent, chronic, recurrent condition characterized by the presence of aphthous stomitis, aphthous genital ulceration, anterior uveitis, cutaneous vasculitis, synovitis, ophthalmologic inflammation, and meningoencephalitis. At least a triad of identifiable changes must be present to reach the diagnosis of Behçet syndrome (44,45).

The diagnosis is clinical. A patient reports recurrent painful ulcers of the vulva and other organs. On physical examination, the vulva is red, and tender muscles and ulcerative lesions can be identified. The lesion itself is approximately 3 to 20 mm in diameter, well-marginated, deep, and very tender. Histology is nonspecific, with dermal inflammation and vasculitis (20).

The differential diagnosis includes herpes, pemphigus, lichen planus, lupus, and Stevens-Johnson syndrome.

Conventional therapy consists of corticosteroids and a high-estrogen dose of oral contraceptives (46). Topical anesthetic, intralesional steroid injection, or systemic cytostatic agents (methotrexate or colchicine) also can be used (43).

Surgery is only indicated when medical conservative management does not provide sufficient symptomatic relief and symptoms are unbearable.

Diabetes Mellitus

Diabetes mellitus vulvitis is commonly associated with recurrent fungal infection and occasionally is the first symptom of diabetes. Pruritis and burning are present, and inspection of the vulva shows edema, erythema, and white opaque patches. Diagnosis of fungal infection can be confirmed by microscopic evaluation with 10% KOH. Appropriate diabetes-controlled treatment and appropriate genitoperineal hygiene are essential therapy. Acute infection can be aborted by applying short-term corticosteroid cream and adequate infection treatment.

Uremia

Uremia can result in a gray-white-brown membrane (uremic frost) of the vulva and mouth that contains urea and uremic acid deposits. A crucial therapeutic approach is to control renal failure and vulvar hygiene.

Blood Dyscrasias

Blood dyscrasias such as agranulocytosis, aplastic anemia and leukemia, and bone marrow depression medication such as methotrexate can cause vulvar ulcerations covered with a gray membrane. Appropriate treatment of the underlying disease will heal the ulcerative process.

Circulatory Abnormalities

The symptomatology of circulatory abnormalities is associated with burning, itching, and heaviness of the vulva; occasionally vulvar swelling also is present. Vulvar varicose veins are observed. Treatment consists of compression of dilated veins, either with sanitary napkins or foam rubber. Surgery is rarely indicated, and intravaricose vein occlusive drug injection treatment also can be applied.

Vitamin Deficiencies

Vitamin deficiencies, particularly of vitamin A, vitamin B_2 (riboflavin), vitamin B_3 (niacin), and vitamin C, can result in vulvitis. Vulvar inspection establishes dry, scaly skin, and occasionally fissures and ulcerative changes. Therapy consists of providing vitamins in a therapeutic dose. Vitamin A overdose can lead to erythematous exudative dermatitis.

Kaposi Sarcoma (AIDS Ulcer)

Kaposi sarcoma (AIDS ulcer) is frequently located in the vulva of patients with immunologically compromised systems. Trivial infections of the vulva (fungal, viral, or bacterial) can recur and present a therapeutic dilemma.

VULVAR ANATOMIC DISORDERS

Hymenal Abnormalities

The imperforate and septate hymen can obstruct vaginal outflow (42). The *imperforate hymen* causes total vaginal obstruction and leads to accumulation of menstrual effluence that may fill up the vaginal pool (hematocolpos) but also can cause retrograde build-up in the uterine cavity (hematometra), and fallopian tubes.

The diagnosis is made based on medical history of delayed menarche, cyclic pelvic pain, urine retention, and constipation (rarely with fecal impaction).

Physical examination shows a bulging bluish membrane at the vaginal introitus. Rectal examination, if possible to perform, may demonstrate a tender pelvic mass, bulging the posterior vaginal wall to the rectum, and the anterior vaginal wall filling the bladder. The bladder can be distended and palpable in the abdominal cavity as a cystic, tender mass.

Pelvic ultrasonography using an abdominal transducer can assist in reaching the diagnosis when the diagnosis cannot be determined by the classic clinical picture.

Conventional therapy consists of surgically opening the imperforated hymen. A stellate incision is made at the 2, 4, 8, and 10 o'clock positions, and clots are removed. Hymenal margins sutured separately with fine absorbable sutures. If the imperforated hymen is diagnosed before puberty, the surgery should be delayed until after tissue estrogenization occurs.

Obstructions may also occur in the septate hymen. The clinical problem begins when a tampon is used or coitus is attempted. The diagnosis is clinical, and the hymenal septum excision with local anesthetic is curative.

Labial Hypertrophy

Labial hypertrophy is enlargement of the labia minora, varying from minimal to extreme, and can be present unilaterally or bilaterally. Two forms of labia minora hypertrophy are clinically observed.

Asymptomatic labial hypertrophy is noticed because of the abnormal appearance, and patients are concerned that male genitalia may be developing. Management of this condition consists of reassurance, patient education on hygiene of the vulvo-perineal-perianal areas, and avoidance of tight clothing.

Symptomatic labial hypertrophy is characterized by the presence of irritation or discomfort associated with compression of the vulva (tight clothing, biking, horseback riding, etc.). Surgery is indicated when reassurance and conservative management for vulvar discomfort have failed, physical appearance is cosmetically unacceptable, or the condition interferes with coitus. Excision of the excess hypertrophic labia with reconstruction usually solves this clinical problem. Postoperative edema can be significant enough to lead to urinary retention that will require a Foley catheter; an ice pack or Dermoplast spray may assist in management.

VULVAR INFECTIOUS AND SEXUAL DISEASES
Sexually Transmitted Infections

Human Papillomavirus (HPV)

Human papillomavirus is a regional viral infection affecting the urogenital-perianal areas. The prevalence of vulvar HPV infection varies significantly and is considered one of the most contagious and prevalent infections (47). Genital tract HPV infections can be caused by over 20 HPV subtypes, and most of them induce subclinical asymptomatic infection. Types 6 and 11 are responsible for external genitalia warts. Vulvar infection is associated with cervical HPV infection in about 30% to 50% of cases (48). Immunocompromised patients (HIV-positive or on immunosuppressant drugs) may present with large, destructive, and locally invasive genitoanal warts. Predisposing factors include poor hygiene, multiple sexual partners, oral contraceptive use, pregnancy, diabetes mellitus, and immunosuppression. HPV infection can occur in multiple sites and frequently affects urogenital-perineal-perianal structures.

There are two clinical forms of HPV clinical manifestation. *Condylomata acuminata* of the vulva (papillary, verrucous skin lesions) can present with or without symptoms. Symptomatic infection manifests with burning, itching, and pain; burning is by far the most prevalent symptom. Condylomata acuminata can be identified on gross inspection as papillary lesions arising from sessile lesions or a central stalk, with an irregular border of multiple locations.

The diagnosis of classic condylomata acuminata is reached on a clinical basis. A colposcopically directed biopsy is performed to look for any deviation from a typical appearance.

Subclinical or flat HPV infection is asymptomatic, although, burning, itching, and pain may occur, particularly postcoitally. Flat HPV infection can be detected by applying 3% to 5% acetic acid for 3 to 5 minutes followed by colposcopic examination or by direct tissue biopsy with histologic verification, or DNA hybridization. Biopsy is indicated when any suspicious lesion is present.

The uro-genital-anal areas should be evaluated using a speculum for vaginal examination and anoscopy for anal canal examination. Patients with HPV infection also should be tested for other sexually transmitted diseases. Overall therapies for HPV infections include the following:

- Patient education is undertaken in reference to the natural history of HPV infection, mode of transmission, likelihood of recurrences, lack of definitive cure and available vaccination, and association with squamous cell carcinoma. Appropriate hygiene of the external genitalia and anal areas should be stressed and monogamous sexual relationships emphasized. Successful removal of warts is considered a lesion-free state, not a cure.
- A condom as a protective measurement is not effective in HPV prevention.
- Topical treatments include podofilox, imiquimod cream (Aldara), trichloroacetic acid (TCA), and bichloroacetic acid. Aldara 5% cream is an immune response modifier and is indicated for external genitalia and perianal warts. Aldara cream is applied three times per week for 6 to 10 hours and should later be washed off with soap and water. Treatment with Aldara cream is continued for 16 weeks.
- Physical destructive therapy (electrocautery, cryotherapy, laser vaporization, infrared coagulation)
- Excisional therapy (cold knife, curettage, electrocautery excision, laser excision)
- Intralesion (alpha-interferon) or general intramuscular beta-interferon injections

If no improvement is noticeable within 6 weeks with one modality, other methods should be implemented.

Posttreatment follow-up should be scheduled 6 to 12 weeks after a completed therapy and every year thereafter, if a patient is lesion-free.

Conventional, complementary and alternative therapies are also described in Chapter 6.

Herpes Simplex Virus

Herpes simplex virus (HSV) is a sexually transmitted viral infection and one of the genital ulcerative diseases. Both type 1 and type 2 cause vulvar disease, but HSV type 2 is predominantly responsible for vulvar infection (48). The prevalence of vulvar infection with HSV in the United States is unknown. The incidence of HSV infection in general is estimated to be 126 per 100,000, with approximately 600,000 new cases per year (20).

Diagnosis of HSV infection is clinically based on local symptoms such as vulvar burning and pain that occasionally can be incapacitating, dysuria and urine retention, and general symptoms, particularly associated with primary infections, such as malaise and fever. Vulvar inspection may reveal all three sequential stages of HSV manifestation on the vulva: vesicles or blisters, pustules, and shallow ulcers. HSV infection can affect an uro-genital-perineal-perianal area. Therefore, similar changes can be observed in the entire region. HSV infection also can be asymptomatic: undetectable or composed of atypical lesions (20). The HSV culture from a vesicle aspirate or an ulcer base smear obtained with a Dacron swab is confirmatory. Direct fluorescent antibody tests also can be used.

Conventional therapy of HSV infection and suppressive treatment for vulvar infection do not differ from perianal conventional and complementary-alternative types of management (see Chapter 6).

Syphilis

Syphilis is a sexually transmitted, ulcerative, painless disease caused by the spirochete *Treponema pallidum* and can be located on the vulva. Details are provided in Chapter 6.

Chancroid

Chancroid is a sexually transmitted ulcerative disease caused by *Haemophilis ducreyi* (a gram-negative bacterium that creates a school-of-fish pattern and is a nonmotile bacillus) with an incubation period of 4 to 10 days. Multiple soft and painful ulcers characterize the condition. Clinical inspection shows ulcers with a necrotic tissue at the base, red edges, and elevated borders. Inguinal unilateral lymphadenopathy can be present with flocculant nodes. The diagnosis is made clinically by excluding other sexually transmitted ulcerative diseases (HSV, syphilis, LGV, and granuloma inguinale). However, approximately 20% of patients with chancroid also have syphilis (syphilitic chancre is painless and indurated) and HSV. Culture (aspirate from lymph nodes or chancroid) is difficult to grow but it provides a definitive diagnosis (50). A

histology or skin test is not reliable, and no serologic test is available.

Conventional therapy consists of oral administration of azithromycin (Zithromax), 1 g in a single dose, or erythromycin, 500 mg four times daily for 7 days, or intramuscular injection of ceftriaxone sodium (Rocephin), 250 mg in a single dose.

Lymphogranuloma Venereum (LGV)

Lymphogranuloma venereum is a sexually transmitted ulcerative vulvar disease caused by the L serovariant of Chlamydia trachomatis. The incubation period is 2 to 5 days but may last up to 4 weeks. There are three phases of clinical manifestation (51):

- Skin erosion, which begins as a papular vulvar skin lesion followed by erosion (ulcer), lasts only a few days. The initial vulvar ulcer is neither indurate nor painful.
- Adenitis is usually painful, with enlarged inguinal nodes that frequently penetrate the skin, rupture, and drain purulent material.
- Fibrosis and stricture of the vulvo-vaginal-anorectal areas occur, creating characteristic genitoinguinal grooves. In this stage external genitalia disfigurement, fistula formation, and edema or (chronic lymphatic obstruction) are present. Lower extremity edema (elephantiasis) may develop.

Diagnosis of LGV is clinical and verified by culture or a serologic test (microimmunofluorescent antibody test or positive complement fixation test). The histology is not diagnostic.

Differential diagnoses include lymphoma, carcinoma, Crohn disease, granuloma inguinale, and other ulcerative vulvar diseases.

Conventional therapy includes local hygiene and cleansing; aspiration of buboes (not incision) may prevent fistula formation. Antibiotics may be administered, such as doxycycline, 100 mg twice daily for 3 weeks, tetracycline, 500 mg four times daily for three weeks, or erythromycin, 333 (E–mycin) mg three times daily for 3 weeks.

Complementary and alternative therapies are not offered.

Granuloma Inguinale

Granuloma inguinale is considered a sexually transmitted ulcerative disease, but gastrointestinal track transmission can occur. *Calymmatobacterium granulomatis* (danovania) is the cause of the condition and occasionally is observed in the United States. It is a tropical disease with an incubation period of 2 to 12 weeks. The initial skin lesions are small, painless, papular, superficial ulcers. These lesions are transformed into red, raised, irregular ulcers. Granuloma inguinale affects the vulva but also may be present on the perineum, anus, and rectum, with enlarged, painless lymph nodes.

Diagnosis is reached by identifying the presence of Donovan bodies on Wright or Giemsa staining of scrapings from the lesion or a tissue specimen for a direct biopsy.

Conventional therapy is with antibiotics [tetracycline, 500 mg four times daily for 3 weeks, erythromycin (E-mycin), 333 mg three times daily for 3 weeks, or trimethoprim/sulfamethoxazole (Bactrim, Septra DS), one tablet twice daily for 3 weeks].

Other Infections

Molluscum Contagiosum

Molluscum contagiosum is transmitted sexually; although, it can be passed through nonsexual contact with a pox type of viral infection that in the majority of cases is asymptomatic. Vulvoperineal pruritis or superimposed secondary bacterial infection with its associated symptomatology may occur. The incubation period ranges from 14 to 50 days.

The multiple vulvar or perineal lesions are found in clusters (but can be single). They are small (3–6 mm in diameter), smooth papules with a central umbilication or dimple. *Diagnosis* can be confirmed by the presence of molluscum bodies (intracytoplasmic inclusion bodies) on cytologic (scrapings from the lesions) or histologic tissue examination (a direct biopsy).

Conventional treatment of symptomatic lesions or for cosmetic purposes is electrocautery excision with a needle. Cantharidin, liquid nitrogen, and chloracetic acid also are recommended.

Complementary-alternative therapies are not available.

Vulvar Shingles

Vulvar shingles or varicella are caused by the herpes zoster virus. Vulvar infection is infrequent. Initially, unilateral vulvar vestibulitis is present that progresses to vesicles and ulcers (both are very painful and sensitive to touch) most commonly affecting postmenopausal women. Vulvar burning, itching, pain, numbness, and tingling may be present. Vulvar vestibulitis, as an independent entity, does not consist of vesicles and ulcers in its clinical characteristics. Eventually, blisters form crusty scabs and the skin peels off. Vulvar pain may continue for months or even years after physical signs disappear.

Diagnosis is based on prodromal symptoms (headaches, fever, chills, and muscle aches 3–4 days before rash appears), and verification of varicella infection is established by cytologic or histologic findings of HSV infection.

Conventional therapy with acyclovir, 200 mg five times daily for a total of 10 days, may reduce pain and recurrence significantly, if the treatment is initiated within 48 hours. Neuralgia and recurrence of vesicular outbreaks are sequelae of this infection.

Complementary and alternative therapies are offered for vulvar shingles as follows:

- Diet includes brewer's yeast, whole grain, garlic, brown rice, and raw fruits and vegetables.
- Nutrients such as L-lysine, 500 mg twice daily with water or juice
- Vitamins
  Vitamin B_6, 50 mg daily for no longer than 6 months
  Vitamin C, 2,000 IU four times daily
  Vitamin D, 1,000 IU daily for 1 week, then 400 IU daily
  Vitamin E, 400 to 800 IU twice daily
  Vitamin A emulsion, 50,000 IU daily for 2 weeks, then 25,000 IU daily
- Minerals
  Zinc, 80 mg daily for 1 week and 50 mg daily thereafter
  Calcium, 1,500 mg daily
  Magnesium, 750 mg daily
- Herbal remedies
  Cayenne (capsicum) is an active component in Zostrix, a topical cream that may relieve pain and aids in healing.
  Goldenseal (*Hydrastis canadensis*) can reduce infection and has antimicrobial properties.
  Chamomile may promote healing.

Alternative therapies are suggested based on anecdotal clinical experience, and no significant proof of their effectiveness and safety are available.

Cytomegalovirus Vulvar Infection

Cytomegalovirus (CVM) vulvar infection is the cause of ulcerative vulvovaginitis. Vulvar ulcers are clinical findings. Culture or specific antibody tests are confirmatory. The differential diagnosis includes all ulcerative vulvar diseases, particularly HSV.

Vulvar Folliculitis

Vulvar folliculitis or vulvar furunculosis is a hair-bearing bacterial skin infection. The most common offending bacteria is *Staphylococcus aureus* (the infection can manifest with irritation, tenderness, and pruritis), and *Pseudomonas aeruginosa* is the most common cause of so called "hot tub folliculitis," which results from contact with contaminated water (the infection distribution coincides with the bathing suit area).

Diagnosis is established based on general symptoms such as headaches, sore throat, and fevers. One or more pustules pierced in the center with hair (2–10 mm in diameter) are observed. In the next stage pustules become red, dome-shaped papules, and in severe cases furuncles ill develop. The clinical diagnosis should be confirmed by a bacterial culture.

Conventional therapy begins with observation, because the condition can be self-limited to oral antibiotics for 10 to 14 days. The most common offending microorganism is *Staphylococcus aureus*; therefore, while waiting for culture results, empiric antibiotic therapy is recommended with semisynthetic penicillin (Dicloxacillin, 250 mg four times daily) or erythromycin (E-mycin, 333 mg three times daily), or cephalexin (Keflex, 500 mg four times daily). When a large fluctuant lesion is present, incision and drainage should be performed, and antibiotic treatment should be instituted.

In recurrent sterile vulvar folliculitis, tetracycline or erythromycin, at the dosage of 500 mg twice daily, is recommended for ongoing treatment.

Complementary and alternative specific treatment for folliculitis are not available.

Impetigo

Impetigo is an autoinoculated (from another part of the body) vulvar skin infection that is caused by *Staphylococcus aureus* or streptococcal bacteria. Bullae and thin-walled vesicles with reddened edges have a crusted surface after rupturing.

The blebs should be incised, and the crusts removed, and topical neomycin or trimethoprim/sulfamethoxazole (Bactrim) applied. Bathing with antibacterial soap also is suggested.

Vulvar Erysipelas

Vulvar erysipelas is a rare disorder caused by beta-hemolytic streptococci. This infection frequently occurs following trauma to the vulva or after surgery.

Diagnosis is based on the presence of systemic symptoms such as malaise, chills, fever, vulvar pain, burning. Erythematous vulvar skin lesions and the occurrence of vesicles and bullae as well as enlargement of erythematous regional lymph nodes make the clinical diagnosis. Culture is confirmatory.

Conventional therapy consists of bed rest, increased fluid intake, and oral penicillin or tetracycline, 500 mg four times daily for 10 to 14 days.

Hidradenitis Suppurativa

Hidradenitis suppurativa is a chronic inflammatory vulvar apocrine gland disorder caused by mixed bacterial infection with organisms such as *Staphylococcus, Streptococcus,* and coliform microorganisms. The condition is seen in women of reproductive age. Keratin obstructs the apocrine sweat gland orifice and creates an environment for bacteria to grow. Therefore, a subcutaneous inflammatory process is responsible for nodule formation, leading to abscesses and eventually to fistulas.

Conventional therapy in an advanced stage requires total excision. Occasionally, skin grafting is necessary (52).

Fox-Fordyce Disease

Fox-Fordyce disease is composed of extravasations of previously plugged sweat glands, which cause severe irritation, pruritis, and skin lesions. It is associated with the menstrual cycle, and this condition may simultaneously affect the vulva and the axilla. Due to its cyclicity, oral contraceptive treatment or topical clindamycin in alcoholic propylene glycol solution is suggested (53).

Necrotizing Fasciitis

Necrotizing fasciitis is a potentially life-threatening polymicrobial (commonly anaerobic streptococci and enterococci) vulvar infection. Predisposing factors include: surgical trauma (episiotomy or vulvovaginal surgery, or even transabdominal surgery), focal infection, diabetes mellitus, previous vulvar surgery, arteriosclerosis, vulvar carcinoma, neutropenia, irradiation, and immunosuppression (54).

Diagnosis is established by the clinical course. Symptoms of severe vulvar pain may, at first, seem unjustified on physical findings. A unique clinical finding is the presence of crepitance associated with vulvar pallor edema, anesthesia, and paresthesia. Inflammation rapidly progresses to cellulites with a fishy smell and a watery discharge (fish water); sepsis may develop shortly thereafter.

Conventional therapy consists of stabilizing the patient with adequate intravenous fluid resuscitation and broad-spectrum systemic antibiotics, and cardiopulmonary monitoring should be instituted. Prompt infected tissue excision with a surgical margin of healthy tissue (bleeding and pink color of tissue) is mandatory. It is equally important not to close the area, because sequential repeat debridement is necessary. Delay in diagnosis and therapy longer that 48 hours result in a 78% mortality rate (54).

Complementary and alternative therapies are not available.

Mycotic Vulvovaginitis

Mycotic vulvovaginitis is discussed in Chapter 15.

BENIGN VULVAR NEOPLASIA

Vulvar benign growths can be divided into following categories:

Cysts

Bartholin Cyst

A Bartholin cyst is a cystic dilatation of the Bartholin gland duct due to obstruction of the duct's vestibular orifice. Such obstruction causes Bartholin gland secretion (mucoid, translucent liquid) to accumulate. Cysts may spontaneously regress; however, they have a tendency to recur. If a cyst is associated with primary infection of the Bartholin gland, marsupialization is recommended with placement of a WARD catheter for 3 weeks (55).

Bartholin Abscess

Bartholin abscess results from acquired infection of the Bartholin gland duct. Polymicrobial organisms (*Staphylococcus* or other anaerobic bacteria) frequently cause the infection. Gonococcal bacteria alone are responsible in about 20% to 30% of cases (56). Sequelae of a Bartholin gland abscess are vaginal dryness and dyspareunia. These complications may require surgical intervention with total Bartholin gland excision to treat the dyspareunia and administration of local lubricant for dryness.

Diagnosis is based on clinical identification of vulvar unilateral severe pain and general symptoms of infection such as malaise and low-grade fever. Inspection reveals the reddened Bartholin gland duct swelling and stretching the surrounding tissue to a balloon-like appearance. It is a tender, a cystic structure with nodularity to palpation.

Conventional Therapy

Conventional therapy consists of incision (to avoid vulvar scarring; incision of the abscess should be made at or behind the hymenal ring) and drainage of the abscess. The procedure can be executed in the office setting. A punch-hole can be created with a 6-mm Keyes-punched instrument and a WARD catheter placed for 3 weeks. The refractory abscess to WARD catheter drainage (in the absence of a WARD catheter, an intrauterine device can be inserted) should be treated with marsupialization (partial excision of the ductal distal wall behind the hymenal ring with the edges of the fenestrated duct sutured to the skin). The neostoma formation with a CO_2 laser requires no catheter insertion for the drainage and can be used to preserve gland function (57). This clinical observational study has not been validated by randomized controlled trial. It has been documented in a prospective randomized controlled study that intracavitary insertion of a silver nitrate ($AgNO_3$) stick is as effective as a classic surgical method with a lower complication rate (58).

Parenteral broad-spectrum antibiotic treatment and pain medication with bath sitz are recommended. When gonorrheal infection is present, therapy for both sexual partners is required.

Epithelial Inclusion Cyst

An epithelial inclusion cyst (keratinous cyst) is a superficial cystic structure (2–5 mm in diameter, but can be larger) that originates from sebaceous glands. It has been observed often among circumcised girls and women (59). Carcinoma may arise from this cyst; even though it is not considered a premalignant lesion. Surgical excision is indicated when a cyst becomes secondarily infected or symptomatic, or interferes with coitus (20).

Cyst of the Canal of Nuck

A cyst of the canal of Nuck arises in the area where the peritoneum inserts into the round ligament of the labia majora (20). The round ligament traverses through the Nuck canal, which can herniate and clinically presents as a cystic structure of the vulva. It is important to recognize that herniorrhaphy may injure the intestine. Hernia of the Nuck canal coexists with inguinal hernia in about 30% of cases (60). Repair of this hernia consists of hernia sac excision, high ligation, and reinforcement of the external inguinal ring. Cyst or hernia drainage is an ineffective clinical approach.

Endometriosis

Endometriosis may create a cystic or partially solid structure following episiotomy or other surgical procedures. Symptoms are cyclic and synchronized with the menstrual cycle. Treatment consists of surgical excision.

BENIGN VULVAR SOLID TUMORS

Squamous Epithelial Origin

Acrochordon

Acrochordon or fibroepithelial polyp or skin tag is predominantly a vulvar hair-bearing lesion, but it also may occur on the labia minora. Clinical manifestation varies from hyperpigmented to hypopigmented papillomatous, pedunculated growths. It may be large at presentation, and for cosmetic purpose can be removed. Otherwise, it is a clinically insignificant condition. Atypical changes within acrochordon can be present (61).

Vulvar Vestibular Papilloma

Vulvar vestibular papilloma is a papillary lesion of the vulva that is located on the lateral-posterior surface of the vulvar vestibulum. The etiology is unknown; HPV has been postulated; although, never positively linked to this condition. This entity usually affects women of reproductive age.

Diagnosis is clinical and is based on the presence of burning and itching, and it occasionally may cause superficial (introital) dyspareunia. This vulvar condition also can be asymptomatic. On inspection, it presents as a small (<5 mm in length and 1–2 mm in diameter) papilla forming clusters without inflammation. Histology will distinguish it from HPV.

Conventional therapy is surgical, electrical, or laser excision.

Keratoacanthoma

Keratoacanthoma is proliferation of the squamous epithelium with overdeposition of keratin. The mass is usually located on the hair-bearing skin of the vulva (20). Surgical excision is usually performed for symptomatic lesions.

Glandular Tumors

Hidradenoma

Hidradenoma is an adenoma of the apocrinic sweat gland. It is located on the labia majora or the lateral aspect of the labia minora. The condition usually occurs in white women of reproductive age. Hidradenoma is a mass less than 2 cm in diameter. It is an asymptomatic tumor, if ulceration does not occur. When ulcerative changes develop, surface bleeding can be observed (62). Because vulvar sweat gland carcinomas can occur, clinical recommendation is to remove all of them, even though a hidradenoma is almost always a benign tumor (63).

Syringoma

Syringoma is an adenoma originating from the eccrinic gland duct and can be located on the vulva, axillae, abdomen, cheeks, and eyelids. The lesions may produce itching or can be asymptomatic. It presents as multiple, clustered, flesh-colored papules. When symptomatic, surgical excision is indicated.

Fibroma

A fibroma is a pedunculated firm lesion of the vulva. It may reach several inches or even feet in size. The tumor is removed when it interferes with coitus or purely for cosmetic effect.

Bartholin Gland Solid Tumor

A Bartholin gland solid tumor may project into the vaginal pool and often presents as a vaginal lesion. Adenoma, nodular hyperplasia, and adenomyoma may present as a solid or cystic structure. Because its mean diameter is 2.3 cm, it is often clinically confused with Bartholin cysts. Bartholin gland solid tumors are usually well circumscribed, with varying degrees of inflammation present. Malignancy may coexist with these tumors. Surgical resection is definitive therapy. When malignant, oncology norms should be applied (64).

Vulvar Tumorlike Lesions

Lipoma

A lipoma arises from the vulvar subcuticular fat pads located on the mons pubis and the labia majora. It is a slow-growing tumor and may reach excessive size, protruding from the inguinal area like a pendulum (usual size 10–12 cm). Although, it is a benign tumor, it should be surgically removed before it interferes with coitus or walking.

Ectopic Breast Tissue

Ectopic breast tissue is located as the extension along the mammary line and can be distributed on the vulva unilaterally or bilaterally. Vulvar ectopic breast tissue may lactate during the postpartum period, and frequently the diagnosis is made at this time or during pregnancy (65). Breast fibrocystic disease, fibroadenomas, lactating adenoma, and intraductal papillomas as well as adenocarcinoma of the breast ectopic tissue can occur (20). Surgical extirpation of ectopic breast tissue is recommended when the patient is not pregnant or lactating.

REFERENCES

1. Association of Professors of Gynecology and Obstetrics. *Medical student educational objectives,* 7th ed. Washington, DC: Association of Professors of Gynecology and Obstetrics, 1997.
2. Council on Resident and Gynecology (CREOG). *Educational objectives core curriculum for residents in obstetrics and gynecology,* 5th ed. Washington, DC: CREOG, 1996.
3. American College of Obstetrician and Gynecologists (ACOG). Technical bulletin No. 241. Washington, DC: ACOG, 1997.
4. American College of Obstetrician and Gynecologists (ACOG). Technical bulletin No. 186. Washington, DC: ACOG, 1993.
5. Warrington SA, de San Lazaro C. Lichen sclerosus et atrophicus and sexual abuse. *Arch Dis Child* 1996;75:512–516.
6. Frederich EG, Kaira PS. Serum levels of sex hormone in vulvar lichen sclerosus and the effect of topical testosterone. *N Engl J Med* 1984;310:488–491.
7. Powell J, Wojnarowska F, Winsey S, et al. Lichen sclerosus premenarche: autoimmunity and immunogenetics. *Br J Dermatol* 2000;142:481–484.
8. Meyric Thomas RH, Kennedy CT. The development of lichen sclerosus et atrophicus in monozygotic twin girls. *Br J Dermatol* 1986;114:377–379.
9. Wallace HJ. Lichen sclerosis et atrophicus. *Trans St Johns Hosp Dermatol Soc* 1971;57:9–30.
10. Berth-Jones J, Graham-Brown RAC, Burns DA. Lichen sclerosus et atrophicus—a review of 15 cases in young girls. *Clin Exp Dermatol* 1991;16:14–17.
11. Meyric Thomas RH, Ridley CM, McGibbsons DH, et al. Lichen sclerosus et atrophicus and autoimmunity—a study of 350 women. *Br J Dermatol* 1988;118:41–46.
12. Dalziel KL, Millard PR, Wojnarowska F. The treatment of vulvar lichen sclerosus with a very potent topical steroid (clobesterol proprionate 0.05%) cream. *Br J Dermatol* 1991;124:461–464.
13. Fischer G, Rogers M. Treatment of childhood vulvar lichen sclerosus with potent topical corticosteroids. *Pediatr Dermatol* 1997;14:235–238.

14. Dalziel KL, Wojnarowska F. Long-term control of vulvar lichen sclerosus after treatment with a very potent steroid cream. *J Reprod Med* 1993;38:25–27.
15. Bracco GL, Carli P, Sonni L, et al. Clinical and histologic effects of topical treatments of vulval lichen sclerosus: a critical evaluation. *J Reprod Med* 1993;38:37–40.
16. Shirer JA, Ray MC. Familial occurrence of lichen sclerosus et atrophicus. *Arch Dermatol* 1987:123:485–488.
17. Shenefelt PD. Hypnosis in dermatology. *Arch Dermatol* 2000; 136:393–399.
18. Kubo M, Matsuda H, Dai Y, et al. Studies on kochiae fructus. I. Antipruritogenic effect of 70% ethanol extract from kochiae fructus and its active component. *Yakugaku Zasshi* 1997;117:193–201.
19. *PDR for herbal medicine,* 2nd ed. Montvale, NJ: Medical Economics Company, 2000.
20. Wilkinson EJ. Benign disease of the vulva. In: Kurman RJ, ed. *Blaustein's pathology of the female genital tract.* New York: Springer-Verlag, 1994:31–86.
21. Lawrence WD. Nonneoplastic epithelial disorders of the vulva (vulvar dystrophies): historical and current perspectives. *Pathol Annu* 1993;28:23–51.
22. Cattaneo A, Bracco GL, Maestrini G, et al. Lichen sclerosus and squamous hyperplasia of the vulva. A clinical study of medical treatments. *J Reprod Med* 1991;36:301–305.
23. Rotsztejn H, Krawczyk T, Bartodziej U. Vulvar squamous cell hyperplasia and lichen sclerosus et atrophicus: clinical picture, morphology and treatment. *Ginekol Pol* 1998;89:67–72.
24. Clark TJ, Etherington IJ, Luesley DM. Response of vulvar lichen sclerosus and squamous cell hyperplasia to graduated topical steroids. *J Reprod Med* 1999;44:958–962.
25. Pelisse M. The vulva-vaginal-gingival syndrome. A new form of erosive lichen planus. *Int J Dermatol* 1989;28:381–384.
26. Eisen D. The vulvovaginal-gingival syndrome of lichen planus: the clinical characteristics of 22 patients. *Arch Dermatol* 1994; 130:1379–1382.
27. Soper DE, Patterson JW, Hurt WG, et al. Lichen planus of the vulva. *Obstet Gynecol* 1988;72:74–76.
28. Ridley CM. *The vulva.* Philadelphia: WB Saunders, 1975.
29. Cirigliano MD, Szapary PO. Chamomile for use as anti-inflammatory, antispasmodic, and sedative. *Alternative Med Alert* 1999; Sept:100–104.
30. Boardman LA, Peipert, MD. Vulvar vestibulitis. Is it a defined and treatable entity? *Clin Obstet Gynecol* 1999;42:945–956.
31. Gibbons JM. Vulvar vestibulitis. In: Steege JS, Metzger DH, Levy BS, eds. *Chronic pelvic pain.* Philadelphia: WB Saunders, 1998:181–187.
32. Wijma B, Jansson M, Nisson S, et al. Vulvar vestibulitis syndrome and vaginismus. A case report. *J Reprod Med* 2000;45:219–223.
33. Nunns D, Mandal D. Psychological and psychosexual aspects of vulvar vestibulitis. *Genitourin Med* 1997;73:541–544.
34. Ashman AM, Ott AK. Autoimmunity as a factor in recurrent vaginal candidiasis and the minor vestibular gland syndrome. *J Reprod Med* 1989;34:264–266.
35. Pagano R. Vulvar vestibulitis syndrome: an often unrecognized cause of dyspareunia. *Aust N Z J Obstet Gynaecol* 1999;39:79–83.
36. Mann MS, Kaugman RH, Brown D, et al. Vulvar vestibulitis: significant clinical variables and treatment outcome. *Obstet Gynecol* 1992;79:122–125.
37. Bornstein J, Pascal B, Abramovici H. Intramuscular beta-interferon treatment for severe vulvar vestibulitis. *J Reprod Med* 1993;38:117–120.
38. Glazer HI, Rodke G, Swencionis C, et al. Treatment of vulvar vestibulitis syndrome with electromyographic biofeedback of pelvic floor musculature. *J Reprod Med* 1995;40:238–290.
39. Solomons CC, Memed MH, Keitler SM. Calcium citrate for vulvar vestibulitis. *J Reprod Med* 1991;36:879–882.
40. Pincus SH. Vulvar dermatoses and pruritis vulvae. *Dermatol Clin* 1992;10:297–308.
41. McKay M, Frankman O, Horowith BJ, et al. Vulvar vestibulitis and vestibular papillomatosis: report of the ISSVD Committee on Vulvodynia. *J Reprod Med* 1991;36:413–415.
42. Tuffnell D, Buchan PD. Crohn's disease of the vulva in childhood. *Br J Clin Pract* 1991;45:159–160.
43. Schroeder B. Vulvar disorders in adolescents. *Obstet Gynecol Clin North Am* 2000;27:35–48.
44. O'Duffy JD, Goldstein NP. Neurologic involvement in seven patients with Behçet's disease. *Am J Med* 1976;61:170–178.
45. Hewitt AB. Behçet's disease. *Br J Vener Dis* 1971;47:52–61.
46. Kaufman RH, Frederich EG Jr, Gardner HL. *Benign disease of the vulva and vagina,* 3rd ed. Chicago: Year Book Medical, 1989.
47. Butler EB, Stanbridge CM. Condylomatous lesions of the lower female genital tract. *Clin Obstet Gynecol* 1984;11:171–175.
48. Walker PG, Colley NV, Grubb C, et al. Abnormalities of the uterine cervix in women with vulvar warts. A preliminary communication. *Br J Vener Dis* 1983;59:120–123.
49. Tayal S, Pattman R. High prevalence of herpes simplex virus type 1 in female anogenital herpes simplex in Newcastle upon Tyne. *Int J STD AIDS* 1994;5:359–361.
50. Oberhofer TR, Back AE. Isolation and cultivation of *Haemophilus ducreyi. J Clin Microbiol* 1982;15:625.
51. Douglas CP. Lymphogranuloma venereum and granuloma inguinale of the vulva. *J Obstet Gynecol* 1962;69:871–875.
52. Bhaha NN, Bergman A, Broen EM. Advanced hidradenitis suppurativa of the vulva: a report of three cases. *J Reprod Med* 1984;29:436–440.
53. Feldman R, Masouye I, Chavaz P, et al. Fox-Fordyce disease: successful treatment with topical clindamycin in alcoholic propylene glycol solution. *Dermatology* 1992;184:310–313.
54. Stephenson H., Dotters DJ, Katz V, Droegemueller W. Necrotizing fasciitis of the vulva. *Am J Obstet Gynecol* 1992;166: 1324–1327.
55. Word B. Office treatment of cyst and abscess of Bartholin's gland duct. *South Med J* 1968;61:514–518.
56. Woodruff JD. The vulva. In: Rosenwaks Z, Benjamin F, Stone ML, eds. *Gynecology principles and practice.* New York: Macmillan Publishing, 1987.
57. Davis GD. Management of Bartholin cyst with the carbon dioxide laser. *Obstet Gynecol* 1985;65:279–280.
58. Mungan T, Ugar M, Yalcin H, et al. *Eur J Obstet Gynecol Reprod Biol* 1995;63:61–63.
59. Junard TA, Thomas SM. Cysts of the vulva and vagina: a comparative study. *Int J Gynecol Obstet* 1981;19:239–243.
60. Kucera PR, Glazer J. Hydrocele of the canal Nuck: a report of four cases. *J Reprod Med* 1985;30:439–442.
61. Carter J, Elliott P, Russell P. Bilateral fibroepithelial polypi of labium minus with atypical stromal cells. *Pathology* 1992;24: 37–39.
62. Basta A, Madej JG Jr. Hidradenoma of the vulva. Incidence and clinical observations. *Eur J Gynecol Oncol* 1990;11: 185–189.
63. Wick M, Goellner JR, Wolfe JT 3rd, Su WP. Vulvar sweat gland carcinomas. *Arch Pathol Lab Med* 1985;109:43–47.
64. Koenig C, Tavassoli FA. Nodular hyperplasia, adenoma, and adenomyoma of Bartholin's gland. *Int J Gynecol Pathol* 1998;17: 289–294.
65. Garcia JJ, Verkauf BS, Hochberg CJ, et al. Aberrant breast tissue of the vulva: a case report and review of the literature. *Obstet Gynecol* 1978;52:225–228.

14

PREMALIGNANT AND MALIGNANT VULVAR DISORDERS

EDUCATIONAL OBJECTIVES

Medical Students (1)
APGO Objective No. 55

Vulvar neoplasia:
  risk factors,
  methods of diagnosis,
  diagnosis and management

Residents in Obstetrics/Gynecology (2)
CREOG Objectives

Vulvar malignancies:
  preinvasive vulvar lesions,
  invasive vulvar carcinoma

Practitioners (3)
ACOG Recommendations

Vulvar cancer:
  squamous cell carcinoma,
  melanoma,
  Bartholin gland carcinoma,
  Paget disease of the vulva,
  verrucous carcinoma

VULVAR PREMALIGNANCY

Vulvar Intraepithelial Neoplasia

Definition

An epithelial vulvar cell loses control of progressive maturation from the basal layer toward the epithelial surface, associated with nuclear atypia.

Incidence

The incidence of vulvar intraepithelial neoplasia (VIN) is difficult to determine due to the recent trend of its increasing occurrence in the younger population (20–35 years). VIN may coexist with cervical neoplasia in about 30% and vaginal neoplasia in approximately 4% of cases. VIN and cervical/vaginal neoplasia occurs in about 3% and concomitant anal neoplasia is estimated in 30% of cases (4). The mean age of a patient diagnosed with invasive vulvar carcinoma is 60 years old, 42 years old for carcinoma *in situ* (5).

Etiology

Human papillomavirus (HPV) infection plays a foremost role in the etiology of VIN in the younger population. Approximately 20% of VIN is associated with lichen sclerosus or squamous cell hyperplasia in patients over 60. HPV type 16 is most commonly associated with VIN-3; types 18 and 31 are less frequently linked. Predisposing factors for VIN development include one or more sexually transmitted diseases, immunosuppression, and anal neoplasia (6).

Classification

Classification of VIN is determined by histology (7):

VIN-1: Mild dysplasia demonstrating dysplastic cellular abnormality involves one third of the epithelium from the base layer (the lower third of the epithelium).
VIN-2: Moderate dysplasia is defined when cellular dysplasia extends through one half to two thirds of the epithelium.
VIN-3: Severe dysplasia or carcinoma *in situ* of the vulva is diagnosed when more than two-thirds the full thickness of the epithelium is occupied by dysplastic changes (upper epithelium).

Diagnosis

Pertinent medical history is related to HPV association or its absence in VIN. When HPV is present, burning is the dominant symptom, along with pruritis or pain. In the absence of HPV, pruritis is the leading symptom and burning may or may not be present. Vulvar pruritis is present with VIN in about 50% of cases. However, asymptomatic VIN can be present not only on the vulva but also on the perineum and anus (8). A medical history of sexually transmitted diseases is positive in about 30% of patients. To a lesser extent, hypertension, diabetes mellitus, and obesity demonstrate an association with VIN (9).

On *physical inspection*, the affected vulvar skin area may be red with inflammation or hypervascularization. Brown lesions may be present due to increased melanin accumulation, or the skin may be white-gray color, which is the most common findings (in about two thirds of cases). Applying 3% to 5% acetic acid for 3 to 5 minutes accentuates the whiteness of the skin. VIN lesions are usually 1 to 3 cm in diameter (varying from a few millimeters to large convergent lesions), slightly raised, sharply distinguished from a surrounding area, and multifocal in younger patients and focal in older patients. On the vulva, the labia minora and vaginal introitus are most commonly affected (10). The clitoris can be affected by lesions in about 18% and the urethral meatus in approximately 2% of patients (8).

Vulvar cytology can be very helpful in the diagnosis of VIN. However, the routine cervical or anal cytobrush technique is not used. Gauze impregnated with sterile normal saline is applied to the vulva for 5 minutes to make the keratin softer, then the keratin is scraped off superficially with a scalpel. Upon reducing the keratin layer, the surface is scraped for cytology materials. When a cytology smear demonstrates atypia, dysplasia, or malignancy, a colposcopically directed biopsy or a direct biopsy is indicated (11).

Colposcopic examination results are more difficult to interpret than cervical results because the keratinized epithelium obscures such changes as punctuation or mosaicism of vessels. Nevertheless, vulvar abnormalities can be identified among approximately 58% of patients (12).

A biopsy should be performed on any suspicious vulvar lesion. Under local anesthesia injected with a 30-gauge needle, a Keyes puncher or other instrument can be used to obtain a specimen. The depth of biopsy usually does not reach the full dermal layer [the thickness of the vulvar epithelium ranges from 0.3 to 0.4 mm (13)], and a full-thickness vulvar biopsy is indicated for suspected melanoma, pigmented nevi, or suspicion for invasive malignancy (irregular counters, ulceration of a lesion, or atypical vessels and their branches) (14).

Differential Diagnosis

- Vulvar pruritis disorders
- Vulvar ulcerative disorders
- HPV infection
- Basal cell carcinoma
- Paget disease
- Malignant melanoma
- Previously applied podophyline

Conventional Therapy

It is widely believed that VIN will not progress to invasive squamous carcinoma. However, it has been documented that untreated VIN-3 can develop invasive squamous carcinoma in young women as well as postmenopausal women (15,16). Nevertheless, spontaneous regression is well documented (8). The dilemma is deciding what patients with VIN-1 to treat, because it is not considered a premalignant state (VIN 2 is considered a premalignant lesion).

Among conventional therapy options for VIN, local destruction techniques include the following:

- Laser vaporization for VIN has almost irreplaceable value for VIN, because
- the epithelial surface can regenerate with a minimal scarring effect. The plane of the epithelium also can be visualized when CO_2 laser is coupled with colposcopy. The first plane of the epithelium is the epidermis; second plane the superficial papillary dermis; third plane the superficial reticular dermis (17).
- Chemosurgery therapy consists of application of 5-fluorouracil (5-FU) before surgery (loosens the neoplastic tissue) and the use of a low-power electrical blade (18).
- Laser ablation, under local anesthesia, for focal vulvar lesions yields satisfactory results (19).

Local excision with primary closure is usually executed when a single VIN lesion is present (20). To execute this procedure, scalpel, scissors, electrocautery, or laser can be used.

Skinning vulvectomy with split-thickness skin grafts is recommended for extensive VIN. Skinning vulvectomy is designed to remove only epidermis and dermis (a depth of approximately 3–5 mm) lateral to the hair line (21). The clitoral epithelium, if not affected, should be conserved (22).

Postoperative care is aimed at decreasing pain and burning, and preventing vulvar agglutination. Unfortunately, analgesic itself does not sufficiently control burning. I recommend sitz baths and application of chamomile extract, Dermoplast spray, and local analgesic; however, using spray too close to the postsurgical area may cause irritation. Dermoplast spray also prevents vulvar agglutination by staying on the surface and requires the patient to separate the vulva for appropriate application. Rinsing the vulva with previously boiled water cooled to body temperature with the addition of chamomile extract helps to maintain hygiene as well as to control the burning sensation.

The overall recurrence rate of VIN is estimated to be about 30% or higher when an immunosuppressive disorder is present. To decrease the likelihood of recurrence, all multifocal lesions must be removed beyond the lesion-free margin. Such an approach will decrease the recurrence rate to approximately 10% (23).

Complementary Therapy

A complementary therapy explicitly for VIN is not offered.

Alternative Therapy

Herbal Medicine

The Ebers Papyrus is one of the oldest documents (1550 b.c.) presenting remedies used in the management of vulvar neoplastic disorders. The recipe consists of garlic, horn, bile, dates, and ass's milk. This mixture has not been tested by modern alternative medicine (24).

Calotropis (*Calotropis procera*)

Traditional folk medicine has recommended the use of this preparation for warts; conceivably, it could also be used to treat VIN. Indeed, the powdered root bark of *Calotropis procera* demonstrates an antitumor effect *in vitro* on human epidermoid carcinoma cells; however, no clinical study has sufficiently supported its safety and effectiveness (25).

Celandine (*Chelidonium majus*)

In Chinese traditional medicine, *Chelidonium majus* is used to treat warts. An oncostatic effect of this remedy in nasopharynx cell cultures has been observed. There is no study conducted on vulvar HPV associated with VIN (25).

Paget Disease

The International Society for the Study of Vulvar Disease Task Force formally classifies extramammary Paget disease as an intraepithelial neoplasia (26). Although Paget disease rarely invades from the epithelium, its association with invasive vulvar adenocarcinoma (10%–15%) is often observed within epithelial lesions. Underneath or remote from Paget lesions, the vulvar carcinoma can be located beneath the epithelial lesion (27).

Definition

Paget disease is defined by the presence of atypical glandular apocrine cell proliferation within the vulvar intraepithelium and by the potential of these cells to invade the dermis layer.

Incidence

Paget disease accounts for less than 1% of vulvar lesions (28).

Etiology

The specific etiologic factor has not been established, and an intraepithelial apocrine origin of Paget cells is one of the most compelling hypotheses (29).

Classification

- Superficial Paget disease of the vulva
- Paget disease associated with invasive adenocarcinoma

Diagnosis

Pertinent medical history includes the following:

- Most commonly a patient is in her seventies (median age at diagnosis is 64 years).
- Long-lasting severe vulvar pruritis
- Vulvar discomfort

Physical examination reveals the following (30):

- Lesions are raised and red or bright pink, with well-demarcated edges on the vulvar epithelium. They are dotted with a white area of hyperkeratosis, desquamated, and eczematous. Sharply delineated borders are elusive because the lesion extends beyond the visible abnormality (28).
- Lesions may arise from any area of the vulva or perineum.
- Paget disease has tendency to occur as multifocal lesions.

Direct biopsy, with a Keyes or excisional puncher, and histologic examination verify the clinical diagnosis. Colposcopic magnification and fluorescein-aided visualization of the margin are recommended (31) because skin penetration is greater than can be seen with the naked eye (28).

Histology demonstrates a positive reaction with intracellular mucopolysaccharide.

Differential Diagnosis

- Superficial amelanotic melanoma

Conventional Therapy

Conventional therapy consists of surgery as follows:

- Wide lesion excision
- Surgical resection of the lesion with a free margin at least 2 cm wide (free margin should be determined by intraoperative frozen section histologic examination)
- The depth of excision should incorporate the fat layer, superficial tendon, and muscular tissue in the absence of a vulvar mass.
- Laser ablation for primary surgery is not recommended. However, recurrent Paget disease can be treated by laser ablation followed by wide local excision, provided the absence of adenocarcinoma has been documented (32).

Occasionally extensive local excision requires skin grafting. Such resection significantly decreases the risk for recurrence of the disease. Paget disease associated with invasive adenocarcinoma will require radical surgery with bilateral inguinal-femoral lymphadenectomy. The overall survival rate of Paget disease associated with underlying adenocarcinoma is estimated to be about 90%.

Complementary Therapy

Complementary therapy has not yet been developed for Paget disease.

Alternative Therapy

No alternative therapy is offered for Paget disease.

VULVAR MALIGNANCY

Vulvar malignancies include invasive squamous cell carcinoma, Paget disease associated with adenocarcinoma, melanomas, Bartholin gland adenocarcinoma, basal cell carcinoma, sarcoma, and verrucous carcinoma. The etiology for vulvar cancer is unknown.

Invasive Squamous Cell Carcinoma

Definition

Invasive squamous cell carcinoma is defined as migration of malignant vulvar squamous cells beneath the epithelium.

Incidence

The incidence of squamous cell carcinoma is estimated at approximately 1.5 in 100,000 women of all ages in the United States, and increases to 20 in 100,000 late postmenopausal women (33). It represents approximately 90% of vulvar malignancies and about 5% of all female genital tract malignancies.

Etiology

The explicit etiology of invasive squamous cell carcinoma is unknown. However, approximately 40% of all vulvar squamous cell carcinomas exhibit an association with HPV infection (type 16 is most commonly found and type 18 also can be present) (34). HPV association is found more often among younger women (mean age 55 years) (35), and lichen sclerosus, squamous cell hyperplasia, and squamous cell carcinoma have exhibited an association with older women (mean age 77 years) (36). Vulvar granuloma inguinale can be associated with this type of vulvar carcinoma (37), and tobacco cigarette smoking is linked to invasive squamous cell carcinoma (38). Diabetes mellitus, immunosuppression, and achlorhydria may be associated with vulvar squamous cell carcinoma (7).

Classification

A classification system for invasive squamous cell carcinoma was introduced by the International Society for the Study of Vulvar Disease Task Force (39):

- Superficially invasive squamous cell carcinoma (depth of invasion ≤1 mm and diameter ≤2 cm)
- Invasive squamous cell carcinoma

Diagnosis

Pertinent medical history includes the following:

- Severe long-lasting vulvar pruritis
- Previous HPV or granuloma inguinale infection
- Diabetes mellitus, immunosuppressive conditions (HIV-positive, drug-induced, transplant recipients) or achlorhydria (absence of gastric hydrochloric acid due to gastric mucosa atrophy)
- Cigarette smoking
- Postmenopausal women at a mean age of 61.1; although, younger women can be affected as well

Physical examination on inspection reveals:

- Predominantly focal single lump with raised surrounding lesion
- Ulcerative lesion, red macule, papule, or white hyperkeratotic plaque is observed in superficially invasive squamous cell carcinoma.
  Palpation will demonstrate:
- Indurated and flimsy adjacent tissues are established in superficially invasive squamous cell carcinoma.
- In an invasive form of squamous cell carcinoma, an exophytic papillomatous tumor with or without ulceration can be appreciated.

Vulvar Carcinoma Staging

The staging of vulvar carcinoma requires surgery and provides the information necessary to determine prognosis, treatment options, and clinical research communication, and for statistical registry. Histologic grading of vulvar squamous cell carcinoma provides prediction of the biologic behavior of this cancer. The grade itself is a ratio between the differentiated and undifferentiated area within the neoplastic tumor.

Grade 1 (well-differentiated) tumors display the absence of undifferentiated cells, and grade 3 (poorly differentiated) tumors show a greater than 50% undifferentiated cell component within the tumor. Grade 2 (moderately differentiated) tumors demonstrate less than 50% undifferentiated cells.

The International Federation of Gynecology and Obstetrics (FIGO) provided a recent modification for the staging classification of vulvar invasive squamous cell carcinoma that is currently used in the United States (Table 14.1) (40):

T is carcinoma *in situ*.

T1, tumor is less than or equal to 2 cm in greatest dimension.

T2, tumor is greater than or equal to 2 cm in greatest dimension.

T3, tumor of any size with a local extension to the vagina, urethra, or anus.

T4, tumor of any size invades the bladder mucosa and/or the rectal mucosa or the upper part of the urethral mucosa, and/or is fixed to the pelvic bone.

N stands for regional lymph nodes.

N0, no lymph node metastasis

TABLE 14.1. VULVAR CARCINOMA STAGING: TNM (TUMOR-NODE-METASTASIS)

Stage 0 T is	Carcinoma *in situ* (intraepithelial carcinoma)
Stage I T1 N0 M0	Tumor confined to the vulva and/or perineum; ≤2 cm in greatest dimension; nodes are negative
Stage II T2 N0 M0	Tumor confined to the vulva and/or perineum; ≥2 cm in greatest dimension; nodes are negative
Stage III T3 N0 M0 T3 N1 M0 T1 N1 M0 T2 N1 M0	Tumor of any size with the following: 1. Adjacent spread to the lower urethra and/or the vagina, or the anus, and/or 2. Unilateral regional lymph node metastasis
Stage IV A T1 N2 M0 T2 N2 M0 T3 N2 M0 T4 any N M0	Tumor invades any of the following: upper urethra, bladder mucosa, rectal mucosa, pelvic bone, and/or bilateral regional node metastasis
Stage IV B Any T Any N M1	Any distant metastasis, including pelvic lymph nodes

N1, unilateral lymph node metastasis
N2, bilateral lymph node metastasis
M stands for distant metastasis
M0, no clinical metastasis
M1, distant metastasis (including pelvic node metastasis)

Surgical staging is based on histologic assessment. The extent of the malignant lesion and lymph node involvement are determined from the surgically obtained specimens. Because vulvar cancer spreads by direct extension to the adjacent structures (the vagina, urethra, perineum, and anus) and lymphatic chains to the regional lymph nodes, lymphadenectomy should be performed (approximately 25% of occult metastases have no palpable node). The prevalence of inguinal node metastasis is related to a patient's age, size of the tumor, node invasion, depth of stromal invasion, grade of the tumor, and prevalence of lymphovascular space involvement. An ultrasonographic study may assist in identifying positive inguinal nodes, but is no substitute for biopsy with histologic verification.

Differential Diagnosis

- Verrucous carcinoma
- Vulvar basal cell carcinoma
- Bartholin gland cancer
- Vulvar sarcoma

Conventional Therapy

Vulvar invasive squamous cell carcinoma is conventionally treated by surgical approach, and radiotherapy is added, if indicated.

When the tumor is *located laterally* and is smaller than 2 cm in greatest dimension (early stage), the following procedure can be performed:

- A radial local excision is made with ipsilateral inguinal node dissection when lymphatic nodes are negative on frozen examination. This approach is just as effective as radical vulvectomy for the prevention of vulvar malignancy recurrences (41).
- If more than two *ipsilateral lymphatic nodes* are positive for malignancy, contralateral selective inguinal lymphadenectomy is recommended. If the surgical margin is within 1 cm, adjuvant radiotherapy of the pelvic nodes, inguinal nodes, and vulva is indicated (42).

When the lesion is *centrally located* and in the early stages of disease, a three-incisions radical vulvectomy is recommended, and adjuvant radiotherapy is added as above (42).

If the lesions of *vulvar microinvasive carcinoma* (grade 1 squamous cell) are less than 1 mm thick and located away from the clitoris and peritoneum, the risk for spread to the inguinal nodes is minimal (43). Wide local excision is sufficient treatment for lesions in this location.

In *advanced vulvar cancer* that extends to the urethra, anus, or vagina, exenteration or a very extensive resection is indicated. Neoadjuvant chemoradiation treatment significantly decreases the size of the tumor, obviating the need for more extensive surgical excision of the tumor. Interstitial brachytherapy, with or without external beam radiotherapy, has offered promising results in the treatment of advanced and recurrent vulvar cancer (44).

Complementary Therapy

No definite therapy for vulvar squamous cell carcinoma has been identified.

Alternative Therapy

General therapies for cancer are widely available, but no distinct treatment specifically for this form of vulvar cancer has been identified.

Verrucous Carcinoma

Verrucous carcinoma is a well-differentiated squamous cell hyperkeratotic epithelial tumor. It is a very slow growing and predominantly locally invasive neoplasia with low potential for metastasis (45). The condition may occur in young women (46). The prevalence is estimated to be approximately 6.5% among malignant lesions of the vulva (47).

Diagnosis is based on extensive vulvar pruritis, similar to squamous cell carcinoma. Physical evaluation typically reveals papillary exophytic growth on the labia. This symptom of verrucous carcinoma clinically resembles broad-based condylomata acuminata. When infected, verrucous carcinoma produces an offensive odor and may lead to lymphadenopathy. Such a clinical picture is similar to that of advanced squamous cell carcinoma. Carcinoma *in situ* of squamous cells, condylomata acuminata of the vulva, and carcinoma *in situ* of the cervix may occur concomitantly with verrucous carcinoma (46). HPV, particularly type 6 but also type 11, may occur in concert with verrucous carcinoma (47).

Differential diagnosis is difficult from both a morphologic and clinical standpoint. This condition should be distinguished from squamous cell carcinoma, condylomata acuminata, and warty carcinoma.

Treatment consists of surgery by wide local excision, and attention should be directed to resection of the lesion with a 2-cm free margin to reduce the risk for recurrence (recurrence is associated with a poor prognosis). Local radiation therapy is contraindicated because radiation may induce anaplastic transformation; however, it can be used in very advanced cases (7).

No complementary or alternative therapeutic modalities are offered for this condition.

Vulvar Malignant Melanomas

Definition

Melanoma is a malignant growth of melanocytes (the cells responsible for melanin synthesis) on the epidermal layer of the skin.

Incidence

Vulvar malignant melanoma constitutes 5% to 10% of all malignant lesions of the vulva (48).These entities are the second most common vulvar malignancy, followed squamous cell carcinoma.

Etiology

The cause of melanomas is unknown. They may evolve from benign preexisting pigmented lesions.

Classification

Classification of melanoma is based on microscopic findings, it is divided into three categories (7):

- Superficial, spreading melanoma tends to grow over a long period.
- Nodular melanoma exhibits rapid growth, with deep invasion of surroundings.
- Acral lentiginous melanoma

Superficial, spreading melanoma and nodular melanoma are the types predominantly found on the vulva.

Diagnosis

Pertinent medical history includes the following:

- Expanding existing vulvar mole located most frequently on the clitoris, labia minora, or labia majora
- Vulvar itching
- Vulvar bleeding
- Discharge

Physical examination may reveal the following:

- Slightly elevated pigmented or nonpigmented lesions or nodular tumors may be observed.
- The melanoma may look like nevi.

The definitive diagnosis is provided by a direct lesional biopsy, and its histology determines the type of melanoma, the thickness of the lesion, and the depth of invasion.

The prognostic value of the level of invasion and the thickness of the malignant melanoma has been modified from the skin to meet variation in thickness of the vulvar skin. The risk of metastasis is low when the lesion is less than 0.76 mm thick and the depth of invasion is superficial (49). Advanced age and inguinal node metastasis, at the time of diagnosis, constitute independent prognostic factors. The prognostic criteria can be summarized as follows:

- Clinical criteria
  Location
  Stage
- Histologic criteria
  Growth pattern
  Ulceration of the lesion
  Thickness of the lesion
  Depth of invasion
  Mitosis rate
  Lymph node metastasis
  Invasion of vessels

The following staging system has been adopted for malignant melanoma (50,51):

- *Level I* corresponds to no measurable thickness (depth of invasion of up to 0.75 mm)

- *Level II* lesions are less than or equal to 1 mm thick (depth of invasion of 0.76–1.49 mm)
- *Level III* lesions are 1 to 2 mm thick (depth of invasion of 1.50–4.00 mm)
- *Level IV* lesions are more than 2 mm thick without extension to subcutaneous fat or structures (depth of invasion of >4 mm)

Differential Diagnosis

- Paget disease
- Pigmented VIN
- Nevi
- Vulvar melanosis
- Nonpigmented squamous cell carcinoma

Conventional Therapy

Conventional therapy consists of surgical resection of the melanoma lesion. The type of operation implemented depends on staging:

Level I: *simple excision* of malignant melanoma is recommended (there is no clinical unity on whether or not to perform inguinal node dissection in this stage).

Level II: *radical local excision* of melanoma with a 2-cm free margin, with regional node sampling

Levels III and IV: *radical local excision* with a 3 cm free margin

As a preventive measure, most new pigmented lesions should be removed from the vulva. Lesions that have been there for many years and have remained unchanged should be observed only.

Because total radical vulvectomy does not prevent vulvar recurrence [lesions recur in about 30%–42% of cases (49)] and has a high risk for postoperative morbidity, the above approaches are recommended.

Posttherapeutic recurrence is associated with a poor prognosis. Two groups of patients can be identified:

- Patients at low risk for melanoma recurrence present with a nonulcerative lump less than 3 mm thick, negative inguinal lymphatic nodes, and histologic documentation of a 2- to 3-cm free margin.
- In patients at high risk for melanoma recurrence, the vulvar melanoma lesion is ulcerative and thicker than 3 mm. No dissection had been performed at the initial surgery, and local excision had been used as a treatment modality.

It is worthwhile to mention that adjuvant therapies such as chemotherapy or immunotherapy are not effective in the treatment of malignant melanoma. This finding has been documented in a well-designed, international multicenter randomized controlled study (52).

Vulvar Basal Cell Carcinoma

Basal cell carcinoma is an epithelial tumor with a low potential for metastasis. However, it has the potential for local invasion and destruction. It is frequently found on the skin exposed to sunlight, but is very infrequently found on the vulva.

Clinical diagnosis is derived from vulvar pruritis and the presence of a tumor. A brown or black mass is usually located on the labia majora, and a central ulcer often is present.

Therapy consists of wide local excision with a histologically documented 2- to 3-cm margin free of disease. Inguinal suspicious lymphatic nodes should be removed. Overall prognosis is good when total tumor resection is accomplished. Vulvar recurrence is estimated at 20% following wide excision (53).

Neither *complementary nor alternative therapy* has been specifically developed for vulvar basal cell carcinoma.

Vulvar Sarcomas

Vulvar sarcoma is a tumor arising from a connective component of the vulva. It may occur at any age, and the prognosis depends on the biologic aggressiveness of the specific sarcoma. Several types of sarcomas can affect the vulva.

Epithelioid Sarcoma

Epithelioid sarcoma occurs at a young age and frequently is located either on the labia majora or in the subclitoral area. It presents as a painless vulvar lesion. It is a relatively aggressive tumor and metastasizes early (54).

A definitive diagnosis is reached by direct biopsy with histologic evaluation.

Conventional therapy consists of wide resection or radical vulvectomy with inguinal node dissection, but these procedures are usually ineffective and prognosis is almost always poor.

No *complementary or alternative* management has been developed.

Leiomyosarcomas

Leiomyosarcomas of the vulva are the most commonly occurring lesions among sarcomas and can affect women from 18 to 66 years of age. They may be present on the labia majora, clitoris, or Bartholin gland. The clinical course is protracted, with distant metastasis and vulvar recurrences.

The diagnosis is established on clinical symptoms of vulvar pain and a noticeably growing mass, which on the average is approximately 5 cm in greatest diameter.

Direct biopsy and histology confirm the clinical diagnosis. It metastasizes most commonly to the lungs and liver (55).

Conventional therapy consists of palliative treatment, including surgery, radiotherapy, and chemotherapy, because a cure is not available and the prognosis is poor.

Complementary and alternative therapies are not clinically offered.

Vulvar Kaposi Sarcoma

Kaposi sarcoma is an endothelial tumor that occasionally occurs on the vulva. Its frequent association with AIDS generates the question of whether this lesion is a malignant process per se or a reactive response to HIV infection. The vulva is not a common site of Kaposi sarcoma. However, due to the increasing incidence of HIV infection, the lesion is being seen more on the vulva. Vulvar skin lesions develop from a skin patch to a skin plaque to a nodule as the final stage.

The clinical diagnosis is determined by the presence of an asymptomatic vulvar mass. When local symptoms present, they relate to nerve compression, traction, or nerve entrapment. The definitive diagnosis achieved via histologic verification and a positive test result for HIV infection.

Conventional therapy consists of radical excision with a histologically documented free margin.

The *complementary and alternative therapy* for Kaposi vulvar sarcoma has not yet been developed.

Bartholin Gland Carcinoma

Malignancy that originates from the Bartholin gland must be determined by criteria of a primary neoplasm (histology is consistent with primary malignancy, not metastasis). Several primary malignancies may arise from the Bartholin gland, with the estimated prevalence of adenocarcinoma 40%, squamous cell carcinoma 40%, adenoid cystic carcinoma 15%, transitional cell carcinoma less than 5% (derives from the Bartholin gland duct wall or mucin-secreting gland cells), and adenosquamous carcinoma less than 5%. The Bartholin gland undergoes a spontaneous involution process (maximum size ≤1 cm) that commences after 30 years. Therefore, the presence of a palpable Bartholin gland or its mass in postmenopausal women should be evaluated regardless of the size. Due to the anatomic location of the Bartholin gland (deep within the vulva), it naturally has access to lymphatic chains and blood vessels—both connections predispose the patient to early metastasis to the inguinal and pelvic nodes (56).

The neoplasm affects women 40 to 70 years of age.

The diagnosis is reached by histology, which verifies clinical suspicions and establishes primary or metastatic sources of Bartholin gland malignancy. A solid tumor is usually present (typically 1–7 cm) and infiltrates the adjacent area.

Several options of *conventional therapy* are available, including *wide excision* to the fascia, simple or partial vulvectomy, and radical hemivulvectomy or total vulvectomy with ipsilateral or bilateral inguinal-femoral and pelvic lymphadenectomy; posterior pelvic exonerations also are recommended in selected cases. The overall absolute 5-year cure rate is approximately 66% (57).

Miscellaneous Information

I have attempted to group certain conditions under similar signs and symptoms. Such an arrangement provides reference points, guiding a health-care practitioner in reaching a definitive diagnosis and achieving a differential analysis of a vulvar entity.

The information provided here will facilitate a practitioner's diagnostic process with reference to the specific vulvar conditions discussed in Chapters 13 and 26 (Tables 14.2 and 14.3).

TABLE 14.2. SYMPTOMS OF VULVAR DISORDERS

Vulvar Symptomatology	Vulvar Condition
Vulvar pruritis	Contact dermatitis
	Vulvar atrophy
	Mycotic infection
	Vulvar malignancy
	HPV infection
	HSV infection
	Eczema
	Vulvar dermatoses
	Lice infestation
	Vulvar squamous cell hyperplasia
	Vulvar intraepithelial neoplasia
Vulvar pain	Bartholin infected cyst or abscess
	Granuloma inguinale
	HSV infection
	HPV infection
	Cellulitis
	Hidradenitis
	Necrotizing fasciitis
	Vulvar intraepithelial neoplasia
	Vulvar malignancy
	Lichen sclerosus
	Pelvic support and/or suspension disorder or functional disorder
Vulvar anesthesia	Necrotizing fasciitis
Vulvar bleeding	Vulvar trauma
	Vulvar ulcerative disorders

HPV, human papillomavirus; HSV, herpes simplex virus.

TABLE 14.3. SIGNS OF VULVAR DISORDERS

Vulvar Signs	Vulvar Conditions
Vulvar papules	Syphilis (chancre or condylomata lata)
	Molluscum contagiosum
	Granuloma inguinale
Vulvar erythema	Contact dermatitis
	Mycotic infection
	Folliculitis
	Cellulitis
	Necrotizing fasciitis
	Lichen sclerosus
	Vulvar Paget disease
	Vulvar atrophy
	Lice infestation
Vulvar edema	Contact dermatitis
	Mycotic infections
	Cellulitis
	Vulvar trauma
Vulvar tenderness	HSV infection
	Bartholin gland infected cyst or abscess
	Folliculitis
	Cellulitis
	Necrotizing fasciitis
	Hidradenitis
	Vulvar carcinoma
	Granuloma inguinale
Vulvar ulceration	HSV infection
	Syphilis
	Chancroid
	Lymphogranuloma venereum
	Contact dermatitis
	Vulvar malignancy
Vulvar vesicles	HSV infection
Vulvar leukoplakia	Vulvar Paget disease
	Lichen sclerosus
	Vulvar atrophy
Vulvar induration	Syphilis
	Hidradenitis
	Necrotizing fasciitis
Vulvar atrophy	Lichen sclerosus
	Senile atrophy
Vulvar mass	Condylomata acuminata
	Vulvar intraepithelial neoplasia
	Nevus
	Bartholin gland abscess or tumor
	Vulvar carcinoma
	Malignant melanomas
	Chancroid
	Lymphogranuloma venereum
	Hidradenitis
Vulvar sinus	Crohn disease
	Lymphogranuloma venerum
	Hidradenitis

REFERENCES

1. Association of Professors of Gynecology and Obstetrics. *Medical student educational objectives,* 7th ed. Washington, DC: Association of Professors of Gynecology and Obstetrics, 1997.
2. Council on Resident and Gynecology (CREOG). *Educational objectives core curriculum for residents in obstetrics and gynecology,* 5th ed. Washington, DC: CREOG, 1996.
3. American College of Obstetricians and Gynecologists (ACOG). Technical bulletin No. 186. Washington, DC: ACOG, 1993.
4. Kaplan AL, Kaufman RH, Birken RH, et al. Intraepithelial carcinoma of the vulva with extension to the anal canal. *Obstet Gynecol* 1981;58:368–371.
5. Woodruff JD. Carcinoma *in situ* of the vulva. *Clin Obstet Gynecol* 1991;34:669–676.
6. Crum CP. Carcinoma of the vulva: epidemiology and pathogenesis. *Obstet Gynecol* 1992;79:448–454.
7. Wilkinson EJ. Premalignant and malignant tumors of the vulva. In: Kurman RJ, ed. *Blaustein's pathology of the female genital tract,* 4th ed. New York: Springer-Verlag, 1994:87–129.
8. Frederich EG Jr, Wilkinson EF, Fu YS. Carcinoma *in situ* of the vulva. A continuing challenge. *Am J Obstet Gynecol* 1980;136:830–843.
9. Powell LC Jr, Dinh TV, Rajaraman S, et al. Carcinoma *in situ* of the vulva. A clinicopathologic study of 50 cases. *J Reprod Med* 1986;31:808–814.
10. Japaze H, Garcia-B, Garcia-Bunnel R, et al. Primary vulvar neoplasia: a review of *in situ* and invasive carcinoma 1935–1972. *Obstet Gynecol* 1977;49:404.
11. Koss LG. *Diagnostic cytology and its histopathologic bases,* 4th ed. Philadelphia: JB Lippincott, 1992.
12. Iversen T, Abeler V, Kolstad P. Squamous carcinoma *in situ* of the vulva: a clinical and histopathologic study. *Gynecol Oncol* 1981;11:224–229.
13. Benedet JL, Wilson PS, Matisic J. Epidermal thickness and skin appendage involvement in vulval intraepithelial neoplasia. *J Reprod Med* 1991;36:608–612.
14. DiSaia PJ, Creasman WT. *Clinical gynecologic oncology,* 4th ed. St. Louis: Mosby Year Book, 1993.
15. Buscema J, Woodruff JD. Progressive histobiologic alterations in the development of vulvar cancer. *Am J Obstet Gynecol* 1980;138:146–150.
16. Jones RW, McLean M. Carsinoma *in situ* of the vulva. A review of 31 treated and five untreated cases. *Obstet Gynecol* 1986;68:499–503.
17. Reid R. Superficial laser vulvectomy. III. A new surgical technique for appendage-conserving ablation of refractory condylomas and vulvar intraepithelial neoplasia. *Am J Obstet Gynecol* 1985;152:504–509.
18. Morrow CP, Townsend DE. *Synopsis of gynecologic oncology,* 3rd ed. New York: Churchill Livingston, 1987:8–14.
19. Ferenczy A. Using the laser to treat vulvar condylomata acuminata and intraepithelial neoplasia. *Can Med Assoc J* 1983;128:135–137.
20. Sillman FH, Sedlis A, Boyce J. A review of lower genital intraepithelial neoplasia and use of topical 5-fluorouracil. *Obstet Gynecol Surv* 1985;40:190–220.
21. Rutledge F, Sinclair M. Treatment of intraepithelial carcinoma of the vulva by skin excision and graft. *Am J Obstet Gynecol* 1968;102:806–808.
22. DiSaia PJ, Rich WM. Surgical approach to multifocal carcinoma *in situ* of the vulva. *Am J Obstet Gynecol* 1981;140:136–145.
23. Kaufman RH, Friedrich EG Jr, Gardner HL. *Benign disease of the vulva and vagina,* 3rd ed. Chicago: Year Book Medical, 1989.
24. Ebbell B. *The papyrus ebers.* London: Oxford University Press, 1937.
25. *PDR for herbal medicines.* Montvale, NJ: Medical Economics Company, 2000.
26. Iversen T, et al. Surgical-procedure terminology for the vulva and vagina. A report of the International Society for the Study of Vulvar Disease Task Force. *J Reprod Med* 1990;35:1033–1034.
27. Koss L, Ladinsky S, Brockunier A. Paget's disease of the vulva: report of 10 cases. *Obstet Gynecol* 168;31:513–525.

28. Gunn RA, Gallager HS. Vulvar Paget's disease: a topographic study. *Cancer* 1980;46:590–594.
29. Bacchi CE, Goldfogel GA, Greer BE, et al. Paget's disease and melanoma of the vulva. Use of a panel of monoclonal antibodies to identify cell type and to microscopically define adequacy of surgical margins. *Gynecol Oncol* 1992;46:216–221.
30. Taylor PT, Stenwig JT, Klausen H. Paget's disease of the vulva. *Gynecol Oncol* 1975;3:46–60.
31. Misas JE, Cold CJ, Hall FW. Vulvar Paget disease: Fluorescein-aid visualization of margins. *Obstet Gynecol* 1991;77:156–159.
32. Ewing TL. Paget's disease of the vulva treated by combined surgery and laser. *Gynecol Oncol* 1991;43:137–140.
33. Henson D, Tarone R. An epidemiologic study of the cancer of the cervix, vagina, and vulva based upon the Third National Cancer Survey in the United States. *Am J Obstet Gynecol* 1977; 129:525–532.
34. Pilotti S, Rotola A, D'Amato L, et al. Vulvar carcinomas: search for sequences homologous to human papillomavirus and herpes simplex virus DNA. *Mod Pathol* 1990;3:442–448.
35. Kurman RJ, Toki T, Schiffman MH. Basaloid and watery carcinoma of the vulva. Distinctive types of squamous cell carcinoma frequently associated with HPV. *Am J Surg Pathol* 1993;17: 133–145.
36. Toki T, Kurman RJ, Park JS, et al. Probable nonpapillomavirus etiology of squamous cell carcinoma of the vulva in older women: a clinicopathologic study using *in situ* hybridization and polymerase chain reaction. *Int J Gynecol Pathol* 1991;10:107–125.
37. Hay DM, Cole FM. Postgranulomatous epidermoid carcinoma of the vulva. *Am J Obstet Gynecol* 1970;108:479–484.
38. Daling JR, Sherman KJ, Hislop TG, et al. Cigarette smoking and the risk of anogenital cancer. *Am J Epidemiol* 1992;135:180–189.
39. Burdick B. Clarifying the "Report of ISSVD Terminology Committee." *J Reprod Med* 1988;33:97–98.
40. International Federation of Gynecology and Obstetrics. *Annual report on the results of treatment in gynecological cancer,* 22nd ed. Stockholm: International Federation of Gynecology and Obstetrics, 1994.
41. Magrina JF, Gonzales-Bosquet J, Weaver AL, et al. Squamous cell carcinoma of the vulva stage IA: long-term results. *Gynecol Oncol* 2000,76:24–27.
42. Hacker NF. Radical resection of vulvar malignancies: a paradigm shift in surgical approaches. *Curr Opin Obstet Gynecol* 1999; 11:61–64.
43. Sedlis A, Homesley H, Bundy BN, et al. Positive groin lymph nodes in superficial squamous cell vulvar cancer. A Gynecologic Oncology Group Study. *Am J Obstet Gynecol* 1987;156:1159–1164.
44. Tewardi K, Cappuccini F, Syed AM, et al. Interstitial brachytherapy in the treatment of advanced and recurrent vulvar cancer. *Am J Obstet Gynecol* 1999;181:91–98.
45. Brisigotti M, Moreno A, Murcia C, et al. Verrucous carcinoma of the vulva. A clinicopathologic and immunohistochemical study of five cases. *Int J Gynecol Pathol* 1989;8:1–7.
46. Dinh TV, Powell LC, Hanninan EV, et al. Simultaneously occurring condylomata acuminata, carcinoma *in situ* of the vulva and carcinoma *in situ* of the cervix in a young woman. *J Reprod Med* 1988;33:510–513.
47. Kondi-Paphitis, Deligeorgi-Politi H, Liapis A, et al. Human papilloma virus in verrucous carcinoma of the vulva: an immunopathological study of three cases. *Eur J Gyneaecol Oncol* 1998;19:319–320.
48. Morrow CP, Rutledge FN. Melanoma of the vulva. *Obstet Gynecol* 1972;39:745–752.
49. Podratz KC, Gaffey TA, Symmonds RE, Johansen KL, O'Brien PC. Melanoma of the vulva: an update. *Gynecol Oncol* 1983; 16:153–168.
50. Chung AF, Woodruff JM, Lewis JL. Malignant melanoma of the vulva: a report of 44 cases. *Obstet Gynecol* 1975;45:638–646.
51. Breslow A. Tumor thickness, level of invasion and node dissection in stage I cutaneous melanoma. *Ann Surg* 1975;182: 572–575.
52. Veronesi U, Adamus J, Aubert C, et al. A randomized trial of adjuvant chemotherapy and immunotherapy in cutaneous melanoma. *N Engl J Med* 1982;307:913–916.
53. Cruz-Jimenez PR, Abel MR. Cutaneous basal cell carcinoma of the vulva. *Obstet Gynecol* 1975;36:1860–1868.
54. Ulbright TM, Brokow SA, Stehman FB, et al. Epithelioid sarcoma of the vulva. Evidence suggesting a more aggressive behavior than extragenital epithelioid sarcoma. *Cancer* 1983;52: 1462–1469.
55. Tavassoli FA, Norris HJ. Smooth muscle tumors of the vulva. *Obstet Gynecol* 1979;53:213–217.
56. Chamilian DL, Taylor HB. Primary carcinoma of the Bartholin's gland. A report of 24 patients. *J Obstet Gynecol* 1973;39: 489–494.
57. Haberthur F, Almendral AC, Ritter B. Therapy of vulvar carcinoma. *Eur J Gynecol Oncol* 1993;14:218–227.

15

VAGINAL DISORDERS

EDUCATIONAL OBJECTIVES

Medical Students (1)
APGO Objective No. 38

Normal vaginal appearance
  and secretions
Evaluation and management:
  vaginitis due to bacteria,
  fungi, trichomonads,
  virus, foreign body, and
  atrophy
Trauma

Residents in Obstetrics/Gynecology (2)
CREOG Objectives

Vaginal infections:
  medical history,
  physical examination,
  diagnostic studies
Diagnosis
Management
Follow-up
Vaginal intraepithelial neoplasia
Vaginal carcinoma

Practitioners (3)
ACOG Recommendations

Vaginal ecosystem
Evaluation of the vagina
Candidal vaginitis
Bacterial vaginosis
Trichomonas vaginalis
Other conditions

VAGINAL EMBRYOLOGY

The embryology of the vagina is not fully understood. The hypothesis of mesodermal (upper vagina) and endodermal (lower vagina) origin is generally accepted (4). Two pairs of genital ducts-the müllerian (paramesonephrotic) ducts and the wolffian (mesonephrotic) ducts—are present before sexual differentiation. In the absence of the Y chromosome, the wolffian ducts regress and the müllerian ducts develop (the absence of müllerian inhibiting factor and androgens promotes this event). At approximately 37 day of embryonic female life, the paramesonephrotic (müllerian) ducts develop in the mesonephrotic ridge as funnel-shaped, contoured openings of the celomic epithelium (5). These pair of ducts expend caudally to join the posterior urogenital sinus. The strait uterovaginal canal with the longitudinal septum is created by midline fusion of the caudal part of the müllerian ducts in approximately 54 postconceptual days. Fusion of the caudal part of the müllerian ducts with the urogenital sinus creates the müllerian tubercle and the sinovaginal bulbs bilaterally. Additional proliferation of these structures eventually creates the vaginal plate, which by growing will move apart the uterocervical canal from the urogenital sinus, creating a space for vaginal plate canalization. In about 5 months (18th–20th weeks of gestation), canalization of the vaginal plate process is accomplished by central cell degeneration and resorption. Hymen formation

separates the vaginal lumen from the urogenital lumen (4,5). According to this dual-duct theory, the upper four fifths of the vaginal canal and its squamous cell epithelium comes from paramesonephric (mesodermal) ducts transformed by a metaplastic process of the columnar epithelium and one fifth of the lower vaginal canal arises from the urogenital sinus (4).

VAGINAL ANATOMY

The vagina is a sheathlike organ. Its walls are created from musculomembranous structures with the ability to distend from a naturally collapsed state.

The vaginal lumen ends are limited by fusion with the cervix and by the hymen (the thin membranous fold at the vaginal orifice). The vagina traverses parallel to the rectum and levator plate in a resting state with the angle approximately 130 degrees. The angle created between the vaginal axis and the cervical angle is about 90 degrees. In a mature woman, the vagina is an average of 9 cm in length (8–10 cm) and has small circumferential folds termed vaginal rugae. The vaginal rugae will become less prominent after childbirth and lose even more prominence in the postmenopausal period. The vagina is surrounded by the urethra and bladder anteriorly and separated by the vesicovaginal and urethrovaginal septum (part of the endopelvic fascia). Posteriorly, the perineal body (at the distal part), rectal ampulla (middle third), and posterior cul-de-sac of Douglas are adjacent to the posterior vaginal wall. These structures are separated from the vagina by the fascia of Denovillieres, which stretches from the perineal body to the posterior cul-de-sac of Douglas, to which the posterior vagina attaches. The upper part of the vagina includes the ectocervix, and both of these structures (the vagina and ectocervix) form four vaginal fornices (two lateral fornices and an anterior and posterior fornix). The posterior fornix is the deepest one and is 3 cm longer than the anterior fornix due to anterior cervical attachment; it serves as a reservoir to collect ejaculate. The cervix aligns perpendicularly to the posterior vaginal wall. Such cervical projection and position place the external os of the cervical canal in direct contact with semen. The lateral vaginal walls exhibit much less flexibility than anterior or posterior walls. The anterior fornix is adjacent to the bladder base and to the proximal urethra, which is loosely connected to the vaginal wall. This loose connection disappears when the urethra inserts distally and fuses with the vaginal wall fascia, creating one structure. The ureters traverse just 1 to 2 cm above the lateral fornices, before piercing the bladder wall. Before opening to the vulvar vestibulum, the vagina is partially enclosed by the bulbocavernosus and the levator ani muscles.

Laterally, the superior vaginal sulci suspend the vaginal walls by attaching to the tendinous arch in the mid-pelvis. Superiorly, the cardinal ligaments support the upper vagina together with the cervix.

At the junction of the lower third and middle part of the vagina, the vagina pierces the hiatus of the levator ani (the pubococcygeal portion) muscle and runs in parallel alignment to the rectum (Fig. 15.1).

Blood supply to the vagina originates from the internal iliac artery (hypogastric artery) and its branches, such as the vaginal artery, uterine artery, middle rectal artery, and the pudendal arteries. The plexus of uterine veins, rectal veins, and pudendal veins conducts blood return, draining into the inferior iliac vein (Fig. 15.2).

The lymphatic system can be divided into the following components:

- The upper anterior vagina or anterior apex drains to the external iliac lymph nodes (the cervical path).
- The posterior vagina drains to the inferior gluteal, sacral, and anorectal lymphatic chain.
- The distal vagina drains into the femoral nodes (Fig. 15.2).

Vaginal innervation comes from pelvic plexus (Fig. 15.3).

The vaginal wall contains the mucosa (superficial layer), which is created by the nonkeratinizing, glucogenated squamous epithelium, which has an irregular surface due to the presence of 2- to 5-mm thick rugae. The framework of the mucosal epithelium demonstrates the presence of the following layers (6).

- Basal layer or stratum cylindricum
- Parabasal layer or deep spinous layer
- Intermediate layer or superficial spinous layer
- Intraepithelial layer or granular cell layer
- Superficial layer or stratum corneum

The epithelium, which lines the vagina, also covers the ectocervix and supposedly has two functions: protecting the underlying tissue and producing glycogen (nourishment for microorganisms and possibly for spermatozoa). The mucosa itself is not equipped with either a glandular component or hair follicles. By the desquamation process, vaginal cells break away from the epithelium, which can be collected and evaluated for hormonal influence, inflammatory reaction, premalignancy, and malignancy.

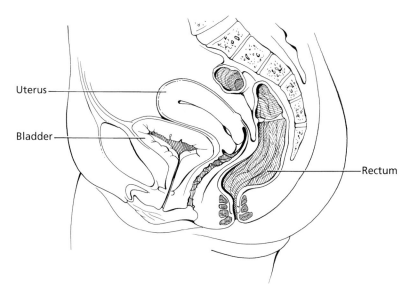

FIGURE 15.1. Vaginal natural position in relationship to adjacent structure.

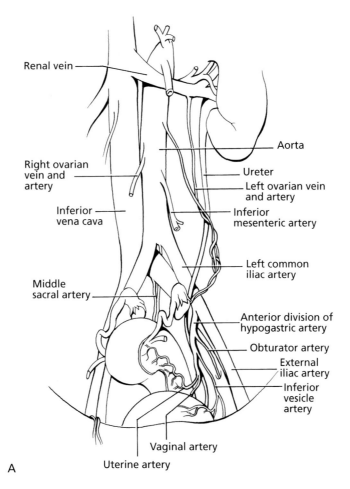

Renal vein

Aorta

Right ovarian
vein and
artery

Ureter

Left ovarian vein
and artery

Inferior
vena cava

Inferior
mesenteric artery

Left common
iliac artery

Middle
sacral artery

Anterior division of
hypogastric artery

Obturator artery

External
iliac artery

Inferior
vesicle
artery

Vaginal artery

Uterine artery

A

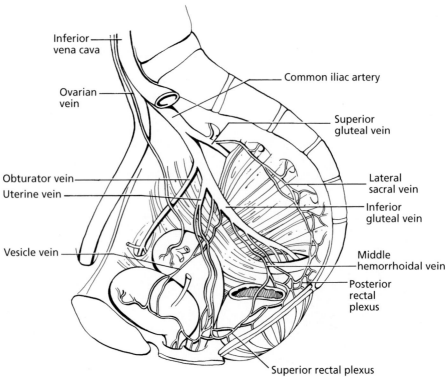

Inferior
vena cava

Common iliac artery

Ovarian
vein

Superior
gluteal vein

Obturator vein

Uterine vein

Lateral
sacral vein

Inferior
gluteal vein

Vesicle vein

Middle
hemorrhoidal vein

Posterior
rectal
plexus

B

Superior rectal plexus

FIGURE 15.2. A: Pelvic artery blood supply. **B:** Pelvic vein blood return.

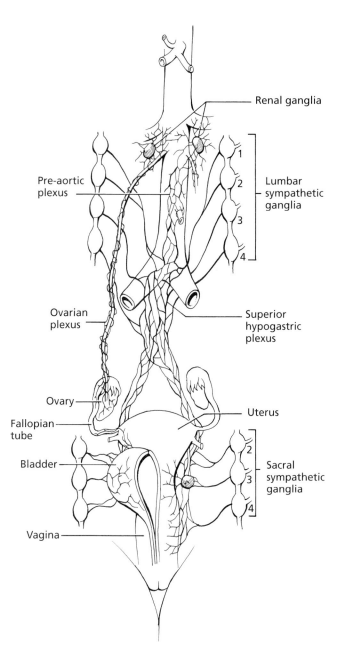

Renal ganglia

1
2 } Lumbar sympathetic ganglia
3
4

Pre-aortic plexus

Ovarian plexus

Superior hypogastric plexus

Ovary

Uterus

Fallopian tube

Bladder

2
3 } Sacral sympathetic ganglia
4

Vagina

FIGURE 15.3. Nerve distribution to female pelvic organs.

The muscularis (mid-layer) is composed of three layers:

■ Outer longitudinal muscles
■ Inner circular muscles
■ The adventitia (deep layer) consists of connective tissue, nerves, and blood vessels.

VAGINAL NATURAL MICROENVIRONMENT

Doderlein first scientifically studied a healthy vaginal ecosystem and he published the results in 1892 (7). The vaginal microenvironment is maintained in a healthy state

of vaginal mucosa, vaginal pH, hormonal milieu, and microorganisms. The vaginal epithelium is rich in estrogen receptors, which respond with proliferation under natural endogenous or exogenous estrogen stimulation (maturation of the stratified epithelium, glycogen storage from the intermediate layer up, and increased tissue blood circulation). Natural vaginal microorganisms coexist commensally, synergistically, or antagonistically. Numerous microorganisms, such as gram-positive and gram-negative aerobic, and facultative and obligate anaerobic bacteria, are natural inhabitants of the vaginal pool.

Disturbances in this natural equilibrium between the vaginal epithelium and microflora can lead to changes in microorganism density and species composition or may allow a new colonization by exogenous microorganisms (8).

Several factors, such as antibiotics, hormonal milieu (including oral contraceptives), coitus or changing sexual partners, barrier contraceptives, vaginal douches, infections, foreign body, stress, and immunologic status, can produce a vaginal ecologic imbalance (9,10).

Lactobacillus acidophilus bacteria use glycogen, present in the cells of intermediate and superficial layers of the vaginal stratified squamous epithelium, to produce lactic acid through a fermentation process. Lactic acid is a part of the vaginal microenvironment that maintains the normal vaginal acidity ranges from pH 3.8 to 4.2 (8,9).

VAGINITIS

Vaginitis is defined as an inflammatory process affecting the vaginal mucosa causing over 10 million office visits in the United States (11). Vaginitis may result from infections [candidiasis, trichomoniasis, and bacterial vaginosis (BV)] or from noninfectious vaginitis that can occur as a local allergic reaction, or mimic vaginitis associated with lower urinary tract infection (UTI) or cervicitis.

Symptomatology of vaginitis is a combination of vaginal discharge, offensive odor, pruritis, burning, and vaginal discomfort. Systemic clinical evaluation of vaginitis includes the following:

■ Inspection may reveal hyperemia and edema of the vaginal introitus and walls on speculum examination.
■ Vaginal culture is often indicated.
■ pH determination is a good predictor of vaginal microenvironment imbalance.
■ Microscopic examination of a wet-mount specimen is helpful in the initial determination of mycotic, bacterial, or *Trichomonas* infection, or a combination of the same. A drop of vaginal discharge is placed on a microscopic glass slide and is separately diluted with a drop of normal saline and a drop of 10% KOH (potassium hydroxide).
■ A cytologic smear from the vaginal or cervical canal may establish the presence of fungal flora. The results of this

examination correspond with mycotic culture in about 80% of cases (12).

■ Palpation can demonstrate tenderness of the vagina.

INFECTIOUS VAGINITIS
Mycotic Vaginal Infection
Definition

Mycotic vaginitis is defined as vaginal inflammation due to fungal infection.

Incidence

The prevalence of fungal infection in women is estimated to be approximately 37.2% (11).

Etiology

Candida albicans is the etiologic cause for mycotic vaginitis in about 85% of cases (11). *Torulopsis globrata, Candida tropicalis* and *pseudotropicalis, Geotrichum candidum, Aspergillus, Trichothecium, Saccharomyces, Rhodotorula,* and Penicillum account for the remainder of the mycotic vaginitis cases (13).

Predisposing factors, such as diabetes mellitus, oral contraceptives, pregnancy, antibiotics, and tight-fitting clothes, are often associated with mycotic vaginitis. Sexual transmission is indicated as a form of contamination in some cases, either vaginal-receptive or oral-genital practices (14). Contrary to popular belief, it has not been proved by scientific clinical study that bathtubs or toilet seats may have a role in the transmission of mycotic flora infection (15).

Classification

■ Saprophytic, asymptomatic presence of mycotic flora in the vaginal pool accounts for 20% to 30% of cases (3,16).

■ Symptomatic mycotic vaginitis is often termed as candidal vaginitis or candidiasis (this nomenclature reflects only *Candida* as the active pathogen, which may not correspond to etiologic factors).

Diagnosis

Pertinent medical history is characteristic for the following:

■ Itching in the vulvovaginal area is a dominant symptom
■ Vaginal "cottage cheese–like" discharge
■ Burning is present at the introitus to the vagina, vulvar vestibulum, and vulva (not a dominant symptom, but gets worse with micturition and coitus).
■ Presence of a predisposing factor is frequently reported.

Physical examination usually discloses the following:

■ Thick, white (cottage cheese–like) discharge
■ Vaginal mucosa is edematous and inflamed. Pseudomembrane of adherent granular debris to the vaginal walls can be noted; when removed, the vaginal mucosa is red with shadow erosion.
■ When color of the discharge changes and an offensive odor occurs, a mixed infection should be suspected.

Laboratory test may confirm the clinical presumption:

■ $pH \leq 4.0$
■ *Wet-mount* from vaginal discharge suspended in 10% KOH under light microscopic examination can identify pseudohyphae and blastospores of mycotic cells in about 50% to 85% of cases (17,18).
■ *Culture* (either Sabaroud agar or Nickerson medium) is used in more difficult cases and is usually confirmatory in 94% of patients (18). However, it is not routinely recommended (3).
■ *Cytology* may identify yeast in approximately 46% of cases (18). This test is not performed for this condition and usually is reported from cervical smear.

Differential Diagnosis

■ Other vaginal infections manifesting with vulvovaginal itching and vaginal discharge
■ Noninfectious vulvovaginal infection presenting pruritis, vaginal discharge, and vaginal discomfort. Further discussion of these conditions is provided in Chapters 13 and 14.

Conventional Therapy

Conventional therapy is effective with administration of suppositories, vaginal cream, or an oral single-dose agent, depending on the preferences of the patient. Medications are often used for mycotic vulvovaginitis and available over the counter, or by prescription for local or oral use.

■ Over-the-counter
Clotrimazole, 5 g of 1% vaginal cream for 7 to 14 days
Clotrimazole, 100-mg vaginal tablet, four times daily for 7 days
Miconazole, 5 g of 2% cream for 7 days
Miconazole, 100-mg vaginal suppositories for 7 days
■ By prescription for local use
Butoconazole, 5 g of 2% vaginal cream for 3 days
Clotrimazole, 500 mg vaginal tablet in a single dose is equally effective as a 3-day trial of clotrimazole 100-mg tablets administered twice daily (19)
Miconazole, 200-mg vaginal suppositories for 3 days
Terconazole, 5 g of 0.4% vaginal cream for 7 days (20)
Terconazole, 5 g of 0.8% vaginal cream for 3 days
Terconazole, 5 g of 6.5% vaginal ointment (single-dose)
Terconazole, 80 mg vaginal suppository for 3 days
■ By prescription for oral use

Fluconazole, 150 mg single oral dose proved to be as effective and safe as intravaginal clotrimazole, 100 mg for 7 days (21).

Intravaginal local antifungal therapy or a single oral dose in no pregnant women is clinically effective treatment. Topical cream should be considered as first-line treatment; however, the single oral dose appears to have better compliance among the patients (22).

Complementary Therapy

Although acupuncture has been used successfully for severe and recurrent oral mycotic mucosal infection (23), no data are available that scientifically validate the use of acupuncture for vulvovaginitis.

Patient Education

Patient education, particularly among women who have recurrent mycotic vaginitis [at least four times per year, estimated to occur in about 5% of cases (24)], should concentrate on self-diagnosis and self-therapy under practitioner supervision. A patient's introduction to mycotic vaginitis, from a holistic approach, should concentrate not only on selection of an appropriate antifungal medication but also on how to improve the local vaginal and systemic immune system functions, to restore normal pH balance and natural vaginal microflora, to decrease vaginal inflammation, and to relieve symptoms. A patient must become a partner in the management of this condition with regard to diet implementation, nutritional supplements, botanical remedies, and personal vulvovaginal hygiene. Patients also should know about the potential of recurrence not necessarily associated with a new infection but with a saprophytic, asymptomatic state of fungal presence in the vaginal pool. Self-diagnosis and self-treatment is crucial so that the patient understands the potential of other infections, mimicking yeast, that may lead to severe clinical sequelae.

Diet

A diet to support the management of mycotic vaginitis should include the following foods:

- Well-balanced whole food low in fat
- Eight ounces unsweetened acidophilus yogurt daily
- Avoidance of fermented food, sugar, refined carbohydrates, and alcohol

Nutritional Supplements

The following nutritional supplements may be used.

Vitamins

- *Vitamin E* in the form of a vaginal suppository or gelatin caps once or twice daily for 7 days. Vitamin E ointment or oil can be applied to the vulva at the same time (25).

- *Vitamin A* supposedly stimulates a vaginal mucosa immune system (26). Vaginal suppositories or gelatin capsules can be taken once daily for 7 days. Suppositories can be alternated with other vaginal remedies.

Alternative Therapy

Herbal Remedies

- *Garlic* (*Allium sativum*) retards the growth of *Candida albicans* and exhibits antifungal properties (27). A garlic clove is peeled and introduced into the vaginal pool for 6 to 8 hours (creating a garlic clove chain helps to remove it from the vagina). Usually, garlic treatment is combined with lactobacillus capsules (e.g., garlic in the morning and lactobacillus at bedtime) (26).
- *Goldenseal* (*Hydrastis canadensis*) can be used in liquid extract form ($^1/_4$ to 1 teaspoon) added to vaginal douching (in conventional gynecology, douching is not recommended) or suppositories. This remedy expresses both antibacterial and antifungal activities; therefore, it can be administered intravaginally in mixed infection in the form of suppositories (solid extract 325–520 mg) (26,28).
- *Orange grape root* (*Berberis vulgaris*) has a similar active antifungal and antibacterial component (berberine sulfate) and is recommended for mixed vaginitis (28).
- *Tea tree* or *Melaleuca alternifolia* is administered in the liquid extract form for vaginal douching for 30 seconds followed by insertion of a tampon saturated with the liquid extract (29).
- *Pau d'arco, lapacho, or taheebo* has antifungal activity when taken as tea, three to six cups daily (30).
- *Solanum nigrescens* vaginal suppositories (50% *S. nigrescens* macerated in ethanol) administered for 15 days yields a beneficial effect similar to that from nystatin vaginal suppositories (31).

No clinical research study has been identified that supports these botanical, traditional medicine approaches.

Other Treatment Agents

Boric acid, 600 mg in a gelatin capsule, is administered intravaginally for 14 days (32). Boric acid is seldom used in the United States owing to lack of a well-designed randomized controlled study documenting its usefulness.

Mycotic forms of vaginitis have been treated with *Lactobacillus* in a lyophilized suspension of live *Lactobacillus acidophilus*. This supportive treatment is administered intravaginally. The natural suspension of lyophilized *Lactobacillus acidophilus* (producing lactic acid) not only has the ability to restore vaginal pH to its normal levels but also inhibits fungal growth. Acidification of the vaginal microenvironment to the expected physiologic norms with a lyophilized form of bacteria promotes natural inhabitants of *Lactobacillus acidophilus* to proliferate in the affected vagina (optimum pH 3.5–4.5) (13,33). The recommended dose of the lyophilized suspension is once daily in combination with an antifungal agent for 7 days in acute mycotic vaginitis. To prevent recurrent infection, it can be administered once or twice weekly (33), and gelatin capsule is recommended once or twice daily (34). During systemic antibiotic therapy, administration of lactobacilli may prevent mycotic vaginitis.

Gentian violet has been used during pregnancy. The speculum must be used to apply gentian violet to the vaginal walls and ectocervix. Without the vaginal speculum and for patient convenience the following compound formula can be prescribed particularly during pregnancy:

- Gentian violet 0.2%
- Lactic acid 3.0%
- Acetic acid 1.0%
- Polyethylene glycol base

Such a formula reportedly provides cure in 78% and significant improvement in about 12% of patients when administered at bedtime once daily for 12 days (35).

Iodine is available for vaginal application in the form of povidone-iodine solution for swabbing, povidone-iodine vaginal gel with an applicator, and povidone-iodine douche. Today, douching is not recommended in clinical practice because it dilutes and washes off natural vaginal microflora, which is essential in maintaining the equilibrium of the vaginal ecosystem. Povidone-iodine can be applied to the ectocervix and vaginal walls under direct visualization using a vaginal speculum. Povidone-iodine gel can be administered intravaginally (5 g per application) at bedtime for 14 days. This mode of therapy is also effective when *Trichomonas* vaginitis coexists with mycotic vaginitis (36).

Bacterial Vaginosis

Definition

Bacterial vaginosis (BV) is defined as disproportional overgrowth of multiple vaginal colonizing bacteria.

Incidence

The prevalence of BV is estimated at 1.6% based on clinical criteria and approximately 4.5% based on Gram stain in a low-risk female population (37). This recent estimate does not correlate with the previously reported 10% to 25% (3).

Etiology

A simultaneous overgrowth of *Gardnerella vaginalis, Bacteroides, Mobiluncus curtisi, Pseudostreptococcus* species, *Mycoplasma hominis, Mobiluncus mulieris,* and other members of Enterobacteria is considered an etiologic factor in BV (3).

Diagnosis

Clinical criteria have been established to reach the diagnosis of BV (38):

- Homogenous, thin, malodorous vaginal discharge
- Vaginal pH more than 4.5
- Vaginal epithelial cells with numerous attached bacteria (clue cells)
- Fishy odor upon alkalization with 10% KOH of vaginal secretion (positive whiff test)

The correlation of clinical criteria with Gram stain appears to be poor and its use has been questioned (37).

Pertinent medical history usually is presented as follows:

- Vaginal offensive, fishy odor and discharge
- Vaginal and vulvar irritation may occur when vaginal discharge is perfused. Such vulvovaginal irritation may clinically express as itching or burning.

Physical examination is usually within normal limits; nevertheless, vaginal discharge in excessive quantity may be observed. Vaginal discharge is homogenous, thin, gray-white or dark, or dull gray.

Laboratory Tests
- *Whiff test:* a drop of vaginal discharge suspended in 10% KOH on a microscopic slide produces a characteristic offensive fishy odor (positive whiff test).
- Wet-mount test: a drop of vaginal discharge suspended in normal saline on a microscopic slide and light microscopic evaluation shows numerous bacteria with different morphologic appearance, clue cells, and absence or significantly reduced *Lactobacillus acidophilus* bacteria.
- Vaginal culture is not routinely recommended, but in selected cases, mycotic or *Trichomonas* vaginitis should be ruled out or BV is refractory to conventional therapy.
- When the diagnosis of BV is established, a patient should be tested for gonorrhea and chlamydia infections. If test results for these conditions are positive, patient should be tested for syphilis, hepatitis B, and HIV infection (3).

Differential Diagnosis

- Mycotic vaginitis
- *Trichomonas* vaginitis

Conventional Therapy

Conventional therapy emphasis is on treatment of the anaerobic microorganism, either with local vaginal treatment or oral administration of medication.

Metronidazole, 250 to 500 mg orally twice daily for 7 days is effective treatment in approximately 90% of patients. A single 2-g dose of metronidazole is as effective as a 7-day course (39,40). However, meta-analysis showed that the single dose may be less effective, with a success rate of 69% to 72% (39). During the course of a metronidazole therapy, alcohol consumption should be avoided, because this combination may cause vomiting.

Metronidazole, 0.75% gel inserted into the vaginal pool twice daily for 7 days, also is recommended. However, a randomized controlled study documented that once-daily intravaginal administration of 0.75% metronidazole gel for a 5-day course yields efficacy, safety, and tolerance equivalent to twice-daily dosing (41).

Clindamycin, orally 300 mg twice daily for 7 days, is also an effective mode of therapy (40).

Clindamycin, 2% vaginal cream applied twice daily, is recommended for BV treatment (40). Clindamycin can be administered either intravenously, orally, or vaginally (3).

Treatment of a symptomatic patient with BV is straightforward; therapy for an asymptomatic patient with documentation of BV is controversial. It has been documented that postoperative infection and complications during pregnancy (e.g., premature rupture of membranes, chorioamnionitis, or postpartum endometritis) are associated with asymptomatic BV (42).

Complementary Therapy

No clinical management suggestion is available for BV therapy.

Patient Education

Patient education is similar to that suggested for mycotic vaginitis, with emphasis on diagnostic process, mode of therapy, and potential sequelae. A preoperative patient may be advised to take medicine and finish before elective surgery is performed. For emergency surgery, either intravenous or oral clindamycin can be administered. Women in early pregnancy and in a symptomatic or asymptomatic state should receive appropriate treatment with clindamycin to prevent development of the severe sequelae of this relatively benign process.

Diet

The general suggestion is to adhere to a diet that enhances the immune system. This approach is described in the section on mycotic vaginitis. Refined food and simple carbohydrates should be avoided. At least 8 ounces of unsweetened yogurt should be consumed daily to increase the population of lactobacilli in the vagina.

Alternative Therapy

Herbal Remedies

Herbal remedies can be used in both mixed and single infections, because some of these remedies express antifungal and antibacterial properties. The following botanical medicine is recommended (26):

- *Goldenseal* (*Hydrastis canadensis*) solid extract, 325 to 352 mg in powder capsule form at bedtime (see also section on mycotic vaginitis)
- *Barbery* or Oregon grape root powder capsule at bedtime
- *Garlic* either fresh or capsules, orally one capsule once or twice daily
- *Povidone-iodine* can be applied to the ectocervix and vaginal walls twice weekly.
- *Sexual abstinence* should be advised for the course of the therapy to eliminate reinfection and microtrauma to the vaginal mucosa.

Trichomonas Vaginitis (Trichomoniasis)

Definition

A vaginal mucosa inflammation induced by *Trichomonas vaginalis* is considered a sexually transmitted infection.

Incidence

The prevalence of symptomatic *Trichomonas* vaginitis among women is estimated to be approximately 3.2% (43). However, in randomly selected women attending a sexually transmitted disease clinic, *Trichomonas vaginalis* organisms can be detected by wet-mount microscopic examination or culture in approximately 15% of cases (44).

Etiology

Trichomonas vaginalis, a parasitic, flagellate, motile protozoan, causes *Trichomonas* vaginitis. It is a sexually transmitted disease, but organisms have been shown to stay alive in chlorinated swimming pools, soapy water, and bath water (14).

Diagnosis

The diagnosis of *Trichomonas* vaginitis is not easy to reach because the symptoms are similar to those of other sexually transmitted diseases and there is no precise method of detection. Patients with multiple sex partners, abnormal vaginal discharge, and more than 10 white blood cells per high-power field on wet-mount preparation are at increased risk for *Trichomonas vaginalis* infection (45). Asymptomatic infestation with *Trichomonas vaginalis* may also occur and is estimated to account for up to 50% of the cases (44). Systemic infection with this protozoon has not been observed.

Pertinent Medical History

- Vaginal discharge is present in about 72% of cases (46)
- Dysuria can be present, because the urethra and bladder mucosa can be affected
- Dyspareunia with temporal exacerbation before menses may occur
- Vulvovaginal itching can be present
- Vulvar irritation may be present

Physical Examination

- A thin, yellow-green vaginal discharge is observed, occasionally with an offensive odor.
- A frothy type of discharge is identified in about 35% of cases (3).
- Physical examination may reveal no vaginal discharge.
- The vaginal mucosa usually is erythematous, with petechia-like striations. The vulva also may be erythematous.
- The ectocervix may have punctate submucosal hemorrhages, also known as strawberry cervix (colpitis macularis), which is observed in fewer than 25% of women with this condition (45).

Laboratory

- Vaginal pH of greater than 4.5 (usually 5.0–6.5)
- A fresh wet-mount direct microscopic examination can establish the diagnosis. A wet-mount microscopic examination of saline vaginal discharge suspension may show the presence of a motile, flagellate organism in 50% to 60% of cases (47). *Trichomonas vaginalis* in its live form is a pear-shaped organism with flagella, which are larger then leukocytes, and move with a snakelike motion.
- Microscopic features characteristic of Papanicolaou stain of a vaginal smear can identify *Trichomonas vaginalis* in about 70% of cases (48).
- Culture media (Trichicult, Diamond, or InPouch TV) have a sensitivity of approximately 89% (47). Culture or direct immunofluorescent staining of vaginal fluid can be used in subclinical (asymptomatic) infestation (44). Culture is indicated when persistent vaginal discharge is present and a fresh wet-mount preparation reveals numerous leukocytes; or when trichomoniasis is refractory to metronidazole therapy (49).

Differential Diagnosis

- BV
- Mycotic vaginitis

Conventional Therapy

Conventional treatment consists of systemic administration of metronidazole, because trichomoniasis may affect not only the vagina but also the bladder and urethra.

In general gynecologic practice, a physician may face the clinical dilemma of the safety of metronidazole during pregnancy. Meta-analysis showed that *in utero* fetal exposure to metronidazole in early pregnancy (first trimester) does not increase the teratogenic risk (50,51).

The following dosages of systemic metronidazole are recommended:

- *Metronidazole*, 250 mg three times daily for a 7-day course
- *Metronidazole*, 500 mg twice daily for a 7-day course
- *Metronidazole*, 2 g in a single dose

It is widely believed that a sexual partner should be treated because trichomoniasis is a sexually transmitted disease.

A specific therapy refractory to metronidazole trichomoniasis has not been developed. The recommended treatment is at least 2.5 g a day or more, with an intravaginal suppository of 500 mg taken once or twice daily for at least 10 days (3).

In selected cases, intravenous metronidazole 500 mg every 8 hours is recommended (52).

Follow-up and additional testing is indicated when both partners comply with the treatment and still are symptomatic. Routine follow-up is not necessary.

Complementary Therapy

Complementary approach to *Trichomonas* vaginitis has not been offered.

Patient Education

Patient education is provided in the context of sexually transmitted diseases. Participating in a monogamous relationship and practicing safe sex are essential. Potential protection against infections may be achieved with condom use, but this is not a fail-safe method of protection from sexually transmitted diseases. Patients should be informed about diagnostic procedures and treatment, and advised about compliance with a management plan to avoid reinfection. Synchronized treatment of both partners is essential. If this is not possible, abstinence from sex should be observed until after both partners complete their treatment regimen.

Diet

No specific diet is recommended in the treatment of trichomoniasis, but avoidance of alcohol, sugar, and refined carbohydrates is suggested, and consumption of 8 ounces of unsweetened yogurt daily for 1 month can provide general support (26).

Alternative Therapy

Herbal Remedies

No scientific data are available that support the use of herbal medicine for the treatment of *Trichomonas vaginalis*. Natural folk medicine offers unproven use of *tea tree oil* (*Melaleuca alternifolia*) (26). A 40% water-miscible emulsified solution is mixed with tea tree, 40% oil, and 13% isopropyl alcohol. This mixture is used to saturate a tampon, which is inserted intravaginally for 24 hours. This medication can be applied on the vulva, if necessary. Vaginal douching with tea tree oil 0.4% in one quart of water can be used.

Other natural botanical remedies also have been used to support the immune system, such as garlic, goldenseal, echinacea, licorice, and myrrh.

LESS COMMON VAGINAL INFECTIONS

Group B Streptococcus

Group B streptococcus is present in the vaginal pool of up to 35% of women (53), and these bacteria can be transmitted either from the intestine or via sexual intercourse (54). This infection carries little risk of morbidity in women. However, an increased obstetric risk for mothers includes intrapartum and postpartum bacteremia, increased abortion and perinatal mortality rates, chorioamnionitis, premature rupture of membranes, and premature delivery. This infection can be vertically transmitted from mother to neonate, who can be affected by early or late onset of disease (53). The Centers for Disease Control and Prevention screening-based guidelines for obstetric care may reduce the early-onset group B streptococcal sequelae significantly when implemented properly (55).

Conventional therapy is penicillin, when treatment is indicated.

Vaginal Actinomycetes

Vaginal actinomycetes (*Actinomyces*) are gram-positive, non–spore-forming anaerobic bacteria that are part of the natural oral flora, but they also are found in the bronchi, gastrointestinal tract, and female genital tract. Occasionally, actinomycetes cause infection of the upper genital tract in association with an intrauterine device. This infection can affect the vagina. The drainage pus sulfur granules, a yellow accumulation of the organisms, can assist in the diagnostic process. Infection occurs when the integrity of the vaginal mucosa is disrupted. The most common clinical findings is "woody" induration of the vaginal wall. Actinomyces can be identified by Papanicolaou stain or by histology. Conventional therapy consists of oral penicillin or amoxicillin for 6 to 12 months (56).

Emphysematous Vaginitis

Emphysematous vaginitis is a benign, self-limited condition of unknown etiology and pathogenesis characterized by countless gas-filled spaces in the subepithelial lining of the vaginal wall. It has been reported to be associated with *Trichomonas* vaginitis and *Gardnerella* vaginitis (BV) (57). It also has been associated with systemic disease or pregnancy (58).

The diagnosis is based on symptoms of popping sounds during coitus. Vaginal discharge is the most common complaint related to this condition. When underlying vaginal infection is identified, specific symptoms can be present representing specific infection. The diagnosis and treatment of any underlying condition assists resolution of emphysematous vaginitis.

The diagnosis of this entity is clinical if the vaginal crepitating sound can be elucidated. Radiographic evaluation provides a characteristic appearance (59).

VAGINAL NONINFECTIOUS INFLAMMATORY DISORDERS

Allergic Reaction to Seminal Fluid

Allergic reaction to seminal fluid is an uncommon allergic response to ejaculate contact. *Symptoms* include local vulvovaginal severe itching and burning during or soon after intercourse, usually lasting for 48 to 72 hours, but these symptoms also may occur in a chronic form. Occasionally, generalized urticaria and bronchospasm with episodic wheezing dyspnea are observed and cause clinical concerns with life-threatening potential (60).

Physical examination shows local vulvovaginal transient edema, redness, and smooth and slightly elevated wheals (patches) (61).

The diagnosis is made clinically by exclusion of other allergens and confirmed by a simple clinical skin prick test (dilutions of seminal plasma or whole semen). Condom use can aid in self-diagnosis (62,63). It is a self-limited condition upon removal of the allergen.

Treatment may include vaginal desensitization (64) or condom use, which is not total protection due to potential rupture and simultaneous allergic reaction to latex and to seminal fluid (65).

Using condoms therapeutically may lead inadvertently to infertility that can be successfully treated with a washing sperm process and separation of sperm from plasma by a continuous-step density gradient centrifugation method (62).

Crohn Disease

Crohn disease can affect the vagina by creating fistulas. Rectovaginal fistulas (65) and fistulas of the sigmoid colon or cecum have been reported (67). Treatment focuses on resolution of the underlying disease and surgical repair of fistulas.

Desquamative Inflammatory Vaginitis

Desquamative inflammatory vaginitis is a vaginal inflammatory reaction to an unknown etiologic factor. It predominantly affects women of reproductive age with preservation of normal ovarian function. It manifests as copious blood-stained purulent vaginal discharge. Vaginal pH is elevated. Papanicolaou stain for cytology evaluation demonstrates increased parabasal cells in an otherwise normal estrogenic state (similar changes are observed in atrophic vaginitis as a response to hypoestrogenism). Gram stain microscopic evaluation of vaginal discharge shows the absence or relative absence of *Lactobacillus acidophilus* bacteria and their replacement by gram-positive cocci (68).

Physical examination may show ulcerative lesions partially covered with pseudomembrane in the upper vagina. Vaginal synechiae and stenosis can develop (69).

Treatment with local or systemic corticosteroids yields unsatisfactory results (69). It was reported that clinically significant improvement (>95%) was achieved with clindamycin 2% suppositories; however, relapse occurred in 30%. A postmenopausal woman also requires estrogen replacement therapy combined with clindamycin (68).

Vaginal Bullous Dermatoses

Vaginal bullous dermatoses are characterized by ulceration of the vaginal mucosa leading to vaginal adhesions, stenosis, or complete obliteration. Vaginal bullous dermatoses result from a severe form of Stevens-Johnson syndrome (bullous erythema multiforme) manifested by oral and genital erosion, ocular inflammation, and skin bullae. They may be induced by bacterial or viral infection, reaction to sulphonamides, allergic reaction, or reaction to other drugs, including antibiotics. This can be a life-threatening condition when general toxicity or fluid loss occurs and renal failure develops (70,71).

Steven-Johnson syndrome is a self-limited condition that requires immediate supportive management with intravenous fluid treatment. It may result in fluid loss, sepsis, and death. Vulvovaginal sequelae such as vaginal mucosal damage, vaginal stenosis, or obliteration can be corrected by surgical reconstruction (71).

OTHER VAGINAL DISORDERS

Atrophic Vaginitis

Atrophic vaginitis is a reflection of the hypoestrogenic state (postmenopausal, premature ovarian failure, either spontaneous or induced by antiestrogen medication), in which the vaginal squamous epithelium become thinner and vaginal pH increases due to decreased *Lactobacillus acidophilus*. Such natural events predispose the patient to colonization of the vaginal pool by other microorganisms, such as streptococci, staphylococci, diphtheroids, and *Escherichia coli*. Microtrauma to the vaginal mucosa creates an environment for infection to develop. Approximately 40% of hypoestrogenic women have symptoms of atrophic vaginitis. The symptoms range from an asymptomatic state, to decreased vaginal lubrication (the earliest symptom), to a watery vaginal discharge that may be blood stained, to light vaginal bleeding, to dyspareunia, to itching, to dysuria. Physical examination provides additional clinical information, such as pale smooth mucose (loss of rugae) with the appearance of petechiae on the vaginal mucosa. Systemic or local treatment with estrogen restores the vaginal ecosystem and relieves the symptoms. Vaginal moisturizers, lubricant, and regular sexual intercourse are beneficial (72). Hormonal therapies are detailed in Chapter 12.

Vaginal Vault Granulation Tissue

Development of vaginal vault granulation tissue is a frequent complication of total hysterectomy. On inspection, one or more small, red, granular or polypoid lesions are observed at the apex of the vaginal vault, usually producing a vaginal discharge. Therapy is observation when the lesion is no larger than 5 mm, because spontaneous regression occurs in about 52% of patients within 20 weeks after hysterectomy (73). If granulation tissue is persistent or vaginal discharge or postcoital vaginal spotting occurs, granulation tissue should be removed. The prevalence of this complication can be reduced by substituting a chromic catgut suture either to a synthetic polymer (74) or absorbable staples (75).

Vaginal Postoperative Pseudosarcoma

Vaginal postoperative pseudosarcoma is an infrequently occurring benign vaginal nodule. It presents clinically with a blood-stained vaginal discharge, usually 1 to 3 months after surgery. Physical examination shows a nodule or polyp. It may occur in any body region where surgery is performed. Histology of the nodule mimics leiomyosarcoma, in which cellular spindle cells proliferate with numerous mitoses and minimal or no cytonuclear atypia present (76,77). *Treatment* is local excision (77,78).

It is essential to distinguish this tumor from leiomyosarcoma to avoid exposing the patient to unnecessary radical surgery such as total hysterectomy or total colpectomy, or to external radiation therapy (78).

Vaginal Radionecrosis

Vaginal radionecrosis may result in stromal fibrosis, small vessel obliteration, vaginal mucosa ulceration, and formation of granulation tissue or polyps. The vulva and vagina should be treated surgically with local excision, radical local excision, or exenteration (79). It has been suggested that hyperbaric oxygen therapy can be beneficial (80).

Vaginal Fistulas

Vaginal fistulas are artificial communications between the vagina and its adjacent organs. They may result from complications of systemic disorders, of obstetric or surgical origin, or from radiation treatment or coital laceration. Vaginal fistulas causing continuous urinary incontinence are discussed in Chapter 25. Fistulas causing fecal incontinence are discussed in Chapter 26.

Conventional therapy for fistulas is surgical correction with removal of granulation, fibrosis, inflammatory tissue, and little, if any, epithelium.

Complementary therapy with hyperbaric oxygen therapy is suggested, based on the results of an observational case clinical study (81).

Vaginal fistula formation may occur in the anterior vaginal compartment, central compartment, or posterior compartment. Fistulas in the *anterior vaginal compartment* have the following features:

- *Urethrovaginal fistulas* may result from all the causes described above. Another cause is associated with periurethral collagen injection for the treatment of urinary incontinence.
- *Vesicovaginal fistulas* may have multifactorial causes. A neglected vaginal silicone Gellhorm pessary eroded in one woman's bladder for several years, forming a fistula (82). It has also been reported that urine components within fistulas may occasionally form calculi (83). Surgical repair is executed via an abdominal or vaginal approach, and a translaparoscopic approach also has been used. However, only one case report is presently available (84).
- *Urethrovaginal fistulas* may cause continuous urinary incontinence, which is discussed in Chapter 25. The treatment is ureteroneocystostomy, most commonly performed with overall satisfactory outcomes (85).
- All fistulas in the anterior location present with urinary incontinence. The diagnosis usually is clinical and can be verified by intravenous pyelography or cystography, or by urethrocystoscopy.

Fistulas in the *central vaginal compartment* have the following features:

- *Uterovaginal fistulas* are usually sequelae of surgical reconstruction or extensive resection in the posterior cul-de-sac and posterior uterine wall. The diagnosis creates a clinical dilemma, and hysterosalpingography may assist in reaching the diagnosis.
- *Tubovaginal fistulas* have been reported after vaginal hysterectomy. Therapy consists of removing the affected fallopian tube with fistula repair (86).

Fistulas of the *posterior vaginal compartment* have the following features:

- *Rectovaginal fistulas* can develop from multiple causes as described above. H-type rectovaginal fistulas can be associated with the Currariono triad (anorectal stenosis, sacral defect, and presacral mass). Feces are usually present in the vaginal pool; symptoms of intestinal subocclusion can be identified. Such cases are seen in pediatric gynecology, and surgical correction of all abnormalities is necessary (87).
- *Anovaginal fistulas* are a rare complication of episiotomy or other obstetric procedures. They can be anocutaneous, anovaginal, suprasphincteric, or transsphincteric. Fistulotomy with sphincteroplasty is a successful therapeutic approach (88).

Fibrin glue application has been used in small clinical series for the treatment of recurrent anorectal fistulas. Preliminary results are appealing, and the procedure can be offered as an alternative approach to conservative surgical management (89).

Fallopian Tube Prolapse

Fallopian tube prolapse is classified as a vaginal condition due to manifestation of predominantly vaginal symptoms. Dyspareunia appears to be the most common symptom in about 44%, vaginal bloody discharge is reported in 39%, vaginal discharge in 28%, and persistent pelvic pain in 28% (90). Fallopian tube prolapse is a complication associated with hysterectomy either via laparotomy or vaginal approach.

The diagnosis is clinical, and cytology findings may help to establish diagnosis (90); histology is not as reliable as would be expected. Laparoscopic verification with salpingectomy at the same time is a reliable paradigm.

Conventional therapy is surgical excision (salpingectomy) of the prolapsed fallopian tube transvaginally, transabdominally, or translaparoscopically.

Spontaneous resolution can be expected in approximately 41% of cases. Therefore, reassurance and observation of the patient should be part of the management plan, particularly when a patient is asymptomatic or minimal symptoms are present (90).

REFERENCES

1. Association of Professors of Gynecology and Obstetrics. *Medical student educational objectives,* 7th ed. Washington, DC: Association of Professors of Gynecology and Obstetrics, 1997.
2. Council on Resident and Gynecology (CREOG). *Educational objectives core curriculum for residents in obstetrics and gynecology,* 5th ed. Washington, DC: CREOG, 1996.
3. American College of Obstetricians and Gynecologists (ACOG). Technical bulletin No. 226. Washington, DC: ACOG, 1996.
4. Cunha GR. The dual origin of the vaginal epithelium. *Am J Anat* 1975;143:387–392.
5. Robboy SJ, Taguchi O, Cunha GR. Normal development of the human female reproductive tract and alternation resulting from experimental exposure to diethylstilbestrol. *Hum Pathol* 1982;13;190–198.
6. Koss LG, Durfee GR. Diagnostic cytology and its histologic bases. Philadelphia: JB Lippincott, 1961.
7. Doderlein A. Die Scheidensekretuntschugen. *Zentralbl Gynakol* 1894;18:10–14.
8. Larsen B. Vaginal flora in health and disease. *Clin Obstet Gynecol* 1993;36:107–121.
9. Mardh PA. The vaginal ecosystem. *Am J Obstet Gynecol* 1991;165:1163–1168.
10. Kent HL. Epidemiology of vaginitis. *Am J Obstet Gynecol* 1991;165:1168–1176.
11. Foxman B, Barlow R, D'Arey H, et al. Candida vaginosis. Self-reported incidence and associated costs. *Sex Transm Dis* 2000;27:230–235.
12. Oriel JD. Genital yeast infections. *BMJ* 1972;4:761–764.
13. Ostrzenski A. An own complex method of treatment in cases of fungal vaginitis. *Pol Tyg Lek* 1975;30:1657–1659.
14. Friedrich EG. Vaginitis. *Am J Obstet Gynecol* 1985;152:247–251.
15. Andrew DE, Bumstead E, Kemptom AG. The role of fomites in transmission of vaginitis. *Can Med Assoc J* 1975;112:1181–1183.
16. Oriel JD. Clinical overview of candidal vaginitis. *Proc R Soc Med* 1977;70(suppl 4):7–10.
17. Pattman RS, Sprott MS, Moss TR. Evaluation of a culture slide in the diagnosis of vaginal candidosis. *Br J Vener Dis* 1981;57:67–69.

18. McLennan MT, Smith JM, McLennan CE. Diagnosis of vaginal mycosis and trichomoniasis: reliability of cytologic smear, wet smear and culture. *Obstet Gynecol* 1972;40:231–234.

19. Fleury F, Hughes D, Floyd R. Therapeutic results obtained in vaginal mycoses after single-dose treatment with 500 mg clotrimazole vaginal tablets. *Am J Obstet Gynecol* 1985;152:968–970.

20. Weisberg M. Terconazole—a new antifungal agent for vulvovaginal candidiasis. *Clin Ther* 1989;11:659–668.

21. Sobel JD, Brooker D, Stein GE, et al. Single oral dose fluconazole compared with conventional clotrimazole topical therapy of *Candida* vaginitis. Fluconazole Vaginitis Study Group. *Am J Obstet Gynecol* 1995;172:1263–1268.

22. Reef SE, Levine WC, McNeil MM, et al. Treatments options for vulvovaginal candidiasis, 1993.*Clin Infect Dis* 1995;20(suppl 1): 80–90.

23. Chopra D, ed. Alternative medicine. The definitive guide. Tiburon, CA: Future Medicine Publishing, 1997:592–593.

24. Faro S. Systemic vs. topical therapy for the treatment of vulvovaginal candidiasis. *Infect Dis Obstet Gynecol* 1994;1:202–208.

25. Ant M. Diabetic vulvovaginitis treated with vitamin E suppositories. *Am J Obstet Gynecol* 1954;67:407–409.

26. Hudson T. *Women's encyclopedia of natural medicine. Alternative therapies and integrative medicine.* Los Angeles: Keats Publishing, 1999.

27. Adetumbi M, Javor G, Lau B. *Allium sativum* (garlic) inhibits lipid synthesis by *Candida albicans. Antimicrob Agents Chemother* 1986;30:499–501.

28. Amin A, Subbaiah T, Abbasi K. Berberine sulfate: antimicrobial activity, bioassay, and mode of action. *Can J Microbiol* 1969;15: 1067–1076.

29. Williams L, Home V. A comparative study of some essential oils for potential use in topical applications for the treatment of the yeast *Candida albicans. Aust J Med Herbal* 1995;7:57–62.

30. Pizzorno JE, Murray MT, eds. A textbook of natural medicine. Seattle, WA: John Bastyr College Publications, 1989.

31. Giron LM, Aguilar GA, Caceres A, et al. Anticandidal activity of plants used for the treatment of vaginitis in Guatemala and clinical trial of a *Solanum nigrescens* preparation. *J Ethnopharmacol* 1988;22:307–313.

32. Van Slyke KK, Michel VP, Rein MF. Treatment of vulvovaginal candidiasis with boric acid powder. *Am J Obstet Gynecol* 1981; 141:145–148.

33. Ostrzenski A. Lyophilized suspension of life *Lactobacillus acidophilus* in supportive treatment of mycotic forms of vaginitis in women. *Pol Tyg Lek* 1974;29:925–926.

34. Hilton E, Rindos P, Isenberg H. Lactobacillus GG vaginal suppositories and vaginitis. *J Clin Microbiol* 1995;33:1433.

35. Waters E, Wager H. Vaginal mycosis in pregnancy: an improved gentian violet treatment. *Am J Obstet Gynecol* 1950;60:885–887.

36. Ratzan J. Monilial and trichomonal vaginitis topical treatment with povidone-iodine preparations. *Calif Med* 1969;110:24–27.

37. Gratacos E, Figueras F, Barranco M, et al. Prevalence of bacterial vaginosis and correlation of clinical to Gram stain diagnostic criteria in low risk pregnant women. *Eur J Epidemiol* 199;15:913–916.

38. Amsel R, Totten PA, Spiegel CA, et al. Nonspecific vaginitis. Diagnostic criteria and microbial and epidemiologic associations. *Am J Med* 1983;74:14–22.

39. Lugo-Miro VI, Green M, Mazur L. Comparison of different metronidazole therapeutic regimens for bacterial vaginosis. A meta-analysis. *JAMA* 1992;268:92–95.

40. Centers for Disease Control and Prevention. 1993 sexually transmitted transmitted diseases guidelines. *MMWR* 1993;42:1–102.

41. Livengood CH 3rd, Soper DE, Sheehan KL, et al. Comparison of once-daily and twice-daily dosing of 0.75% metronidazole gel in the treatment of bacterial vaginosis. *Sex Transm Dis* 1999;26: 137–142.

42. Thomason JL, Gelbert SM, Scaglione NJ. Bacterial vaginosis: current review with indications for asymptomatic therapy. *Am J Obstet Gynecol* 1991;165:1210–1217.

43. Soszka S, Kazanowska W, Kuczynska K, et al. *Trichomonas vaginitis* at different life stages of women. *Wiad Parazytol* 1990; 36:211–217.

44. Wolner-Hanssen P, Krieger JN, Stevens CE, et al. Clinical manifestations of vaginal trichomoniasis. *JAMA* 1989;261: 571–576.

45. McLellan R, Spence MR, Brockman M, et al. The clinical diagnosis of trichomoniasis. *Obstet Gynecol* 1982;60:30–34.

46. Imandel K, Aflatoni M, Behjatnia Y. Clinical manifestation of female trichomoniasis and comparison of direct microscopy and culture media in its diagnosis. *Bull Soc Pathol Exot Filiales* 1985; 78:360–367.

47. Eschenbach DA, Hillier SL. Advances in diagnosis testing for vaginitis and cervicitis. *J Reprod Med* 1989;34:555–564.

48. Lossick JG, Kent HL. Trichomoniasis: trends in diagnosis and management. *Am J Obstet Gynecol* 1991;165:217–222.

49. Lossick JG, Muller M, Gorell TE. *In vitro* drug susceptibility and doses of metronidazole required for cure in the cases of refractory vaginal trichomoniasis. *J Infect Dis* 1986;153:948–955.

50. Burtin P, Taddio A, Arburnu O, et al. Safety of metronidazole in pregnancy: a meta-analysis. *Am J Obstet Gynecol* 1995;172: 525–529.

51. Caro-Paton T, Carvajal A, Martin de Diego I, et al. Is metronidazole teratogenic? A meta-analysis. *Br J Clin Pharmacol* 1997;44:179–182.

52. Larsen B, Wilson AH, Glover DD, et al. Implications of metronidazole pharmacodynamics for therapy of trichomoniasis. *Gynecol Obstet Invest* 1986;21:12–18.

53. Yow MD, Leeds LJ, Thompson PK, et al. The natural history of group B streptococcal colonization in the pregnant woman and her offspring. I. Colonization studies. *Am J Obstet Gynecol* 1980; 137:34–38.

54. Hill SL. Group B streptococcal infections. In: Holmes KK, Mardh PA, Sparling PF, et al., eds. *Sexually transmitted diseases.* New York: McGraw-Hill, 1984:397–407.

55. Brozanski BS, Jones JG, Krohn MA, et al. Effect of a screening-based prevention policy on prevalence of early-onset group B streptococcal sepsis. *Obstet Gynecol* 2000;95:496–501.

56. Curtis EM, Pine L. Actinomyces in the vaginas of women with and without intrauterine contraceptive devices. *Am J Obstet Gynecol* 1981;140:880–884.

57. Gardner HL, Fernt P. Etiology of vaginitis emphysematosa. Report of ten cases and review of literature. *J Obstet Gynecol* 1964;88:680–694.

58. Settnes A, Engel PJ, Kringelbach M. Vaginitis emphysematosa. *Ugeskr Laeger* 1992;154:2088–2089.

59. Laing FC, Shanser JD, Salmen BJ. Vaginitis emphysematosa. Importance of its radiologic recognition. *Arch Surg* 1978;113: 156–158.

60. Ebo DG, Stevens WJ, Bridts CH, De Clerck LS. Human seminal plasma anaphylaxis (HSPA): case literature review. *Allergy* 1995;50:747–750.

61. Levine BB, Sriaganin RP, Schenkein I. Allergy to human seminal plasma. *N Engl J Med* 1973;288:894–896.

62. Kroon S. Allergy to human seminal plasma: a presentation of six cases. *Acta Derm Venereol* 1980;60:436–439.

63. Iwahashi K, Miyazaki T, Kuji N, et al. Successful pregnancy in a women with human seminal plasma allergy. A case report. *J Reprod Med* 1999;44:391–393.

64. Nusam D, Gva A, Kalderon I, et al. Intravaginal desensitization to seminal fluid. *Allergy* 1999;54:765.

65. Presti ME, Druce HM. Hypersensitivity reactions to human seminal plasma. *Ann Allergy* 1989;63:477–481.

66. Faulconer HT, Muldoon JP. Rectovaginal fistula in patients with colitis: review and report of a case. *Dis Colon Rectum* 1975; 18:413–415.

67. Bacon PM, Ross ST, Malvar P. Sigmoidovaginal and cecovaginal fistulas as a complication of peridiverticulitis. *Dis Colon Rectum* 1972;15:41–48.

68. Sobel JD. Desquamative inflammatory vaginitis: a new subgroup of purulent vaginitis responsive to topical 2% clindamycin therapy. *Am J Obstet Gynecol* 1994;171:1215–1220.

69. Oats JK, Rowen D. Desquamative inflammatory vaginitis. A review. *Genitourin Med* 1990;66:275–279.

70. Graham-Brown RA, Cochrane GW, Swinhoe JR, et al. Vaginal stenosis due to bullous erythema multiforme (Stevens-Johnson syndrome). Case report. *Br J Obstet Gynecol* 1981;88:1156–1157.

71. Wilson EE, Malinak LR. Vulvovaginal sequelae of Stevens-Johnson syndrome and their management. *Obstet Gynecol* 1988;71:478–480.

72. Bachmann GA, Nevadunsky NS. Diagnosis and treatment of atrophic vaginitis. *Am Fam Physician* 2000;61:3090–3096.

73. Saropala N, Ingsirorat C. Conservative treatment of vaginal vault granulation tissue following total abdominal hysterectomy. *Int J Gynecol Obstet* 1998;62:55–58.

74. Manyonda IT, Welch CR, McWhinney NA, et al. The influence of suture material on vaginal vault granulation following abdominal hysterectomy. *Br J Obstet Gynaecol* 1990;97:608–612.

75. Kalbfleisch RE. Prospective randomized study to compare a closed vault technique using absorbable staples at the time of abdominal hysterectomy versus open vault technique. *Surg Gynecol Obstet* 1992;175:337–340.

76. Guillou L, Gloor E, De Grandi P, et al. Post-operative pseudosarcoma of the vagina. A case report. *Pathol Res Pract* 1989; 185:245–248.

77. Guillou L, Costa J. Postoperative pseudosarcomas of genitourinary tract. A diagnostic trap. Presentation of 4 cases of which 2 were studied immunohistochemically and review of the literature. *Ann Pathol* 1989;9:340–345.

78. Tariel D, Body G, Fetissof F, et al. Postoperative vaginal pseudosarcoma. Apropos of a case. *J Gynecol Obstet Biol Reprod (Paris)* 1986;15:769–771.

79. Roberts WS, Hoffman MS, LaPolla JP, et al. Management of radionecrosis of the vulva and distal vagina. *Am J Obstet Gynecol* 1991;164:1235–1238.

80. Farmer JC, Shelton DL, Angelillo JD, et al. Treatment of radiation-induced tissue injury by hyperbaric oxygen. *Ann Otol Rhinol Laryngol* 1978;87:707–715.

81. Douhgomori H, Arikawa K, Nobori M, et al. Hyperbaric oxygenation for rectovaginal fistula: a report of two cases. *J Obstet Gynecol Rep* 1999;25:343–344.

82. Grody MH, Nyirjesy P, Chatwani A. Intravesical foreign body and vesicovaginal fistula: a rare complication of a neglected pessary. *Int Urogynecol J Pelvic Floor Dysfunct* 1999;10: 407–408.

83. Ueno Y, Hosaka K, Takezaki T. A case of vesicovaginal fistula with vaginal stone. *Hinykika Kiyo* 1999;45:763–765.

84. Miklos JR, Sobolewski C, Lucente V. Laparoscopic management of recurrent vesicovaginal fistula. *Int Urogynecol J Pelvic Floor Dysfunct* 1999;10:116–117.

85. Akman RY, Sargin S, Ozdemir G, et al. Vesicovaginal fistulas: a review of 39 cases. *Int Urol Nephrol* 1999;31:321–326.

86. Rivlin ME. Tubovaginal fistula after vaginal hysterectomy complicated by a tobo-ovarian abscess and diffuse peritonitis. *Obstet Gynecol* 1999;94:858.

87. Nanni L, Valasciani S, Perrelli L. H-type rectovaginal fistula associated with the Currariono triad. *Chir Ital* 1999;51: 409–412.

88. Barranger E, Hassad B, Paniel BJ. Fistula in ano as a rare complication of mediolateral episiotomy: report of three cases. *Am J Obstet Gynecol* 2000;182:733–734.

89. Venkatesh KS, Ramanujam P. Fibrin glue application in the treatment of recurrent anorectal fistulas. *Dis Colon Rectum* 1999;42: 1136–1139.

90. Ramin SM, Ramin KD, Hemsell DL. Fallopian tube prolapse after hysterectomy. *South Med J* 1999;92:963–966.

16

BENIGN, PREMALIGNANT, AND MALIGNANT VAGINAL NEOPLASMS

EDUCATIONAL OBJECTIVES

Medical Students (1) *APGO Objective*	*Residents in Obstetrics/Gynecology (2)* *CREOG Objectives*	*Practitioners (3)* *ACOG Recommendation*
No specific recommendation	Vaginal intraepithelial neoplasia Vaginal carcinoma	No specific recommendation

BENIGN VAGINAL DISORDERS

Vaginal Cysts

A vaginal cyst is a formation of cystic structure; it results from entrapment of the mucosal epithelium within the vaginal walls, or it can be a remnant of the mesonephric ducts. The most frequent cyst types are discussed.

Müllerian Cyst

A müllerian cyst is most commonly a benign mucus-producing cyst and accounts for approximately 44% of vaginal cysts (2). When the cyst is lined by columnar mucin-secreting endocervical type cells, it will produce mucous; although, other linings can be observed such as endometrial or ciliated Fallopian tube–type cells within the cyst's wall (3). A müllerian cyst can be located anywhere within the vaginal walls. Usually, it is <2 cm in diameter; nevertheless, it may become extremely large (4). Clinically, on gross examination, a müllerian cyst resembles a Gartner's duct cyst; histology can distinguish one from the other.

Diagnosis is reached on a clinical basis. A patient may complain of a vaginal mass or vaginal swelling, dyspareunia, and pelvic pressure; however, an asymptomatic case can occur, when the cyst is small.

Pelvic examination by inspection and palpation provides enough information to make the diagnosis.

Conventional therapy may include observation when the cyst is asymptomatic and does not interfere with coitus. A symptomatic or large cyst requires surgical resection (vaginal cystectomy) and vaginal reconstruction.

Complementary or alternative therapies are not offered.

Epithelial Inclusion Cyst

Epithelial inclusion cyst, also known as epidermal inclusion cyst or squamous inclusion cyst, is the second most common vaginal cyst and is estimated to account for 23% of such cysts (2). This cyst arises from the entrapment of vaginal mucosa as a result of surgery (episiotomy, obstetrical trauma, or vaginoplasty) or injury. Clinically, the lesion is small (it ranges from a few millimeters to several centimeters in diameter), is located in the lower third of the posterior vaginal wall, and is usually asymptomatic and clinically insignificant. Histological examination is required for a definitive diagnosis, since on gross examination it is difficult to distinguish the epithelial inclusion cyst from Gartner's cyst; however, a cheese-like substance (which results from the degenerative process of the buried vaginal epithelium) within the cyst can provide a diagnostic clue.

Conventional therapy includes observation when the cyst is asymptomatic. Vaginal cystectomy is recommended when the cyst becomes symptomatic.

Conventional and alternative therapies have not been developed.

Gartner's Duct Cyst

Gartner's duct cyst arises from incomplete regression of the vaginal portion of the Wolffian (mesonephric) ducts. Gartner's ducts are determined by the presence of persistent remnants of mesonephric ducts. Since the mesonephric ducts have secretory properties, cysts can develop. Gartner's duct cysts account for approximately 11% of vaginal cysts (2).

Usually, cysts located along the anterior-lateral vaginal wall, matching the Wolffian duct path, are ≤2 cm in size and asymptomatic. Occasionally, they can grow larger, to 16 cm in diameter, and cause dyspareunia and birth canal obstruction during parturition (5). The vagina is not the only location of the Gartner's duct cyst; it can be found within the leaves of the broad ligament or mesosalpinx.

The diagnosis is clinical; sonographic or magnetic resonance imaging (MRI) can confirm the clinical diagnosis. Histology provides the definitive diagnosis.

Conventional therapy is observation only, when the cyst is small and asymptomatic. A symptomatic cyst is surgically removed, or marsupialization is performed, if the cyst penetrates deeply into the paravaginal area.

Bartholin's Duct Cyst

Bartholin's duct cyst is often discussed as a vaginal condition, although it is located, in actuality, in the vulvar vestibulum. Therefore, this condition as well as abscess of the Bartholin's duct cyst are presented in Chapter 13.

Vaginal Endometriotic Cyst

Vaginal endometriotic cyst is defined as endometrial tissue functioning within the vaginal wall. It has been estimated that endometriotic vaginal cysts account for 7% of all cystic vaginal masses.

Clinical diagnosis is reached by a patient history of vaginal spotting and increased dyspareunia before menses. Gross examination of the lesions reveals, most commonly, a bluish color (other colors can be identified also) and a slightly tender cyst. Histological examination provides verification and a differential diagnosis.

Conventional therapy depends upon the severity of symptoms. Conservative medical therapy, which will prevent cyclic bleeding within the endometriotic implant, can be recommended. The regression of the cyst can be expected, but the conservative therapy probably will not be adequate to eliminate the cyst completely (6).

Surgical excision or laser vaporization of the lesion is usually definitive therapy. Since malignant transformation can occur, excisional biopsy is recommended, particularly in recurrent endometriosis (7).

Benign Solid Tumors of the Vagina

In general, benign solid tumors of the vagina arise from vaginal connective tissue such as fibrous muscle, smooth muscle, and skeletal muscle tissues. These tumors are rare clinical occurrences. The definitive diagnosis is established by histological examination, which also rules out malignancy.

Condylomata Acuminata

The condylomata acuminata condition is described in Chapters 13 and 26. This vaginal condition is similar, both biologically and pathologically, to the vulvar and anal conditions. Therefore, the discussion of diagnosis and therapy found in those other chapters for the condylomata acuminata condition also applies here.

Vaginal Polyps

Vaginal polyps are benign tumors composed of loose connective tissue. The most common symptoms are postcoital vaginal spotting or bleeding, or a vaginal lump. Gross clinical evaluation discloses polypoid structures within the vagina, which ooze blood when touched. Therapy is vaginal polypectomy; histology verifies the clinical diagnosis (8).

Vaginal Fibromyoma

Vaginal fibromyoma are benign solid masses of smooth muscle that occur infrequently. The most common symptoms are dyspareunia and/or urinary symptoms, and vaginal bleeding; they may, alternatively, occur as asymptomatic masses.

Pelvic examination of the vaginal wall may reveal a circumscribed, nontender, mobile vaginal mass-located anywhere in the vaginal wall. The consistency of the tumor is variable and may confound clinical interpretation.

The clinical diagnosis can be supported by needle biopsy and ultrasonography, both transabdominal and transvaginal.

Conventional therapy is enucleation of the tumor, which is a relatively easy procedure, since there is a cleavage line present (9,10).

Vaginal Leiomyomata

Vaginal leiomyomata can be located anywhere within the submucosa of the vaginal wall. Their size ranges from 0.5 to 15 cm in diameter (the average size is about 3 cm). No symptoms are present when the tumor is small.

Diagnosis is made based on symptoms, which will occur as the tumor increases in size, including vaginal discomfort, vaginal bleeding, and dyspareunia.

Physical examination will reveal the presence of a firm and well-circumscribed mass of variable size. Ultrasonography or MRI will further establish the clinical diagnosis, and histology will provide the final diagnosis.

Conventional therapy is surgical resection (11–13).

Vaginal Rhabdomyoma

Vaginal rhabdomyoma differentiates from skeletal muscle. Clinically, it presents as a pedunculated polypoid structure with intact, overlying vaginal mucosa, measuring from 1 to 11 cm (14). Microscopic examination establishes the definitive diagnosis (15). Vaginal rhabdomyoma can also be found on the ectocervix. However, vaginal rhabdomyoma and cervical rhabdomyomata are vary rare lesions (16).

Local excision is usually curative, although recurrence of this benign lesion has been reported (17).

Mixed Tumors of the Vagina

Mixed tumors of the vagina are composed predominantly of spindle cells, often mixed with minor glandular and focal areas of squamous differentiation (18). These mixed tumors are painless and slow growing, and reach the size of 1.5 to 5.0 cm. Clinically, they are finger-like protruded polypoid structures, well-circumscribed, nonencapsulated within the submucosa, and unconnected to the surface of epithelium tumors, mainly located near the hymenal ring; however, they may be found in any location within the vagina.

Conventional therapy is surgical local excision; recurrence has not been reported (19–21).

Vaginal Adenosis

Vaginal adenosis is characterized as the presence of columnar endocervical epithelium, or tubo-endometrial or embryonic tissue within the vaginal wall. These lesions can occur spontaneously or can be induced by *in utero* exposure to diethylstilbestrol (DES) in a female fetus (22); they can also occur as a result of CO_2 laser or 5-fluorouracil treatments of condylomata acuminata (23). Spontaneous vaginal adenosis occurs in about 10% in adult women and is mostly an insignificant coincidental finding. In women who were exposed prenatally to DES, vaginal adenosis can be identified in about 90% and is associated with clear cell adenocarcinomas of the vagina (24). However, progress of vaginal adenosis to malignancy has not been proven (25).

It has been documented that vaginal adenosis, in women born prior to the DES era, is microscopically identical (of three types: mucinous, tuboendometrial, and embryonic) to that encountered in women exposed *in utero* to DES (26). DES is not a complete carcinogen. The risk of developing vaginal and cervical cancer is 0.5 to 2.0 cases per 1,000 for women exposed *in utero* to DES (27,28). Vaginal and cervical intraepithelial neoplasms occur at a rate of 15.7 per 1,000 woman-years in women exposed to DES and at a rate of 7.9/1,000 woman-years in women who were not exposed to DES *in utero* (28).

Diagnosis is arrived at clinically, but in most instances the condition is asymptomatic. Occasionally, mucus-type vaginal discharge or bloodstain discharge can be present. Vaginal examination may reveal a diffuse granular thickening. It may also reveal irregular or rugose mucoid lesions and the cervical hood may be apparent.

Colposcopy is useful in identifying the particular pattern present: the columnar epithelium pattern appears in 94.4% of cases, the mosaic pattern in 85.5%, and a white appearance in 68.0% (29). Although it is less accurate in identifying adenocarcinoma, a colposcopically directed biopsy and tissue histology yield a definitive diagnosis.

Conventional therapy is closely followed-up by employing cytology and colposcopic examination, with biopsy when indicated. Intraepithelial neoplasia or symptomatic vaginal adenosis can be treated by tissue destruction using electrocautery, cryosurgery, or laser technology(22).

PREMALIGNANT VAGINAL DISORDERS
Vaginal Intraepithelial Neoplasia (VAIN)
Definition

Epithelial vaginal cells lose control of progressive maturation from the basal layer towards the epithelial surface and are associated with nuclear atypia.

Incidence

The incidence of VAIN is unknown but is lower than cervical intraepithelial neoplasia.

Etiology

The etiologic factors behind VAIN have not been determined. The risk factors that may increase the chance of developing VAIN include the following (30–32):

- HPV infection
- Presence of squamous neoplasia in the lower genital tract other than in the vagina
- Immunosuppression
- Pelvic radiation therapy for either benign or malignant lesions
- DES exposure *in utero*

Although most VAIN (70%–78%) will regress after initial therapy and only 5% to 9% of cases will progress to invasive carcinoma, VAIN is considered a premalignant condition of the vagina (30,32).

Classification

The Bethesda System for reporting cervical/vaginal cytologic diagnoses (33) presents an alternative to the previously recognized classification for VAIN. The new cytology reporting system as applied to VAIN can be characterized as follows:

- VAIN-1 reflects mild dysplasia (the lower third of the squamous epithelium is affected by dysplastic cells) and/or HPV lesions, which corresponds to low-grade squamous intraepithelial lesions (LSILs); VAIN-1 is the most common form of VAIN occurring about 52.6% of the time(34).
- VAIN-2 reflects moderate dysplasia (the middle third of the squamous epithelium is affected by dysplastic cells), which has been described as high-grade squamous intra-

epithelial lesion (HSIL); VAIN-2 occurs about 19.1% of the time (34).

- VAIN-3 reflects severe dysplasia (the upper third of the squamous epithelium is affected by dysplastic cells) or vaginal carcinoma *in situ*, which corresponds to HSIL; it spreads among VAIN lesions approximately 28.9% of the time(34).

Therefore, VAIN-2, VAIN-3, and carcinoma *in situ* have been combined into one HSIL group.

Diagnosis

Vaginal lesions are predominantly multifocal in young women and associated with HPV infection. In older women, a single lesion, more biologically aggressive than those found in younger women, is normally observed (32,35). One-half of VAIN coexists with cervical or vulvar intraepithelial neoplasia (32); therefore, the cervical, vulvar, perineal, and perianal areas should be included in the clinical investigation.

- *Pertinent medical history* may include vaginal discharge or postcoital vaginal spotting; however, VAIN is, for the most part, an asymptomatic lesion.
- *Physical examination* is usually negative; although, a clinically skillful practitioner may appreciate vaginal mucosal lesions, where the epithelium is white or pink, raised, and roughened (36), which are, most commonly, located in the upper third of the vagina.
- *Cytological screening* is an initial diagnostic step to prove clinical diagnosis in VAIN evaluation; the sensitivity of the vaginal cytological smear is 83% when compared with histology. An inflammatory process in the vagina may compromise the results and lead to a false negative diagnosis (37). Fine needle aspiration of various lesions from the vaginal cuff for cytology study appears to be an accurate procedure (38).
- *Colposcopic examination* with 3% to 5% iodine solution previously applied to the vaginal walls for 5 minutes (a Schiller's test will reveal light dysplastic cells, which have lower glycogen cellular content) will assist in identifying suspicious lesions, for which biopsy should be performed and histological verification obtained(39).

Differential Diagnosis

- Inflammation
- Trichomoniasis
- Cervical intraepithelial neoplasia

Conventional Therapy

Several therapeutic choices are offered depending upon the histologically documented grade of lesion:

- VAIN-1 can be observed for 1 year, with follow-up visits every 3 months. Lesions can spontaneously regress or can

persist, or progress to the more advanced form, VAIN-2. When VAIN-1 is persisting and HPV is present, topical Efudex, 5% cream (5-fluorouracil), can be applied (using a vaginal applicator filled to one-third of its volume) high in the vagina (a tampon and petroleum jelly to prevent vulva irritation should be used) every other night for 7 to 10 days with a 2-week off interval or weekly application at bedtime for 10 weeks. A regimen can be repeated as needed, but one course usually is sufficient (40,41). CO_2 laser vaporization of a VAIN-1 lesion to a depth of 1.5 mm, including the zone of thermal necrosis, is sufficient to destroy the vaginal epithelium affected by VAIN-1 (42). Most of the reported CO_2 surgery is not as successful as expected, and failure up to 50% has been reported. Electrocautery failure occurs in approximately 25% of cases; surgical excision provides the best results (43).
- VAIN-2 and VAIN-3 require wide local excision, because local therapy (electrocautery, topical chemotherapy or a laser) is unsafe since residual, recurrent, or occult invasive malignancy can be missed (44).

Complementary therapy for VAIN is not available. It is worthwhile to mention that, contrary to vulvar HPV, local therapy with *herbal medicine* such as Podophyline is contraindicated for local vaginal therapy.

- Also, vaginal douching with folk medicine remedies should be discouraged, since douching itself has been shown to be associated with increased risks of bacterial vaginosis and pelvic inflammatory disease, and an increased ectopic pregnancy rate (45).

MALIGNANT VAGINAL NEOPLASMS

Primary or secondary malignancies can involve the vaginal walls. Primary vaginal cancers are the least common primary cancers of the female genital tract; squamous cell cancers are the most common malignancy of the vagina. It must be stressed that early diagnosis is the most important factor affecting outcome of the disease; selection of a therapeutic paradigm is the next most important factor.

Vaginal Squamous Cell Carcinoma
Definition

The presence of malignant squamous cells originating from the vagina walls, when clinical and histological examination has confirmed the absence of cervical or vulvar participation (primary vaginal cancer).

Incidence

The incidence of squamous cell carcinoma of the vagina is 0.42 per 100,000 Caucasian women and 0.93 per 100,000 African-American women (46). This carcinoma constitutes about 1% of all malignant squamous cell carcinomas of the genital tract in women (47). Overall, squamous cell carcinoma accounts for approximately 90% of primary vaginal invasive malignancies in the general population of women and 95% of these malignancies in the population of women older than 55 years (with a mean age of 64) (48). A surgically created neovagina can also be affected by vaginal carcinoma, usually between 8 to 25 years after the initial operation (49).

Vaginal squamous cell carcinoma occurring within 5 years of therapy for cervical cancer is considered recurrent cervical carcinoma and not primary vaginal carcinoma (50).

Etiology

The etiology of vaginal squamous cell carcinoma has not been established. One hypothesis postulates that chronic vaginal mucosal exposure to irritants may lead to this malignancy (51).

Classification

- Primary vaginal squamous cell carcinoma
- Secondary vaginal squamous cell carcinoma

Diagnosis

Pertinent medical history of vaginal cancer can range from the asymptomatic (20%) to the symptomatic, including the following (52,53):

- Offensive smell; blood-stained vaginal discharge
- Postcoital vaginal bleeding
- Postmenopausal (painless) vaginal bleeding—the most frequently observed symptom
- Postdouching vaginal bleeding
- Urinary frequency, urgency, dysuria, and blood in the urine may occur when the anterior vaginal wall is affected by cancer.
- Tenesmus, melena, or dischasia may occur when the posterior vaginal wall is affected by cancer.

Physical examination with vaginal speculum may identify mucosal lesions at the upper third of the vagina in about 40% to 50% of cases; the posterior vaginal wall is affected in 57%, and 27% can be found on the anterior vaginal wall. The size of the tumors range from occult to >10 cm; therefore, they can be identified by palpation in some cases. The mass itself is bulky and can extend to the cervix.

Vaginal cytology may display abnormality and can be helpful in clinically occult tumor diagnosis.

Colposcopic evaluation and colposcopically directed biopsy is indicated whenever a suspicious small vaginal lesion is identified or cytology is abnormal. A direct biopsy should be carried out when a lesion is visible. Histology provides definitive diagnosis of vaginal squamous cell carcinoma.

Cystoscopic and proctoscopic evaluation is necessary when a tumor is bulky. Upon accomplishing clinical staging, all patients with stage II or higher should undergo *metastasis* evaluation, which usually includes the following:

- Chest x-ray
- Intravenous pyelography
- Barium enema: a recent study on the accuracy of barium enema revealed a 35% overall rate of detection, a 24% rate when lesions are 2.1 to 2.5 cm, and a 2% rate when lesions are 0.1 to 0.5% (54,55).
- Computed tomography (CT) with intravenous and oral contrast
- MRI may provide information that can distinguish between fibrotic tissue and cancer infiltration
- Lymphangiography in obese cases may be helpful; nevertheless, it is not routinely performed.

Evaluation under anesthesia for appropriate clinical staging is recommended.

Clinical staging of vaginal carcinoma has been recommended by the International Federation of Gynecology and Obstetrics (FIGO) and is widely accepted. The following clinical stages of vaginal carcinomas are recognized (56):

- Stage 0: Carcinoma *in situ*; intraepithelial carcinoma
- Stage I: Carcinoma limited to vaginal mucosa (wall)
- Stage II: Carcinoma infiltrates to subvaginal tissue (parametrium), not extending to the pelvic wall
- Stage III: Carcinoma extends to the pelvic wall
- Stage IV: Carcinoma extends beyond the true pelvis and involves the bladder mucosa or rectum
- Stage IVA: Carcinoma spreads to adjacent organs and/or directly extends beyond the true pelvis
- Stage IVB: Carcinoma spreads to distant organs

In some institutions, stage II has been divided into stage IIA (parametrial extension) and stage IIB (parametrial involvement) (57). Also, microinvasive carcinoma has been postulated as a distinct clinical entity, when invasion is <2.5 cm as measured from the surface, where there is a lack of involvement of the lymph-vascular space, and when microinvasions arise from carcinoma *in situ* (58).

Differential Diagnosis

- Cervical squamous cell carcinomas
- Vulvar squamous cell carcinomas
- Metastasis from other organs

Conventional Therapy

Management of vaginal squamous cell carcinoma should take into account several factors such as the extent of cancer (stage), sexual activity, general health, and preservation of childbearing capacity. Early detection and appropriately selected treatment play essential roles.

■ In stage I disease (lesion of <1 cm or occult), a small, localized lesion can be treated with radical surgery. When a cancer lesion is thick, external beam radiation can be added. Involvement of the upper third of the vagina may require a radical hysterectomy, i.e., vaginectomy with bilateral pelvic node dissection. Positive nodes will indicate external beam irradiation (59).

The 5-year survival rate in stage I vaginal squamous cell carcinoma is between 72% and 90% (58). Recently, clinical data suggest that a survival rate even higher than 90% can be achieved by using a combination of external radiotherapy and brachytherapy in the form of either vaginal cylinders or uterine tandems with vaginal cylinders (60,61).

The therapeutic modalities for vaginal carcinoma in stage I and stage II disease, excluding malignant melanoma, are surgery alone, surgery and radiotherapy, and radiotherapy alone. Overall outcome yielded a 5-year survival rate of 82% with stage I and a 53% rate with stage II disease. Statistical analysis of survival according to treatment modality did not produce significant differences (62).

In general, most patients with superficial stage I vaginal carcinoma can be managed surgically. Also, for central non-metastatic stage IV disease or central recurrence following radiotherapy, surgical exenteration can be considered (62).

Patients with *Surgically inoperable carcinoma* of the vagina (stage I cancer with mid vagina involvement, stage II cancer, or more advanced cancer) are routinely treated with radiotherapy. Nevertheless, all stages of vaginal carcinoma may be subjected to irradiation (57).

■ Stage 0 cancer will be controlled with intracavitary therapy alone; 10-year disease-free survival is 94%.
■ Stage I 10-year disease-free survival rate is 80% with interstitial and/or intracavitary and external-beam irradiation; a total prevalence of distant metastasis in stage I disease is about 13%.
■ Stage IIA (paravaginal extension) 10-year disease-free survival rate is 55% with a combination of brachytherapy and external-beam irradiation; a total incidence of distant metastasis in stage IIA disease is about 30%.
■ Stage IIB (paravaginal involvement) 10-year disease-free survival rate is 35% with the same irradiation that is applied in stage IIA; a total prevalence of distant metastasis in stage IIB of disease is about 52%.
■ Stage III favorably responds to irradiation with a 38% 10-year disease-free survival rate; a total prevalence of distant metastasis in stage III disease is about 50%.
■ Stage IV 10-year disease-free survival rate is 0%; a total prevalence of distant metastasis in stage IV disease is about 47%.

Radiotherapy for vaginal squamous cell carcinoma is initiated with external radiation to the whole pelvis at 4,000 cGy, with total doses of 5,000 to 6,000 cGy to the parametrium. The dose of irradiation delivered to the primary tumor or the parametrial extension of interstitial and intracavitary insertions is 6,500 cGy (63,64).

Radiotherapy complications are related to the dose: the higher the dose, the more often complications will occur, including proctitis, cystitis, vaginal strictures, and/or vaginal fistulas.

Chemotherapy is used infrequently (65). Overall outcomes of this modality are difficult to judge because its use is infrequent; thus, published clinical studies are not numerous enough to provide conclusions as to safety and efficacy.

Complementary Therapy

No complementary therapy is offered for vaginal squamous carcinoma.

Alternative Therapy

There is no specific alternative therapy for vaginal carcinomas, although for malignancies in general, a number of clinically unproven alternative remedies can be found in the literature.

Vaginal Adenocarcinoma
Definition

The presence of malignant glandular cells originating from the vagina walls, with clinical and histological confirmation of the absence of a cervical or vulvar origin (primary vaginal cancer), is defined as vaginal adenocarcinoma.

Incidence

The incidence of vaginal adenocarcinoma is not known. The prevalence of clear cell adenocarcinoma is 0.014% to 0.14% in women exposed to DES (66). In 1991, a total of 23 new cases and eight recurrences of vaginal clear cell adenocarcinoma were reported in the United States; however, a question remains as to whether or not the system of registry for this rare disease is adequate (67).

Etiology

The etiology of vaginal adenocarcinoma is unknown. Vaginal clear cell adenocarcinoma appears to be associated with exposure to DES *in utero* in the female fetus (68). Vaginal endodermal sinus tumor (69) and vaginal adenocarcinoma arising from endometriosis have been reported (70).

Classification

■ Primary vaginal adenocarcinoma
■ Secondary vaginal adenocarcinoma

Diagnosis

Pertinent medical history may range from asymptomatic, when the tumor is small, to malodorous vaginal discharge, bloodstain, and vaginal bleeding.

On *physical examination*, most vaginal adenocarcinomas are found to be located on the upper third of the anterior vagina, reflecting the most common adenosis site, although it may be present anywhere on the vagina walls. "Kissing lesions" on opposing vaginal walls, are frequently present. Polypoid, nodular, or both of these types of lesions can be present, and in some cases, flat, ulcerated, or indurated lesions may be appreciated. The lesions may extend to the cervix.

Diagnostic procedures are the same as has been described for vaginal squamous cell cancer.

Cytologic examination to screen for adenocarcinoma of the vagina is the recommended technique to establish whether the disease is in an early or advanced stage. The importance of yearly clinical and cytological examinations should be stressed, particularly in a patient who has been exposed to DES *in utero* (71,72).

Colposcopy and colposcopically directed biopsy provides material for histological verification, which is usually diagnostic. When lesions are visible, direct biopsy is recommended.

Metastatic evaluation is similar to those presented for squamous cell carcinoma in the vagina.

Clinical staging of vaginal adenocarcinoma is identical to that presented for squamous cell carcinoma in the vagina.

Endodermal sinus tumors may secrete alpha-fetoprotein (AFP), which can be used for diagnosis as well as for post-therapeutic monitoring. AFP has good predictability; therefore, the response to therapy or recurrence can be monitored (69).

Differential Diagnosis

- Cervical ectopic pregnancy
- Cervical adenocarcinoma
- Bartholin's gland adenocarcinoma
- Adenocarcinoma of müllerian duct cyst
- Vaginal metastatic adenocarcinoma

Conventional Therapy

Conventional therapy can be divided into two categories:

- Preservation of childbearing capacity is a clinical dilemma in clear cell adenocarcinoma, since this disease affects women during their reproductive years (range, 7–42 years of age). Reproductive potential can be preserved when there is a solitary lesion with a size of <2 cm and less than 3 mm of invasion. Wide local excision with node dissection and local radiation can be offered. Conservative

surgery (partial vaginectomy) followed by chemotherapy (vincristine, actinomycin D, cyclophosphamide [VAC], or bleomycin, etoposide, cisplatin [BEP]; BEP is recommended as the second line of therapy) has been reported to be a successful treatment in children (69).
- When preservation of the childbearing capacity is not an issue, radical hysterectomy, i.e., upper vaginectomy with pelvic node dissection (50% of pelvic nodes are affected in stage II), is an acceptable approach.

The 5-year and 10-year survival rates for patients with vaginal clear cell adenocarcinoma of stage I and stage II are approximately 93% and 87%, respectively (73). Pregnancy at the time of diagnosis does not seem to negatively affect overall results (74).

Complementary Therapy

No specific complementary therapy for vaginal adenocarcinoma is recommended.

Alternative Therapy

No particular alternative treatment for this malignancy is available.

Malignant Vaginal Melanomas

Malignant vaginal melanomas arise from vaginal melanophore cells. It is a very rare malignancy. The biological aggressiveness of this entity results in an extremely poor prognosis, with a 5-year survival rate of 14% (57). A tumor's size at the time of diagnosis appears to influence the survival rate, whereas the thickness of a vaginal malignant melanoma does not significantly affect a patient's survival unless the thickness is >8 mm (75).

The *clinical diagnosis* of asymptomatic or symptomatic (vaginal discharge, bleeding, or a tumor) melanotic lesions (dark vaginal lesions), frequently located in the anterior vaginal wall (though they may arise anywhere within the vaginal walls), is verified by histology (76).

Conventional therapy falls into five categories (75):

- Wide local excision
- Radical surgery, including radical hysterectomy with radical vaginectomy and lymphadenectomy [recently, radioactive agents have been developed and used preoperatively and intraoperatively to identify the affected iliac basin of lymphatic nodes (77)] or exenterations
- Radiation therapy
- Combination of wide excision and radiotherapy
- Other treatment such as chemotherapy has been used, but it appears ineffective.

These treatments represent a wide range of approaches, and great disagreement exists as to the optimal treatment. The most frequent treatment for primary vaginal malignant melanoma has been radical surgery, although recent clinical findings do not support such an approach. The current recommendation, supported by clinical observational studies, is wide local excision followed by radiotherapy (75,78,79).

For prevention and early diagnosis of vaginal malignant melanoma, dark lesions of the vagina should be excised and histological examination should be performed (80). This is particularly important, since the size of a lesion at diagnosis affects a patient's survival (75).

Vaginal Sarcomas

Vaginal sarcomas are very infrequent malignancies. Taking age into consideration, two distinctive categories apply:

1. *Girls under the age of 5* are often affected by sarcoma botryoides (embryonal rhabdomyosarcomas). It is the most common malignancy of the vagina in girls, accounting for approximately 90% of all known cases (81). On average, the diagnosis is reached at age 2.

   Diagnosis is based on symptoms such as vaginal bleeding and a vaginal mass. Clinically, the tumor arises from the anterior wall of the vagina and presents itself in a "grape-like" appearance (papillae, small nodule sessile, or pedunculated lesion covered with intact vaginal mucosa). Histology verifies the clinical diagnosis.

   Conventional therapy is a combination of chemotherapy (vincristine, dactinomycin, cyclophosphamide) and local excision or local radiation, which preserves future reproductive capacity (82).

2. *Adult women* are affected by the following forms of vaginal sarcomas:

   ■ Rhabdomyosarcoma of the vagina in adult women is an exceedingly rare occurrence and usually is diagnosed in the postmenopausal period. Vaginal bleeding and the presence of a characteristic vaginal mass may suggest this form of malignancy. Direct biopsy with histological examination makes the definitive diagnosis. Suggested therapy is local wide excision of the tumor with total hysterectomy and salpingo-oophorectomy. Postsurgical irradiation is recommended (83).

   ■ *Leiomyosarcoma* of the vagina is an extremely uncommon tumor, which clinically may manifest with odorous vaginal discharge, vaginal bleeding, and dyspareunia. The tumor can occur at age 25 to 85. It is very aggressive and spreads by local extension and a hematogenous route. The safety and efficacy of treatment are difficult to assess due to the extreme rarity of this tumor. Radical surgery or exenteration is the first line of therapy, complemented by pelvic irradiation. The 5-year survival rate is approximately 35% (84).

   ■ *Other forms of vaginal sarcoma* such as mixed mesodermal tumors, stromal sarcoma, neurofibrosarcoma, and adenosarcoma arising from endometriosis are such rare tumors that specific management is not available; the therapy used for leiomyosarcoma is usually offered (84,85).

Secondary Vaginal Carcinoma

Secondary vaginal carcinoma may be the result of spreading—by extension, by lymphatic metastasis, or by hematogenous metastasis. The most common secondary vaginal carcinoma is a result of cervical carcinoma (32%), of endometrial carcinoma (18%), of colorectal carcinoma (9%), of vulvar carcinoma (6%), of ovarian carcinoma (6%), and of the urinary tract (4%) (86).

REFERENCES

1. Council on Resident Education in Obstetrics and Gynecology (CREOG). *Educational objectives core curriculum for residents in obstetrics and gynecology,* 5th ed. Washington, DC: CREOG, 1996.
2. Pradhan S, Tobon H. Vaginal cysts: a clinicopathological study of 41 cases. *Int J Gynecol Pathol* 1986;5:35–46.
3. Deppisch LM. Cyst of the vagina: classification and clinical correlation. *Obstet Gynecol* 1975;45:632–637.
4. Lucente V, Benson JT. Vaginal müllerian cyst presenting as an anterior enterocele: a case report. *Obstet Gynecol* 1990;76:906–908.
5. Hagspiel KD. Giant Gartner duct cyst: magnetic resonance imaging findings. *Abdom Imaging* 1995;20:566–568.
6. Brosens IA. Endometriosis. Current issues in diagnosis and medical management. *J Reprod Med* 1998;43:281–286.
7. Judson PL, Temple AM, Fowler WC Jr, et al. Vaginal adenosarcoma arising from endometriosis. *Gynecol Oncol* 2000;76:123–125.
8. Chirayil SJ, Toban H. Polyps of the vagina: a clinicopathologic study of 18 cases. *Cancer* 1981;47:2904–2907.
9. Marinetti C, Comiti J. Vaginal fibromas. *J Chir (Paris)* 1980;117:321–325.
10. Yound SB, Rose PG, Peuter KL. Vaginal fibromyomata: two cases with preoperative assessment, resection, and reconstruction. *Obstet Gynecol* 1991;78:972–974.
11. Tazvassoli FA, Norris HJ. Smooth muscle tumors of the vagina. *Obstet Gynecol* 1979;53:689–693.
12. Tramier D, Marinetti C, Jouve MP. Leiomyoma of the vagina. *J Gynecol Obstet Biol Reprod* 1980;9:367–368.
13. Ruggieri AM, Brody JM, Curhan RP. Vaginal leiomyoma. A case report with imaging findings. *J Reprod Med* 1996;41:875–877.
14. Lopez JI, Brouard I, Eizaguirre B. Rhabdomyoma of the vagina. *Eur J Obstet Gynecol Reprod Biol* 1992;45:147–148.
15. Iversen UM. Two cases of benign vaginal rhabdomyoma. Case reports. *APMIS* 1996;104:575–578.
16. Hanski W, Hagel-Lewicka E, Daniszewski K. Rhabdomyomas of female genital tract. Report on two cases. *Zentralbl Pathol* 1991;137:439–442.
17. Losi L, Choreutaki T, Nascetti D, et al. Recurrence in a case of rhabdomyoma of the vagina. *Patholgica* 1995;87:704–708.
18. Barton PA, Tavassoli FA. Spindle cell epithelium, the so-called mixed tumor of the vagina. A clinicopathologic, immunohistochemical, and ultrastructural analysis of 28 cases. *Am J Surg Pathol* 1993;17:509–515.
19. Sirota RL, Dickersin GR, Scully RE. Mixed tumors of the vagina. A clinicopathological analysis of eight cases. *Am J Surg Pathol* 1981;5:413–422.
20. Nakashima Y, Sueishi K, Morishita Y. A case report of mixed tumor arising in the vagina. *Fukuota Igaku Zashi* 1992;83:333–337.

21. Fukunaga M, Endo Y, Ishikawa E, et al. Mixed tumor of the vagina. *Histopathology* 1996;28:457–461.

22. Ostergard DR. DES-related vaginal lesions. *Clin Obstet Gynecol* 1981;24:379–394.

23. Bornstein J, Sova Y, Atad J, et al. Development of vaginal adenosis following combined 5-fluorouracil and carbon dioxide laser treatments for diffuse vaginal condylomatosis. *Obstet Gynecol* 1993;81:896–898.

24. Kranl C, Zegler B, Kofler H, et al. Vulval and vaginal adenosis. *Br J Dermatol* 1998;139:128–131.

25. Ghosh TK, Cera PJ. Transition of benign vaginal adenosis to clear cell carcinoma. *Obstet Gynecol* 1983;61:126–130.

26. Robboy SJ, Hill EC, Sandberg EC, et al. Vaginal adenosis in women born prior to the diethylstilbestrol era. *Hum Pathol* 1986;17:488–492.

27. Edelman DA. Diethylstilbestrol exposure and the risk of clear cell cervical and vaginal adenocarcinoma. *Int J Fertil* 1989;34:251–255.

28. Vessey MP. Epidemiological studies of the effects of diethylstilbestrol. *IARC Sci Publ* 1989;96:335–348.

29. Burke L, Antonioli D. Vaginal adenosis. Factors influencing detection in a colposcopic evaluation. *Obstet Gynecol* 1976;48:413–421.

30. Sillman FH, Fruchter RG, Chen YS, et al. Vaginal intraepithelial neoplasia: risk factors for persistence, recurrence, and invasion and its management. *Am J Obstet Gynecol* 1997;176:93–99.

31. Minucci D, Cinel A, Insacco E, et al. Epidemiological aspects of vaginal intraepithelial neoplasia (VAIN). *Clin Exp Obstet Gynecol* 1995;22:36–42.

32. Aho M, Vesterinen E, Meyer B, et al. Natural history of vaginal intraepithelial neoplasia. *Cancer* 1991;6:195–197.

33. The Bethesda System for reporting cervical/vaginal cytologic diagnoses. *Acta Cytol* 1993;37:115–124.

34. Audet-Lapointe P, Body G, Vauclair R, et al. Vaginal intraepithelial neoplasia. *Gynecol Oncol* 1990;36:232–239.

35. Micheletti L, Zanotto Valentino MC, Barbero M, et al. Current knowledge about the natural history of intraepithelial neoplasms of the vagina. *Minerva Ginecol* 1994;46:195–204.

36. Gallup DG, Morely GW. Carcinoma *in situ* of the vagina: a study and review. *Obstet Gynecol* 1975;46:334–340.

37. Davila RM, Miranda NC. Vaginal intraepithelial neoplasia and the Pap smear. *Acta Cytol* 2000;44:137–140.

38. Pisharodi LR, Attal H. Fine needle aspiration cytology of vaginal cuff lesions. *Acta Cytol* 2000;44:147–150.

39. Nguyen HN, Nordqvist SR. The Bethesda system and evaluation of abnormal Pap smears. *Semin Surg Oncol* 1999;16:217–221.

40. Kirwan P, Naftalin NJ. Topical 5-fluorouracil in the treatment of vaginal intraepithelial neoplasia. *Br J Obstet Gynecol* 1985;92:287–291.

41. Krebs HB. Treatment of vaginal intraepithelial neoplasia with laser and topical 5-fluorouracil. *Obstet Gynecol* 1989;73:657–660.

42. Benedet JL, Wilson PS, Mastisic JP. Epidermal thickness measurements in vaginal intraepithelial neoplasia. A basis for optimal CO_2 laser vaporization. *J Reprod Med* 1992;37:809–812.

43. Lenehan PM, Meffe F, Lickrish GM. Vaginal intraepithelial neoplasia: biologic aspects and management. *Obstet Gynecol* 1986;68:333–337.

44. Cheng D, Ng TY, Ngan HY, et al. Wide local excision (WLE) for vaginal intraepithelial neoplasia (VAIN). *Acta Obstet Gynecol Scand* 1999;78:648–652.

45. Merchant JS, Oh K, Klerman LV. Douching: a problem for adolescent girls and young women. *Arch Pediatr Adolesc Med* 1999;153:834–837.

46. Cramer DW, Cutler SJ. Incidence and histopathology of malignancies of the female genital organs in the United States. *Am J Obstet Gynecol* 1974;118:443–460.

47. Daw E. Primary carcinoma of the vagina. *J Obstet Gynecol Br Commonwealth* 1971;78:853–856.

48. Kurman RJ, Norris HJ, Wilkinson E. Tumors of the vagina. In: *Atlas of tumor pathology. 3rd series, Fascicle 4. Tumors of the cervix, vagina, and vulva.* Washington, DC: Armed Forces Institute of Pathology, 1992:141–178.

49. Hopkins MP, Morley GW. Squamous cell carcinoma of the neovagina. *Obstet Gynecol* 1987;69:525–527.

50. Peters WA, Kumar NB, Morley GW. Carcinoma of the vagina. Factors influencing treatment of outcome. *Cancer* 1985;55:892–997.

51. Schraub S, Sun XS, Maingon P, et al. Cervical and vaginal cancer associated with pessary use. *Cancer* 1992;69:2505–2509.

52. Al-Kurdi M, Monaghan JM. Twenty-two years experience in management of primary tumors of the vagina. *Br J Obstet Gynecol* 1981;88:1145–1150.

53. Anderen ES. Primary carcinoma of the vagina: a study of 29 cases. *Gynecol Oncol* 1989;33:317–320.

54. Winawer SJ, et al. A comparison of colonoscopy and double-contrast barium enema for surveillance after polypectomy. *N Engl J Med* 2000;342:1766–1772.

55. Fletcher RH. The end of barium enema? *N Engl J Med* 2000;342:1823–1824.

56. The International Federation of Gynecology and Obstetrics (FIGO). *Annual report on the results of treatment in gynecologic cancer,* 22nd ed. Stockholm: FIGO, 1994.

57. Creasman WT, Phillips JL, Menck HR. The National Cancer Data Base report on cancer of the vagina. *Cancer* 1998;83(5):1033–1040.

58. Peters WA III, Kumar NB, Marley GW. Microinvasive carcinoma of the vagina: a distinct clinical entity. *Am J Obstet Gynecol* 1985;153(5):505–507.

59. Ball HG, Berman ML. Management of primary vaginal carcinoma. *Gynecol Oncol* 1982;14:154–163.

60. Spirtos NM, Doshi BP, Kapp DS, et al. Radiation therapy for primary squamous cell carcinoma of the vagina: Stanford University experience. *Gynecol Oncol* 1989;35:20–26.

61. Dixit S, Singhal S, Baboo HA. Squamous cell carcinoma of the vagina: a review of 70 cases. *Gynecol Oncol* 1993;48:80–87.

62. Davis KP, Stanhope CR, Garton GR, et al. Invasive vaginal carcinoma: analysis of early-stage disease. *Gynecol Oncol* 1991;42:131–136.

63. Lindeque BG. The role of surgery in the management of carcinoma of the vagina. *Baillieres Clin Obstet Gynaecol* 1987;1:319–329.

64. Perez CA, Grigsby PW, Garipagaoglu M, et al. Factors affecting long-term outcome of irradiation in carcinoma of the vagina. *Int J Radiat Oncol Biol Phys* 1999;44:37–45.

65. Urbanski K, Kojs Z, Reinfuss M, et al. Primary invasive carcinoma treated with radiotherapy: analysis of prognostic factors. *Gynecol Oncol* 1996;60:16–21.

66. Horowitz RI, Viscoli CM, Merino M, et al. Clear cell adenocarcinoma of the vagina and cervix: incidence, undetected disease, and diethylstilbestrol. *J Clin Epidemiol* 1988;41:593–597.

67. Trimble EL, Rubinstein LV, Menck HR, et al. Vaginal clear cell adenocarcinoma in the United States. *Gynecol Oncol* 1996;61:113–115.

68. Herbst AL, Cole P, Norusis MJ, et al. Epidemiologic aspects and factors related to survival in 384 registry cases of clear cell adenocarcinoma of the vagina and cervix. *Am J Obstet Gynecol* 1979;135:876–886.

69. Hwang EH, Han SJ, Lee MK, et al. Clinical experience with conservative surgery for vaginal endodermal sinus tumor. *J Pediatr Surg* 1996;31:219–222.

70. Orr JW Jr, Holimon JL, Sisson PF. Vaginal adenocarcinoma

developing in residual pelvic endometriosis: a clinical dilemma. *Gynecol Oncol* 1989;33:96–98.

71. Hanselaar AG, Boss EA, Massuger LF, et al. Cytologic examination to detect clear cell adenocarcinoma of the vagina or cervix. *Gynecol Oncol* 1999;75:338–344.

72. Burnett AF. Atypical glandular cells of undetermined significance Pap smears: appropriate evaluation and management. *Curr Opin Obstet Gynecol* 2000;12:33–37.

73. Herbst AL. Vaginal clear cell cancer: incidence, survival and screening. In: *Long-term effects of exposure to diethylstilbestrol (DES). NIH Workshop.* Falls Church, VA, 1992:19–20.

74. Senekjian EK, Hubby M, Bell DA, et al. Clear cell adenocarcinoma (CCA) of the vagina and cervix in association with pregnancy. *Gynecol Oncol* 1986;24:207–219.

75. Buchanan DJ, Schlaerth J, Kurosaki T. Primary vaginal melanoma: thirteen-year disease-free survival after wide local excision and review of recent literature. *Am J Obstet Gynecol* 1998;178:1177–1184.

76. Chung AF, Casey MJ, Flannery JT, et al. Malignant melanoma of the vagina—report of 19 cases. *Obstet Gynecol* 1980;55:720–727.

77. Rodier JF, Janser JC, David E, et al. Radiopharmaceutical-guided surgery in primary malignant melanoma of the vagina. *Gynecol Oncol* 1999;75:308–309.

78. Petru E, Nagle F, Czerwenka K, et al. Primary malignant melanoma of the vagina: long-term remission following radiation therapy. *Gynecol Oncol* 1998;70:23–26.

79. Irvin WP Jr, Bliss SA, Rice LW, et al. Malignant melanoma and locoregional control: radical surgery revisited. *Gynecol Oncol* 1998;71:476–480.

80. Heim K, Hopfl R, Muller-Holzner E, et al. Multiple blue nevi of the vagina. A case report. *J Reprod Med* 2000;45:42–44.

81. Hilgers RD, Malkasian GD Jr, Soule EH. Embryonal rhabdomyosarcoma (botryoid type) of the vagina: a clinicopathology review. *Am J Obstet Gynecol* 1970;107:484–502.

82. Hicks ML, Piver MS. Conservative surgery plus adjuvant therapy for vulvovaginal rhabdomyosarcoma, diethylstilbestrol clear cell adenocarcinoma of the vagina, and unilateral germ cell tumors of the ovary. *Obstet Gynecol Clin North Am* 1992;19:219–233.

83. Shy SW, Lee WH, Chen D, et al. Rhabdomyosarcoma of the vagina in a postmenopausal woman: report of a case and review of the literature. *Gynecol Oncol* 1995;58:395–399.

84. Peters WA, Kumar NB, Anderson WA, et al. Primary sarcoma of the adult vagina: a clinicopathological study. *Obstet Gynecol* 1985;65:699–704.

85. Judson PL, Temple AM, Fowler WC Jr, et al. Vaginal adenosarcoma arising from endometriosis. *Gynecol Oncol* 2000;76:123–125.

86. Fu YS, Reagan JW. *Pathology of the uterine cervix, vagina, and vulva.* Philadelphia: WB Saunders, 1989:336–379.

17

BENIGN CERVICAL DISORDERS

EDUCATIONAL OBJECTIVES

EMBRYOLOGY

Cervical embryological development commences at 12 weeks of fetus life. Following the vaginal lumen formation, transformation of pseudostratified epithelium to the stratified squamous epithelium occurs. Most authorities suggest that the transformation originates from the müllerian epithelium (4), although it is possible that the transformation may originate from the sinus epithelium (5).

The stratified squamous epithelium migrates upwards and eventually transforms into the columnar endocervical epithelium (6).

Remnants of mesonephric ducts, present as small tubules, can be identified in the lateral aspect of the cervical walls (7). The clinical significance of these structures is determined by their potential to grow out of ordinary cervical masses.

ANATOMY

The uterine cervix is one of the uterine segments (the corpus uterus, isthmus, and the cervix) that protrude into the upper vaginal pool; this is termed the vaginal portion (portio vaginalis, exocervix, ectocervix, or anatomical portio) of the cervix. The upper part of the cervix is called the supravaginal portion, which is adjacent to the bladder and is separated by the endopelvic fascia and pubovesicocervical fascia. The cervix fuses with the vagina, forming fornices. The length of the cervix is 2.5 to 3.0 cm, measured from the external os to the anatomical internal os of the cervical

canal, which divides the exocervix into the anterior and posterior lips. The external os of the cervical canal is circular in the nulligravida woman and is slit-like in a parous woman. The cervical canal is 8 mm wide in greatest diameter and has longitudinal mucosal ridges and plicae palmatae. The function of the cervical canal is to connect the ectocervix with the isthmic part (the part of the uterus that distally is limited by the histological os of the uterus, the area in which endocervical glands meet endometrial glands and the anatomical internal os of the cervical canal is located, adjacent to the endometrial cavity) (Fig. 17.1).

Suspension and support of the cervix from the latero-posterior aspect is provided by the cardinal ligament (Mackenrodt's ligament). Posteriorly, the uterosacral ligaments (which arise from the posterior supravaginal portion of the cervix and attach to the second and the fourth sacral vertebrae) suspend the cervix. Anteriorly, the endopelvic fascia and pubovesicocervical fascia support the cervix. The cervix finds additional support by fusing with the vagina.

The *cervical blood supply* comes from the descending branch of the uterine artery, and *blood return* is secured by the venous drainage (which runs parallel to the artery distribution); this has anastomosis between the cervical plexus and the bladder base.

Cervical innervation arrives from the pelvic autonomic system and the superior, middle, and inferior hypogastric plexuses; this innervates the endocervix and runs deep into the periphery of the ectocervix (8).

The cervical lymphatic system has two chains of distribution: submucosal distribution and deep distribution in the fibrous stroma (9).

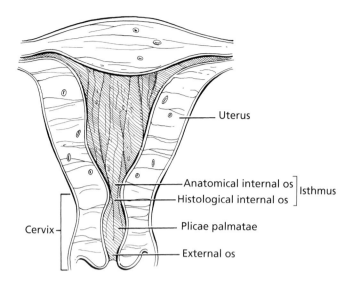

FIGURE 17.1. The cervix and its structures.

The cervical function is multifactorial: the channel providing exit for menstrual flow, the route for sperm migration (facilitated by mucus secretion), a barrier against the passage of microorganisms (the mucosal plug produced by endocervical glands), a mechanical support for pregnancy, and the passive segment of the birth canal. Mucus secretion is affected by changes in estrogen levels during a menstrual cycle. From the eighth day of the menstrual cycle, the amount of mucus production and secretion increases while simultaneously the viscosity decreases and the mucus becomes very elastic (spinnbarkeit is a reflection of elasticity and is measured in centimeters). Such changes are designed to provide an environment for good sperm penetration. In the days following ovulation, the quality of the mucus becomes progressively worse for sperm penetration. At the peak of mucosal secretion, in the days just prior to ovulation, the mucus is shiny, transparent, and very elastic.

The cervix, a unique part of the uterus, distinguishes itself from the rest of the uterus by the following:

- Dual locations: intraperitoneal (the intraabdominal part is covered by the vesicouterine peritoneal reflexion) and extraperitoneal
- Dual epithelia that participate in covering the ecto- and endocervical structures (the stratified squamous epithelium and the mucin-secreting columnar epithelium)
- Dual response to cyclic hormonal fluctuations when no menstrual phase occurs (proliferative phase, an estrogen domineering effect and secretory-phase, a progesterone domineering effect, particularly in cervical mucus production)
- Fibrous connective tissue makes up to 85% of the cervical structure, in contrast to the uterine corpus, which is made up of muscle tissue predominantly
- Venous blood return occurs in the absence of venous sinuses

The cervical transformation zone is the area in which the endocervical columnar epithelium meets the ectocervical stratified squamous epithelium. From a clinical point of view, it is a significant structure, since, most commonly, neoplasia arises from this area (two different types of cells with two different functions—the mucin-secreting columnar cell epithelium and the squamous cell epithelium—coexist).

The mucin-secreting columnar epithelium usually covers the ectocervix at birth; the presence of columnar epithelium on the ectocervix at reproductive age is termed ectropion (cervical ectopy). Ectropion may remain on the ectocervix until puberty in about 43% of girls; thereafter, squamous cell epithelium replaces columnar epithelium in approximately 57% of cases (10). At two periods in a woman's life—at the time of menarche and during pregnancy (when natural enlargement of the uterus occurs)—a reverse replacing process takes place: to a lesser extent, squamous cell epithelium is substituted by columnar epithelium. Therefore, cervical ectopy is a natural process in these two periods. Ectropion is predominantly located on the anterior cervical lip, although the posterior cervical lip or both lips can be affected. Progestins (a component of oral contraceptives) can potentiate ectropion. Ectropion is often incorrectly called cervical erosion or confused with true cervical erosion, which is denudation of the epithelium. Since ectropion is a natural, physiological occurrence, it will not require therapeutic intervention, and with time, spontaneous replacement of ectropion with squamous cell epithelium takes place. This process will create a new squamocolumnar junction, also termed as functional, or physiologic new squamocolumnar junction.

The area between the original squamocolumnar junction (from the neonatal period) and the functional squamocolumnar junction (from the postpubertal period)—is named the *transformation zone*. The clinical importance of the transformation zone is recognized, since cervical squamous cell neoplasia is associated with the new squamocolumnar junction. The transformation zone is not visible by the naked eye. Colposcopic examination with 3% to 5% acetic acid will disclose a smooth, translucent, white area. Such colposcopic findings characterize squamous cell metaplasia, which is a natural process of replacing the columnar epithelium by the squamous epithelium.

The *cervical Nabothian cyst* is created when mucin-secreting columnar cells are covered by the metaplastic squamous epithelium. Outflow of the secretion is blocked, leading to glandular distention.

Cervical squamous metaplasia is a natural restorative process, in which the stratified squamous epithelium substitutes for the mucin-secreting columnar epithelium. The replacement can be achieved by two mechanisms (11):

- Squamous epithelialization is defined as expansion of the stratified squamous epithelium to the neighboring columnar epithelium.

- Squamous metaplasia (epidermidization or squamous prosoplasia) is characterized as differentiation of sub-columnar reserve cells (undifferentiated) into the squamous epithelium.

BENIGN CERVICAL DISORDERS

Cervicitis

Infectious Cervicitis

The etiologic factors in *mucopurulent cervicitis (MPC)* are varied.

Chlamydia trachomatis Cervicitis
Definition
Chlamydia trachomatis cervicitis is an inflammatory process of the cervix due to *C. trachomatis,* an obligate intracellular bacterial parasite of the columnar and transitional epithelium.

Incidence
C. trachomatis cervicitis is the most common sexually transmitted disease (STD) worldwide (12). Prevalence is estimated to be 3% to 5% among asymptomatic women and reaches 40% among women seeking assistance in STD clinics (13).

Etiology
C. trachomatis is the most common etiologic agent in MPC.

Classification

- Acute *C. trachomatis* cervicitis
- Chronic *C. trachomatis* cervicitis

Diagnosis
Pertinent medical history consists of symptoms of *C. trachomatis* cervical infections (present in about one-third of affected women); in up to 80% of affected women, asymptomatic clinical infection can be present (14).

The most commonly reported symptoms are as follows:

- Persistent, yellow-green vaginal discharge
- Postcoital or postdouche vaginal spotting

Physical examination is not specific for *C. trachomatis* cervicitis, but reveals the general clinical manifestations of MPC:

- Visible, yellow-green discharge from the cervical external os; a clinical Q-tip test can be positive (a green stain on the cotton tip)
- On speculum examination, the presence of cervical edema, erythema, and friability of the cervix (on touch, the cervix bleeds with ease)
- Hypertrophy of the cervix observed
- Central cervical eversion or ectopy with mucorrhea, and oozing blood when touched
- Cervical tenderness elicited by palpation and/or motion

A recent study has established that a visual indicator such as yellowish vaginal discharge and easily induced cervical bleeding into the mucous are more indicative of *C. trachomatis cervicitis* than is opacity of the endocervical discharge (15).

The presence of dysuria, urinary urgency, urinary frequency, and the presence of >10 white blood cells per high power field with negative bacterial culture is highly suggestive of *C. trachomatis* infection.

Laboratory tests are as follows:

- Utilizing the cytobrush endocervical sampling technique for microbiological material and the Polymerase Chain Reaction (*PCR*) method, *C. trachomatis* cervicitis can be detected with a sensitivity of 93.8% (16); however, the difference between culture and PCR from cervical specimen is not significant (17). The cytobrush endocervical sampling technique can be considered an opportunistic screening, since the cytobrush can be used for cervical cytology sampling and, thereafter, the same cytobrush can be placed in the transport medium for subsequent *C. trachomatis* detection by PCR (16).
- Utilizing a cytobrush endocervical sampling technique for microbiological material and the *culture method, C. trachomatis* cervicitis can be detected with a sensitivity of 87.5% (16).
- *Cervical wet mount* has been postulated as a negative predictor for *C. trachomatis*–induced cervicitis in a pregnant woman. A count of <10 polymorphonuclear lymphocytes per × 400 high-power field is considered as predictive of the absence of *C. trachomatis*–induced cervicitis (18). It is a very promising finding; however, this observation requires clinical validation.

Since *Neisseria gonorrhoeae* frequently is associated with *C. trachomatis*–induced cervicitis (10%–50%), testing for both pathogens is highly recommended.

High prevalence of an asymptomatic occurrence with significant morbidity and its sequelae suggest that screening programs are of paramount importance in prevention, since diagnosis and therapies are easily accessible.

A recent study has postulated that at the time when genital infection is present, opportunistic cytology should be performed, since it does not increase the rate of incorrect or inadequate diagnosis (19).

Differential Diagnosis The following infections may cause MPC:

- *Neisseria gonorrhoeae*
- *Trichomonas vaginalis*
- Bacterial vaginosis
- Group B streptococcus
- Mycosis
- *Mycoplasma hominis*
- *Ureaplasma urealyticum*

Conventional Therapy

In response to a diagnosis of *C. trachomatis* cervicitis, one of the following agents can be instituted for therapy (20):

- Doxycycline, 100 mg orally twice daily for 7 days
- Azithromycin (Zithromax), 1 g orally in a single dose
- Ofloxacin, 300 mg orally twice daily for 7 days
- Erythromycin base, 500 mg orally four times daily for 7 days
- Erythromycin ethylsuccinate, 800 mg four times daily for 7 days

A recent double-blind study revealed that, in uncomplicated *C. trachomatis* infection, *Trovafloxacin*, 200 mg orally once daily for 5 days, was as clinically and bacteriologically effective as doxycycline given orally at 100 mg twice daily for 7 days (21).

All patients who are symptomatic or who present risk factors (a new male partner with urethritis, multiple sexual partners within the preceding 2 months, exposure to gonorrhea, or a clinical picture of urethritis) should be tested for *C. trachomatis* (21). Silent or asymptomatic chlamydia infection may compromise tubal function and may lead to infertility or tubal ectopic pregnancy, or may develop into pelvic inflammatory disease (PID). Taking into consideration the clinical sequelae of chlamydia infection, it seems reasonable to initiate therapy for all those who are symptomatic and in a high-risk group while waiting for laboratory results (22).

Retesting for *C. trachomatis* should be scheduled routinely within 3 to 4 weeks following the conclusion of the treatment course. To prevent reinfection, sexual partners should be evaluated and treated.

Complementary Therapy and Alternative Therapy

Antibiotics are essential in the treatment of *C. trachomatis* infection, but an alternative treatment can be offered to complement conventional therapy (23) as well.

Patient education in prevention of this disease is as follows:

- Monogamous sexual practice
- Learning the sexual disease history of prospective sexual partners
- Avoiding sexual activities with frequently changing partners or multiple partners
- Testing for other STDs when one STD test result is positive
- Compliance with prescribed medication for STD
- Condom protection is not a guarantee against STD, although it may provide some degree of disease protection (24,25).

Vitamins recommended are as follows:

- Vitamin A, 50,000 IU orally, daily for 1 week and a reduced dose of 25,000 IU for 1 additional week.
- Vitamin C, 500 mg orally every 2 hours for 2 days and 1,000 mg orally three times per day for 2 weeks

- Carotenoids, 50,000 IU orally, daily for 2 weeks

The only *mineral* recommended is zinc, 30 mg orally, daily for 2 weeks.

As to *diet*, yogurt at 4 to 8 oz daily for 2 weeks is recommended.

With respect to an *herbal remedy*, Echinacea exhibits antiinflammatory properties and has been used in *C. trachomatis*, although there is no scientific data to support its use. If used, the recommended course is an oral dose of 2 capsules every 2 hours for 2 days and thereafter 2 capsules three times daily for 2 weeks.

Neisseria gonorrhoeae
Definition

Neisseria gonorrhoeae is an inflammatory process of the cervix due to *N. gonorrhoeae* bacteria.

Incidence

The true incidence of gonorrhea infection is difficult to establish due to underreporting of this condition. It is estimated that each year in the United States about 2 million cases occur (26). Gonorrhea has declined since its 1975 peak (27), although a rise in gonorrhea is observed in some countries at an alarming rate (28–31).

Etiology

N. gonorrhoeae is an identified pathogen in gonorrhea. It is a gram-negative aerobic diplococcus with the ability to invade the columnar and transitional epithelium.

Classification

- Acute gonorrheal cervicitis
- Chronic gonorrheal cervicitis

Diagnosis

Pertinent medical history is similar to that which has been presented for *C. trachomatis* cervicitis.

Physical examination is based upon the same criteria that are presented for *C. trachomatis* cervicitis, since there is no specific sign for gonorrhea infection (27).

As to *laboratory* tests, isolation of *N. gonorrhoeae* by *culture* on selective media such as Thayer-Martin (the antibiotic component inhibits other forms of bacteria and mycotic flora) is diagnostic in 80% to 90% of women with a single swab from the endocervical canal (32).

Gram stain of material from the infected site in women yields positive findings in about 60%; therefore, culture is a standard clinical approach in making the diagnosis (33).

Differential Diagnosis

Differential diagnosis includes the following conditions:

- *Chlamydia trachomatis*
- *Trichomonas vaginalis*
- Bacterial vaginosis
- Group B streptococcus

- Mycosis
- *Mycoplasma hominis*
- *Ureoplasma urealyticum*

Conventional Therapy

Conventional therapy is indicated while waiting for culture results with one of the following antibiotics for uncomplicated gonococcal endocervicitis (20):

- Ceftriaxone sodium (Rocephin), 125 mg intramuscularly in a single dose
- Ofloxacin (Floxin), 400 mg orally in a single dose
- Cefixime (Suprax), 400 mg orally in a single dose
- Ciprofloxacin (Cipro), 500 mg orally in a single dose

Recent sexual partners need to be treated as well. Also, it is recommended the patient abstain from coitus until after therapy concludes and symptoms subside. Potentially coexisting *C. trachomatis* infection should be treated with one of the effective regimens presented above.

Antibacterial resistance may cause failure of gonorrheal therapy. Fluoroquinolone-resistant gonococcal strains are now prevalent in Australia and Asia. Nevertheless, no clinically significant resistance to broad-spectrum cephalosporins has been identified (34).

Complementary Therapy and Alternative Therapy

Complementary-alternative therapies for gonococcal treatment can be offered as an adjunctive approach to antibiotics therapy. The same modalities that are suggested for chlamydia cervicitis can be administered.

Other Pathogens Causing Mucopurulent Cervicitis

Pathogens affecting the vagina, vulva, or anus may cause MPC. Clinical management of these conditions is described in their respective chapters. The following pathogens may be responsible for MPC:

- Protozoal disease *(Trichomonas vaginalis)*
- Parasitic infection of the cervix: (a) *Amebiasis* clinically presents as multiple small ulcerative and friable lesion; wet mount microscopic examination of cervico-vaginal smear shows typical *Entamoeba histolytica* trophozoites; metronidazole, 750 mg orally three times daily for 7 days is the recommended therapy (35,36). (b) *Echinococcosis cyst* has been reported as a pathogen responsible for MPC; however, there is scarce information about this entity; the diagnosis can be established on a clinical basis and through a specific immunodiagnostic test (37,38). The therapy is surgical excision or cyst drainage with mebendazole, a broad-spectrum anthelmintic agent, which is administered as chewable tablets, at 100 mg twice daily for 3 days (39).
- Bacterial vaginosis
- Group B streptococcus
- Mycosis

- *Mycoplasma hominis* (this pathogen may cause PID or infertility; the diagnosis is reached either by culture or antibody titer; therapy with clindamycin or tetracycline is effective)
- *Ureoplasma urealyticum* (culture or antibody titer is diagnostic; tetracycline and erythromycin are effective modes of therapy)
- Actinomycosis
- Viral infections

The management of each of these conditions is similar to vaginal and vulvar modalities; more detailed information can be found in their respective chapters.

Noninfectious Cervicitis

A nonspecific inflammatory response of the cervix to chemical substances, mechanical microtrauma, or iatrogenic cases is considered noninfectious cervicitis. This medical entity may clinically manifest in an acute or chronic form. The most commonly observed noninfectious cervicitis is associated with chemical substances introduced into the vagina by douching. Mechanical microtrauma is commonly inflicted by tampons, diaphragms, pessaries, IUDs, or surgical procedures.

Diagnosis is based on symptoms such as malodorous yellowish vaginal discharge, bloodstain discharge, lower back pain, and dyspareunia. These symptoms may follow douching, insertion of a foreign body, or surgery.

Physical examination may find cervical erythema, areas that bleed when touched and decreased mucosal secretion.

As to *laboratory* tests, on wet mount examination no pathogen is identified. Cervical cultures are negative.

Colposcopic examination will reveal epithelial erosion with hyperemic cervical mucosa.

Conventional therapy is removal of the irritating chemical substance or foreign body. Prophylaxis Sultrin vaginal cream (triple-sulfa cream) can be administered twice daily for a 5-day course.

Benign Cervical Lesions

Nabothian Cyst

Squamous metaplasia that replaces the columnar epithelium within the transformation zone may trap and obliterate endocervical mucin-producing glands and result in the formation of cervical cysts. The Nabothian cyst (retention cyst of the cervix) is a superficial cyst; although, deep location within the cervix occurs, which presents a clinical differential diagnosis dilemma (mucin-producing adenocarcinoma or Nabothian cyst?). Recently, magnetic resonance imaging (MRI) has been recognized as a valuable tool in diagnosis (40). The differential diagnosis includes mesonephric duct cysts or cervical cysts of inclusion, along with mucin-producing adenocarcinoma. Nabothian cysts vary in size from 6 to 20 mm, and in most cases, are present in groups. The location of a Nabothian cyst within 1 cm of the external os of the cervical canal is classified as a low location and above 1 cm a high location. Single or multiple cysts cause cervical enlargement (41). Clinically, a Nabothian cyst is either white or yellow in appearance and usually is asymptomatic. This cervical condition is clinically insignificant and in most cases will not require any therapeutic intervention. When a Nabothian cyst is the result of chronic cervicitis, the underlying pathogen or cause should be determined and subjected to an appropriate therapy.

Cervical Endometriosis

Cervical endometriosis is implantation of the endometrium tissue on the ecto- or endocervix. Cervical endometriosis can be observed in 5% to 15% of menstruating women following cervical procedures. Procedures such as electrocautery, trachelorrhaphy, and cervical cone biopsy cause 43% of all cervical endometriosis (42). There is a potential of adenocarcinoma arising from cervical endometriosis (43–45), and for this reason, direct biopsy should be performed.

Diagnosis is clinical and verified by histology, which documents the presence of endometrial glands and stroma.

This condition may manifest *symptoms* of premenstrual spotting and occasionally may produce dysmenorrhea and/or dyspareunia, and infertility. In most instances, cervical endometriosis is asymptomatic. If cervical endometriosis is symptomatic, symptoms will get worse premenstrually, within 2 weeks of the next menses, and will ease with menses. When endometriotic implant is large, vaginal bleeding may occur.

In the majority of cases, the *signs* of cervical endometriosis are present as small (a few millimeters in diameter) red or reddish-blue nodular lesions. Large endometriotic implants may be nodular or cystic in appearance.

Therapy includes the following modalities:

- Hormonal treatment
- Destructive treatment, by (a) classical excision, (b) deep cauterization, and (c) laser vaporization

These therapeutic methods are presented in Chapter 16.

Cervical Polyps

Cervical polyps can be defined as a local overgrowth of the endocervical epithelium. This cervical entity is frequently associated with chronic cervicitis.

Diagnosis is established on clinical and histological grounds [all cervical polypoid lesions should be subjected to microscopic evaluation (46), since, occasionally, carcinoma may arise from endocervical polyps (47)].

Symptoms may include perfuse vaginal discharge, postcoital spotting, or bleeding, with severity of bleeding usually corresponding to the degree of ulceration.

The *signs* of cervical polyp are characterized by the presence of a single lesion that is a red, soft, elongated, globular, and lobular mass. The size of this lesion usually varies from a few millimeters up to 3 cm; although, a giant cervical polyp may occur (48).

Differential diagnosis of cervical polyp includes the following:

- Adenomyoma
- Adenocarcinoma
- Condylomata acuminata
- Decidua or retained product of conception
- Fibroadenoma
- Granulation tissue
- Leiomyomata or prolapsing endometrial submucosal myomata
- Microglandular endocervical hyperplasia
- Papillary adenofibroma
- Sarcomas
- Squamous cell carcinoma
- Squamous papilloma

Surgical removeal of the cervical polyp by twisting (cervical polypectomy) is a recommended mode of *therapy*. Endocervical curettage (ECC) following polypectomy is customarily performed and considered an essential part of managing cervical polyps. The Kovorkian curette is used to perform ECC, which can improve the accuracy of diagnosing premalignant and malignant cervical lesions (49). A randomized controlled clinical study documented that the endocervical brush, following ECC sampling, significantly increased the likelihood of obtaining sufficient material for histological evaluation (50).

Cervical Leiomyomata

Leading gynecological textbooks present the opinion that the prevalence of cervical leiomyomata is approximately 8% of all uterine myomata; however, a recent study has documented that cervical leiomyomata occurs in only about 0.6% (51). Small cervical myomata are asymptomatic. Larger tumors may produce local symptoms such as dyspareunia or symptoms that may result from tumor compression on adjacent organs such as the bladder or rectum. Very scattered information exists in the literature in reference to the risk of malignant transformation; although, benign cervical leiomyomata leading to disseminated fatal malignancy has been presented in one report (52). That report highlights the rare potential for malignant transformation in histologically documented benign leiomyomata with no microscopic indications for such potential.

Diagnosis is clinical, and sonography or MRI may provide verification of this extremely rare condition. The definitive diagnosis is established by histological examination.

Conventional therapy for symptomatic cervical leiomyomata is myomectomy, but definitive treatment will only be accomplished by performing a total hysterectomy.

Cervical Adenomyomata or Fibroadenoma

Cervical adenomyomata and fibroadenoma are mixed tumors; assigning one name or the other is dependent upon the preponderance of fibrous or muscular tissue. Limited clinical experience, due to an extremely rare occurrence of the tumor, does not allow the establishment of a meaningful diagnostic process or therapy.

Cervical Leukoplakia

A keratinization process of the cervical squamous cell epithelium is viewed as an abnormal occurrence. Clinically, hyperkeratosis and parakeratosis appear on the ectocervix as white, elevated plaques. Leukoplakia itself is not considered a premalignant lesion; nevertheless, it can be associated with cervical neoplasia. Due to this fact, a direct biopsy of each leukoplakia lesion should be performed. If there is premalignancy or malignancy histologically documented, appropriate management should be undertaken.

Cervical Ectopic Pregnancy

Implantation of an embryo within the cervical canal (below the internal os) is considered a cervical pregnancy. Such a clinical event is extremely rare and often confused with a low uterine intracavitary location. A cervical pregnancy can be associated with perfuse bleeding and is a life-threatening condition with approximately a 5% maternal mortality rate. Today in industrialized countries, these rates are declining, probably due to progress in early diagnosis, conservative therapies, and improved surgical techniques. Conservative surgical interventions may induce excessive hemorrhaging from the descending uterine vessels. Both viable and nonviable types of cervical pregnancies are potentially life-threatening conditions.

Early diagnosis is an essential factor in conservative medical and surgical management of an ectopic cervical pregnancy.

Diagnosis is arrived at clinically, if a changing menstrual pattern or oligomenorrhea are present (in neglected cases, secondary amenorrhea may be present). Vaginal spotting or bleeding, which can intensify after coitus, the presence of bloodstain vaginal discharge, and deep dyspareunia may also be reported.

With respect to *laboratory* tests, a serum beta–human chorionic gonadotropin (hCG) serial level is crucial in diagnosing ectopic pregnancy. The same general criteria are utilized in establishing the diagnosis of ectopic pregnancy as in an intrauterine pregnancy; when an hCG levels reaches 1,200 to 1,500 IU/L, intrauterine pregnancy can be reliably visualized by ultrasonography. Also, it has been suggested that progesterone levels of ≤17.5 ng/mL (55.7 nmol/L) may indicate ectopic pregnancy (53).

Imaging studies with transvaginal ultrasonography (54) or three-dimensional power Doppler ultrasonography have extraordinary value in the diagnosis of cervical ectopic pregnancy (55).

Conventional therapy for cervical ectopic pregnancy falls into several categories:

- Hysterectomy is considered a definitive treatment.
- *Conservative medical treatment* with methotrexate is successful in 91% of cervical pregnancies, either viable or nonviable (56). Methotrexate can be administered either intramuscularly in a single 50-mg dose (57,58) or via intraamniotic instillation of 50 mg. Both routes of administration are equally effective; although, intraamniotic instillation should be guided ultrasonographically (57). Monitoring of serum beta-hCG treatment effects is not a reliable paradigm, and no guidelines are available to practitioners for predicting treatment failures of methotrexate in patients with cervical ectopic pregnancy (59). Prognostic factors have been offered, based upon quantitative literature review, for satisfactory primary methotrexate treatment of cervical pregnancy. The following data may suggest an unsatisfactory outcome of primary methotrexate treatment of cervical pregnancy (60): (a) cervical ectopic pregnancy that initially presented with serum beta-hCG of ≥10,000 IU/mL, (b) gestational age of ≥9 weeks, and (c) ultrasonographically determined crown-rump length of >10 mm.
- *Simple selective uterine artery embolization* with or without methotrexate therapy has been reported to be a successful treatment (55,56). Also, this technique has been used preoperatively for cervical pregnancy to decrease intraoperative hemorrhage during pregnancy evacuation from the cervical location (61).
- *A Foley catheter balloon* compression within the cervical canal or the performance of cervical cerclage before cervical pregnancy evacuation is effective (62,63).
- *Fetal reduction with a KCl solution* treats a heterotopic cervical pregnancy with preservation of an intrauterine pregnancy. Under transabdominal ultrasonographic guide, a 6-inch 20-gauge spinal needle is inserted transcervically into the thorax of the embryo. Such an approach selectively terminates the cervical pregnancy, allowing the intrauterine pregnancy progress to term (64).

REFERENCES

1. Association of Professors of Gynecology and Obstetrics (APGO). *Medical student educational objectives,* 7th ed. Washington, DC: Association of Professors of Gynecology and Obstetrics, 1997.
2. Council on Resident Education in Obstetrics and Gynecology (CREOG). *Educational objectives core curriculum for residents in obstetrics and gynecology,* 5th ed. Washington, DC: CREOG, 1996.
3. American College of Obstetricians and Gynecologists (ACOG). *Technical bulletin no. 183.* Washington, DC: ACOG, 1996.
4. Koff AK. Development of the vagina in the human fetus. *Contrib Embryol Carnegie Inst* 1993;24:54–59.

5. Bulmer D. The development of the human vagina. *J Anat* 1957; 91:490–495.
6. Fluhmann CF. Developmental anatomy of the cervix uteri. *Obstet Gynecol* 1960;15:62–57.
7. Huffman J. Mesonephric remnants in the cervix. *Am J Obstet Gynecol* 1948;56:233–238.
8. Krantz KE. The anatomy of the human cervix, gross and microscopic. In: Blandau RJ, Moghissi K, eds. *The biology of the cervix.* Chicago: University of Chicago Press, 1973.
9. Reiffenstuhl G. *The lymphatics of the female genital organs.* Philadelphia: JB Lippincott, 1964.
10. Linhartova A. Extent of the columnar epithelium on the ectocervix between the ages of 1 and 13 years. *Obstet Gynecol* 1978; 52:451–456.
11. Feldman D, Romaney SL, Edgcomb J, et al. Ultrastructure of normal, metaplastic and abnormal human uterine cervix: use of montages to study the topographical relationship of epithelial cells. *Am J Obstet Gynecol* 1984;150:573–688.
12. Paavonen J, Eggert-Kruse W. *Chlamydia trachomatis:* impact on human reproduction. *Hum Reprod Update* 1999;5:433–447.
13. Stamm WE, Holmes KK. *Chlamydia trachomatis* infections of the adult. In: Holmes KK, Mardh PA, Sparling PF, et al., eds. *Sexually transmitted diseases.* New York: McGraw-Hill, 1984:258–269.
14. Harrison HR, Costin M, Meder JB, et al. Cervical *Chlamydia trachomatis* infection in university women: relationship to history, contraception, ectopy, and cervicitis. *Am J Obstet Gynecol* 1985;153:244–251.
15. Sellors JW, Walter SD, Howard M. A new indicator of chlamydial cervicitis? *Sex Transm Infect* 2000;76:46–48.
16. Wandall DA, Ostergaard L, Overgaard L, et al. Opportunistic screening for Chlamydia screening for *Chlamydia trachomatis* cervicitis: the value of cytobrush specimens for detection by PCR compared with cell culture. *APMIS* 1998;106:580–584.
17. Labau E, Henry S, Bennet P, et al. Direct diagnosis of *Chlamydia trachomatis* genital infections: culture or PCR? *Pathol Biol (Paris)* 1998;46:813–818.
18. Bohmer JT, Schemmer G, Harrison FN Jr, et al. Cervical wet mount as a negative predictor for gonococci– and *Chlamydia trachomatis*–induced cervicitis in a gravid population. *Am J Obstet Gynecol* 1999;181:283–287.
19. Edwards SK, Sonnex C. Influence of genital infection on cervical cytology. *Sex Transm Infect* 1998;74:271–273.
20. Centers for Disease Control and Prevention. Sexually transmitted diseases guidelines. *MMWR* 1993;42:51–57.
21. McCormack WM, Dalu ZA, Martin DH, et al. Double-blind comparison of trovafloxacin and doxycycline in the treatment of uncomplicated chlamydia urethritis and cervicitis. Trovafloxacin Chlamydial Urethritis/Cervicitis Study Group. *Sex Transm Dis* 1999;26:531–536.
22. Handsfield HH, Jasman LL, Roberts PL, et al. Criteria for selective screening for *Chlamydia trachomatis* infection in women attending family planning clinics. *JAMA* 1986;255:1730.
23. Hudson T. *Women's encyclopedia of natural medicine. Alternative therapies and integrative medicine.* Los Angeles: Keats Publishing, 1999:257–264.
24. Crosby R, Leichliter JS, Brackbill R. Longitudinal prediction of sexually transmitted diseases among adolescents (1). *Am J Prev Med* 2000;18:312–317.
25. Wong ML, Chan RK, Koh D, et al. Factors associated with condom use for oral sex among female brothel-based sex workers in Singapore. *Sex Transm Dis* 2000;27:39–45.
26. Sweet RL, Gibbs RS. *Infectious diseases of the female genital tract,* 3rd ed. Baltimore: Williams & Wilkins, 1995:134.
27. Emmert DH, Kirchner JT. Sexually transmitted diseases in women. Gonorrhea and syphilis. *Postgrad Med* 2000;107: 181–184,189–190.
28. Martin IM, Ison CA. Rise in gonorrhoea in London, U.K. London Gonococcal Working Group. *Lancet* 2000;355:623.
29. Hughes G, Andrews N, Catchpole M, et al. Investigation of the increased incidence of gonorrhoea diagnosed in genitourinary medicine in England, 1994–6. *Sex Transm Infect* 2000;76:18–24.
30. Panchaud C, Singh S, Feivelson D, et al. Sexually transmitted diseases among adolescents in developed countries. *Fam Plann Perspect* 2000;32:24–32.
31. Epidemiology of syphilis and gonorrhea in eastern Poland in the years 1988–1997. *Int J STD AIDS* 1999;10:680–684.
32. Thin RN, Shaw EJ. Diagnosis of gonorrhea in women. *Br J Vener Dis* 1979;55:10–13.
33. Hook EW III, Handsfield HH. Gonococcal infections in the adult. In: Holmes KK, Mardh PA, Sparling PF, et al., eds. *Sexually transmitted diseases.* New York: McGraw-Hill, 1990: 149–165.
34. Fox KK, Knapp JS. Antimicrobial resistance in *Neisseria gonorrhoeae. Curr Opin Urol* 1999;9:65–70.
35. Cohen C. Three cases of amoebiasis of the cervix uteri. *J Obstet Gynecol Br Commonw* 1973;80:476–479.
36. Nopdonrattakoon L. Amoebiasis of the female genital tract: a case report. *J Obstet Gynaecol Res* 1996;22:235–238.
37. Kammerer WS, Schantz PM. Echinococcal disease. *Infect Dis Clin North Am* 1993;7:605–618.
38. Langley FG. Primary echinococcal cyst of the uterus. *Br J Surg* 1943;30:278–281.
39. Smago DR, Smago RA Jr. Hydatid cyst: preoperative sterilization with mebendazole. *South Med J* 1986;79:900–901.
40. Li H, Sugimura K, Okizuka H, et al. Markedly high signal intensity lesions in the uterine cervix on T_2-weighted imaging: differentiation between mucin-producing carcinomas and Nabothian cysts. *Radiat Med* 1999;17:137–143.
41. Fogel SR, Slasky BS. Sonography of Nabothian cysts. *AJR Am J Roentgenol* 1982;138:927–930.
42. Ismail SM. Cone biopsy causes cervical endometriosis and tuboendometrioid metaplasia. *Histopathology* 1991;18:107–114.
43. Marzullo F, Damiani N. Anatomo-clinical and histologic consideration of endometrial adenocarcinoma of the cervix uteri. *Riv Anat Patol Oncol* 1965;28:791–807.
44. Chang SH, Maddox WA. Adenocarcinoma arising within cervical endometriosis and invading the adjacent vagina. *Am J Obstet Gynecol* 1971;110:1015–1017.
45. Giana M, Ripamonti N, Giudici M. A case of primary adenocarcinoma of the cervix of probable origin from an area of endometriosis. *Minerva Med* 1985;76(6):221–223.
46. Shirumizu K, Ryou E, Tsukagoshi T, et al. Diagnostic problems relating to uterine cervical polyps with malignancy. *Asia Oceania J Obstet Gynecol* 1993;19:257–260.
47. Nishida T, Sugiyama T, Miyoshi T, et al. A carcinoma *in situ* arising in an endocervical polyp—a case report. *Kurume Med J* 1994; 41:37–40.
48. Duckman S, Suarez JR, Sese LQ. Giant cervical polyp. *Am J Obstet Gynecol* 1988;159:852–854.
49. Toki T, Fujii S, Yajima A. Clinical significance of endocervical curettage (ECC) in predicting neoplastic lesions of the cervix. *Nippon Sanka Fujinka Gakkai Zasshi* 1994;46:265–270.
50. Tate KM, Strickland JL. A randomized controlled trial to evaluate the use of the endocervical brush after endocervical curettage. *Obstet Gynecol* 1997;90:715–717.
51. Tiltman AJ. Leiomyomas of the uterine cervix: a study of frequency. *Int J Gynecol Pathol* 1998;17:231–234.
52. O'Connell MP, Jenkins DM, Curtain AW, et al. Benign cervical leiomyoma leading to disseminated fatal malignancy. *Gynecol Oncol* 1996;62:119–122.
53. McCord ML, Muram D, Buster JE, et al. Single serum progesterone as a screen for ectopic pregnancy: exchanging specificity

and sensitivity to obtain optimal test performance. *Fertil Steril* 1996;66:513–516.

54. Amor F, Vaccaro H, Martinez J, et al. Cervical pregnancy. Three clinical cases. *Rev Chil Obstet Gynecol* 1995;60:181–183.

55. Su YN, Shih JC, Chiu WH, et al. Cervical pregnancy: assessment with three-dimensional power Doppler imaging and successful management with selective uterine artery embolization. *Ultrasound Obstet Gynecol* 1999;14:284–287.

56. Kung FT, Chang SY. Efficacy of methotrexate treatment in viable or nonviable cervical pregnancies. *Am J Obstet Gynecol* 1999;181: 1438–1444.

57. Hung TH, Jeng CJ, Yang YC, et al. Treatment of cervical pregnancy with methotrexate. *Int J Gynaecol Obstet* 1996;53: 243–247.

58. Goldberg JM, Widrich T. Successful management of a viable cervical pregnancy by single-dose methotrexate. *J Womens Health Gend Based Med* 2000;9:43–45.

59. Hajenius PJ, Roos D, Ankum WM, et al. Are serum human chorionic gonadotropin clearance curves of use in monitoring methotrexate treatment in cervical pregnancy? *Fertil Steril* 1998; 70:362–365.

60. Hung TH, Shau WY, Hsieh TT, et al. Prognostic factors for unsatisfactory primary methotrexate treatment of cervical pregnancy: a quantitative review. *Hum Reprod* 1998;13:2636–2642.

61. Lobel SM, Meyerovitz MF, Benson CC, et al. Preoperative angiographic uterine artery embolization in the management of cervical pregnancy. *Obstet Gynecol* 1990;76:938–941.

62. Bernstein D, Holzinger M, Ovadia J, et al. Conservative treatment of cervical pregnancy. *Obstet Gynecol* 1981;58:741–742.

63. Thomas R, Gingold BR, Gallagher MW. Cervical pregnancy: a report of two cases. *J Reprod Med* 1991;36:459–462.

64. Carreno CA, King M, Johnson MP, et al. Treatment of heterotopic cervical and intrauterine pregnancy. *Fetal Diagn Ther* 2000; 15:1–3.

18

PREMALIGNANT AND MALIGNANT NEOPLASIA OF THE CERVIX

EDUCATIONAL OBJECTIVES

Medical Students (1) *APGO Objective No. 56*	*Residents in Obstetrics/Gynecology (2)* *CREOG Objectives*	*Practitioners (3)* *ACOG Recommendations*
Risk factors for cervical disease and neoplasia	Preinvasive cervical disease Diagnosis	Frequency of cytology screening Techniques of cytology screening
Indications for screening	Management	Reporting of cytology diagnosis
Symptoms and physical findings of cervicitis and neoplasia	Invasive carcinoma of the cervix Diagnosis	HPV detection in diagnosis and management
Evaluation and management of the patient with an abnormal Pap smear	Management Follow-up	Diagnostic procedures Guidelines for management
Impact of staging on management and prognosis		Therapy

Early detection for cervical premalignant or malignant lesions is an essential factor in controlling these conditions. Cervical squamous cell cancer was the number one cause of death for women in the United States in 1930; today it is number 12. On average, 13,700 new cervical cancers are diagnosed and 5,000 deaths occur each year in the United States. The most important factor responsible for this decline is screening with Papanicolaou cervico-vaginal smears (Pap smear) (4); although, it has been estimated that approximately 2.5 million women in the United States have never had a Pap smear (5). This unquestionable success is obvious among women with squamous cell cervical carcinoma; however, similar decreases have not been observed in the incidence of adenocarcinoma of the cervix (6). Nonsquamous cervical carcinoma constitutes approximately 23% of all cervical invasive cancers (7).

Documentation proves that it is not only the accessibility and affordability of the Pap smear, which accounts for delaying the diagnosis of cervical cancer. But, it is also inadequately executed Pap smear sampling or errors in interpretation that are responsible for about 30% of cervical squamous cell carcinoma (8), and for approximately 24% to 25% of all invasive cervical carcinomas (8,9). In addition, inappropriate management and follow-up of abnormal Pap smears account for 9.6% of all new cases of cervical cancer.

The highest rate of occurrence happening within 3 years from the last Pap smear and estimated at approximately 34.3% (8).

CERVICAL CYTOLOGY AS A SCREENING TOOL

Cervical cytology tests or Pap smears have been credited with early detection of cervical precancerous or cancerous lesions leading to a reduced death rate among women from cervical cancer. The false-negative Pap smear is one of several factors, within the issue of quality, that is associated with sampling errors (which accounts for the majority of mistakes) or interpretative errors. In order to decrease the interpretative errors of Pap smears, a new technology, ThinPrep, has been developed and approved by the U.S. Food and Drug Administration (FDA). In clinical trials, the new technology has been proved significantly more effective than the conventional Pap smear by reducing the false-negative rate from 5.6% to 2.2%. Also, the ThinPrep identifies more high-grade squamous intraepithelia (10). After improving these aspects of the Pap smear by introducing ThinPrep technology, it becomes obvious that attention should now be turned to advance the average practitioner's skills in clinical management and effective follow-up of abnormal Pap smears to achieve further reduction in false-negative Pap smear results. Clinical training of medical personnel, population-based education on the importance of such screening, compliance with screening recommendations, and finding a way to attract women who have never had a Pap smear to participate in screening programs; should provide additional reductions in invasive cervical cancer.

Recently, neural network-based screening has been compared with conventional light-microscopic screening techniques. The results of this study documented that network-based screening was more effective than conventional screening in the diagnosis of invasive cervical cell carcinoma, even in smears with a small number of cancer cells (11). These preliminary clinical data will need validation.

The FDA approved a computer-based automated technology system that reduces false-negative results by the rescreening of negative smears. The accuracy of automated technology for Pap smears is significantly improved when compared to the results of conventional manual screening (12).

Women who participate in universal, well-organized, population-based screening and have negative result Pap smears will have a low risk of invasive cervical cancer for more than 10 years. Also, the relative risk of a preinvasive lesion after an initial negative smear is decreased for more than 5 years. Based upon this information, it has been postulated that a 5-year screening interval is appropriate (13). These data are in sharp contrast with the American College of Obstetrics and Gynecology (ACOG) recommendation (3):

- All women who are or who have been sexually active, or who have reached the age of 18 years should have an annual cervical smear and pelvic examination.
- In women who have three or more consecutive yearly Pap smears and pelvic examination, the Pap smear can be performed less frequently at the discretion of the practitioner.
- Women with any identifiable *high-risk factor* (previous abnormal Pap smear, history of human papilloma virus (HPV), or human immunodeficiency virus (HIV) infection, cigarette smokers, or those who have multiple sex partners) should have a Pap smear annually.
- Following preinvasive lesion treatment, a Pap smear should be performed every 3 to 4 months for 1 year; if these cervical cytology test results are negative, an annual Pap smear is recommended
- Following treatment of invasive cervical carcinoma, cytological evaluation should be scheduled every 3 to 4 months for 2 years and every 6 months thereafter.

The U.S. Preventive Service Task Force recommendation calls for intervals of Pap smears (14) of between 1 and 3 years depending on the presence or absence of risk factors for cervical cancer.

In reviewing results of a case-controlled clinical study, comparing organized mass-screening Pap smears with spontaneous Pap smear for cervical cancer indicates that the organized mass screening provides significant decreases in the incidence of invasive cervical cancer and mortality (15).

The prevalence of *cervical adenocarcinoma* has not significantly decreased with Pap smear screening. When atypical glandular cells of undetermined significance on Pap smears are present, a prompt and aggressive workup can identify approximately 32% preinvasive or invasive cervical lesions and 13% benign lesions (16). Therefore, a high index of suspicious and appropriate ecto- and endocervical evaluation may produce early-detection results.

To perform a Pap smear and to obtain suitable material for cytological evaluation, the following steps should be undertaken (3):

- A Pap smear test should be performed before pelvic examination or cervical culture.
- When lubricant is used for speculum insertion, contamination of the specimen with lubricant should be avoided.
- Complete visualization of the cervical portio vaginalis is necessary.
- The cervical portio vaginalis should be sampled first, followed by the endocervical smear (obtained by gently rotating a brush).
- A microscopic slide is prepared by uniform distribution of the smear without clumping material, and it is rapidly fixed.
- Spray fixatives should be applied at least 10 inches (25 cm) from a specimen.
- An upper two-thirds vaginal smear should be obtained circumferentially in patients exposed to DES *in utero*.
- Vaginal discharge does not contradict the performance of a Pap smear. Gentle removal of excessive discharge from the cervix without inducing cervical blood is advocated.

The Bethesda Reporting System

The Bethesda System for Reporting Cervical/Vaginal Cytologic Diagnoses has been introduced to improve the reporting of cytological findings (17).

The Bethesda system institutes the following reporting criteria:

- *Specimen adequacy* for cytological interpretation
- *New cytology terminology*
  1. Atypical squamous cells of undetermined significance (ASCUS)
  2. Atypical glandular cells of undetermined significance (AGCUS)
  3. Inclusion changes associated with HPV infection (i.e., koilocytosis)
  4. Low-grade squamous intraepithelial lesion (LSIL)
  5. High-grade squamous intraepithelial lesion (HSIL)
- Descriptive diagnoses
  1. Benign cellular changes

a. Infection
b. Reactive changes
c. Hormonal changes
2. Epithelial cell abnormalities
3. Glandular cell abnormalities
a. Endometrial cells
b. Atypical glandular cells of undetermined significance
c. Endocervical adenocarcinoma
d. Endometrial adenocarcinoma
e. Extrauterine adenocarcinoma
f. Nonspecified adenocarcinoma
4. Hormonal evaluation of vaginal smear
a. Hormonal pattern compatible with age and history
b. Hormonal pattern incompatible with age and history
c. Hormonal evaluation not possible due to: Specify (17)

In general, the Bethesda System, in contrast to previous classification, differs in the following aspects:

■ Old numerical Pap smear classification is disregarded.
■ New nomenclature is introduced.
■ Atypia or inflammatory atypia was substituted with ASCUS or AGCUS.
■ Cervical intraepithelial neoplasia classification (CIN) was changed.
a. LSIL incorporates inclusion changes associated with HPV infections and previous CIN I grade (mild dysplasia).
b. HSIL encompasses previous CIN II (moderate dysplasia) and CIN III [severe, including carcinoma *in situ* (CIS)].
■ Specimen adequacy evaluation is required.

Abnormal Pap Smear Management

The objective of abnormal Pap smears evaluation is to determine the presence or absence of cervical cancer and its potential advance. The ecto- and endo–cervical assessment falls into the following steps (3):

■ *Visual inspection* of the vagina and cervix is used to identify any abnormality.
■ *Repeat cytology* is controversial and the clinical conviction is not to repeat, since repeated tests may result in false-negative results, which may lead to false clinical security; nevertheless, they can be performed from a visualized cervical/vaginal lesion. It is particularly important to pursue colposcopic evaluation when the cytological diagnosis predicts SIL.
■ *Colposcopically directed biopsy* is performed (after applying 3% to 5% acetic acid for 5 min) from the abnormal changes that are illustrated in the following:
a. Atypical vessels

b. Mosaic cell area
c. Punctation
d. White epithelium

Usually, punch biopsy (single or multiple) is performed from each lesion, unless a practitioner is skillful in a colposcopic grading system of cervical, vaginal, and vulvar lesions. The colposcopically directed biopsy's accuracy rate is 85% to 95% (3). The lesion location, from which the specimen is obtained, should be clearly mapped by using o'clock hours to communicate with the pathologist.

■ *Endocervical curettage (ECC)* is a generally accepted and performed procedure; although, during pregnancy it is not recommended. ECC should be executed under colposcopic view with a specially designed curette (i.e., the Kovarkain's curette).
■ *Cervical conization* is designed to remove the entire transformation zone and the nearly complete endocervical canal. Such an extensive procedure inadvertently may lead to postoperative bleeding and compromised future fertility. If positive conization margins are present, the procedure should be repeated. Cervical cone biopsy is not executed as an initial diagnostic procedure and is indicated in the following conditions:
a. Existing discrepancy between cytological and histological diagnosis
b. Colposcopically, the transformation zone not visualized completely
c. Histologically, documented microinvasive cervical cancer from punched biopsy
d. Histology of endocervical curettage specimen determining an intraepithelial lesion or microinvasive carcinoma
e. Premalignant or malignant glandular epithelium established either by cytologic or histological evaluation
■ *Dilatation and fractional curettage* (the cervical canal and the endometrium) is performed when the following is present:
a. Atypical glandular cells (AUCUS) of endocervical origin are present, which should be evaluated by colposcopically directed biopsy and ECC, and when preinvasive or invasive adenocarcinoma is documented, cervical conization with ECC above the conization area and endometrium sampling is performed.
b. Abnormal endometrial cells are present on an endometrial biopsy specimen.

Guidelines For Management Of Abnormal Pap

The following management guidelines are offered for an abnormal Pap smear (3).
1. *ASCUS* can be managed by either of the following:
a. Follow-up with Pap smear alone, every 6 months. If

two or more reports document the presence of ASCUS, colposcopic evaluation with biopsy and ECC is recommended.

    b. Initial colposcopic evaluation with biopsy and ECC can be performed if a patient's compliance with follow-up is called into question.

2. *LSIL* clinical management is based upon conviction that most of the lesions will spontaneously reverse to normal and the following approach is suggested:

    a. Repeat Pap smears every 4 to 6 months with no therapy and proceed with colposcopically directed biopsy and ECC if lesion persists. If the lesion persists for over 1 year with no follow-up or treatment by ablation or excision, one of the therapeutic modalities should be recommended.

    b. Colposcopic evaluation with biopsy and ECC should be done upon initial LSIL documentation.

    c. If the lesion is entirely visible, focal, and the transformation zone clearly is delineated, ablation or simple excision can be offered.

    d. If a patient's complaints with follow-up are uncertain, lesion ablation or excision can be carried out (15% of LSIL will progress to HSIL).

    e. LSIL limited to the endocervical canal can be followed with a Pap smear taken with a cytobrush and ECC.

2. *HSIL* lesion evaluation requires the following:

    a. Colposcopically directed biopsy

    b. ECC

    c. If histology verifies the presence of HSIL lesion, cervical cone biopsy should be performed and considered as a diagnostic–therapeutic modality at the same time. Ablation or excision of the lesions is indicated when an ECC specimen histological result is negative.

Abnormal Pap smear evaluation during pregnancy should not depart from the established diagnostic process, such as colposcopic evaluation with directed biopsy. Shortly after postpartum (about 6 weeks), reevaluation with ECC should be carried out. A frequent cytobrush Pap smear may be an efficient tool for follow-up. If stromal microinvasion is present during pregnancy, the definitive therapy can be deferred until after delivery. An invasive form of cervical cancer therapy during pregnancy depends upon the trimester in which the diagnosis is reached.

There are several therapeutic modalities for local eradication of intraepithelial lesions. To select a therapeutic option, the following criteria should be considered:

1. The lesion affects the ectocervix and is entirely visible.
2. The endocervix is free from intraepithelial lesion, which is documented by ECC and histological verification.
3. The cytological, colposcopical, and histological results are correlated; when discrepancies are noticed, further evaluation such as repeat direct biopsy or cervical cone biopsy should be offered.

When these criteria are met, one of the following therapeutic modalities can be utilized:

1. *Cryotherapy destruction* of the lesion to 4 to 5 mm beyond the edge of the probe will provide a 90% to 95% success rate. Optimal results with cryotherapy are achieved when a small ectocervical lesion and no endocervical gland involvement are documented by histology. Cryotherapy of the cervix is based upon the crystallizing effect of the intracellular water leading to cell lysis. It is accomplished by freezing tissue with a temperature between −20°C and −30°C.

2. *Local excision* with punch biopsy or loop electrode excision, or laser excision can be applied. The loop electrosurgical excision procedure (LEEP) is a relatively new technology. The effect of thermoenergy inadvertently leads to thermal artifact in electrosurgical and laser technologies. The excised specimen margin makes histological interpretation more difficult. Using a 0.5-mm diameter of wire and delivering 35 to 55 W of cutting electrical current can minimize this effect. The most common cervical complication following LEEP is cervical stenosis, which occurs in approximately 1% and postoperative bleeding. Therefore, LEEP, with minimal complication and good therapeutic effect, is favored over laser ablation and cervical conization; although, the high incidence of HSIL after LEEP highlights the need for vigilant follow-up, since the readable post-LEEP margin is present in about 32.4% (18).

3. *Laser lesion destruction* is executed under direct colposcopic visualization that should reach 7 mm in depth. The laser technology is based on water absorption from extracellular and intracellular cervical tissues by laser energy with temperatures of >1000°C. At this temperature; the cervical cells will vaporize. The success rate of laser therapy is similar to that with cryotherapy.

4. *Total hysterectomy* is definitive therapy for HSIL when maintaining future reproductive capacity is not a patient's desire.

In patients with immune-compromised conditions, a recurrent rate is high after standard treatment for high-grade cervical dysplasia. Vaginal 5-fluorouracil (5-FU) cream for high-grade cervical dysplasia in HIV infection following surgical treatment effectively reduced recurrence of cervical intraepithelial neoplasia. In a randomized controlled unmasked multicenter study, 5-FU cream, 2 g, was administered twice weekly for 6 months. This mode of therapy was significantly more effective in preventing recurrence (28% recurrence), when compared to the control group (47% recurrence) (19).

CERVICAL PREMALIGNANCY

A cervical lesion with potential progression to malignancy defines cervical premalignant or precancerous lesion. In general, this process is also termed a "cervical neoplasia" (progressive multiplication of the abnormal cells that eventually may replace multiplication of normal cells). Malignant spontaneous transformation of a premalignant lesion within the cervical epithelium is one of the possible options, and spontaneous regression of the lesion to the normal cervical epithelium is another possibility. Which patient's lesion will eventually progress and which one will regress is an open question; therefore, adequate diagnosis and appropriate treatment can help to promote regression. The cervical epithelium has the natural potential to transform one form of the epithelium to another form (squamous cells replacing columnar cells), which is called a "metaplastic event." Metaplastic transformation is controlled growth of the new tissue, and uncontrollable tissue growth occurs in a neoplastic process. Neoplastic growth can express a benign character or malignant character (ability to invade and to metastasize). These two conditions differ from each other by demonstrating greater degrees of anaplastic changes within the cells in malignancy (less differentiation, less orientation to one another, and departure from original framework of the cells).

Cervical Squamous Intraepithelial Lesion

Cervical squamous intraepithelial lesion (SIL), natural history of progression to CIS, or regression to the normal cervical epithelium are well-known processes. *LSIL* (CIN I) and *HSIL* (CIN II and CIN III) progression to CIS is a continuous process with a variable mean transit time of transformation to CIS (Table 18.1).

It is clear that, the more advanced the grade of cervical SIL, the shorter the time needed to progress to CIS. Histology of cervical dysplasia and its grade are defined as follow:

1. Mild dysplasia or CIN I: dysplastic cells involve the lower third of the epithelium
2. Moderate dysplasia or CIN II: dysplastic cells present in two-thirds of the epithelium or the middle of the epithelium
3. Severe dysplasia or CIN III: dysplastic cells involve the upper third of the epithelium or full-thickness of the epithelium

The natural history of cervical intraepithelial neoplasia falls into three basic categories of the likelihood of regression, persistence, and progression (Table 18.2).

The natural history of SIL indicates that the probability of intraepithelial neoplasia becoming invasive cervical cancer increases with the grade of severity of SIL; even though, this does not occur in every case. Also, HSIL regresses in a significant proportion of cases. Unfortunately, histology by itself is not able to predict the regressive, progressive, or persistence behavior of squamous intraepithelial lesion. Until such time that a predictor factor of progression from SIL to CIS, other than tissue morphology, will become available for clinicians, the natural history knowledge of progression should be incorporated into practice.

There is no clinical scientific study that will determine either the time of progression or the natural history of ASCUS to CIS. Nevertheless, a recent morphological study indicates that 48% of women with ASCUS diagnosis on Pap smears had SIL (43% low grade SIL, 4% high grade HSIL, and 1% CIS) (22).

These clinicopathological findings concurred with previously published results of the Pathology Panel Review under the auspice of the National Cancer Institute. The panel determined that, among patients diagnosed with ASCUS, in fact, 24% have HSIL and recommended "ASCUS, rule out HSIL" in patient management (23).

Both these findings strongly suggest that ACUS cytological diagnosis warrants further colposcopic evaluation with biopsy and ECC to rule out SIL or CIS (22,23).

An additional qualification of atypical squamous cells of undetermined significance by cytological determination of the presence of either an epithelial lesion or a reactive cell process may predict occurrence of SIL. The likelihood of the presence of SIL is greater in women with ASCUS and with cytological suggestion of the presence of an intraepithelial lesion, than in women with ASCUS and with cytological suggestion of a reactive process (24,25).

The diagnosis of ASCUS does not require performing routinely endometrial sampling as a part of evaluation; although, AGCUS may require such sampling. All other tests such as colposcopically directed biopsy, ECC, and cervical cone biopsy are similarly indicated in both ASCUS and AGCUS.

TABLE 18.1. TIME OF PROGRESSION FROM SIL TO CIS

	LSIL		HSIL	
	Very Mild Dysplasia (CIN I)	**Mild Dysplasia (CIN I)**	**Moderate Dysplasia (CIN II)**	**Severe Dysplasia (CIN III)**
Time of progression from SIL to CIS	85 months (7 years)	58 months (4.8 years)	38 months (3.1 years)	12 months (1 year)

SIL, squamous intraepithelial lesion; CIS, carcinoma *in situ*; LSIL, low-grade squamous intraepithelial lesion; HSIL, high-grade squamous intraepithelial lesion; CIN, cervical intraepithelial neoplasia classification.
Data from Richart RM, Barron BA. A follow-up study of patients with cervical dysplasia. *Am J Obstet Gynecol* 1969;105:386–393.

TABLE 18.2. NATURAL HISTORY OF SIL

| | LSIL | HSIL | |
	Mild Dysplasia (CIN I)	Moderate Dysplasia (CIN II)	Severe Dysplasia (CIN III)
Regression	60%	40%	33%
Persistence	30%	40%	55%
Progression	10%	20%	12%

SIL, squamous intraepithelial lesion; LSIL, low-grade squamous intraepithelial lesion; HSIL, high-grade squamous intraepithelial lesion; CIN, cervical intraepithelial neoplasia classification.
Data from Ostor AG. Natural history of cervical intraepithelial neoplasia: a cervical review. *Int J Gynecol Pathol* 1993;12:186–192.

Conventional therapy for a cervical intraepithelial lesion is excision or destruction of the lesion, or total hysterectomy for HSIL or CIS.

Cervical Glandular Intraepithelial

Similar to atypical glandular cells of undetermined significance (AGCUS) need further cytological qualification as to whether they originate from either a reactive or a neoplastic process (25). Patients with a subclassification of ASCUS cytological indication favoring neoplastic cells have a greater proportion of significant histopathological findings in about 72% as compared to AGCUS favoring reactive cytology in approximately 20%. Cytological AGCUS diagnosis, when verified by histology, yields about 21.3% of SIL, invasive cervical adenocarcinoma in 3.5%, cervical adenocarcinoma *in situ* (ACIS) in 1.1%, endometrial hyperplasia in 11.8%, endometrial adenocarcinoma in 5.9%, and ovarian cancer in 1.1% (26). These findings and others (27) demonstrate the high prevalence of not only cervical pathology but also the presence of endometrial neoplasia and, to a lesser degree, ovarian lesions. Therefore, these data heighten the potential of the presence of significant gynecological neoplasia and call for the need of aggressive AGCUS evaluation that includes the following (25–31):

1. *Colposcopic evaluation with biopsy*
2. *Obtaining endocervical cytology* specimen with a cytobrush; however, the accuracy of this technique has not yet been determined in AGCUS
3. *Endocervical curettage* (ECC); effectiveness has to be established in AGCUS
4. *Endometrial biopsy*, particularly in postmenopausal women
5. *Cervical cone biopsy* is not as effective in AGCUS as it is in ASCUS due to frequently multifocal location, particularly in cervical ACIS (or AIS). Therefore, free cone margins or negative conization margins are not as good a predicting factor as it is in squamous cell CIS or HSIL. It has been documented that up to 40% with negative conization margins in patients with ACIS will have residual lesions upon removal. Therefore, in light of

these data, it is not surprising that recurrent glandular cervical lesion occurs in approximately 47%. Traditionally, cervical cytology, ECC, or both modalities are used in follow-up for cervical glandular cell abnormality; although, ECC is positive in only 43% (32).

Conventional initial treatment of high-grade glandular lesions falls into two categories:

1. *Conservative surgical therapy*, i.e., cone biopsy, is offered when a patient wants to preserve reproductive capacity, although the safety and adequacy of therapeutic conization as conservative management of patients with cervical high-grade glandular intraepithelial lesion, including ACIS, is called into question (32). In view of the absence of a reliable paradigm for postconization follow-up, the tendency of the lesions to be commonly multifocal, and because the cervical conization margins are not practical to forecast the presence of residual lesions; it seems reasonable to perform total hysterectomy as soon as a patient's reproductive desire is accomplished.
2. *Definitive surgical therapy* for cervical high-grade glandular cell lesion, including ACIS, is total hysterectomy.

Complementary Therapy

Patient Education

Patient education can complement either conventional or alternative therapeutic approaches, and by simple life changes, cervical cancer prevalence can be reduced. The following risk factors for cervical cancer should be a complementary part of routine gynecologic visits:

1. *Sexual behavioral factors* such as multiple sexual partners in vaginal receptive coitus and first sexual intercourse before the age of 18 years are agents implicated in causing an increased risk of cervical premalignancy and malignancy. It is hypothesized that HPV is the major factor in cervical intraepithelial neoplasia or cancer development. HPV virus can be transmitted either by the semen or by invisible, subclinical flat HPV lesions, which can be contracted by women during sexual intercourse. There is a remote potential of transmitting and

contracting HPV infection through oral sex, and theoretically transmission and contraction of the virus is possible through lesbian sex. Early education among school children and continuation among the adolescent population may prove to be fruitful. Avoiding genital-to-genital direct contact is required if the virus affects a sexual partner. In education of women, male high-risk sexual behavior and its prevention are very important aspects of the educational program (34). Also, monogamous relationships and no extramarital sexual relationships coincide with a low prevalence of cervical cancer (35). Sexual behavior as a risk factor in *cervical adenocarcinoma* has also been indicated in reference to the number of sexual partners, particularly before the age of 20 years (36).

2. *Cigarette smoking* increases the prevalence of cervical intraepithelial lesions. There is also a statistically significant correlation between the number of cigarettes smoked per day, the duration of smoking (years of exposure), and the grade of intraepithelial lesions or cervical squamous cancer (37). Cigarette smoking, however, is not significantly associated with developing adenocarcinoma (36). Unfortunately, only 49% of cigarette-smoking women are aware of the existing relationship between smoking and an increased risk of potential squamous intraepithelial lesion or cancer occurrence. Prevention can be greatly enhanced if the opportunity of a routine gynecologic visit is fully utilized for educational aspects of cigarette smoking and for promotion of smoking cessation (38), since nonsmoking women have a substantially lower risk for cervical squamous carcinoma (35).

3. *Oral contraceptives* in long-term use (>10 years), in both types of cervical cancer (squamous cell cancer and glandular cell adenocarcinoma), increase the risk of cervical premalignancy and malignancy (36,39). For both types combined, risk increases with the duration of oral contraceptive use and has the highest prevalence among recent and current users. It declines with the time of cessation of use. Also, it has been documented that the risk is strongly associated with a low progestin potency of oral contraceptive pills (40).

4. *Weight gain* in women should be considered an increased risk for cervical adenocarcinoma (36); such correlation has not been documented in squamous cell carcinoma.

In brief, a combination of factors such as the number of sexual partners, smoking habits, and uses of contraceptive are common risk factors in both types of cervical cancer. There is no data available linking alcohol consumption to an increased risk of cervical cancer (40).

The proper and frequent use of female and/or male condoms may provide protection in the transmission and contraction of sexually transmitted diseases, particularly HPV. Although condom protection is not as reliable a method as one might hope due to incomplete coverage of the penis and the scrotum, and the tendency to break easily. Long-time diaphragm use appears to be protective of cervical adenocarcinoma (36).

Diet

In general, frequent consumption of green-yellow vegetables (oranges, carrots, yellow squash, cantaloupe, peaches, corn, etc.) may provide protection, and reduce cervical dysplasia and cancer (41). A vegetarian diet is also recommended by folk medicine for 3 months.

Acupuncture

Acupuncture singly or in combination with herbal remedies can provide good results in cervical dysplasia regression within 6 months of therapy (33). Scattered scientific and anecdotal information will not allow for deep analysis in reference to safety, effectiveness, and which grade of cervical dysplasia regresses, persists, or progresses with acupuncture treatment.

Nutritional Supplements

Carotenes

Beta-carotene deficiency levels in exfoliated cervicovaginal epithelial cells in cervical intraepithelial neoplasia and cervical cancer have been suggested to play etiologic roles in the pathogenesis of these conditions (42). Preliminary clinical study supports the notion that a derivative of vitamin A can reverse or suppress epithelial preneoplasia; therefore, cervical cancer is potentially preventive (43). The currently available clinical data does not support preliminary findings that beta-carotene (even in a high dose, 30 mg/day orally) will increase the likelihood of regression or will decrease the progression of minor atypia and CIN (44–46). In subsequent clinical trials, beta-carotene has not only been proved to be ineffective but also has been demonstrated to be harmful (47,48); although, the natural medicine view is that carotenes are not toxic, while vitamin A is toxic in high doses (49).

In spite of this controversy, natural medicine suggests *carotenes* (mixed natural), 150,000 IU orally, daily, for 3 months (skin pigment may turn an orange tint); carotenes at 25,000 to 50,000 IU orally, daily, is recommended for prevention (49).

Vitamins

Vitamin A is recommended in the form of a suppository for 6 nights (commercially available in the United States). Topically, vitamin A can also be administered via a cervical cap or collagen sponge, with a 50% cure rate in mild and moderate cervical dysplasia (50). However, the effectiveness of Vitamin A is questionable, since established results show the rate of potential spontaneous regression of squamous intraepithelial lesions is 60% (21). It appears that no difference exists between local treatment with vitamin A and no therapy at all.

Vitamin C participates in collagen synthesis, in detoxification of carcinogens, and in modulation of the immune system. For these reasons, it is recommended for SIL or as preventive therapy. It has been demonstrated that vitamin C levels were significantly decreased in patients with SIL (51). Recent randomized, double-blind, placebo-controlled study results on vitamin C supplementation at the oral dose of 500 mg daily in cervical squamous intraepithelial neoplasia did not support the notion that it may increase the regression or decrease the progression of CIN (44). In this study, 500 mg of vitamin C was used; this does not correspond to the doses recommended by natural medicine (49):

1. *Vitamin C, in a therapeutic oral dose,* 2,000 to 6,000 mg per day for 3 months
2. *Vitamin C, in a preventive dose,* 1,000 to 2,000 mg per day

Folic Acid

It has been postulated that folate deficiency may play a role in inducing an initial process of developing cervical dysplasia (52). An oncogenic type of HPV is associated with some cases of cervical cancer; although, HPV infection alone is an insufficient cause of cervical cancer. The combination of folic acid deficiency and HPV infection might commence neoplastic induction; therefore, nutrients had been indicated in this neoplastic process (53). Clinical randomized controlled studies of folic acid supplementation demonstrated that folic acid supplementation is not able to alter the course of already induced cervical neoplastic processes (52,54). Nevertheless, natural medicine recommends the following folic acid regimen (49):

1. *Folic acid, in a therapeutic dose* in SIL, 2.5 to 10 mg orally, daily, for 3 months
2. Folic acid, in a preventive dose, 800 to 2,400 mcg orally, daily

Alternative Therapy

Herbal Remedies

Lack of clinical scientific data to support folk medicine in using traditional herbal remedies makes it impossible to express views on the safety and effectiveness of such an approach. The concept behind botanical treatment rests on enhancing the immune system and utilizing the herbs' antiviral properties.

The following compound, herbal suppository formulas are recommended (49):

1. *Compound formula 1:*
■ *Red clover, 1 oz*
■ *Dandelion root, 1.5 oz*
■ *Licorice root, 1 oz*
■ *Goldenseal root, 0.5 oz*

2. Compound formula 2:
■ Thuja, 1 oz
■ Echinacea, 1.5 oz
■ Goldenseal root, 1 oz

One of these formulas can be used alternately with vitamin A suppositories for a total of 4 weeks.

CERVICAL MALIGNANCY

Invasive Cervical Squamous Cell Carcinoma

Definition

Invasive cervical squamous cell carcinoma is defined as a transformation of normal squamous cells into malignancy that migrated beyond the epithelial limit.

Incidence

The invasive cervical cancer incidence in the United States is not uniformly distributed and varies among ethnic groups, from 4.5 per 100,000 Japanese-American women, to 7.2 per 100,000 Caucasian women, to 12.2 per 100,000 African-American women, to a high of 18.4 per 100,000 Hispanic American women (55). This difference among ethnic groups is not due to variance in risk factors only but also to the degree of access to preventive services.

Etiology

Cervical squamous cell cancer etiology is unknown; although, there is a strong association with HPV infection. The presence of high-risk HPV genital subtypes increases the risk of cervical malignant transformation (56). Also, genetic susceptibility to HPV infection may play an important role in determining the individual risk to develop this type of cancer (57).

Classification

Progress of Invasion

1. *Cervical malignancy classification is based upon:*
■ Microinvasive squamous cell carcinoma is also called HSIL, or frank clinical invasive cervical carcinoma. Microinvasive squamous cell carcinoma is defined as cancer invasion of the cervical stroma of <3 mm beneath the basement membrane, and the absence of blood vessels or lymphatic channel infiltration (58).
■ *Invasive squamous cell carcinoma* (see cervical cancer staging; Table 18.3).
2. *Histological type* of squamous cell carcinoma, include the following:
■ *Keratinizing* squamous cell carcinoma is determined by the presence of focal keratinization, which creates epithelial cornification with a pearl-like appearance.

TABLE 18.3. STAGING FOR CERVICAL CARCINOMA

Stage	Description	Therapy	Survival 5-Year	10-Year
0	Carcinoma *in situ;* intraepithelial carcinoma	Surgery	99%	99%
I	Carcinoma is strictly confined to the cervix			
IA	Preclinical carcinoma microscopically diagnosed only with depth of invasion of ≤5 mm and width of ≤7 mm			
IA$_1$	Minimal microscopical stromal invasion	Surgery	98%	98%
IA$_2$	Microscopical stromal invasion 3–5 mm and width ≤7 mm	Surgery	98%	98%
IB	Preclinical carcinoma with invasion greater than stage 1A or clinical lesions is confined to the cervix			
IB$_1$	Clinical lesions of <4 cm	Surgery or irradiation	90%	90%
IB$_2$	Clinical lesions of >4 cm	Surgery or irradiation	73%	?
II	The carcinoma extends beyond the cervix but has not extended to the pelvic wall. The carcinoma involves the vagina but not as far as the lower third			
IIA	No obvious parametrial involvement	Irradiation	83%	79%
		Surgery	78%	75%
IIB	Obvious parametrial involvement	Irradiation	67%	57%
III	The cancer has extended to the pelvic wall. On rectal examination, there is no cancer-free space between the tumor and the pelvic wall; the tumor involves the lower third of the vagina; all cases with hydronephrosis or nonfunctional kidney are included, unless they are known to be due to other causes.			
IIIA	No extension to the pelvic wall	Irradiation	45%	40%
IIIB	Extension to the pelvic wall and/or hydronephrosis	Irradiation	36%	30%
IV	The carcinoma has extended beyond the true pelvis or has clinically involved the bladder or rectal mucosa; a bullous edema, as such, should not permit a case to be assigned to stage IV			
IVA	Spread of the growth to adjacent organs	Irradiation	14%	14%
IVB	Spread to distant organs			

Data from International Federation of Gynecology and Obstetrics (FIGO). *Annual report on the results of treatment in gynecological cancer,* 22nd ed. Stockholm: FIGO, 1994.

- *Nonkeratinizing* squamous cell carcinoma is defined by the absence of a pearl-like cornification.
- *Small-cell* squamous cell carcinoma is a poorly differentiated neoplasm and mass border with small, round, or spindle-shape cells. It constitutes 1% to 2% of all cervical cancers.

Diagnosis

As to *pertinent medical history*, there are no specific symptoms present in cervical carcinoma, but the following symptoms are often associated with this condition:

- Pink and odorous postcoital vaginal discharge
- Vaginal bleeding in different degrees, ranging from postcoital spotting, prolonged menses, intermenstrual bleeding, menorrhagia, postmenopausal vaginal bleeding, and gross hemorrhage
- A sciatic pain distribution (back of the buttock, thigh, knee), which is usually a late symptom of cervical cancer (it may suggest extension of cancer to the pelvic side wall)
- Pelvic pain

- Symptomatology associated with cervical cancer infiltration of adjacent organs (the bladder, the rectum)

Physical examination may identify the following:

- In early invasive cervical cancer, local granular indurated and/or ulcerative lesions can be present
- In late invasive cervical cancer, the following abnormalities can be identified: (a) An exophytic or proliferative lesion that resembles a polypoid or papillary (cauliflower-like) tumor of the cervix, which has a tendency to grow and invade outward from the cervix. (b) An endophytic lesion, which is usually a nodular and/or ulcerative tumor and is predominantly observed within the endocervical canal. It may produce a barrel-shaped cervix (this lesion proliferates upward from the cervical canal, infiltrating the lower segment of the uterus, and extends to the parametrium and/or the uterosacral ligament faster than exophytic cervical lesion. When this happens, the infiltrated area is indurated and dense to palpation).

Direct biopsy is performed from a suspicious, visible or palpable cervical mass. Histology verification provides definitive diagnosis. Neither cold-knife cervical cone biopsy, nor loop electrical, nor laser excision is indicated for the presence of a gross cervical lesion.

Colposcopic evaluation with biopsy and endocervical curettage is considered a routine examination of an abnormal Pap smear when clinically no lesion is identifiable.

As to *cervical cone biopsy*, its indication is discussed above.

Histological Grading of Cervical Cancer

Histological grating of squamous cell carcinoma is based upon the degree of maturation and is categorized as follows:

- Grade 1 or well-differentiated tumor
- Grade 2 or moderately differentiated tumor
- Grade 3 or poorly differentiated tumor

The prognostic influence of this grading scheme has very little value; although, the less that tumor is differentiated, the higher the incidence of pelvic node metastasis. Also, the more anaplastic (undifferentiated tumor) the cancer cells,

the larger the mass has the tendency to grow when compared to well-differentiated squamous cell carcinoma (59).

Clinical staging for cervical cancer is derived from the pelvic evaluation, including inspection with a vaginal speculum and palpation of the vagina, cervix, parametrium, and the pelvic side walls. The physical clinical findings (pelvic and general) are appropriately matched with those proposed by FIGO with respect to the degree of cervical cancer advances in the true pelvis and extrapelvic areas (Table 18.4).

Other tests can be performed to establish the extent of cervical cancer as indicated:

- *Chest x-ray*
- *Intravenous pyelography* (excretory urography)
- *Cystoscopy*, when there is suspicion of cervical cancer extending to the bladder mucosa (hematuria, cervical cancer infiltration of the anterior abdominal wall)
- *Flexible sigmoidoscopy* needs to be performed when cervical cancer infiltrates the posterior vaginal wall or when

TABLE 18.4. CERVICAL CANCER THERAPY ACCORDING TO CLINICAL STAGING

Stage	Treatment Options
0 CIS	1. Cervical conization alone is considered only when a patient desires to preserve reproductive capacity. 2. Total simple hysterectomy with bilateral preservation of the ovaries.
IA₁ microinvasion (≤3 mm)	1. Cervical conization alone is indicated when it is desirable to preserve reproductive capacity, when cone margins are free of disease, when patient's compliance with a follow-up is expected. 2. Total simple hysterectomy with the preservation of the ovaries. 3. Radiotherapy alone.
IA₂ microinvasion (3–5 mm)	1. Total simple hysterectomy with pelvic node dissection with the preservation of the ovaries. 2. Radical hysterectomy with pelvic lymphadenectomy. 3. Radiotherapy alone.
IB₁ (tumor of ≤4 cm)	1. Radical hysterectomy with pelvic and paraaortic lymphadenectomy. 2. Radiotherapy alone.
IB₂ (tumor of >4 cm)	1. Radical hysterectomy with pelvic and paraaortic lymphadenectomy. 2. Radiotherapy alone.
IIA	1. Radical hysterectomy with pelvic and paraaortic lymphadenectomy. 2. Radiotherapy alone. 3. Combination of surgery and radiation therapy, when pelvic nodes are positive (which appears to increase likelihood of pelvic control of disease).
IIB	Radiotherapy alone.
IIIA	Radiotherapy alone.
IIIB	Radiotherapy alone.
IVA	Radiotherapy alone.
IVB (distant metastasis)	Chemotherapy.
IVB (distant metastasis)	Chemotherapy.

Recurrent cervical carcinoma	1. For central recurrence occurred after:
	  a. Radical hysterectomy, where treatment is usually with radiation (salvage rates in about 50%); if tumor is large, neoadjuvant chemotherapy can be recommended.
	  b. Radiotherapy, where therapy is radical pelvic surgery such as radical hysterectomy or exonerations.
	2. Chemotherapy.

Occult invasive cervical carcinoma at the time of simple total hysterectomy	1. When cancer confined to the cervix (early-stage), radical reoperation is offered (parametrectomy, upper vaginectomy with node dissection; the 5-year absolute survival estimated is about 82–89%) (81,82); a similar procedure is suggested in treating stump cancer 2. Radical radiotherapy can be applied in all the stages of the disease (83).

CIS, carcinoma *in situ*.

rectal examination suggests the presence of cancer. Also, sigmoidoscopy should be performed if symptoms of rectal bleeding, the presence of excessive mucus in stools, rectal pressure, or tenesmus are reported.

- *Computed tomography (CT) or magnetic resonance imaging (MRI)* may assist in determining the extent of cancer in the pelvis. In spite of the lack of FIGO recommendations as a measure for clinical staging, a new trend of utilizing MRI in the clinical staging of cervical carcinoma is emerging; lately, MRI is often considered a diagnostic tool (61,62).
- *Lymphangiography* can be a very helpful paradigm in determining sentinel lymph node status in cervical cancer. Nevertheless, interpretation is difficult, and the method does not have much practical implication. FIGO clinical staging does not require lymphangiography. Recently, preoperative lymphatic mapping with paracervical injection of isosulfan blue day for node sampling in the cervical cancer has been proposed (63). Clinical validation of this method is needed before the adoption of this practice.

Differential Diagnosis

Differential diagnosis includes the following clinical entities:

- Cervical polyps
- Papillary endocervicitis
- Cervical papillomas

Direct cervical lesion biopsy usually provides the definitive diagnosis and must be performed on any suspicious cervical lesion.

Conventional Therapy

Modern conventional therapy for invasive cervical squamous cell carcinoma is strictly related to the stage of the disease and can be categorized as follows:

1. Surgical treatment
   a. *Cervical conization* is indicated in young women, who desire to preserve reproductive capacity. This conservative surgery can be performed when cervical stromal invasion is 3 mm and when lymphovascular space is free of cancer infiltration (64,65). Cervical conization can yield similar results when executed either with the cold-knife technique or electrical loop excision (66). Laser conization will excise completely the lesion in microinvasive stromal infiltration and is a good tool in early invasive cervical carcinoma (67).
   b. *Simple total hysterectomy* with pelvic node dissection and ovary preservation is a therapeutic modality for invasive cervical cancer when cancer infiltration is 3 to 5 mm and there is lymphovascular space invasion

(63,64). Total abdominal hysterectomy with pelvic lymphadenectomy can be executed abdominally, laparoscopic lymphatic node dissection can be combined with vaginal hysterectomy (68–70), or total laparoscopic hysterectomy can be undertaken with pelvic node dissection and with no vaginal approach (71).
   c. *Radical hysterectomy* with lymphadenectomy requires uterine extirpation, removal of the proximal and distal portions of the parametrial tissue, and upper vaginal amputation. Pelvic node dissection is executed from the bifurcation of the iliac vessels down, reaching the proximity of the inguinal ligament and including the obturator lymphatic chains. The common iliac and para-aortic lymphadenectomy is usually preserved for a bulky cervical mass (72). Radical hysterectomy with lymphadenectomy can be executed via an abdominally or laparoscopically assisted Schauta vaginal operation (73), or a total laparoscopic abdominal hysterectomy with pelvic and para-aortic node dissection, with no transvaginal approach, can be undertaken (71).
   d. *Pelvic exenteration* with reconstructive surgery usually is preserved for young patients with centro-pelvic recurrence of the cervical carcinoma. Improved surgical technique and better understanding of the long-term side effects makes pelvic exenteration for palliation a more accepted approach due to the substantial improvement in quality of life. In appropriately selected patients, significant palliation of physical and emotional symptoms can be accomplished by implementing this procedure (72,74).
2. *Radiotherapy* for invasive cervical carcinomas has been used either as a primary or an adjuvant therapeutic modality and can be used in all stages. It is delivered as an external beam to the whole pelvis in divided doses, within 4 to 5 weeks (single doses of 180 to 200 cGy, until the total dose reaches 4,500 to 5,000 cGy). It is also delivered as transvaginal intracavitary cesium (after cervical dilatation, a tandem [a hollow tube] is inserted into the cervical canal. Two ovoids [rounded applicators] are placed in the lateral vaginal fornices, with 10,000 to 15,000 cGy.) Radiotherapy is not free of complications, and, among them, cystitis and proctitis are commonly observed. Occasionally, vesicovaginal and or rectovaginal fistulas, vaginal stenosis, bone marrow suppression, late small intestine obstruction, or hot flashes and sweats resulting from the cessation of ovarian function (3) may occur (estrogen replacement therapy is safe and is recommended). Radiotherapy is the primary therapy for stages IIB, III, and IVA. Intraoperative radiation therapy increases the pool of patients for whom surgical salvage therapy is an option (65). Irradiation is carried out in the operating room setting, followed by maximal surgical debulking of the tumor. Recently, evidence-based data indicate that concurrent chemotherapy with pelvic radi-

ation may become the new standard of care for bulky and advanced cervical cancer (75). Hydroxyurea or a combination of cisplatin and 5-fluoruracil (5-FU) has the ability to enhance responsiveness of a tumor to radiation therapy. It has yet to be determined which chemotherapy regimen is most effective and safest (76), although hydroxyurea as a single agent is favored as a sensitizer to radiation therapy and presents promising results (77).

3. *Combination of surgery and radiotherapy* is often used in stage IIA with positive lymph nodes; however, there is a lack of medical evidence that such an approach will influence survival rates.

4. *Chemotherapy* offers some benefits in the primary treatment of advanced or recurrent cervical cancers. Chemotherapy as a primary mode of either neoadjuvant therapy or a radiation sensitizer can be utilized.

Neoadjuvant treatment is used to reduce the cervical cancer tumor volume before radical surgery. Cisplatin with various agent combinations such as vincristine mitomycin C, bleomycin, and 5-FU or cisplatin and epirubicin, etoposide and bleomycin holds promising results in initial clinical studies. Other combinations have been also clinically tested with equal clinical results (78,79). It has been documented that small cell cervical cancer may clinically respond even though microscopic residual tumor is frequently present. This behavior of small cell cervical cancer creates the need for local treatment after chemotherapy (80).

In disseminated cervical carcinomas, chemotherapy is administered as a *primary* therapy. Cisplatin, Ifosfamide, Dibromodulcitol (Mitolacol), and Adriamycin (Doxyorubicin) are the most commonly used agents in cervical carcinomas. A combination of cisplatin and ifosfamide provides therapeutic results in approximately 33% of an objective response rate (78).

Pregnancy and Cervical Cancer

Pregnancy and cervial cancer are a rare occurrence, estimated at 0.01%. The diagnosis should be reached without delay, and clinical management depends upon the following facts:

1. Patient's desire to continue pregnancy
2. The stage of cervical cancer is the domineering factor in clinical management decision making prior to the third trimester of pregnancy. There is no difference in the overall management of a pregnant versus a nonpregnant woman, although when radiation therapy is planned, pregnancy termination can be executed either before or shortly after irradiation (postradiation spontaneous abortion may occur).
3. Gestational age and clinical management
   a. *The third trimester* pregnancy will allow vaginal delivery as soon as fetal maturity is documented. Cesarean section can be performed, followed by radical hysterectomy with lymphadenectomy; nevertheless, surgery during pregnancy is more technically demanding than in a nonpregnant state.
   b. *The late second trimester* pregnancy may continue until after fetal viability is reached. In the same setting, classic cesarean section can be executed and radical surgery performed according to the clinical cervical cancer stage. When a surgical approach is not recommended due to the advanced stage of cervical cancer, radiation is usually postponed for 10 days, allowing the abdominal wall incision to heal.
   c. *The first and early second trimester* will require pregnancy termination and therapy according to the clinical stage of cervical cancer.

Complementary Therapy

Patient Education

Patient education is the focus of prevention to reduce the prevalence of cervical cancer by promoting lifestyle changes. One of these changes is to avoid cigarette smoking. Another is to promote sexual behavior that will minimize the risk of cervical cancer, such as safe sex strategies (monogamous sexual relationships, use of condoms, later age of first coitus and avoiding or reducing multiple sex partners). One of the major risk factors for cervical cancer is HPV; therefore, an educational program that targets all socioeconomic groups, with particular emphasis on socially disadvantaged women, is indicated. Such a program should be designed to provide necessary information and to develop sexual negotiation skills that can reduce sexual risk behavior (84). Particular attention should be given to adolescent and young females. Study has documented that 52% of females sexually active at the ages of 15 to 23 did not know that cigarette smoking increased the risk for cervical cancer; 42% believed that HPV contraction is always symptomatic; and 22% did not know that condoms decreased the transmission and contraction of HPV. Health providers should tailor educational objectives and strategies to the functional level of adolescents when discussing prevention (85).

Almost half of all invasive cervical cancer is diagnosed at a late stage (regional or distant). The likelihood of a late stage of diagnosis is recognized among elderly, unmarried, and uninsured women (86). To identify this group of patients and to furnish them with basic education and access to a screening program may increase the early diagnoses of premalignant and malignant cervical cancer.

The need to participate in appropriately frequent Pap smear screenings and to change lifestyles should be promoted at every occasion, including, but not limited to, office visits.

Alternative Therapy

Alternative natural medicine addresses cancer prevention strategy and does not offer a specific approach to cervical cancer (49).

Cervical Adenocarcinoma

The prevalence of adenocarcinoma has increased, within the last twenty-five years, from approximately 5% to over 10% of all cervical cancer. The most common histological type is mucinous cervical adenocarcinoma (57%), followed by endometrioid adenocarcinomas (30%), clear cell adenocarcinomas (11%), and other types (3%) (87).

Diagnosis is based upon the clinical symptom of copious mucoid vaginal discharge and a visible lesion; although, the classic clinical picture of cervical adenocarcinoma often takes an unusual course, making timely diagnosis is difficult and delayed. Therefore, experience and vigilance play a role in reaching the diagnosis. Rates of a false-negative Pap smear may reach as high as 80% due to perfuse vaginal mucoid discharge. Also colposcopy, cervical biopsy, and ECC are not as informative here as in squamous cell cancer (88). The multifocal location of adenocarcinoma makes cervical cone biopsy, even with the margin free, not as reliable a test as would be expected. Residual disease occurs in approximately 31% with negative margins and in 56% with positive margins. LEEP cones have the highest rate of positive endocervical margins (75%), followed by laser cone (57%); cold-knife cervical conization has the lowest rate (24%) (89). The natural clinical tendency is to treat a patient's chief complaint of vaginal discharge as a presumptive cervicitis or vaginitis condition. Such an approach may delay the diagnosis and optimal timing for appropriate treatment (90).

Clinical staging is presented above and does not differ from squamous cell carcinoma. Also metastatic clinical investigation is similar to that presented above.

Conventional therapy includes the following:

1. FIGO staging of ACIS (89) treatment options are:
   a. *Cervical conization* should be considered with great caution, since high rates of residual disease occur. Cervical conization can be recommended if a patient wants to preserve reproduction capacity. Among LEEP cones, laser cones, cold-knife cones, and cold-knife cervical conization, the latter promises the least residual disease, even though it is not free of residual cancer.
   b. *Simple hysterectomy* is usually definitive treatment for cervical adenocarcinoma.
2. *Early invasive cervical adenocarcinoma* by FIGO clinical staging can be treated by the following modalities (91):
   a. *Stage IB1* cervical adenocarcinoma is treated by radical hysterectomy with lymphadenectomy and upper vaginal amputation.
   b. *Stage IB2 to IIA* disease is treated by primary radiotherapy.
   c. Similar therapy is recommended in higher clinical staging, since cervical adenocarcinoma and squamous cell carcinoma extend in a similar pattern by local infiltration and lymph node spread.

Cervical Clear Cell Adenocarcinoma

DES-exposed *in utero* carcinoma and adenosis have been described in Chapter 16.

Conventional therapy is similar to that described for cervical squamous cell carcinoma. When surgery is performed on young women, ovarian conservation is advocated with radical hysterectomy and lymphadenectomy. Vaginectomy is executed when the lesion extends to the vagina. At the time of vaginectomy, vaginal reconstruction is recommended. The overall survival rate in cervical clear cell carcinoma is 80%. The survival rate in stage I is 90% (92). For FIGO stage IB to IIB clear cell carcinoma (in women not exposed *in utero* to DES), the 5-year survival rate is 67% (93). Both early and late recurrences are well established. Metastases to the lungs and the subclavicular nodes are recorded. If exenteration is considered, positive pelvic or para-aortic nodes constitute contraindications for this operation (92).

Other Types Of Cervical Cancer

Occasionally, other cervical malignant neoplasia can occur. It has been reported following original cervical cancer:

1. *Cervical verrucous carcinoma* is a very rare variant of squamous cell carcinoma and is a slowly growing, locally invasive, nonmetastatic tumor, which demonstrates strong association with viral infection. Usually, it is located on the posterior lip of the cervical portio. The definitive diagnosis is made by wide excisional biopsy, followed by histological verification. The therapy is either wide local excision or simple total hysterectomy or exenterations (when primary tumor is large and infiltrates adjacent organs). Radiation therapy is contraindicated due to radioresistant and postradiotherapy anaplastic transformation (94–96).
2. *Cervical lymphoma* (non-Hodgkins's lymphoma) is a malignant disease arising from extranodal tissue; primary lymphoma (which can be a part of a systemic lymphoma) is more frequently seen in the cervix than in the uterine corpus. Primary cervical lymphoma is a very rare condition. Clinically, postcoital vaginal bleeding is an initial symptom. Abnormal Pap smear can suggest SIL, although negative cytology can be present. Cervical biopsy is diagnostic. Staging of the disease is usually performed utilizing the Ann Arbor classification. Conventional therapy includes a combination of chemotherapy and radiotherapy (97–99).
3. *Cervical carcinoid* is a neuroendocrinologically aggressive malignant tumor, which, even in a low stage, metastasizes early (to the liver); therefore, prompt diagnosis and appropriate treatment are essential to improve survival. Occasionally, a tumor of any location, including the cervix, may produce the classic triad: cutaneous flushing, diarrhea, and valve heart disease. This triad, when

present, constitutes the carcinoid syndrome. *Diagnosis* is established by histology and documentation of urine secretion of more than 15 mg of 5-hydroxyindoleacetic acid (5-HIAA). Octreotide scintigraphy can identify metastatic disease. *Conventional therapy* for primary cervical carcinoid is surgery and adjuvant chemotherapy. Symptoms can be controlled with histamine blockers and Octreotide, 150 to 1,500 mg daily, in three doses (100,101).

4. *Cervical malignant melanoma* is an extremely rare condition. *Diagnosis* is reached by evaluating the main symptom of vaginal bleeding (83%) and is verified by histology from a cervical biopsy specimen. The majority of patients are diagnosed in stage I or II of the disease. Diagnostic steps do not differ from squamous cell carcinoma evaluation. *Conventional therapy* is surgery, ranging from simple wide excision of cervical lesion to radical hysterectomy with pelvic/para-aortic lymph node dissection and partial vaginectomy with margins free of disease at about 2 cm. Adjuvant radiation or chemotherapy is also recommended (102,103).

5. *Cervical sarcomas* should be viewed as a complex group of cervical tumors within the endocervical stroma. These malignancies, affecting the uterine cervix, are rare. There are no well-established diagnostic criteria, and therapy varies, with an overall poor prognosis. Surgical treatment ranges from wide excision to total hysterectomy with oophorectomy combined with chemotherapy (104–106). Diagnosis and therapy of these tumors are based upon case presentation, with no prospective or retrospective results published to date; therefore, consulting case reports on individual tumors can be helpful.

Cervical Metastatic Cancer

In general, cervical metastatic cancer may originate from adjacent pelvic organs or distant different organs, and can be categorized as follows:

1. Local direct extension from the endometrium, vagina, rectum, and the bladder
2. Pelvic malignancy extension
3. Hematogenous metastasis from organs such as the breast or lungs

Conventional therapy is targeted to the organ from which metastasis originated.

REFERENCES

1. Association of Professors of Gynecology and Obstetrics. *Medical student educational objectives,* 7th ed. Washington, DC: APGO, 1997.
2. Council on Resident Education in Obstetrics and Gynecology (CREOG). *Educational objectives core curriculum for residents in obstetrics and gynecology,* 5th ed. Washington, DC: CREOG, 1996.
3. American College of Obstetricians and Gynecologists (ACOG). *Technical bulletin no. 183.* Washington, DC: ACOG, 1996.
4. Papanicolaou G, Traut HF. The diagnostic value of vaginal smears in carcinoma of the uterus. *Am J Obstet Gynecol* 1941; 42:193–206.
5. Anderson LM, May DS. Has the use of cervical, breast, and colorectal cancer screening increased in the United States? *Am J Public Health* 1995;85:840–842.
6. Nieminen P, Kallio M, Hakama M. The effect of mass screening on incidence and mortality of squamous and adenocarcinoma of cervix uteri. *Obstet Gynecol* 1995;85:117–121.
7. Platz CE, Benda JA. Female genital tract cancer. *Cancer* 1995; 75:270–294.
8. Janerich DT, Hadjimichael O, Schwartz PE, et al. The screening histories of women with invasive cervical cancer, Connecticut. *Am J Public Health* 1995;85:791–794.
9. Mitchell HS, Giles GG. Cancer diagnosis after a report of negative cervical cytology. *Med J Aust* 1996;164:270–273.
10. Linder J, Zahniser D. ThinPrep Papanicolaou testing to reduce false-negative cervical cytology. *Arch Pathol Lab Med* 1998; 122:139–144.
11. Kok MR, Boon ME, Schreiner-Kok PG, et al. Cytological recognition of invasive squamous cancer of the uterine cervix: comparison of conventional light-microscopical screening and neural network-based screening. *Hum Pathol* 2000;31:23–28.
12. Ku NN. Automated Papanicolaou smear analysis as a screening tool for female lower genital tract malignancies. *Curr Opin Obstet Gynecol* 1999;11:41–43.
13. Viikki M, Pukkala E, Hakama M. Risk of cervical cancer after a negative Pap smear. *J Med Screen* 1999;6:103–107.
14. U.S. Preventive Service Task Force. Screening for cervical cancer. In: *Guide to clinical preventive services: an assessment of the effectiveness of 169 interventions.* Baltimore: Williams and Wilkins, 1989:57–62.
15. Nieminen P, Kallio M, Anttila A, et al. Organized vs. spontaneous Pap-smear screening for cervical cancer: a case-control study. *Int J Cancer* 1999;83:55–58.
16. Veljovich DS, Stoler MH, Andersen WA, et al. Atypical glandular cells of undetermined significance: a five-year retrospective histologic study. *Am J Obstet Gynecol* 1998;179:382–390.
17. National Cancer Institute Workshop. The 1988 Bethesda system for reporting cervical/vaginal cytological diagnoses. *JAMA* 1989;262:931–934.
18. Hanau CA, Bibbo M. The for cytology follow-up after LEEP. *Acta Cytol* 1997;41:731–736.
19. Maiman M, Watts DH, Andersen J, et al. Vaginal 5-fluorouracil for high-grade cervical dysplasia in human immunodeficiency virus infection: a randomized trial. *Obstet Gynecol* 1999;94: 954–961.
20. Richart RM, Barron BA. A follow-up study of patients with cervical dysplasia. *Am J Obstet Gynecol* 1969;105:386–393.
21. Ostor AG. Natural history of cervical intraepithelial neoplasia: a cervical review. *Int J Gynecol Pathol* 1993;12:186–192.
22. Lousuebsakul V, Knutsen SM, Gram IT, et al. Clinical impact of atypical squamous cell of undetermined significance. A cytohistologic comparison. *Acta Cytol* 2000;44:23–30.
23. Sharman ME, Tabbara SO, Scott DR, et al. "ASCUS, rule out HSIL": cytologic features, histologic correlates, and human papillomavirus detection. *Mod Pathol* 1999;12:335–342.
24. Vlahos NP, Dragisic KG, Wallach EE, et al. Clinical significance of the qualification of atypical squamous cells of undetermined significance: an analysis on the basis of histologic diagnosis. *Am J Obstet Gynecol* 2000;182:885–889.
25. Nguyen HN, Nordqvist SR. The Bethesda system and evaluation of abnormal Pap smear. *Semin Surg Oncol* 1999;16: 217–221.

26. Cheng RF, Hernandez E, Anderson LL, et al. Clinical significance of a cytologic diagnosis of atypical glandular cells of undetermined significance. *J Reprod Med* 1999;44:922–928.

27. Korn AP, Judson PL, Zaloudek CJ. Importance of atypical glandular cells of uncertain significance in cervical cytologic smears. *J Reprod Med* 1998;43:774–778.

28. Zweizig S, Noller K, Reale F, et al. Neoplasia associated with atypical glandular cells of undetermined significance on cervical cytology. *Gynecol Oncol* 1997;65:314–318.

29. Kennedy AW, Salmieri SS, Wirth SL, et al. Results of the clinical evaluation of atypical cells of undetermined significance (SGCUS) detected on cervical cytology screening. *Gynecol Oncol* 1996;63:14–18.

30. Manetta A, Keefe K, Lin F, et al. Atypical glandular cells of undetermined significance in cervical cytology findings. *Am J Obstet Gynecol* 1999;180:883–888.

31. Obenson K, Abreo F, Grafton WD. Cytohistologic correlation between AGCUS and biopsy-detected lesions in postmenopausal women. *Acta Cytol* 2000;44:41–45.

32. Poynor EA, Barakat RR, Hoskins WJ. Management and follow-up of patients with adenocarcinoma *in situ* of the uterine cervix. *Gynecol Oncol* 1995;57:158–164.

33. Maciocia G. *Obstetric and gynecology Chinese medicine.* London: Churchill Livingstone, 1998.

34. Niruthisard S, Trisukosol D. Male sexual behavior as risk factor in cervical cancer. *J Med Assoc Thai* 1991;74:507–512.

35. Gardner JW, Sanborn JS, Slattery ML. Behavioral factors explaining the low risk for cervical carcinoma in Utah Mormon women. *Epidemiology* 1995;6:187–189.

36. Ursin G, Pike MC, Preston-Martin S, et al. Sexual, reproductive, and other risk factors for adenocarcinoma of the cervix: results from a population-based case-control study. *Cancer Causes Control* 1996;7:391–401.

37. Kalograki A, Tamilakis D, Tzardi M, et al. Cigarette smoking as a risk factor for intraepithelial lesion of the cervix uteri. *In Vivo* 1996;10:613–616.

38. McBride CM, Scholes D, Grothaus L, et al. Promoting smoking cessation among women who seek cervical cancer screening. *Obstet Gynecol* 1998;91:719–724.

39. de Vet HC, Knipschild PG, Sturmans F. The role of sexual factors in the aetiology of cervical dysplasia. *Int J Epidemiol* 1993; 22:798–803.

40. Oral contraceptives and invasive adenocarcinomas and adenosquamous carcinomas of the uterine cervix. The World Health Organization Collaborative Study of Neoplasia and Steroid contraceptives. *Am J Epidemiol* 1996;144:281–289.

41. Hirose K, Hamajima N, Takezaki T, et al. Smoking and dietary risk factors for cervical cancer at different age group in Japan. *J Epidemiol* 1998;8:6–14.

42. Palan PR, Mikhail MS, Basu J, et al. Beta-carotene levels in exfoliated cervicovaginal epithelial cells in cervical intraepithelial neoplasia and cervical cancer. *Am J Obstet Gynecol* 1992; 167:1899–1903.

43. Meyskens FL Jr, Urwit E, Moon TE, et al. Enhancement of regression of cervical intraepithelial neoplasia II (moderate dysplasia) with topically applied all-trans-retinoic acid: a randomized trial. *J Natl Cancer Inst* 1994;86:539–543.

44. Mackerras D, Irwig L, Simpson JM, et al. Randomized double-blind trial of beta-carotene and vitamin C in women with minor cervical abnormalities. *Br J Cancer* 1999;79:1448–1453.

45. Christen WG, Buring JE, Manson JE, et al. Beta-carotene supplementation: a good thing, a bad thing, or nothing? *Curr Opin Lipidol* 1999;10:29–33.

46. Romney SL, Ho GY, Palan PR, et al. Effects of beta-carotene and other factors on outcome of cervical dysplasia and human papillomavirus infection. *Gynecol Oncol* 1997;65:483–492.

47. Potter JD. Beta-carotene and the role of intervention studies. *Cancer Lett* 1997;114:329–331.

48. Palan PR, Chang CJ, Mikhail MS, et al. Plasma concentrations of micronutrients during nine-month clinical trial of beta-carotene in women with precursor cervical cancer lesions. *Nutr Cancer* 1998;30:46–52.

49. Hudson T. *Women's encyclopedia of natural medicine. Alternative therapies and integrative medicine.* Los Angeles: Keats Publishing, 1999:49–69.

50. Graham W, Surwite E, Weiner S, et al. Phase II trial of beta-all-trans-retinoic acid for cervical intraepithelial neoplasia delivered via a college sponge and cervical cap. *West J Med* 1986; 145:192–195.

51. Romney SL, Duttagupta C, Basu J, et al. Plasma vitamin C and uterine cervical dysplasia. *Am J Obstet Gynecol* 1985;151: 976–980.

52. Butterworth CE Jr, Hatch KD, Soong SJ, et al. Oral folic acid supplementation for cervical dysplasia: a clinical intervention trial. *Am J Obstet Gynecol* 1992;166:803–809.

53. Giulioano AR, Gapstur S. Can cervical dysplasia and cancer be prevented with nutrients? *Nutr Rev* 1998;56:9–16.

54. Meyskens FL Jr, Manetta A. Prevention of cervical intraepithelial neoplasia and cervical cancer. *Am J Clin Nutr* 1995;62: 1417S–1419S.

55. American Cancer Society (ACS). *Cancer facts and figures.* Atlanta: ACS, 1995.

56. Canavan TP, Doshi NR. Cervical cancer. *Am Fam Physician* 2000;61:1369–1376.

57. Magnusson PK, Gyllesten UB. Cervical cancer: is there a genetic component? *Mol Med Today* 2000;6:145–148.

58. American Cancer Society (ACS). *Cancer facts and figures—1997.* Atlanta: ACS, 1997.

59. Chung CK, Stryker JA, Ward SP, et al. Histologic grade and prognosis of carcinoma of the cervix. *Obstet Gynecol* 1981;57:636–642.

60. International Federation of Gynecology and Obstetrics (FIGO). *Annual report on the results of treatment in gynecological cancer,* 22nd ed. Stockholm: FIGO, 1994.

61. Querleu D, Leblanc E, Castelain B, et al. New trends in management of carcinomas of the cervix. *J Gynecol Obstet Biol Reprod (Paris)* 2000;29:254–257.

62. Viala J. Imaging of cancer of the uterine cervix. *Cancer Radiother* 2000;4:109–112.

63. Medl M, Peters-Engl C, Schultz P, et al. First report of lymphatic mapping with isosulfan blue dye and sentinel biopsy in cervical cancer. *Anticancer Res* 2000;20:1133–1134.

64. Sevin BU. Management of microinvasive cervical cancers. *Semin Surg Oncol* 1999;16:228–231.

65. Chi DS, Gemiganani ML, Curtin JP, et al. Long-term experience in the surgical management of cancer of the uterine cervix. *Semin Surg Oncol* 1999;17:161–167.

66. Duggan BD, Felix JC, Muderspach LI, et al. Cold-knife conization versus conization by the loop electrictrosurgical excision procedure: a randomized prospective study. *Am J Obstet Gynecol* 1999;180:276–282.

67. Okamoto Y, Ueki K, Ueki M. Pathological indications for conservative therapy in treating cervical cancer. *Acta Obstet Gynecol Scand* 1999;78:813–823.

68. Possover M, Krause N, Plaul K, et al. Laparoscopic para-aortic and pelvic lymphadenectomy: experience with 150 patients and review of the literature. *Gynecol Oncol* 1998;71:1 9–28.

69. Dottio PR, Tobias DH, Beddoe A, et al. Laparoscopic lymphadenectomy for gynecologic malignancies. *Gynecol Oncol* 1999;73:383–388.

70. Leblanc E, Querleu D, Castelain B, et al. Role of laparoscopy in

management of uterine cervix cancer. *Cancer Radiother* 2000;4:113–121.

71. Ostrzenski A. A new laparoscopic abdominal radical hysterectomy: a pilot trial. *Eur J Surg Oncol* 1996;22:602–606.

72. Lindegaard JC, Thranow IR, Engelholm SA. Radiotherapy in the management of cervical cancer in elderly patients. *Radiother Oncol* 2000;56:9–15.

73. Sardi J, Vidaurreta J, Bermudez A, et al. Laparoscopically assisted Schauta operation: learning experience at the Gynecologic Oncology Unit, Buenos Aires University Hospital. *Gynecol Oncol* 1999;75:361–365.

74. Vergote IB. Exenterative surgery. *Curr Opin Obstet Gynecol* 1997;9:25–28.

75. Thomas GM. Concurrent chemotherapy and radiation for locally advanced cervical cancer: the new standard of care. *Semin Radiat Oncol* 2000;10:44–50.

76. Resbeut M, Haie-Meder C, Alzieu C, et al. Radiochemotherapy of uterine cervix cancers. Recent data. *Cancer Radiother* 2000;4:140–146.

77. Haie-Meder C, Fervers B, Chauvergne J, et al. Standards, options and recommendations: concomitant radiochemotherapy for cancer of the cervix: a critical analysis of the literature and update of SOR. *Bull Cancer* 1999;86:829–841.

78. Nguyen HN, Nordqvist SR. Chemotherapy of advanced and recurrent cervical carcinoma. *Semin Surg Oncol* 1999;16:247–250.

79. Panetta A, Angelelli B, Martoni A. Pilot study on induction chemotherapy with cisplatin and epirubicin, etoposide and bleomycin in cervical cancer stage Ib, IIa and IIb. *Anticancer Res* 1999;19:765–768.

80. Chang TC, Hsueh S, Lai CH, et al. Phase II trial of neoadjuvant chemotherapy in early-stage small cell cervical carcinoma. *Anticancer Drugs* 1999;10:641–646.

81. Kinney WK, Egorshin EV, Ballard DJ, et al. Long-term survival and sequelae after surgical management of invasive cervical carcinoma diagnosed at the time of simple hysterectomy. *Gynecol Oncol* 1992;44:24–27.

82. Chapman JA, Mannel RS, DiSaia PJ, et al. Surgical treatment of unexpected invasive cervical cancer found at total hysterectomy. *Obstet Gynecol* 1992;80:931–934.

83. Orr JW Jr, Ball GC, Soong SJ, et al. Surgical treatment of women found to have invasive cervical cancer at the time of total hysterectomy. *Obstet Gynecol* 1986;68:353–356.

84. Shephard J, Weston R, Peersman G, et al. Interventions for encouraging sexual lifestyle and behaviours intended to prevent cervical cancer. *Cochrome Database Syst Rev* 2000;2:CD001035.

85. Gerhard CA, Pong K, Kollar LM, et al. Adolescents' knowledge of papillomavirus and cervical dysplasia. *J Pediatr Adolesc Gynecol* 2000;13:15–20.

86. Ferrante JM, Gonzalez EC, Roetzheim RG, et al. Clinical and demographic predictors of late-stage cervical cancer. *Arch Fam Med* 2000;9:439–445.

87. Saigo PE, Cain JM, Kim WS, et al. Prognostic factors in adenocarcinoma of the uterine cervix. *Cancer* 1986;57:1584–1593.

88. Tay EH, Yew WS, Ho TH. Management of adenocarcinoma *in situ* (ACIS) of the uteri cervix—a clinical dilemma. *Singapore Med J* 1999;40:36–39.

89. Azodi M, Chambers SK, Rutherford TJ, et al. Adenocarcinoma in situ of the cervix: management and outcome. *Gynecol Oncol* 1999;73:348–353.

90. Nguyen HN, Averette HE. Special problems in cervical cancer management. *Semin Surg Oncol* 1999;16:261–266.

91. Schorege JO, Lee KR, Lee SJ, et al. Early cervical adenocarcinoma: selection criteria for radical surgery. *Obstet Gynecol* 1999;94:368–390.

92. Reich O, Tamussino K, Lahousen M, et al. Clear cell carcinoma of the cervix: pathology and prognosis in surgically treated stage IB–IIB disease in women not exposed *in utero* to diethylstilbestrol. *Gynecol Oncol* 2000;76:331–335.

93. Knopp RC. Clear cell carcinoma of the vagina. In: Heintz APM, Griffitths CT, Trimbos JB, eds. *Surgery in gynecological oncology.* The Hauge, 1984.

94. Kawagoe K, Yoshikawa H, Kawana T, et al. Verrucous carcinoma of the uterine cervix. *Nippon Sanka Fujinka Gakkai Zasshi* 1984;36:617–672.

95. Wong WS, Ng CS, Lee CK. Verrucous carcinoma of the cervix. *Arch Gynecol Obstet* 1990;247:47–51.

96. Degefu S, O'Quinn AG, Lacey CG, et al. Verrucous carcinoma of the cervix: a report of two cases and literature review. *Gynecol Oncol* 1986;25:37–47.

97. Nasu K, Yoshimatsu J, Urata K, et al. A case of primary non-Hodgkin's lymphoma of the uterine cervix. *J Obstet Gynaecol Res* 1998;24:157–160.

98. Grace A, O'Connell N, Byrne P, et al. Malignant lymphoma of the cervix. An unusual presentation and rare disease. *Eur J Gynaecol Oncol* 1999;20:26–28.

99. Amichetti M, Chiappe E, Mussari S, et al. Primary non-Hodgkin's lymphoma of the female genital tract. *Oncol Rep* 1999;6:651–654.

100. Seidel R Jr, Steinfeld A. Carcinoid of the cervix: natural history and implications for therapy. *Gynecol Oncol* 1988;30:114–119.

101. Koch CA, Azumi N, Furlong MA, et al. Carcinoid syndrome caused by an atypical carcinoid of the uterine cervix. *J Clin Endocrinol Metab* 1999;84:4209–4213.

102. Canturia G, Angioli R, Nahmias J, et al. Primary malignant melanoma of the uterine cervix: case report an review of literature. *Gynecol Oncol* 1999;75:170–174.

103. Takehara M, Ito E, Saito T, et al. Primary malignant melanoma of the uterine cervix. A case report. *J Obstet Gynaecol Res* 1999;25:129–132.

104. Rotmenshch J, Rosenshein NB, Woodruff JD. Cervical sarcoma. *Obstet Gynecol Surv* 1983;38:456–460.

105. Vlahos NP, Matthews R, Veridiano NP. Cervical sarcoma botryoides. A case report. *J Reprod Med* 1999;44:306–308.

106. Amr SS, Sheikh SM. Polypoid endocervical stromal sarcoma with heterologous elements. Report of a case with review of the literature. *Eur J Obstet Gynecol Reprod Biol* 2000;88:103–106.

BENIGN UTERINE DISORDERS

EDUCATIONAL OBJECTIVES

Medical Students (1) *APGO Objective No. 57*	*Residents in Obstetrics/Gynecology (2)* *CREOG Objectives*	*Practitioners (3)* *ACOG Recommendations*

Uterine leiomyomas
  Prevalence of uterine leiomyomas
  Symptoms and physical findings
  Methods to confirm the diagnosis
  Indications for medical and
    surgical treatment
	Pelvic mass
	  History
	  Physical examination
	  Diagnostic studies
	  Diagnosis
	  Management
	  Follow-up
		Uterine leiomyomata
		  Etiology
		  Clinical features
		  Evaluation
		  Treatment
		  Management guidelines

UTERINE EMBRYOLOGY

The myometrium and endometrium originate embryologically from the mesoderm. Fusion of the müllerian ducts occurs between 8 and 9 weeks postovulatory weeks, creating the beginning of the uterus, a muscular, hollow organ (2). In about 20 weeks of gestational age, the endometrium is formed from a single layer of columnar epithelium, which transforms into glandular structure lengthening under the myometrium. This newly created endometrium bears a close resemblance to the atrophic, inactive postmenopausal endometrium with a thickness of <0.5 mm.

From the neonatal period until the pubertal period, the uterus and endometrium remain inactive. An average neonatal uterine size is approximately 4 cm in length; two-thirds is composed of the cervix. Puberty activates growth of the uterus, which attains 8 cm in length, 5 cm in width, and 2.5 cm in thickness of the fundus. The weight of the uterus ranges from 40 to 100 g in a mature nulliparous woman of reproductive age. Each delivery of a child will cause the uterine to grow. The multigravida (four deliveries) uterus on average will measure 10 to 12 cm × 5 to 7 cm × 2.5 cm, with a weight up to 250 g. Upon reaching reproductive maturity, the endometrium is transformed from an inactive to a functionally active and integral part of the uterus (4).

UTERINE ANATOMY

The uterus anatomically is divided into two parts: the corpus of the uterus and the cervix. *The corpus* of the uterus is the muscular, hollow organ, its cephalic segment connects intra–abdominal space via the Fallopian tubes bilaterally. The caudal segment connects the vagina through the cervical canal. Three segments—*the fundus, the cornua*, and *the isthmus*—can be identified within the corpus of the uterus. *The cornua* represent the upper lateral aspect of the uterine corpus bilaterally, in which the Fallopian tubes traverse and open to the uterine cavity. The portion of the cornua in which the Fallopian tubes run is known as *the interstitial part* of the Fallopian tubes. The corpus of the uterus is pear-shaped with a narrow part caudally that is termed the isthmus. *The isthmus* becomes constricted enough to fuse, and to connect with the cervix and the cervical canal, which opens to the uterine cavity (average depth is about 6 cm, with a capacity of 3 to 8 mL). The visceral peritoneal envelope encompasses the uterus and is also called *the uterine serosa*, which is the external part of the uterus. Anteriorly, the uterine peritoneum extends to the bladder part of the peritoneum. This transient peritoneal area between the bladder and the uterus is known as *the vesicouterine peritoneal* reflection. *The visceral peritoneum* fuses firmly with the uterine muscular layer; although, it does not cover the isthmus and has a loose connection with the vesicouterine peritoneal reflection. This loose union is utilized during surgery, when separation of the bladder from the uterine cervix is required. The uterine visceral peritoneum changes into the parietal peritoneum and lines the anterior cul-de-sac. *The anterior cul-de-sac* is the space between the bladder and the anterior uterine wall. Contrary to the anterior, loose peritoneal connection with the bladder reflection, posteriorly the visceral peritoneum completely invests the myometrium and covers the cervix, the upper portion of the posterior vaginal wall, and the uterosacral ligaments. The space between the uterosacral ligaments is also covered by peritoneum that reflects over the rectum and the lower segment of the sigmoid colon, and is termed *the posterior cul-de-sac or the pouch of Douglas*. Laterally, the anterior and posterior uterine visceral peritoneum creates the leaves of *the broad ligaments* on both sides of the uterus. Laterally, the broad ligaments extend to the pelvic wall and the upper part covers the Fallopian tubes (the mesosalpinx or the tubal mesentery). From the ovaries, they cover the infundibulopelvic ligament; their middle part covers the round ligaments; and the inferior segment grows thicker and becomes a part of *the cardinal ligaments* (transverse cervical ligament of Mackenrodt). The mesosalpinx comprises small blood vessels, the vestigial remnants of mesonephric tubules, and ducts; they are termed the *epoophoron* (lateral segment of the tubules) and *paroophoron* (medial segment of the tubules). The *uterine arteries* (ascending and descending), accompanied by veins, traverse within the leaves of the broad ligaments and the cardinal ligaments (Figs. 19.1–19.3). This part of the *uterine lymphatic system* courses within the broad ligament leaves.

Uterine suspension, support, and functional anatomy are elaborated in Chapter 24.

Uterine blood supply is delivered from two sources: the uterine artery, which is a branch of the anterior hypogastric artery (the internal iliac artery), and the ovarian artery (Fig. 19.4). *The uterine artery*, after branching from the hypogastric artery, creates the uterine artery arch, under which the ureter traverses. At the level corresponding to the internal os of the cervical canal, the uterine artery splits into the descending and ascending uterine artery, which runs tortuously. The descending limb provides blood supply to the cervix and the lateral vagina, and the ascending uterine artery limb provides blood supply to the uterine corpus. When the uterine artery reaches the attachment of the round ligament, it sends a branch to the round ligament (*the Sampson's artery*). The main ascending uterine artery runs upward to the mesosalpinx, where anastomosis with the ovarian artery takes place. *The anterior uterine vein*, which drains directly to the hypogastric vein, provides uterine blood return from the anterior uterine surface. The posterior aspect of the uterus blood return is directed to the *short and long trunk*, which empties to either the hypogastric vein or the obturator vein. It is worthwhile to mention that collateral circulation to the pelvis can be established from the aorta, the femoral artery and the external iliac artery upon hypogastric artery ligation, which allows uterine function.

The uterine lymphatic system can be divided into the upper uterine corpus lymphatics and the lower uterine corpus lymphatics. The upper segment drains to the ovarian lymphatics, which opens to para-aortic lymphatics. Also, this segment communicates with the superficial inguinal lymphatic nodes alongside the round ligaments. The lower segment of the uterine corpus connects with the cervix lym-

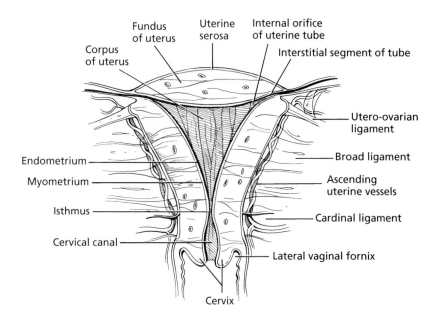

FIG. 19.1. The uterine structures.

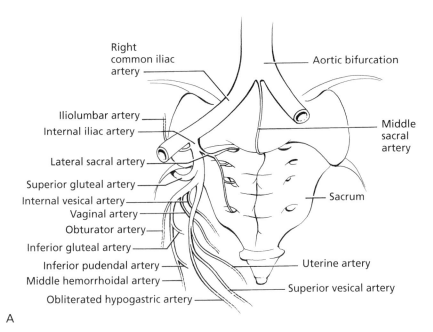

A

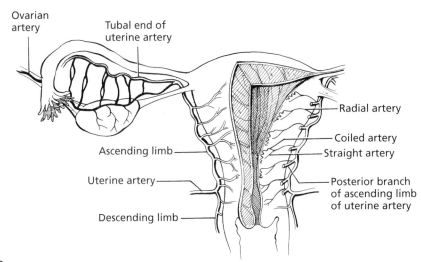

B

FIG. 19.2. A: The internal iliac artery divisions.
B: Uterine blood distribution.

phatics and drains to the pelvic lymphatic nodes (sacral, iliac, hypogastric, and obturator nodes).

The uterine myometrium is located between the serosa (outer peritoneal uterine layer) and the endometrium. The myometrium itself is composed of three layers of smooth muscles. The outer muscle of the myometrium runs in *longitudinal arrangements,* and a small portion of this layer goes into the broad and round ligaments. The middle layer of the myometrium is arranged in a *circular fashion* and is the thickest among the layers. Within this muscle layer, the stratum vasculare is present. The inner layer is arranged in *oblique and longitudinal patterns.* Such myometrial layers

create a unique system allowing compressing vessels to stop bleeding.

Uterine innervation comes from the following sources:

1. Frankenhäuser's cervical ganglion (the pelvic plexus) provides motor fibers to the uterine muscular layers. The fibers enter the myometrium from the posterior aspect of the cervix alongside the uterosacral ligaments.
2. The aortic and hypogastric plexuses, as visceral afferent sensory fibers, innervate the cervix. The fibers run via the sacral parasympathetic nerve bundle and reach the second, third, and fourth sacral nerves.

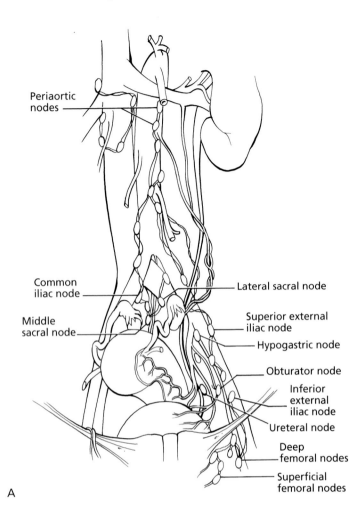

Periaortic nodes

Common iliac node

Lateral sacral node

Middle sacral node

Superior external iliac node

Hypogastric node

Obturator node

Inferior external iliac node

Ureteral node

Deep femoral nodes

Superficial femoral nodes

A

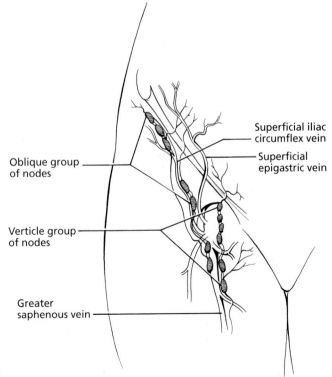

Superficial iliac circumflex vein

Superficial epigastric vein

Oblique group of nodes

Verticle group of nodes

Greater saphenous vein

B

FIG. 19.3. A: Pelvic lymphatic system. **B:** The oblique and vertical groups of the superficial inguinal nodes.

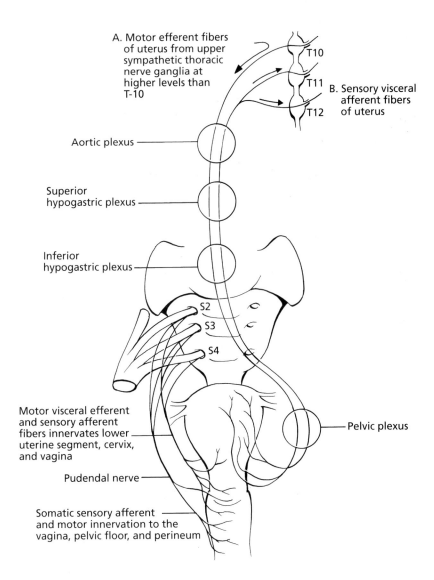

A. Motor efferent fibers of uterus from upper sympathetic thoracic nerve ganglia at higher levels than T-10

B. Sensory visceral afferent fibers of uterus

Aortic plexus

Superior hypogastric plexus

Inferior hypogastric plexus

Motor visceral efferent and sensory afferent fibers innervates lower uterine segment, cervix, and vagina

Pudendal nerve

Somatic sensory afferent and motor innervation to the vagina, pelvic floor, and perineum

Pelvic plexus

FIG. 19.4. Uterine innervation. **A:** Motor efferent fibers of uterus from upper sympathetic thoracic nerve ganglia at higher levels than T-10. **B:** Sensory visceral afferent fibers of uterus.

3. The sympathetic and parasympathetic plexuses deliver sensory and motor fibers, which innervate the cervix and the lower uterine part

Endometrium (its structure and function) is presented in Chapters 1 and 3.

MYOMETRIAL BENIGN DISORDERS

Uterine Anomalies

Uterine congenital anomalies are presented in Chapter 4.

Uterine Leiomyomas

Definition

Uterine leiomyoma (leiomyomata, myomata, myoma, fibroids, and fibromyomata) is a benign tumor of smooth myometrial muscles (mesenchymal tumor).

Incidence

The prevalence of uterine leiomyomata in women over 30 years of age in their reproductive years is estimated to be 20% to 30% and is uncommon in women under the age of 30 years and in older women (5). Postmenopausal *de novo* formation and prepubertal occurrence has not been reported, although uterine myomas in adolescence, even symptomatic myomas, are well documented (6).

Etiology

The etiology of the initiation of growing leiomyomata is not known. It has been hypothesized as follows:

1. *One cell* of smooth muscle starts off the entire process of *de novo* tumor formation (7).
2. *Thymidine phosphorylase inhibition activity* is greater within uterine leiomyomata than in uterine muscles (8).

3. *Cytogenetic abnormalities* include deletions and translocations located within several chromosomes (most frequently chromosome 12) (9,10).
4. *Steroid hormones* express their activity by the presence of estrogen and progesterone receptors (there is no unity on the view that leiomyoma contains greater number of receptors than healthy myometrium). Additional clinical information supporting the theory that hormonal milieu influences myoma clinical behavior and induces a hypoestrogenic state has been documented; this leads to significant reduction in myoma size (11). Also, clinical observation points out that uterine fibroids occur in reproductive years and regress in the postmenopausal period. Steroid hormones may influence myoma clinical behavior (12,13).
   a. Estrogen stimulates leiomyoma to increase in size.
   b. Progesterone may rapidly increase myometa, in size and may lead to leiomyomata hemorrhagic degeneration.
5. *Growth factors*, including several peptide growth factors, may play a role in the etiology of leiomyoma (14).
6. *Other factors* such as progestins, clomiphene citrate or pregnancy, may stimulate the rapid growth of uterine leiomyomata.

Predisposing factors for the development of uterine leiomyomata include the following:

1. Elevated adult body mass index (15)
2. Radiation exposure (16)
3. Early normal menstrual cycle (17).
4. Oral contraceptive use at a young age (13 to 16 years of age) influences the risk of uterine leiomyomata among premenopausal women (18).

Recently, study has been initiated to establish the role of genes in the pathogenesis of uterine leiomyomata. The research tries to identify the susceptibility of genes for myoma by performing a genome-wide screen (19).

Classification

Classification of leiomyomata is based upon the tumor's location, and uterine myomata can develop in any uterine location:

- *Subserosal leiomyomata* can grow and become pedunculated, which may lead to torsion and necrosis, causing symptoms. Occasionally, subserosal myoma can separate from the uterus and live on other abdominal or pelvic organs as parasitic leiomyomata.
- *Intramural leiomyomata* is the most common form of uterine leiomyoma and is located within the myometrium.
- *Submucosal leiomyomata* is observed in about 5% of leiomyomata (3). This tumor can compress the endometrium and can protrude into the uterine cavity; when pedunculated, it can prolapse via the cervical canal to the vaginal pool. Ulceration of leiomyoma is often observed in this location.

Diagnosis

Pertinent medical history associated with uterine leiomyomata is present in about 20% to 50% and will include the following:

- *Abnormal endometrial bleeding* is present in a form of menorrhagia (>80 mL of bleeding during menses). Modern scientific clinical data indicates that the risk of developing anemia from heavy menstrual bleeding usually occurs at a menstrual blood loss level of 120 mL. Abnormal endometrial bleeding, however, is the most common symptom of myoma, reported in about 30% of the cases (21,22).
- *Pelvic pain* related directly to leiomyoma is an infrequent event. Usually, other pelvic pathology can be present causing pelvic pain (ovarian, Fallopian tube pathology, pelvic endometriosis, adenomyosis, or intestinal disorders). When torsion and necrosis of pedunculated leiomyoma or red degeneration occur, an acute pain can be observed. Partial ureter obstruction, symptomatic or asymptomatic, can also occur occasionally, with an unknown clinical significance (3). Acute urinary retention can be associated with pelvic pain due to a large uterine myoma (23).
- *Pelvic pressure* from anterior uterine wall myoma compression may produce urine urgency or frequency, or incontinence; the posterior wall tumor location may produce rectal pressure (3).
- *Interference of leiomyoma with reproductive capacity* has been postulated by several observational and anecdotal clinical reports; even though, uterine fibroids alone very seldom cause infertility, spontaneous abortion, or premature or preterm labor (24). These data are in contrast with a successful outcome of myomectomy (>40%) for infertility or pregnancy losses (15,16). Therefore, it seems that treatment of fibroids in infertility patients is useful, but this has not yet been proven scientifically (25,26).

Physical examination may reveal a pelvic-abdominal mass when a tumor is large enough (corresponding to >12 weeks' gestational size) to move above the brim of the pelvis and is palpable above the symphysis pubis.

Pelvic examination provides sufficient information to arrive at an initial clinical impression of uterine leiomyoma in approximately 95%. A typical bimanual examination will identify the enlarged, irregular (often asymmetrical), nodular uterus, nontender to motion and palpation. In acceptable clinical practice, uterine size is determined by establishing a corresponding gestational uterine size, since it correlates well with the actual weight of the uterus (i.e., 12 weeks' gestational size is about 280 g) (27). Low-grade body core temperature, uterine tenderness, and mild peritoneal signs can be identified when uterine leiomyomata undergoes either a degenerative or necrotic or both processes.

Laboratory tests for leiomyomata and their potential sequelae include the following:

- Hemoglobin or hematocrit is indicated when menometrorrhagia is present.
- Bleeding time and coagulation profiles are performed when bleeding diathesis is suspected.
- Endometrial sampling should be performed when abnormal endometrial bleeding is identified.
- *Imaging studies* such as ultrasonography, computed tomography, and magnetic resonance imaging are useful techniques; although, those studies do not significantly influence management and are not recommended for routine assessment (3). Ultrasound and computed tomography will not distinguish leiomyomata from adenomyomas. Magnetic resonance imaging has been postulated to be a tool that will assist in providing the adenomyosis and adenomyomas diagnosis (28). Imaging studies can be utilized in certain clinical situations such as when a practitioner is uncertain of the diagnosis, for differential diagnosis, particularly when there are ovarian or other pelvic masses, and when the patient is morbidly obese. Also, the submucosal location of uterine leiomyomata can be diagnosed by utilizing hysterosalpingography. Uterine artery Doppler velocimetry with leiomyomas has been suggested for the diagnosis of uterine myoma (29). Additional study in this field is currently being conducted to determine the validity of this diagnostic modality.
- *Endoscopic studies* can assist in reaching a definitive diagnosis. Laparoscopic, hysteroscopic, or both evaluations in uncertain diagnosis may establish the source of a mass or endometrial lesions responsible for a patient's complaints.

Differential Diagnosis

- Adenomyosis
- Ovarian mass
- Endometriosis
- Other pelvic organ mass
- Intestinal disorders

Conventional Therapy

Uterine leiomyomata can be managed conservatively and/or surgically. When a clinical decision is made to manage this condition, it is advisable to document the number and location of myomata. Modern technology such as ultrasound or magnetic resonance imaging may substantially enhance the reliability of follow-up. Prophylactic intervention is hardly ever recommended for this condition.

Conservative Management

I. *Expectant management* is recommended, when leiomyomata that are asymptomatic and smaller than 12 weeks' gestational size are present. Initial clinical observation within 1 to 2 years should follow leiomyomata of a slow-growing nature (i.e., <6 weeks' gestational size within 1 year, fast or established mass size, and presenting symptomatology). It usually requires 1 to 2 years of clinical evaluation, in intervals of 3 to 6 months. If no significant changes in clinical behavior are observed, a patient can be scheduled for follow-up assessment on a yearly basis. Women with asymptomatic uterine leiomyomata who desire pregnancy should be advised to try to get pregnant for 1 year before myomectomy is suggested. Myomectomy itself may cause a mechanical type of infertility due to formation of abdominal-pelvic adhesions (3).

II. *Medical management* is indicated when symptomatic uterine leiomyomata are present [10% to 40% among women (15,16)], using the following approaches:

A. *Nonsteroidal anti-inflammatory drugs* (prostaglandin synthesis inhibitors) are recommended by ACOG to control menorrhagia and dysmenorrhea. This recommendation is in contrast with the clinical effectiveness of these forms of medication. Idiopathic menorrhagia can be reduced approximately 30% to 50% by administering nonsteroidal antiinflammatory drugs (30); although, neither myoma-induced menorrhagia nor coagulation defect–associated menorrhagia can be treated with these drugs (31,32). The use of these agents in menorrhagia and in secondary dysmenorrhea is presented in Chapters 3 and 5.

B. *Low-dose oral contraceptives* have been postulated by ACOG to control menorrhagia associated with uterine myoma. There are no convincing data available to support such a recommendation. Some of the research results suggest that oral contraceptives are contraindicated to use, and other results postulate that uterine leiomyomata should not be considered a contraindication for the use of oral contraceptives (33).

C. *Progestins* are also recommended in the treatment of menorrhagia, as recommended by ACOG; although, there is surprisingly scant convincing clinical scientific data to support such a clinical approach. It has been reported that a patient responded to progestin therapy with a significant increase in size of uterine leiomyomata, even in combination with concomitant antiestrogen medication (34). *An antiprogesterone agent (RU 486)* is able to reduce uterine leiomyomata volume in about 80% (35); therefore, such data indicate that progestins can be counterproductive.

D. *Gonadotropin-releasing hormone agonists (GnRH)* suppress the pituitary–ovarian axis and lead to decreased estradiol and progesterone circulating levels. Low levels of steroidal hormones will cause uterine leiomyomata to shrink (a 50% reduction). In order to decrease significant bone loss, add-back therapy can be administered (following an initial 12 weeks of therapy with GnRH, cyclic or continuous estrogen, and progesterone are added). Treatment should continue for 3 to 6 months. The maximum reduction of myoma size is observed at 12 to 24 weeks of therapy (11,36,37). This mode of therapy should be used before myomectomy; however, the risk of recurrence of uterine leiomyoma is higher when GnRH is used (38). More detail about GnRH therapy is presented in Chapters 10 and 11.

E. *Selective estrogen receptor modulators (SERM)* such as Raloxifene are currently being tested for the treatment of uterine leiomyomata. Preliminary data indicate that Raloxifene can be effective as leiomyomata treatment (35,39).

F. *Antiprogesterone (RU 486 or Mifepristone)* in initial results at a dose of 25 mg three times daily for a 12-week course can cause significant regression of uterine leiomyomata volume (76.3%) (35,40).

Surgical Management

I. *Conservative surgical management* is designed to remove uterine leiomyomata with uterus preservation. Myomectomy or myolysis plays an essential role in conservative surgical management.

A. *Myomectomy* is performed when reproductive capacity is to be preserved. ACOG recommends the following criteria for myomectomy (3).

1. *Indications* include female infertility or recurrent pregnancy loss due to uterine leiomyomata.
2. *Confirmation* of the indication for myomectomy requires documentation of the presence of leiomyomata of sufficient size or specific location to be a probable cause of female infertility or recurrent pregnancy loss. In light of such confirmation, it should be established that there is no more likely an explanation for the failure to conceive or for recurrent pregnancy loss.
3. *Action prior to myomectomy* includes the following:
   a. Evaluate other potential causes of male and female infertility or recurrent pregnancy loss.
   b. Document the discussion that the complexity of the disease process may require hysterectomy.

ACOG's criteria for myomectomy, limits indications to cases of infertility and recurrent pregnancy losses. Symptomatic leiomyomata, without infertility aspects, is disregarded as an indication for myomectomy by ACOG. The emotional consequences for the patient are usually disregarded. This; however, should not be the case according to the current knowledge of the psychological aspects of uterine preservation versus hysterectomy. The uterus should be preserved, not only for the purpose of reproduction, but because the patient's sexual identity, body image, self-esteem, lifestyle, and social life will not be compromised (41).

Data have been available since 1994, when the ACOG criteria were published, to support the view that the presence and severity of myoma-related symptoms, and not the size of the uterus, should be the most important consideration in establishing surgical criteria (42).

Classical myomectomy can be executed either transabdominally or transvaginally.

Laparoscopic myomectomy provides very satisfactory results, although we cannot neglect the fact that it is a lengthy and technically demanding procedure. The size of myoma or multiple locations should be taken under consideration and matched with a surgeon's skill (it is a general consensus that one leiomyomata between 5 and 8 cm, or more than two myoma should be reserved for laparotomy) (43). Even intramural leiomyomata penetrating to the endometrial cavity can be safely removed by utilizing a laparoscopic tourniquet, suturing in layers, and employing extra- and intracorporeal knots (44).

Hysteroscopic resection of submucosal myoma is a procedure recognized by ACOG (45). The procedure is very effective and relatively easy to perform when leiomyomata are mainly located in the submucosal area. When submucosal myomata are predominantly in the intramural location, the resection of myoma should be continued until after healthy myometrium is identified. The overall hysteroscopic resection long-term effectiveness rate is approximately 84% (46).

Recurrence of myomas after myomectomy is greater when the total number of myoma exceeds four or more tumors. Leiomyomata recurrence is not associated with preoperative medical therapy, preoperative uterine volume, or resected myoma mass (47).

Laparoscopic or hysteroscopic myolysis (leiomyomata coagulation), either with laser or a bipolar needle, is utilized. A laparoscopic approach for intramural and a hysteroscopic approach for submucosal leiomyomata have been applied (43,48). It has been postulated that a combination of myolysis with endometrial ablation or resection performed for perfuse endometrial bleeding due to the presence of myoma is quite an effective technique. Such a combined clinical approach requires 12% subsequent surgery and 38% for ablation alone (49). It is a controversial approach, since endometrial ablation/resection should be performed only where there is no existing uterine or endometrial pathology. Additional clinical research is needed to establish the validity of this combined technique of myolysis with endometrial ablation or resection.

I. *Definitive surgical management* is either total or supracervical hysterectomy. ACOG-established criteria for hysterectomy for uterine leiomyomata executed via either an abdominal or a vaginal approach (3):

A. *Confirmation of indication*:

1. Asymptomatic leiomyomata of such size that they are palpable abdominally and are a concern to the patient

2. Excessive uterine bleeding evidenced by either of the following:
   a. Profuse bleeding with flooding, clots, or repetitive periods lasting for more than 8 days,
   b. Anemia due to acute or chronic blood loss
3. Pelvic discomfort caused by myomata (a or b or c)
   a. Acute and severe
   b. Chronic lower abdominal or low back pressure
   c. Bladder pressure with urinary frequency not due to urinary tract infection

B. *Action prior to procedure*
   1. Confirmation of the absence of cervical malignancy
   2. Elimination anovulation and other causes of abnormal bleeding
   3. Confirmation of the absence of endometrial malignancy when abnormal bleeding is present
   4. Assessment of surgical risk from anemia and need for treatment
   5. Evaluation of the patient's medical and psychological risks from hysterectomy

C. *Contraindications:*
   1. Desire to maintain fertility, in which case myomectomy should be considered
   2. Asymptomatic leiomyomata of size less than 12 weeks' gestation determined by physical examination or ultrasound examination

Unless otherwise stated, each item (except contraindications) must be present.

Although ACOG criteria for hysterectomy for leiomyomata has been established for either the abdominal or the vaginal approach, laparoscopic total hysterectomy without transvaginal surgery can be applied (50). Also, laparoscopically assisted vaginal hysterectomy can be utilized (51); laparoscopic supracervical uterine corpus amputation (subtotal abdominal hysterectomy) has also been advocated (52).

Complementary Therapy

Complementary medical therapy is usually used to accompany either conventional or alternative therapies and consists of changing one's lifestyle, getting more rest, avoiding the use of tampons, and appropriate nutrition (taking nutritional supplements such as vitamin C, beta-carotene, selenium, and zinc; along with a deit including fresh vegetables, fruits, nuts, seeds, and whole grain; while avoiding dairy products, red meat, fried fat, sugar, salt, caffeine, and alcohol). In some cases acupuncture can be helpful for pelvic pain associated with fibroids.

Alternative Therapy

Alternative medical treatment includes a basic mixture of tinctures in equal proportion of Blue cohosh, Chasteberry,

Cranesbill, and Wild yam; in addition to this mixture, Bark tincture may assist in pain management.

Asherman's Syndrome

The Asherman's syndrome is described in the Abnormal Endometrial Bleeding chapter.

REFERENCES

1. Association of Professors of Gynecology and Obstetrics (APGO). *Medical student educational objectives,* 7th ed. Washington DC: APGO, 1997.
2. Council on Resident Education in Obstetrics and Gynecology (CREOG). *Educational objectives core curriculum for residents in obstetrics and gynecology,* 5th ed. Washington, DC: CREOG 1996.
3. American College of Obstetrician and Gynecologists (ACOG). *Technical bulletin no. 192.* Washington, DC: ACOG, 1994.
4. Langlois PL. The size of the normal uterus. *J Reprod Med* 1970;4:220–228.
5. Cramer SF, Patel A. The frequency of uterine leiomyomas. *Am J Clin Pathol* 1990;94:435–438.
6. Fields KR, Neinstein LS. Uterine myomas in adolescents: case report and a review of the literature. *J Pediatr Adolesc Gynecol* 1996;9:195–198.
7. Townsend DE, Sparkes RS, Baluda MC, et al. Unicellular histogenesis of uterine leiomyomas as determined by electrophoresis by glucose-6-phosphate dehydrogenase. *Am J Obstet Gynecol* 1970;107:1168–1173.
8. Miszczak-Zaborska E, Wozniak K. The activity of thymidine phosphorylase obtained from uterine leiomyomas and studied in the presence of pyrimidine derivatives. *Z Naturforsh* 1997; 52:670–675.
9. Nilbert M, Heim S. Uterine leiomyoma cytogenetic. *Genes Chromosome Cancer* 1990;2:3–13.
10. Pandis N, Heim S, Bardi G, et al. Chromosome analysis of 96 uterine leiomyomas. *Cancer Genet Cytogenet* 1991;55:11–18.
11. Friedman AJ, Hoffman DI, Comite F, et al. Treatment of leiomyomata with leuprolide acetate depot: a double-blind, placebo controlled, multicenter study. *Obstet Gynecol* 1991;77:720–725.
12. Soules MR, McCarty KS Jr. Leiomyoma: steroid receptors content. Variation within normal menstrual cycles. *Am J Obstet Gynecol* 1982;143:6–11.
13. Tamaya T, Fujimoto J, Okada H. Comparison of cellular levels of steroid receptors in uterine leiomyoma and myometrium. *Acta Obstet Gynecol Scand* 1985;64:307–399.
14. Fayed YM, Tsibris JCM, Langenberg PW, et al. Human uterine leiomyoma cells: binding and growth responses to epidermal growth factor, platelet-derived growth factor, and insulin. *Lab Invest* 1989;60:30–37.
15. Marshall LM, Spiegelman D, Manson JE, et al. Risk of uterine leiomyomata among premenstrual women in relation to body size and cigarette smoking. *Epidemiology* 1998;9:511–517.
16. Kawamura S, Kasagi F, Kodama K, et al. Prevalence of uterine myoma detected by ultrasound examination in the atomic bomb survivors. *Radiat Res* 1997;147:753–758.
17. Sato F, Miyake H, Nishi M, et al. Early normal menstrual cycle pattern and the development of uterine leiomyomas. *J Womens Health Gender Based Med* 2000;9:299–302.
18. Marshall LM, Spiegelman D, Goldman MB, et al. A prospective study of reproductive factors and oral contraceptive use in relation to the risk of uterine leiomyomata. *Fertil Steril* 1998; 70:432–439.
19. Gross K, Morton C, Stewart E. Finding genes for uterine fibroids. *Obstet Gynecol* 2000;95:S60.

20. Janssen CA, Scholten PC, Heintz AP. Reconsidering menorrhagia in gynecological practice. Is a 30-year-old definition still valid? *Eur J Obstet Gynecol Reprod Biol* 1998;78:69–72.

21. Buttram VC Jr, Reiter RC. Uterine leiomyomata: etiology, symptomatology, and management. *Fertil Steril* 1981;36:433–445.

22. Ploszynski A, Gniadek R, Adamcio-Deptulska M, et al. Surgical treatment of uterine myoma: need for surgery and long-term results. *Ginecol Pol* 1997;68:423–426.

23. Melilli GA, DiGesu G, Loizzi V, et al. Acute urinary retention in uterine myoma: description of a case. *Arch Ital Urol Androl* 1998; 70:163–164.

24. Vollenhoven BJ, Lawrence AS, Healy DL. Uterine fibroids; a clinical review. *Br J Obstet Gynaecol* 1990;97:285–298.

25. Willemsen WN, de Kruif JH, Velthausz MB, et al. Fibroids and fertility. *Ned Tijdschr Geneeskd* 2000;144:789–791.

26. Sudik R, Husch K, Steller J, et al. Fertility and pregnancy outcome after myomectomy in sterility patients. *Eur J Obstet Gynecol Reprod Biol* 1996;65:209–214.

27. Reiter RC, Wagner PL, Gambone DO. Routine hysterectomy for large asymptomatic leiomyomata: a reappraisal. *Obstet Gynecol* 1992;79:481–484.

28. Reinhold C, Tafazoli F, Mehio A, et al. Uterine adenomyosis: endovaginal US and MR imaging features with histopathologic correlation. *Radiographics* 1999;19:S147–160.

29. Farmakides G, Stefanidis K, Paschopoulous M, et al. Uterine artery Doppler velocimetry with leiomyomas. *Arch Gynecol Obstet* 1998;262:53–57.

30. Van Eijkeren MA, Christiaens GC, Geuze HJ, et al. Effects of mefenamic acid on menstrual hemostasis in essential menorrhagia. *Am J Obstet Gynecol* 1992;166:1419–1428.

31. Ylikorkala O, Pekonen F. Naproxen reduces idiopathic but not fibromyoma-induced menorrhagia. *Obstet Gynecol* 1986;68:10–12.

32. Makarainen L, Ylikorkala O. Primary and myoma-associated menorrhagia: role of prostaglandins and effects of ibuprofen. *Br J Obstet Gynaecol* 1986;93:974–978.

33. Chiaffarino F, Parazzini F, La Vechia C, et al. Use of oral contraceptives and uterine fibroids; results from a case-control study. *Br J Obstet Gynaecol* 1999;106:857–860.

34. Harrison-Woolrych M, Robinson R. Fibroid growth in response to high-dose progestogen. *Fertil Steril* 1995;64:191–192.

35. Murphy AA, Morales AJ, Kettel LM, et al. Regression of uterine leiomyomata to the antiprogesterone RU486: dose response effect *Fertil Steril* 1995;64(1):187–190.

36. Nowak RA. Fibroids: pathophysiology and current medical treatment. *Baillieres Best Pract Res Clin Obstet Gynecol* 1999;13: 223– 238.

37. Amiel C, Mollard J, Cravello L, et al. Treatment of uterine fibromas. *Ann Chir* 1996;50:40–50.

38. Fedele L, Vercellini P, Bianchi S, et al. Treatment with GnRH agonists before myomectomy and the risk of short-term myoma recurrence. *Br J Obstet Gynaecol* 1990;97:393–396.

39. Dhingra K. Antiestrogen—tamoxifen, SERMS and beyond. *Invest New Drugs* 1999;17:285–311.

40. Mahajan DK, London SN. Mifepristone (RU 486): a review. *Fertil Steril* 1997;68:967–976.

41. Ostrzenski A. Psychological impact of pelvic surgery: a comparison of laparoscopy versus laparotomy. In: Grochmal S, ed. *Minimal access gynecology.* New York: Radcliffe Medical Press, 1995:16–22.

42. Friedmen AJ, Haas ST. Should uterine size be an indication for surgical intervention in women with myomas? *Am J Obstet Gynecol* 1993;168:751–755.

43. Dubuisson JB, Chapron C, Fauconnier A, et al. Laparoscopic myomectomy and myolysis. *Curr Opin Obstet Gynecol* 1997;9:233–238.

44. Ostrzenski A. A new laparoscopic myomectomy technique for intramural fibroids penetrating the uterine cavity. *Eur J Obstet Gynecol Reprod Biol* 1997;74:189–193.

45. American College of Obstetrician and Gynecologists (ACOG). *Technical bulletin no. 191.* Washington, DC: ACOG, 1994.

46. Derman SG, Rehnstrom J, Neuwirth RS. The long-term effectiveness of hysteroscopic treatment of menorrhagia and leiomyomas. *Obstet Gynecol* 1991;77:591–594.

47. Friedman AJ, Daly M, Juneau-Norcross M, et al. Recurrence of myomas after myomectomy in women pretreated with leuprolide acetate depot or placebo. *Fertil Steril* 1992;58:205–208.

48. Goldfarb HA. Myoma coagulation. *Obstet Gynecol Clin North Am* 2000;27:421–430.

49. Goldfarb HA. Combining myoma coagulation with endometrial ablation/resection reduces subsequent surgery rates. *JSLS* 1999;3:253–260.

50. Ostrzenski A. Laparoscopic total abdominal hysterectomy by suturing technique, with no transvaginal surgical approach: a review of 276 cases. *Int J Gynecol Obstet* 1996;247–257.

51. Garcia-Padial J, Osborne NG, Sotolongo J, et al. Laparoscopic-assisted vaginal hysterectomy compared with abdominal hysterectomy. *J Natl Med Assoc* 1995;87–91.

20

MALIGNANT UTERINE AND TROPHOBLASTIC NEOPLASIA

EDUCATIONAL OBJECTIVES

Medical Students (1) *APGO Objective No. 58*	*Residents in Obstetrics/Gynecology (2)* *CREOG Objectives*	*Practitioners (3)* *ACOG Recommendations*

Endometrial carcinoma
  Risk factors
  Symptoms
  Physical findings
  Management of the patient with
    postmenopausal bleeding
  Impact of staging on management
    and prognosis
  Management of
    endometrial carcinoma
Trophoblastic neoplasia
  Symptoms and physical findings
  Diagnostic methods
  Management and follow-up
	Uterine sarcoma
	Endometrial carcinoma
	  History
	  Physical examination
	  Diagnostic studies
	  Diagnosis
	  Management
	  Follow-up
	Hydatidiform mole and malignant
	    gestational trophoblastic disease
	  History
	  Physical examination
	  Diagnostic studies
	  Diagnosis
	  Management
	  Follow-up
		Endometrial carcinoma
		  Risk factors
		  Diagnosis
		  Management
		Hydatidiform mole classification
		  Diagnosis
		  Management
		Malignant gestational
		    trophoblastic disease
		  Histologic consideration
		  Clinical diagnosis
		  Classification
		  Management (of nonmetastatic
		    and metastatic carcinoma)

ENDOMETRIAL HYPERPLASIA

Endometrial hyperplasia is presented in Chapter 10.

ENDOMETRIAL CANCER

Definition

Endometrial cancer is defined as uterine malignancy originating from the endometrial tissue.

Incidence

Endometrial cancer is the most common gynecologic malignancy in the United States. The incidence is about 0.7 per 1,000 women, and it has been estimated that 37,400 new cases and 6,400 deaths occurred in 1999 (4). The incidence of endometrial cancer is higher in the industrialized countries of Europe and North America (5). The most common age in which endometrial cancer affects women is between 50 and 59 years, with the median age of diagnosis at 61 years. About one-fourth of cases of endometrial carcinoma are diagnosed before menopause.

Etiology

The etiology of endometrial cancer is unknown. Preliminary genetic study shows that a series of genetic imbalances occurs in precursor lesions of endometrial cancer detected by stepwise comparative genomic hybridization. This genetic mechanism is suggested as the mode of tumorigenesis (6).

Based upon two different, contrasting forms of endometrial cancer development, a dual model of endometrial carcinogenesis is offered (7):

1. *A classic model of an estrogen-driven pathway* is based on the theory that unopposed estrogenic (hyperestrogenic state) stimulation of the endometrium (e.g., polycystic ovary syndrome [PCOS]) can induce the development and growth of endometrial cancer (endometrioid adenocarcinoma) even in younger women.

2. *An alternative model of an estrogen-unrelated pathway* hypothesizes that endometrial cancer develops and grows independently of influence by the sex steroids (e.g., serous carcinoma). Genetic abnormality of p53 gene overexpression also is suggested as a model for the development of postmenopausal endometrial cancer (8).

Risk factors associated with endometrial cancer fall into the following categories:

- *A family history* of endometrial cancer (endometrial cancer risks increase among immediate family members) (9)
- *A reproductive history* that may influence endometrial cancer development includes (9,10) the following:
  a. Early menarche (a longer period of an anovulatory menstrual cycle is present, causing hyperestrogenism)
  b. Late menopause (a longer anovulatory cycle)
  c. Nulliparity [less exposure to progesterone; each full-term pregnancy results in a decrease in the risk of endometrial cancer by 16% (11)]
  d. Infertility (often anovulatory cycles are present, i.e., polycystic ovarian disease [PCOD] or frequently irregular menstrual cycles)
- *Unopposed estrogen,* either exogenous (e.g., estrogen replacement therapy without or with not enough progesterone or progestin) or endogenous (hyperestrogenism or overweight women in the sixth decade of life), can stimulate proliferation and hyperplasia of the endometrium, which may transform to endometrial cancer (12,13). To add progesterone or progestin to estrogen does not eliminate completely the risk of endometrial cancer. Yet, the reduction in risk of endometrial cancer is greater the more days each month that progesterone or progestin is used. The longer the period of use of hormone replacement therapy, the greater the likelihood of excess incidence of endometrial cancer (14); however, the limited scientific evidence cannot unequivocally support this view. Particularly, the use of oral contraceptives (combination of estrogen/progestins) offers long-lasting protection against endometrial cancer (1-year use of oral contraceptives extends protection for at least 10 years) (15,16).
- *Race* plays a role in endometrial cancer. Caucasian women are more frequently affected than African-American women (16); however, among uniformly treated patients with endometrial carcinoma, therapeutic outcomes for African-American women are significantly worse when compared to those for Caucasian women (17).
- *Other risk factors* include the following:

  a. *Hypertension* in otherwise asymptomatic women may harbor occult endometrial cancer in about 1.3% (18).
  b. *Diabetes mellitus* may also harbor occult endometrial cancer in approximately 6.3% (18). Recently, contrary to prevailing views that overweight, hypertension, and diabetes mellitus are independent risk factors for endometrial cancer development, research results failed to establish any statistical significance of these parameters. The only risk factor of statistical significance is a delay in the onset of menopause past 49 years of age (19).
  c. *Better-educated women* are more frequently affected by endometrial cancer than less-educated women (16).
  d. *Tamoxifen* is an estrogen agonist/antagonist agent used in breast cancer therapy. It displays effects on the endometrium (no effects on vasomotor symptoms or vaginal atrophic changes associated with menopause) and may lead to endometrial hyperplasia and cancer (20,21). Although tamoxifen-induced endometrial cancer may have a different path from those associated with hyperestrogenism, it still presents a risk for high-grade endometrial cancers associated with poor prognosis (20).

Classification

Endometrial cancer classification is based upon histological types as outlined below (22):

1. *Endometrioid adenocarcinoma* accounts for more than three-fourths of all carcinomas and may present with very distinct histology, making it possible to establish subtypes:
   a. Villoglandular
   b. Secretory
   c. Ciliated cell
   d. Endometrioid adenocarcinoma with squamous differentiation
2. *Serous carcinoma* [papillary serous carcinoma of the endometrium represents only 3% to 4% of all endometrial cancers, yet it is of particular interest due to the aggressive clinical natural course and poor prognosis associated with this type of endometrial cancer (4)]
3. *Clear cell carcinoma*
4. *Mucinous carcinoma*
5. *Squamous carcinoma*
6. *Mixed types of carcinoma*
7. *Undifferentiated carcinoma*

Diagnosis

Pertinent medical history includes the following:

- Abnormal endometrial bleeding is the most common symptom, occurring in approximately 80%.

- Postmenopausal women represent about 75% of all cases.
- Irregular perimenopausal bleeding, as long as it is lighter and less frequent, is a normal event associated with approaching menopause. Any deviation from such a menstrual pattern (prolonged, heavy, or intermenstrual bleeding) during this period should be considered as abnormal and warrants further clinical evaluation.
- History of overweight, infertility, anovulatory cycle, high blood pressure, excessive alcohol consumption, and diabetes mellitus should evoke suspicion.

Physical examination may establish an increased body mass index; elevated blood pressure; oily skin, skin stries, acne, and hirsutism.

Pelvic examination may reveal enlarged, firm, nontender ovaries bilaterally, suggesting PCOS, obesity, and elevated blood pressure.

Endometrial biopsy is an in-office procedure and is a reliable method if sufficient sample for histological diagnosis is obtained. In the general outpatient clinical population, Pipelle sampling yields up to 33% insufficient samples, and in about 3%, the Pipelle cannot pass through the cervical canal (23).

Dilatation and curettage is recommended when atypical hyperplasia is documented, since concomitant endometrial cancer may coexist.

Pap smear is not an efficient tool for endometrial cancer screening; although, when endocervical cells are present on a postmenopausal woman's Pap smear, they constitute an indication for further evaluation (24).

Endometrial cytology has been introduced but has not been well received in clinical practice due to interpretive difficulties (25)

Vaginal ultrasonography has been suggested as a tool in the diagnosis of endometrial cancer. The thickness of the endometrium—with a 5-mm cutoff point of endometrial thickness—can suggest endometrial abnormality. It has been postulated that the positive predictive value for identifying endometrial abnormality in such a setting is 87.3% (26). Recently, researchers suggested that the cutoff point should be lowered to 3 mm, and others argued that 8 mm or 10 mm of endometrial thickness should trigger further evaluation, at least with endometrial biopsy. Since abnormal endometrial bleeding, in most instances, is evaluated by endometrial sampling, ultrasound evaluation will not provide sufficient information to substitute for histological verification.

The high index of clinical suspicion for endometrial cancer is still the best clinical approach for early diagnosis, since currently there is no screening modality available for endometrial cancer (27).

Magnetic resonance imaging has emerged as an accurate modality for the evaluation of pathologic conditions, including endometrial cancer. It provides unique diagnostic information and may guide the therapeutic management of endometrial carcinoma (28).

Hysteroscopy with direct biopsy of endometrial lesions is considered an effective and safe method; although, precision of the diagnosis largely depends on the practitioner's operative skill. There is a legitimate clinical concern about facilitating tumor cell dissemination, with potential spreading of endometrial cancer. Recently, it has been documented that approximately 9% of endometrial cell carcinoma could be disseminated to the peritoneal cavity during hysteroscopic examination with fluid used as the destination media (29). Whether such positive peritoneal endometrial cancer cytology dissemination automatically guarantees the growth of malignant cells on the peritoneum has yet not been determined; although, such a possibility cannot be ruled out.

Other studies are usually performed when the presence of endometrial cancer is established:

- Test for occult blood in stool
- Two-view chest x-ray (anterior-posterior and lateral)
- Complete blood count
- Urinalysis
- Serum electrolytes
- Renal and hepatic function
- Baseline serum CA125 oncologic marker

Staging of endometrial carcinoma is surgical and incorporates histological verification, grade, depth of myometrial invasion, lymphatic node involvement, and adnexal and/or peritoneal extension. Staging is based upon the International Federation of Gynecology and Obstetrics (FIGO) recommendations and includes the following steps:

- Appropriate abdominal incision
- Upon entering the abdominal-pelvic cavity, free pelvic fluid aspiration for cytology evaluation is obtained. If free fluid is absent, saline washings should be performed for a cytology study (right colonic region, hepatic colonic flexure, splenic flexure, left colonic region, and posterior cul-de-sac). Palpation of the intestinal mesentery, para-aortic lymphatic nodes, and the diaphragm should be accomplished (the diaphragm should be directly inspected with laparoscopic visualization at laparotomy). Total simple hysterectomy and bilateral salpingo-oophorectomy remain standard surgical therapy, and a surgical uterine specimen is examined for the depth of myometrial invasion, either by gross evaluation and/or frozen section microscopic evaluation. Since preoperatively the histological cell types and grades (the degree of differentiation) are usually determined, establishing myometrial depth of infiltration completes the characterization of endometrial cancer. These parameters (histology type, grade of differentiation, and the depth of myometrium penetration) provide information for the potential risk of lymphatic node extension. Stage I, grade 1 disease with minimal

invasion of the myometrium presents a remote potential for pelvic or para-aortic node extension. Stage I, grade 3 with deep myometrial invasion strongly suggests a potential for pelvic and para-aortic lymphatic node involvement (up to 45%). Therefore, in such a clinical scenario, the decision whether or not to proceed with pelvic and para-aortic node dissection can be made. Lymphadenectomy is recommended not only for diagnostic purposes, but also for the therapeutic potential.

Total simple extrafascial hysterectomy with bilateral adnexectomy, and para-aortic and pelvic node dissection is indicated.

Since surgical staging was first introduced in 1988 by FIGO, preoperative radiation has not been a part of therapy as previously recommended (Table 20.1). Also, preoperative fractional dilatation and curettage have been abandoned due to the introduction of surgical staging.

Prognosis of the endometrial cancer is based on multiple factors that include the age (the younger a patient the better prognosis), histological type, stage of the disease, grade, and depth of invasion. Additional clinical data such as hormonal receptors, endometrial ploidy, and S-phase fractions may be used as prognostic characteristics.

Grade (G) refers to the degree of histological differentiation of tumor cells and is determined as follows:

- G1 has 5% nonsquamous or nonmorular solid growth pattern
- G2 has 6% to 50% nonsquamous or nonmorular solid growth pattern
- G3 has >50% nonsquamous or nonmorular solid growth pattern

TABLE 20.1. FIGO STAGING OF THE UTERINE CORPUS

Stage	Grade "G"	Description
IA	G 123	Tumor limited to the endometrium
IB	G 123	Invasion to less than half of the myometrium
IC	G 123	Invasion to more than half of the myometrium
IIA	G123	Endocervical glandular involvement only
IIB	G 123	Cervical stromal invasion
IIIA	G123	Tumor invades serosa and/or adnexa, and/or positive peritoneal cytology
IIIB	G123	Vaginal metastases
IIIC	G123	Metastases to pelvic and/or paraaortic lymph nodes
IVA	G123	Tumor invasion of bladder and/or bowel mucosa
IVB	—	Distant metastases including intraabdominal and/or inguinal lymph nodes

Data from International Federation of Gynecology and Obstetrics (FIGO). Annual report on the results of treatment in gynecologic cancer. *Int J Gynecol Obstet* 1989;28:189–190.

Differential Diagnosis

Endometrial cancer differential diagnosis includes the following:

- Cervical cancer
- Cervical polyp
- Endometrial polyp
- Endometrial atypical hyperplasia (see Chapter 10)
- Secondary endometrial cancer
- Submucosal uterine leiomyomata
- Chronic endometritis

Conventional Therapy

Early clinical manifestations of endometrial cancer allow the establishment of a diagnosis, in most instances, of stage I disease. Such early detection provides an opportunity for optimal treatment with surgery alone.

Stage I disease management (confined to the uterine corpus), of grade 1 or grade 2 with no myometrial or superficial (inner third) invasion, requires surgical exploration with total hysterectomy and bilateral salpingo-oophorectomy [abdominal, vaginal or laparoscopic total hysterectomy (31)]. Endometrial cancer characteristics of myometrial invasion and intraoperative findings establish an indication for lymphadenectomy (4). A randomized controlled study documented that postoperative radiotherapy in stage I, grade 1 to 2 endometrial carcinoma reduces local/regional recurrence but has no impact on overall survival. Consequently, postoperative radiotherapy is not indicated in patients younger than 60 years of age with stage I endometrial carcinoma and or in patients with grade 2 tumors with superficial invasion (32).

Grade 3 endometrial carcinoma will require lymphadenectomy due to extension often to the pelvic and para-aortic lymph nodes. The procedure can be performed either through laparotomy or through a laparoscopic approach (hysterectomy and adnexectomy can be performed at the same time) that provides 3-year survival and recurrence rates, which are comparable to the rates of the traditional abdominal approach (33,34).

If a patient presents with a medical condition contraindicating surgery, radiotherapy alone is recommended. The 5-year survival rate is approximately 50% when this therapeutic modality is instituted (35).

Stage II endometrial cancer management combines surgical exploration, total hysterectomy with bilateral salpingo-oophorectomy, and lymphadenectomy. Due to a great inclination for lymph node extension in this stage, postoperative radiotherapy is the standard approach.

Stage III and IV endometrial cancer treatment is surgery followed by postoperative pelvic radiotherapy. Hormonal therapy (megestrol acetate) or adjuvant chemotherapy (cisplatinum and doxorubicin) has not been proven to be effective (36).

Recurrent endometrial cancer predictability has been increased since histological measurement of the tumor microvessel density was introduced, allowing us to identify patients at high risk for recurrence (4). Tumor recurrence in the vaginal vault is treated either by surgery alone or surgery combined with radiotherapy. When the lower vagina is affected, the outcome is poor. In distant metastatic disease, hormonal therapy with progestins (megestrol acetate) may provide response in about 15% to 20% in well-differentiated cancer. Chemotherapy appears to have a very limited therapeutic response.

Postoperative follow-up is orchestrated based on the risk of recurrence of endometrial cancer (37,38). Postoperative surveillance will include an updated medical history, a general physical and pelvic examination, a serum CA 125 level, and one of the imaging techniques, such as transvaginal ultrasonography, magnetic resonance imaging, or color Doppler. Such an approach may ultimately improve the early detection of endometrial cancer recurrence (4). Postoperatively, the following group of patients can be identified for management (39):

- *Low-risk group* (stage I, grade 1 or 2, and superficial myometrial infiltration) management will require no additional postsurgical treatment, and periodic routine follow-up evaluation is sufficient. The overall survival rate is approximately 96% (40).
- *Intermediate-risk group* (stage I, grade 1 or 2, and middle third invasion with no extrauterine extension of the disease) management may require postoperative irradiation to the whole pelvis or intracavitary vaginal brachytherapy, which appears to reduce local/regional recurrence.
- *High-risk group* (tumor extension to adnexal, pelvic nodes, outer third myometrial infiltration, cervical invasion, or grade 3 tumors with any invasion) postoperative management includes whole-pelvis radiation (4,000 to 5,000 cGy). Positive para-aortic nodes without other distant metastasis will require extended field irradiation. A 5-year survival rate is estimated at approximately 40% (41).
- *Positive peritoneal cytology* management is controversial and includes the following approaches (39):
  1. Intraperitoneal ^{32}P installation (may cause significant side effects)
  2. Radiation therapy to the whole abdomen, with or without a progestin agent
  3. Chemotherapy

Health-related quality of life in survivors of endometrial cancer is poor. To improve the patient's quality of life, early psychological counseling and treatment should be offered. Young and single women require particular attention. Menopausal symptoms will strongly affect young women shortly after the surgical removal of ovaries. Endometrial cancer is considered a hormone-dependent malignancy; therefore, hormone replacement therapy is not suitable for this group of patients; even though, hormonal replacement therapy may be considered, with caution, in a very selective group of patients who are at low risk of endometrial cancer recurrence. The prevalence of somatic symptoms is higher in the older woman survivors of endometrial cancer, and special care should be provided in the early stages of this condition (42). Hormonal and nonhormonal management of menopausal symptoms is presented in Chapter 12.

Specific complementary and alternative therapies are not available for endometrial cancer, although a general approach for cancer supportive therapy is offered in several publications. This general information does exceed the scope of this publication.

UTERINE SARCOMAS

Definition

Uterine sarcoma is an extremely aggressive malignant tumor, which may arise either from the uterine muscle (leiomyosarcomas), endometrial glands and stroma (endometrial sarcomas), or supporting tissue.

Incidence

The incidence of uterine sarcoma is estimated to be 2.3 in 100,000 in the United State. It is a rare malignancy that constitutes approximately 2% of all uterine neoplastic tumors (43).

Etiology

The etiology of uterine sarcoma is unknown. The risk factor associated with development of uterine sarcomas is a history of irradiation to the pelvic region, predominantly for benign pelvic conditions (44). This malignant entity occurs on average 16 years after initial radiotherapy to the pelvis (45).

Classification

Uterine sarcoma is classified based upon histology:

1. Pure uterine sarcoma comprises one cell type
2. Mixed uterine sarcoma consists of more than one cell type

Uterine sarcoma classification is a controversial issue, and regardless of the type of sarcoma, most represent very aggressive malignant biology.

The following clinical classification is most commonly accepted (46):

A. *Pure homologous uterine sarcomas*
- Leiomyosarcoma
- Endometrial stromal sarcoma

- Endolymphatic stromal meiosis
- Angiosarcoma
- Fibrosarcoma

B. *Pure heterologous uterine sarcomas*
- Rhabdomyosarcoma
- Chondrosarcoma
- Osteosarcoma
- Liposarcoma

C. *Mixed uterine sarcoma*
- Mixed homologous
- Mixed heterologous

D. *Malignant mixed Mullerian tumors*
- Homologous type
- Heterologous type

Leiomyosarcoma constitutes about 25% of all uterine sarcomas. It arises from the uterine muscles; although, it controversial whether or not leiomyosarcoma originate from malignant transformation (malignant degeneration) of uterine myoma or *de novo* formation from uterine muscles. It appears that more data support *de novo* formation.

This condition is diagnosed almost exclusively on the mitotic index. The overall 5-year survival rate for patients with leiomyosarcoma is approximately 39%, and 10-year survival is about 27% (47). Early tumor stage, age of <50 years, and the absence of vascular space involvement are independently associated with better prognosis. The mitotic index appears to be a strong prognostic factor in early tumor stage; even though, it failed to act as an independent prognostic factor in patients with tumors of stage II to IV disease (48).

Endometrial stromal sarcomas are divided into two categories: a low-grade (<10 mitoses/10 high-power fields and a high-grade tumor (>10 mitoses/10 high-power fields).

A low-grade mass has sluggish biological behavior and expresses hormonal dependability (most commonly seen in a young woman). Due to this propensity, this tumor requires bilateral oophorectomy and progestin therapy (49).

A high-grade mass is an extremely aggressive malignant lesion and clinically may present as a fleshy and polypoid tumor (50). The 5- and 10-year survival rate is 61% and 37%, respectively (48).

Mixed Mullerian sarcomas are the most common uterine sarcomas. They originate from the endometrial stroma or undifferentiated cell rests and they are aggressive tumors (50). The overall 5- and 10-year survival rates are about 33% and 14%, respectively (48).

Diagnosis

Pertinent medical history includes menorrhagia or postmenopausal abnormal endometrial bleeding. Also, abdominal-pelvic pain is often associated with uterine sarcomas.

Physical examination may establish the presence of abdominal mass, when a tumor is large enough to pass the pelvic brim (the size corresponding to a 12 weeks' gesta-

tional uterus). Parasitic leiomyosarcoma can be present in the abdominal area connected by long pedicle to the uterus with the absence of symptoms (unpublished observations, A. Ostrzenski).

Pelvic examination can reveal a polypoid mass protruding from the dilated cervical canal. The tumor bleeds with ease to the touch. The rapidly enlarging uterus, particularly when this event is present during the postmenopausal period may suggest the diagnosis of uterine sercoma. Yet, an enlarged, asymmetrical, nontender, freely movable uterus can be encountered.

Diagnosis is determined by microscopic mitotic index (the number of mitosis per 10 high-power fields). This mitotic index is performed from permanent histological section, since frozen section has a limited usefulness in this respect. At least 10 mitoses per 10 high-power fields are considered diagnostic for leiomyosarcoma.

Differential Diagnosis

Differential diagnosis includes the following:

- Uterine leiomyomata
- Intravenous leiomyomatosis
- Disseminated leiomyomatosis

Conventional Therapy

Essentially, uterine sarcoma therapy is surgery. Total abdominal hysterectomy with bilateral salpingo-oophorectomy is the recommended procedure. Due to hematogenous dissemination, lymphadenectomy is not indicated.

Adjuvant chemotherapy has a limited role in the treatment of this condition. Radiation therapy does not improve the survival rate.

Recurrent uterine sarcoma is usually approximately 90% outside of the pelvis within 2 years of initial diagnosis and treatment. The therapy for this clinical form is the use of a single cytostatic agent such as doxorubicin. Hormonal treatment with progestational drugs is also recommended; the palliative modalities do not seem to increase a disease-free survival rate.

There are no designated complementary and alternative therapies for uterine sarcomas.

GESTATIONAL TROPHOBLASTIC NEOPLASIA

Due to the scope of this book, only basic clinical data for gestational trophoblastic disease will be presented.

Gestational trophoblastic neoplasia (GTN) is either a benign or a malignant tumor arising from trophoblastic tissue of the placenta. GTN is characterized by the presence of the following:

- Symptoms and signs of pregnancy

- High levels of serum human chorionic gonadotropin (hCG) hormones
- Genetic characteristics
- High responsiveness to cytotoxic agents
- Potential risk of malignant transformation

In general, GTN is classified as follows:

- Molar pregnancy (hydatidiform mole)
- Complete mole (complete hydatidiform mole)
- Partial mole (partial hydatidiform mole)
- Persistent GTN
- Histologically benign neoplasia
- Persistent histologically benign neoplasia
- Persistent histologically malignant neoplasia

Hydatidiform Mole

Hydatidiform mole (molar pregnancy) is clinically characterized by the presence of placenta villi vesicular swelling (hydropic) associated with a microscopic syncytiotrophoblastic and cytotrophoblastic proliferation (hyperplasia and dysplasia of the trophoblast is present to a varying degree).

Incidence in the United States is estimated to be between 0.6 and 1.1 per 1,000 pregnancies, and is one per 200 pregnancies in Asia.

Etiology of molar pregnancy is unknown. Hydatidiform mole predominantly affects women in early or late reproductive periods.

Classification of hydatidiform mole is divided into two forms based upon the presence or absence of fetal formation within the neoplasia:

1. *Complete hydatidiform* mole is characterized by the absence of a fetus, fetal membranes, or fetal erythrocytes. Its karyotype corresponds to that of a normal female karyotype 46,XX; although, it derives from fertilization by a haploid (23,X) sperm, which reaches 46,XX by its own duplication (totally replacing the maternal genetic make-up). Infrequently, the composition of 46,XY may occur as a result of dispermic fertilization of an empty ovum. In brief, complete mole chromosomal composition comes from the paternal origin, with mitochondrial DNA derivatives from the maternal site. Complete hydatidiform mole constitutes approximately 90% of all molar pregnancies. It displays greater predisposition to malignant degeneration (invasive mole or choriocarcinoma is estimated to occur in about 15% to 20% and is commonly associated with the heterozygotic chromosomal makeup of 46,XY) than does partial mole (the 4% to 11% uncommon metastatic predisposition and choriocarcinoma has not been reported in partial mole).
2. *Partial hydatidiform* mole distinguishes itself from complete mole by the presence of an embryo or fetus associated with chromosomal aberrations (frequently triploidy 69,XXY, which is composed from one maternal chromosomal haploid set [23,X] and two paternal haploid sets). The presence of fetal membranes or fetal erythrocytes and the absence of embryo or fetus will still constitute the basis for partial mole diagnosis.

Diagnosis is reached based upon clinical symptoms and signs, which are similar for complete or partial mole (partial mole symptoms occur usually after 20 weeks of gestation).

Symptoms directly related to pregnancy mole can be characterized by:

1. The presence of oligomenorrhea or amenorrhea
2. Pregnancy complicated by excessive nausea and vomiting (hyperemesis gravidarum in about 8%)
3. Abnormal painless uterine bleeding at 6 to 16 weeks of gestational age (80% to 90%)
4. Passing tissue mixed with blood and often identified by a patient
5. Lower abdominal-pelvic pain usually present in association with bilateral theca lutein cysts and estimated in approximately 15%

Associated symptomatology can also be present as follows:

1. Visual disturbances
2. Hyperthyroidism
3. Tachycardia
4. Shortness of breath

Signs associated with hydatidiform mole are as follows:

1. Uterine enlargement is greater than expected for the current age of pregnancy, uterine size too small for gestational age occasionally has been reported.
2. Uterine bleeding with the passing of grape-like tissue
3. Bilateral adnexal mass present in about 15% of cases
4. Fetal heart tone usually absent

Signs associated with hydatidiform mole are usually related to the following:

1. Early pregnancy preeclampsia
2. Hypertension
3. Hyperreflexia

Laboratory testing in hydatidiform mole is essential not only for diagnostic purposes, but also for evaluating treatment progress (hCG is a sensitive tumor marker in follow-up). The laboratory tests include the following:

1. Serum hCG levels are customarily elevated, frequently >100,000 mIU/mL. In partial mole, only 10% of patients will exceed 100,000 mIU/mL, and the serum hCG levels in partial mole are usually lower when compared with complete hydatidiform mole.
2. Proteinuria is occasionally present in association with early pregnancy preeclampsia.

3. Elevated serum thyroid gland hormone levels are observed infrequently when symptoms of hyperthyroidism are present.
4. Hemoglobin and hematocrit must be obtained.

Imaging studies, mainly ultrasonography findings, are considered pathognomonic in complete moles when the intrauterine "snowstorm" pattern is present, which is a result of diffused chorionic villi hydropic swelling. Such an ultrasonographic picture is confirmatory for a clinical diagnosis of hydatidiform mole, yet definitive diagnosis is provided by histological verification. In partial moles, ultrasonographic studies may demonstrate focal cysts within the placenta and increase the diameter of the gestational sac.

A baseline chest x-ray is usually requested to eliminate the possibility of metastasis.

Differential diagnosis includes the following:

- Physiological uncomplicated intrauterine pregnancy
- Multiple gestation
- Physiological uncomplicated intrauterine pregnancy associated with uterine leiomyomata
- Placental enlargement in association with intrauterine infection or erythroblastosis

Conventional therapy is surgical uterine evacuation. Preoperative tests are recommended as follows:

- Serum hCG level
- Complete blood and platelets counts
- Serum chemistries
- Blood type and Rh and screen for antibodies and cross-match
- Coagulation profile
- Urine analysis
- Pelvic ultrasonography
- Chest x-ray
- Electrocardiography

The classic conventional treatment for hydatidiform mole is surgery, which can be divided into the following categories:

1. *Conservative surgery* with uterine evacuation by the suction technique is followed by gentle sharp curettage and accompanied by an oxytocic agent at the end of the procedure (the oxytocic agent should be maintained for several hours following the evacuation procedure). During and after the procedure, appropriate crystalloid fluid, administered intravenously, is recommended to reduce potential pulmonary complications. For those women who are D-negative, D (Rho [D]) immune globulin should be administered by the end of the evacuation procedure or shortly thereafter. The overall evacuation curative rate is approximately 80%.
2. *Definitive treatment* is total hysterectomy with ovarian preservation even in the presence of theca lutein cysts.

Hysterectomy can be offered to those patients whose reproductive capacity is not a concern. Although the risk of persistent benign molar pregnancy following hysterectomy is low (3% to 5%), the follow-up with serum hCG is mandatory.

Follow-Up

Follow-up comprises the following:

1. Pelvic evaluation following successful uterine evacuation should reveal appropriate uterine involution, ovarian cyst regression, and subsiding uterine bleeding. Inadequate clinical progress raises suspicion of persistent hydatidiform mole.
2. Ultrasonography may produce evidence of retained molar tissue.
3. Quantitative serum hCG is considered as the standard follow-up tool for monitoring the progress of treatment; the following schedule is generally accepted:
   a. Every 1 to 2 weeks until after three consecutive negative results are obtained (usually the lapsed time from initial evacuation to the first negative serum quantitative hCG is 9 to 11 weeks).
   b. Every 3 months for the next 6 to 12 months

It is important to offer a reliable contraceptive method, including but not limited to oral contraceptives. The mechanism of oral contraceptives, among others, has the ability to suppress luteinizing hormone (LH), and this may compromise the effects of hCG when the levels are low.

Particular attention should be given to those patients who present risk factors for postmolar trophoblastic tumor such as the following:

1. Age over 40 years at the time of diagnosis
2. Elevated hCG over 100,000 mIU/mL
3. Preevacuation uterine size larger than expected for gestational age
4. Preevacuation uterine size larger than 20 weeks
5. Preevacuation medical complications present (e.g., preeclampsia or hyperthyroidism)

This group of high-risk patients can be considered for prophylactic chemotherapy shortly after uterine evacuation. Also, patients who present the following hCG parameters should be considered for postuterine evacuation chemotherapy:

1. Plateau of elevated serum hCG levels for 3 consecutive weeks
2. Rising serum hCG levels for 2 consecutive weeks
3. Elevated levels over 20,000 mIU/mL after 4 weeks following uterine evacuation
4. Persistently elevated serum hCG levels for 4 to 6 months
5. The presence of metastatic disease

GESTATIONAL TROPHOBLASTIC TUMORS

Gestational trophoblastic tumors are categorized as follows:

1. *Invasive* mole is a benign hydatidiform mole mass with the ability to invade the myometrium by direct infiltration, and/or it exhibits potential for distant metastasis (approximately 15% of all cases with frequent metastatic site involve the lungs or vagina). Microscopic examination reveals *hyperplastic and dysplastic changes* within the trophoblastic tissue. Incidence is estimated to be one per 15,000 pregnancies. Diagnosis is based on increasing serum hCG levels following uterine evacuation for hydatidiform mole. Histological confirmation of the uterine or metastatic lesion is not required, since the definitive diagnosis is established before initial uterine evacuation, and the high response of invasive hydatidiform to chemotherapy.
2. *Choriocarcinoma* is a malignant tumor that histologically displays *hyperplastic and anaplastic changes,* absence of chorionic villi, hemorrhage, and necrosis within the lesion. The incidence of choriocarcinoma is estimated to be approximately one per 40,000 pregnancies and is identified in 25% of term pregnancies and in 25% of ectopic pregnancies or abortions. Remaining cases arise from malignant degeneration of pregnancy mole (2% to 3% hydatidiform mole transforms to choriocarcinoma). The tumor has the ability to invade the myometrium by direct extension from the primary lesion. Distant metastasis is commonly identified in the lung, liver, central nervous system, pelvis, vagina, kidney, spleen, and intestines.
3. *Placental-site trophoblastic tumor* derives from the placental implantation site. The tumor histology resembles syncytial endomyometritis; although, placenta-site trophoblastic tumor invades the vessels and syncytial endomyometritis does not. Serum quantitative hCG levels are lower here than in choriocarcinoma. The clinical course of this tumor is often benign, even though mortality in advanced cases has been reported due to a poor response of the tumor to chemotherapy. Therefore, surgery is the treatment of choice.

Diagnosis of gestational trophoblastic tumors is based on the following:

1. Increase or plateau of serum quantitative hCG following uterine evacuation for hydatidiform mole with or without the presence of metastasis.
2. Persistent uterine bleeding following any pregnancy or uterine evacuation for pregnancy mole.
3. Uterine enlargement associated with bilateral adnexal cystic mass may suggest hydatidiform mole transformation to trophoblastic tumor. Infrequently, vaginal metastasis of trophoblastic tumor can be identified and biopsied.

Staging of trophoblastic tumors is based upon the FIGO recommendations, and its delineation is presented in Table 20.2.

To determine the clinical extent of the disease, the following are used:

1. Chest x-ray
2. The cerebrospinal fluid hCG level should be determined if central nervous symptoms are present.
3. Pelvic ultrasonography

Conventional Therapy

Conventional therapy is typified by the following:

TABLE 20.2. FIGO STAGING FOR GESTATIONAL TROPHOBLASTIC TUMORS

Stage	Description
I	Disease is confined to the uterus.
IA	Disease is confined to the uterus with no risk factor[a].
IB	Disease is confined to the uterus with one risk factor.
IC	Disease is confined to the uterus with two factors.
II	Gestational trophoblastic tumor extends outside uterus but is limited to genital structures (adnexa, vagina, broad ligament).
IIA	Gestational trophoblastic tumor involves genital structures with no risk factor.
IIB	Gestational trophoblastic tumor extends outside uterus but is limited to genital structures with one risk factor.
IIC	Gestational trophoblastic tumor extends outside uterus but is limited to genital structures with two risk factors.
III	Gestational trophoblastic tumor extends to lungs with or without known genital tract involvement.
IIIA	Gestational trophoblastic tumor extends to lungs with or without genital tract involvement and with no risk factor.
IIIB	Gestational trophoblastic tumor extends to lungs with or without genital tract involvement and with one risk factor.
IIIC	Gestational trophoblastic tumor extends to lungs with or without genital tract involvement and with two risk factors.
IV	Included are all other metastatic sites.
IVA	Included are all other metastatic sites without risk factor.
IVB	Included are all other metastatic sites with one risk factor.
IVC	Included are all other metastatic sites with two risk factor.

[a]High risk factors affecting staging are as follows: (a) serum hCG levels >100,000 mIU/mL; (b) duration of disease >4 months from termination of antecedent pregnancy; (c) brain or liver metastasis; (d) prior chemotherapy; and (e) antecedent term pregnancy.
Data from International Federation of Gynecology and Obstetrics (FIGO). *Annual report on the results of treatment in gynecological cancer,* 22nd ed. Stockholm: FIGO, 1994.

I. Treatment for *nonmetastatic tumor*, for those patients who desire to preserve childbearing capacity, involves single-agent sequential chemotherapy (Methotrexate, 0.4 mg/kg, intramuscularly or intravenously per day for 5 days per treatment course; or Dactinomycin, 300 mg per day intravenously every day for 5 days, is indicated for patients with renal, hepatic, or effusion disease or patients who have serum hCG levels that are unchanged or rising). Multiple-agent chemotherapy is implemented in nonmetastatic cases if meaningful serum hCG elevation is documented or metastasis occurs. A single-agent or multiple-agent treatment (Methotrexate and Etoposide) is administered until after two consecutive normal hCG levels are documented. Hysterectomy is uncommonly required (<5%) for cure in this group and is recommended for patients associated who are chemotherapy resistant or to shorten the duration of therapy. Overall cure rate in nonmetastatic gestational trophoblastic tumors is approximately 85% to 90% with initial chemotherapy and a majority of remaining patients responding to multiple-agent chemotherapy.

II. *Metastatic tumor* treatment depends upon the presence of the following:
   A. Low-risk metastatic disease treatment is similar to that for nonmetastatic tumor.
   B. High-risk metastatic disease therapy includes the following:
      1. Multiple-agent chemotherapy (Etoposide along with Methotrexate is the most common protocol recommended)
      2. Combination of chemotherapy and radiation
      3. Combination of chemotherapy, radiotherapy, and surgery

Overall cure rate in appropriately managed patients is estimated to be about 80% to 90%.

Follow-up is based upon serum quantitative hCG levels and is obtained at 1- to 2-week intervals for 3 months and at 1-month intervals thereafter for 1 year. General physical evaluation with pelvic examination is performed at 6-month intervals. Other laboratory tests and imaging studies are ordered as indicated.

At the time of commencement of initial therapy, oral contraceptive or barrier methods, if oral contraceptive is contraindicated, are usually prescribed. Contraception is advised for at least 1 year following completion of therapy.

A subsequent pregnancy creates an increased potential risk of developing trophoblastic disease. An ultrasonography is usually performed during the first trimester to exclude trophoblastic disease. Histological examination must be performed either on the placenta or on the product of conception if abortion occurs. Serum quantitative hCG levels should be determined at the 6th week after delivery or following abortion.

REFERENCES

1. Association of Professors of Gynecology and Obstetrics (APGO). *Medical student educational objectives,* 7th ed. Washington, DC: APGO, 1997.
2. Council on Resident Education in Obstetrics and Gynecology (CREOG). *Educational objectives core curriculum for residents in obstetrics and gynecology,* 5th ed. Washington, DC: CREOG, 1996.
3. American College of Obstetricians and Gynecologists (ACOG). *Technical bulletin no. 162.* Washington, DC: CREOG, 1991.
4. Bristow RE. Endometrial cancer. *Curr Opin Oncol* 1999;11:388–393.
5. Doll R, Muir C, Waterhouse J. *Cancer incidence in five continents. International Union against Cancer.* Berlin: Springer-Verlag, 1970.
6. Kiechle M, Hinrichs M, Jacobson A, et al. Genetic imbalances in precursor lesions of endometrial cancer detected by comparative genomic hybridization. *Am J Pathol* 2000;156:1827–1833.
7. Sherman ME. Theories of endometrial carcinogenesis: a multidisciplinary approach. *Mod Pathol* 2000;13:295–308.
8. Niwa K, Imai A, Hashimoto M, et al. A case-control study of pre-and post-menopausal women. *Oncol Rep* 2000;7:89–93.
9. Hemminski K, Vaittinen P, Dong C. Endometrial cancer in the family-cancer database. *Cancer Epidemiol Biomarkers Prev* 1999;8:1005–1010.
10. Parslov M, Lidgaard O, Klintorp S, et al. Risk factors among young women with endometrial cancer: a Danish case-control study. *Am J Obstet Gynecol* 2000;182:23–29.
11. Pettersson B, Adami HO, Bergstrom R, et al. Menstruation span—a time-limited risk factor for endometrial carcinoma. *Acta Obstet Gynecol Scand* 1896;65:247–255.
12. Hagen A, Morack G, Grulich D. Evaluation of epidemiologic risk factor for endometrial carcinoma based on a case-control study. *Zentralbl Gynakol* 1995;117:368–374.
13. Persson I, Weiderpass E, Bergkvist L, et al. Risk of breast and endometrial cancer after estrogen and estrogen-progestin replacement. *Cancer Causes Control* 1999;10:253–260.
14. Beral V, Banks E, Reeves G, et al. Use of HRT and the subsequent risk of cancer. *J Epidemiol Biostat* 199;4:191–210.
15. Weiderpass E, Adami HO, Baron JA, et al. Use of oral contraceptives and endometrial cancer risk (Sweden). *Cancer Causes Control* 1999;10:277–284.
16. Kelsey JL, LiVolsi VA, Holford TR, et al. A case-control study of cancer of the endometrium. *Am J Epidemiol* 1982;116:333–342.
17. Connell PP, Rotmensch J, Waggoner SE, et al. Race and clinical outcome in endometrial carcinoma. *Obstet Gynecol* 1999;94:713–720.
18. Gronroos M, Salmi TA, Vuento MH, et al. Mass screening for endometrial cancer directed in risk groups of patients with diabetes and patients with hypertension. *Cancer* 1993;71:1279–1282.
19. Cardosi RJ, Fiorica JV. Surveillance of the endometrium in tamoxifen treated women. *Curr Opin Obstet Gynecol* 2000;12:27–31.
20. Magriples U, Naftolin F, Schwartz PE, et al. High-grade endometrial carcinoma in tamoxifen-treated breast cancer patients. *J Clin Oncol* 1993;11:485–490.
21. Koss LG. Detection of occult endometrial carcinoma. *J Cell Biochem Suppl* 1995;23:165–173.
22. Nordstrom B, Strang P, Lindgren A, et al. Carcinoma of the endometrium: do the nuclear grade and DNA ploidy provide more prognostic information than do the FIGO and WHO classification. *Int J Gynecol Pathol* 1996:15:191–201.

23. Gordon SJ, Westgate J. The incidence and management of failed Pipelle sampling in a general outpatient clinic. *Aust NZ J Obstet Gynaecol* 1999;39:115–118.

24. Runowicz CD, Fields AL. Screening for gynecologic malignancies: a continuing responsibility. *Surg Oncol Clin North Am* 1999; 8:703–723.

25. Meisels A, Jolicoeur C. Criteria for the cytologic assessment of hyperplasias in endometrial samples obtained by the Endopap Endometrial Sampler. *Acta Cytol* 1985;29:297–302.

26. Granberg S, Wikland M, Karlsson B, et al. Endometrial thickness as measured by endovaginal ultrasonography for identifying endometrial abnormality. *Am J Obstet Gynecol* 1991;164:47–52.

27. Zucker PK, Kasdon EJ, Feldstein ML. The validity of Pap smear parameters as predictors of endometrial pathology in menopausal women. *Cancer* 1985;56:2256–2263.

28. Kier R. Magnetic resonance imaging of the uterus. *Magn Reson Imaging Clin North Am* 1994;2:189–210.

29. Obermair A, Geramou M, Gucer F, et al. Does hysteroscopy facilitate tumor cell dissemination? Incidence of peritoneal cytology from patients with early stage endometrial carcinoma following dilatation and curettage (D&C) versus hysteroscopy and D&C. *Cancer* 2000;88:139–143.

30. International Federation of Gynecology and Obstetrics (FIGO). Annual report on the results of the treatment in gynecologic cancer. *Int J Gynecol Obstet* 1989;28:189–190.

31. Ostrzenski A. Laparoscopic total abdominal hysterectomy by suturing technique, with no transvaginal surgical approach: a review of 276 cases. *Int J Gynecol Obstet* 1996;55:247–257.

32. Creutzberg CL, van Putten WL, Koper PC, et al. Surgery and postoperative radiotherapy versus surgery alone for patient with stage-1 endometrial carcinoma: multicenter randomized trial. PORTEC Study Group. Post Operative Radiation Therapy in Endometrial Carcinoma. *Lancet* 2000;355:1404–1411.

33. Ostrzenski A. A new laparoscopic abdominal radical hysterectomy: a pilot phase trial. *Eur J Surg Oncol* 1996;22:602–606.

34. Magrina JF, Mutone NF, Weaver AL, et al. Laparoscopic lymphadenectomy and vaginal or laparoscopic hysterectomy for endometrial cancer: morbidity and survival. *Am J Obstet Gynecol* 1999;181:376–381.

35. Varia M, Rosenman J, Halle J, et al. Primary radiation therapy for medically inoperable patients with endometrial carcinoma—stage I–II. *Int J Radiat Oncol Biol Phys* 1987;13:11–15.

36. Nelson G, Randall M, Sutton G, et al. FIGO stage IIIC endometrial carcinoma with metastases confined to pelvic lymph nodes: analysis of treatment outcomes, prognostic variables, and failure patterns following adjuvant radiation therapy. *Gynecol Oncol* 1999;75:211–214.

37. Delaloye JF, Pampallona S, Coucke PA, et al. Effect of grade on disease-free survival and overall survival in FIGO stage I adenocarcinoma of the endometrium. *Eur J Obstet Gynecol Reprod Biol* 2000;88:75–80.

38. Gatta G, Lasota MB, Verdecchia A. Survival of European women with gynecological tumors, during the period 1878–1989. EUROCARE Working Group. *Eur J Cancer* 1998;34:2218–2225.

39. Marrow CP, Bundy BN, Kurman RJ, et al. Relationship between surgical-pathological risk factors and outcome in clinical stage I and II carcinoma of the endometrium: Gynecologic Oncology Group study. *Gynecol Oncol* 1991;40:55–65.

40. Hording U, Hansen U. Stage I endometrial carcinoma: a review of 140 patients primary treated by surgery only. *Gynecol Oncol* 1985;22:51–58.

41. Potish RA, Twiggs LB, Adcock LL, et al. Paraaortic lymph node radiotherapy in cancer of the uterine corpus. *Obstet Gynecol* 1985;65:251–256.

42. Li C, Samsioe G, Iosif C. Quality of life in endometrial cancer survivors. *Maturitas* 1999;31:227–236.

43. Harlow BL, Weiss NS, Lofton S. The epidemiology of sarcomas of the uterus. *J Natl Cancer Inst* 1986;76:399–402.

44. Meredith RF, Eisert DR, Kaka Z, et al. An excess of uterine sarcomas after pelvic irradiation. *Cancer* 1986;58:2003–2007.

45. Doss LL, Llorens AS, Henriquez FM. Carcinosarcoma of the uterus: a 40-year experience from the state of Missouri. *Gynecol Oncol* 1984;18:43–53.

46. Atman KH. Uterine sarcomas. In: Knapp RC, Berkowitz RS, eds. *Gynecologic oncology.* New York: McGraw-Hill, 1993.

47. Kahanpaa KV, Wahlstrom T, Grohn P, et al. Sarcomas of the uterus: a clinicopathologic study of 119 patients. *Obstet Gynecol* 1986;67:417–424.

48. Mayerhofer K, Obermair A, Windbichler G, et al. Leiomyosarcoma of the uterus: a clinicopathologic multicenter study of 71 cases. *Gynecol Oncol* 1999;74:196–201.

49. Gloor E. Endolymphatic stromal meiosis. Surgical and hormonal treatment of extensive abdominal recurrence 20 years after hysterectomy. *Cancer* 1982;50:1888–1893.

50. Atman KH. Malignancy of the uterine corpus. In: Knapp RC, Berkowitz RS, eds. *Gynecologic oncology.* New York: Macmillan Publishing, 1986.

51. Norris HJ, Taylor HB. Mesenchymal tumors of the uterus: I. A clinical and pathologic study of 53 endometrial stromal tumors. *Cancer* 1966;19:755–766.

52. The International Federation of Gynecology and Obstetric (FIGO). *Annual report on the results of treatment in gynecological cancer,* 22nd ed. Stockholm: FIGO, 1994.

21

FALLOPIAN TUBE DISORDERS

EDUCATIONAL OBJECTIVES

Medical Students (1)
APGO Objective No. 40

Salpingitis
Pathogenesis
Common organisms
Signs and symptoms
Methods of diagnosis
Treatment
Sequelae:
1. Tuboovarian abscess
2. Chronic salpingitis
3. Ectopic pregnancy
4. Infertility

Residents in Obstetrics/Gynecology (2)
CREOG Objectives

Fallopian tube carcinoma
History
    Physical examination
    Diagnostic studies
    Diagnosis
    Management
    Follow-up

Practitioners (3)
ACOG Recommendation

No specific recommendation

FALLOPIAN TUBE EMBRYOLOGY

In the seventh week of gestation, the unfused segments of the Müllerian ducts (paramesonephric ducts) create the Fallopian tubes (the fused portion of paramesonephric ducts form the uterus and upper part of the vagina). The Müllerian ducts traverse within the mesosalpinx, parallel to and in the proximity of the remnants of Wolffian ducts (mesonephric ducts). These remnants comprise 10 to 15 of the mesonephric tubules, which join the mesonephric ducts (4).

FALLOPIAN TUBE ANATOMY

The Fallopian tubes (oviducts) are the muscular canalized structures that extend from the anterior-medial aspect of the ovary (with no direct attachment to the ovaries) to the posterior-superior-lateral area of the uterine fundus. The oviduct is the essential connection between the ovary and the uterine cavity. The ovarian segment opens to the pelvic-peritoneal cavity. The uterine portion of the Fallopian tube stretches out directly to the uterine cavity. The entire Fallopian tube length is 9 to 12 cm, with an average of 10.5 cm. The oviduct is divided into the following segments (Fig. 21.1):

1. *The fimbriae* are the parts of the Fallopian tube closely located near the ovary. They consist of fingerlike (25 in the average) structures; fine folds, which are fused with the infundibulum (1 cm in diameter and 1 cm long). One of the fimbriae is elongated and connected to the mesosalpinx, termed the "fimbria ovarica."
2. *The infundibulum* resembles a funnel-shaped composition that progressively narrows towards the uterus, reaching the tubal ampulla in about 4-mm-reduced diameters. Some authorities suggest that the fimbriae and the infundibulum should be analyzed as one inseparable unit, and some believe that these are two distinctive tubal formations.
3. *The ampulla* is minimally convoluted and thin, and approximately 6 cm long (the longest portion of the tube).
4. *The isthmus* is the thick, straight, and narrow part of the Fallopian tube, which fuses with the cornual area of the uterine corpus and is about 2 cm in length. Upon entering the myometrium, it traverses about 1 cm to reach the endometrial cavity.

The arterial blood supply is provided by the following:

1. The tubal branch of the ascending uterine artery departs from the lateral cornual area of the uterus and runs in the mesosalpinx.

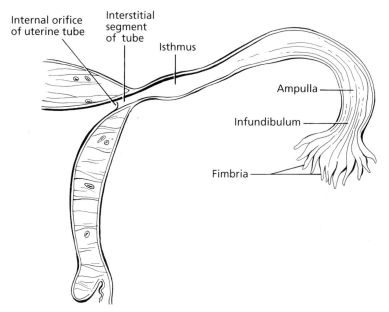

FIG. 21.1. Fallopian tube anatomical division.

2. The tubal branch of the ovarian artery anastomosizes with the tubal branch of the uterine artery in the meso-salpinx.

Veins run parallel to the arteries and return blood to the uterine and ovarian veins. Similar to the tubal arteries, the veins traverse within the mesosalpinx, where they create an anastomosis between the tubal branches (uterine and ovarian) and the uterine and ovarian veins.

Tubal lymphatic chains are divided as follows:

1. *The right side* of the oviduct of lymphatic nodes drains to nodes in the area of the right renal vein and to the inferior vena cava.
2. *The left side* of the oviduct lymphatic nodes drains to the nodes located between the left ovarian vein and the left renal vein.

Tubal innervation comes from both sympathetic and parasympathetic systems. The sympathetic system arises from T10 through L2 synapses in the aortic, celiac, renal, inferior mesenteric, presacral, and cervicovaginal plexus.

The parasympathetic system delivers fibers from the vagus nerve to the extrauterine portion of the oviduct. The intramural part of the Fallopian tube is supplied by S2–S4 parasympathetic fibers, which provide synapses within the pelvic plexus. Sensory fibers conduct tubal impulses that terminate in T10 and T4 (5).

The Fallopian tube outer layer is covered by the peritoneum (the tubal serosa), which extends from the uterine broad ligaments and covers all the segments of the oviduct, except the intramural portion and the attachment of the mesosalpinx. Under the serosa, the muscular layer comprises the longitudinal smooth muscles. The inner layer consists of a circular arrangement of muscles. The tubal mucosa lines of the oviduct canal are arranged in a plicae pattern, which gets thicker towards the fimbriae and is termed "plicae tubaria." The mucosa contains the columnar epithelium with ciliated and nonciliated (secretory) cells, which together with intercalary (peg) cells, create the endosalpinx. The endosalpinx expresses morphological fluctuation in harmony with the changing hormonal milieu of the menstrual cycle (6). It has been documented that, in a postmenstrual follicular phase, estrogens stimulate the endosalpinx to grow and create a new ciliated epithelium (ciliogenesis). Progesterone influences the endosalpinx to regress with deciliation. The process of endosalpinx regression occurs in the late luteal phase and the menstrual bleeding phase of the menstrual cycle. Expeditious regeneration of the endosalpinx commences in the proliferative phase (in process similar to that in the endometrium) (7). A post-menopausal endosalpinx atrophic state is present. The space between the serosa and the outer layer of the tube is filled with connective tissue, within which the blood supply and return vessels, as well as nerves, traverse.

The *function of the Fallopian tubes* is the primary element in human reproduction. It is a multifunctional organ responsible for the following fertility processes (8,9):

- *The ovum pick-up and transport* following ovulation is guided by fimbria ovarica and requires healthy fimbria to complete this event. After ovum/preembryo retention, the ovum is transported to the ampulla of the Fallopian tubes.
- *Upward migration of sperm, storage, activation, and collection in a reservoir* occur in the isthmic segment of the oviduct.
- *Fertilization* (sperm penetration of the ovum) usually occurs in the ampulla of the Fallopian tube.

■ *Embryo transport* depends upon a healthy endosalpinx. An embryo is propelled from the ampulla to the endometrial cavity by endosalpinx cilia movement, neuromuscular activity, and synchronized and appropriate endocrine function. This process is usually completed by the third postovulatory day.

BENIGN DISORDERS

Fallopian Tube Congenital Anomalies

Fallopian tube congenital anomalies are an infrequent occurrence and are often associated with uterine congenital abnormalities such as bicornuate uterus or rudimentary uterine horn (10,11).

Fallopian congenital tube anomalies fall into the following categories:

■ *Absence of the tubes* is usually part of uterine and vaginal agenesis. The ovaries are present and suspended from the broad ligament in these cases. The absence of one tube is associated with ipsilateral ovarian, ureteral, or renal agenesis or congenital abnormalities (12).
■ *Absence of the ampullary muscularis* has been reported as a complete lack of the muscular layer of the segment of the ampulla of the oviduct (13).
■ *Absence of a segment of the tube* of the proximal tube also has been reported (14).
■ *Accessory tubes* may originate from any segment of the Fallopian tube, although they do not connect with the oviduct lumen. The abdominal osmium of the accessory tubes usually is found in the vicinity of the primary oviduct (15).
■ *Anomalies associated with Diethylstilbestrol (DES)* in an in utero–exposed female may present with the Fallopian tube pinpoint ostium, constricted fimbriae, short, sacculated, or convoluted oviduct. Such a clinical condition may cause female infertility and cannot be detected by hysterosalpingogram, which is usually normal (16). Also, it has been postulated that salpingitis isthmica nodosa may follow DES exposure during gestation.
■ *Duplication of the tube* is considered by some clinicians as a form of accessory tube; although, in the literature, it exists as a separate condition (17).

Conventional therapy is surgical reconstruction. Pregnancy can be achieved with assisted reproductive technology in cases of absent or dysfunctional Fallopian tubes when the uterus is present. When the uterus and/or vagina are absent, embryo transfer to a surrogate can be utilized.

Torsion of the Tube

Definition

Torsion of the tube is a rotation of the oviduct along the long axis that causes blood supply obstruction.

Incidence

The incidence or prevalence of tubal torsion has not been established; it is an uncommon clinical occurrence.

Etiology

Etiology of tubal torsion is unknown; although, there are some identifiable predisposing factors (18–22):

■ Ipsilateral ovarian mass (ovarian cyst or solid tumor)
■ Paraovarian cyst
■ Prior tubal ligation
■ Prior pelvic surgery
■ Hydro- or pyosalpinx

Classification

Tubal torsion can occur as follows:

■ Isolated, unilateral tubal torsion with ovarian sparing (20)
■ Isolated, bilateral tubal torsion with ovarian sparing (21)
■ Adnexal torsion (ovarian and tubal involvement) (23)

Diagnosis

Diagnosis is reached based upon symptoms of acute and sudden onset lower quadrant abdominal and pelvic pain. Pain is usually present in reproductive aged women [pediatric (24) and adolescent (25) as well as postmenopausal (26) cases have been reported] and is located on the side of the affected tube or bilaterally, if both tubes are twisted. Nausea and vomiting are associated with pain due to peritoneal irritation (20,25). Although, these symptoms are not specific for tubal or adnexal torsion, a high index of suspicion may provide guidance for establishing the diagnosis and potential salvage of the tube or adnexa. Diagnosis is often delayed because of the rarity of clinical occurrence, and prolonged investigations to rule out more common causes of acute abdominal-pelvic pain often take place (25). Torsion of accessory or duplication of the Fallopian tubes also can occur with similar symptomatology (27).

Imaging technology is utilized for abdominal-pelvic pain evaluation. Ultrasound examination can reveal a unilateral or bilateral lobulated inhomogeneous mass, adjacent to the uterus (25,27). Magnetic resonance imaging (MRI) identifies a pseudo-encapsulated mass with inhomogeneous area (27). Also, the use of computed tomography has been reported. None of these techniques can distinguish torsion of the Fallopian tube from other pelvic masses, e.g., endometrioma.

Diagnostic laparoscopy provides the definitive diagnosis. Early diagnosis is paramount to improve the likelihood of salvage of the Fallopian tube or adnexa (25,28). Particularly important is to stress that Fallopian tube torsion symptoms, physical examination (including pelvic evaluation), and imaging studies have a very poor diagnostic correlation; therefore, the value of diagnostic laparoscopy is irreplaceable.

Differential Diagnosis

- Appendicitis
- Endometrioma
- Hemorrhagic ovarian cyst
- Cryptomenorrhea (severe pelvic pain at the first few menstrual cycles; usually a pelvic mass is present)
- Congenital abnormality

Conventional Therapy

Conventional therapy is surgery with tubal preservation; therefore, early diagnosis before any irreversible process within the tube (e.g., tissue necrosis or thrombosis) takes place is paramount. Early diagnosis and therapy can be achieved with the laparoscopic approach. Laparoscopic direct tubal inspection usually reveals the swollen, edematous-tubes, congested with hemorrhagic infarction, and gangrenous.

Through laparoscopy, untwisting (detortion) of the Fallopian tube can be successfully executed (20,21).

Exploratory laparotomy still remains an option, with salvage of the oviducts, if possible. If the tube is beyond salvage, extirpative surgical intervention is necessary. Salpingectomy can be performed either via laparotomy or laparoscopy.

Undiagnosed and untreated torsion of the tube may lead to spontaneous resorption or a calcification process (29). Recurrence of Fallopian tube torsion affecting the same oviduct has been reported (20); however, literature on the prevention of recurrences is scant. Adolescent patients in particular are vulnerable to recurrence of isolated tubal torsion. If predisposing risk factors are present, such as paraovarian cyst or hydrosalpinx, treatment should be offered at the time of initial diagnostic and/or operative laparoscopy or laparotomy. Paraovarian cystectomy can be executed at the time of the initial operation. Hydrosalpinx can be treated by fimbrioplasty, which will establish permanent fluid drainage. Any pelvic surgery should be executed by exercising the best technique, appropriate suturing material, gentle tissue handling, and meticulous hemostasis to minimize postsurgical adhesion formation. Particular attention should be paid, when tubal ligation is performed, to using the appropriate segment of tube and selecting the correct type of operation may provide prevention against tubal torsion.

Complementary Therapy

Patient Education
Patient education should involve all necessary information about symptomatology and the importance of early contact with a health care practitioner. The complexity of the diagnostic process and the clinical (even lifetime) sequelae of delayed diagnosis and appropriate surgical intervention should be presented. The importance of avoiding potential tubal damage by infection, leading to hydro- or pyosalpinx formation, should be explained.

Alternative Therapy

In general, there is no specific recommendation for herbal or homeopathic therapies; although, nutritional supplements and spiritual-body harmony exercises are usually advisable. If pelvic pain or dysmenorrhea persists after treatment, management can be accomplished with alternative approaches for pain (see respective chapters).

Tubal Prolapse

Definition

Tubal prolapse is defined as the presence of the Fallopian tube within the vaginal cuff or within the vaginal pool following total hysterectomy.

Incidence

The incidence of oviduct prolapse is unknown, although it is an uncommon complication (30).

Etiology

Tubal prolapse is considered an iatrogenic condition induced by total abdominal or vaginal hysterectomy. Recent clinical data suggest that tubal prolapse follows abdominal hysterectomy in about 65% of cases with preexisting risk factors identified as cuff cellulitis, cuff infection, cuff hematoma, postextubation pulmonary edema, and elevated temperature (30).

Diagnosis

The *pertinent medical history* for tubal prolapse consists of post–hysterectomy symptoms (30):

- Dyspareunia is present in approximately 44%.
- Vaginal bleeding or vaginal bloody discharge is present in about 39%.
- Vaginal discharge (leukorrhea) is present in 28%.
- Abdominal pain is present in approximately 28%.

On the other hand, an asymptomatic clinical course is present in approximately 28%.

Physical examination will document an abdominal scar if total hysterectomy has been executed via laparotomy.

Pelvic examination can reveal the absence of the cervix and can identify a tender mass or protruding lesion from the vaginal cuff.

Cytology of the vaginal cuff can be obtained directly from the lesion. An exfoliative cytological smear can be helpful in establishing diagnosis in the case of tube prolapse with the presence of a distinctive appearance of the small, regular, and occasionally ciliated columnar cells with granular nuclei and prominent nucleoli (31).

Direct biopsy with histological verification will provide the definitive diagnosis, but postbiopsy bleeding can complicate the procedure, and extreme care should be exercised to prevent such an event.

Differential Diagnosis

Differential diagnosis of Fallopian tube prolapse includes the following:

- Vaginal cuff (vault) granulations or granuloma (31)
- Small bowel prolapse through the vaginal vault, following hysterectomy, which is a very serious complication with a potentially fatal result. The immediate surgical replacement of the small intestine loops is a life-saving approach. Severe infection can complicate this clinical occurrence (32).
- Vaginal adenocarcinoma can masquerade as Fallopian tube prolapse in a postmenopausal patient (33).

Conventional Therapy

Conventional therapy for posthysterectomy Fallopian tube prolapse is total salpingectomy, which can be executed through the following approaches (30,34):

- Laparotomy alone
- Transvaginal approach alone
- Combined transabdominal and transvaginal approaches
- Combined transvaginal and laparoscopic approaches

Spontaneous resolution of tubal prolapse with no surgical therapy or other treatment modality can be expected in up to 41% of cases.

A specific complementary or alternative therapy is not available for tubal prolapse.

OTHER FALLOPIAN TUBE DISORDERS

- *Tubal intussusception* is spontaneous migration and entrapment of the fimbriated segment of the Fallopian tube within the ampulla of the oviduct. This condition can be associated with paraovarian cyst, which may engulf the oviduct. Treatment of this entity is achieved with cystectomy and eversion of fimbriae with tubal preservation (35).
- *Tubal endometriosis* may affect the oviduct serosa, wall, and lumen, and can have devastating effects on reproductive capacity. The tubal damages can range from an innocent superficial endometriosis implant present on the tubal serosa, through peritubal adhesions, which may compromise Fallopian tube function, to complete occlusion of the oviduct lumen (36). MRI, based on morphologic features, can provide sufficient information to

detect the presence of Fallopian tube endometriosis (37). Treatment varies depending upon the stage of the disease. For more detail, see Chapter 9.

- *Endosalpingiosis* is the extratubal presence of tubal-like epithelium. It can be found as peritoneal, omental, intestinal, or other organ implants (38–40). Until recently, endosalpingiosis has been considered to be a clinically innocent pathology; today, this clinical condition has been linked to pelvic pain similar to that of endometriosis (41,42). The pelvic distribution of endosalpingiosis, in association with pelvic pain, is consistent with that generally observed in endometriosis (43). *Conventional therapy* is similar to that for endometriosis and consists of oral contraceptives, danazol, or a GnRH agonist. Surgical excision in selective cases is another option (41).
- *Salpingitis isthmica nodosa (SIN)* is the spontaneous pathological development of variable sized sacs within the isthmic section of the tubal epithelium (isthmic diverticula). The prevalence of SIN in healthy, fertile women ranges from 0.6% to 11%; it is significantly higher in women with infertility or an ectopic pregnancy. It is considered a progressive disease with deleterious effects on female infertility because it causes proximal tubal occlusion that accounts for 20% of tubal infertility (44), (45). The etiology is unknown; although, two theories have been postulated as potential mechanisms of SIN: (a) the adenomyosis-like process, which is the more frequently accepted and convincing concept (46,47); and (b) the postinflammatory process (48). This condition is not observed in prepubertal girls; the age of initial diagnosis of SIN is between 25 and 60 years of age, with an average age of 30 years (45). Concomitant distal bilateral tubal occlusion with or without hydrosalpinx can be present in approximately 17% of cases (49). *The diagnosis* is suggested by the presence of distinctive pathological changes on hysterosalpingographic study. *Diagnostic laparoscopy* with a tubal day perfusion study may confirm the radiographic diagnosis. A laparoscopic view is consistent with the presence of smooth serosa with identifiable nodular lesions, one or more at 1 to 2 cm in diameter (subserosal diverticula not connected with serosa).

Differential diagnosis (44) includes the following:

1. *Nonnodular proximal tubal occlusion* is true fibrotic proximal tube occlusion. This condition will benefit from microtuboplasty. Recanalization, followed by GnRH-analog conservative treatment, has not proven successful (on the other hand, nodular proximal occlusion such as salpingitis isthmica nodosa can benefit from GnRH—analog post-recanalization therapy).

2. *Pseudo-proximal tubal occlusion* can be caused by tubal spasmodic contraction, endosalpinx polyp, transient mucus plague, or hypoplastic tube.

Conventional Therapy

Conventional therapy is either of the following:

1. *Microtubal surgery (microtuboplasty)* (45) is the preferable surgical approach. *Transcervical fluoroscopic Fallopian tube recanalization* or Fallopian tube recanalization (FTR) is an outpatient technique that can be utilized as an alternative to *in vitro* fertilization or microsurgical reanastomosis of the proximal tube. *Transcervical tubal catheterization* is performed with the assistance of flexible hysteroscopy (falloposcope) under real-time fluoroscopic visualization of the tube. This procedure not only establishes the diagnosis of proximal tubal occlusion but also provides treatment at the same time (50). The definitive diagnosis, however, is provided by histological verification. The success rate of achieving tubal patency (technical success) is between 68% and 72%, with 18% to 32% live births and 4.5% to 10% tubal pregnancies (50,51). There are no studies comparing tubal surgery for proximal tubal occlusion with hysteroscopic or radiologically controlled recanalization.
2. *The use of assisted technology* is often preferred over surgical intervention since the advent of this modality.

No specific complementary or alternative therapy is currently available in the literature.

TUBAL INFECTION (SALPINGITIS)

Acute Salpingitis

Definition

Acute salpingitis is a purulent inflammatory response of the Fallopian tube epithelium to micropathogens.

Incidence

The incidence of acute salpingitis alone (not as a part of pelvic inflammatory disease) is unknown.

Etiology

Acute salpingitis is caused by microorganisms. *Neisseria gonorrhea* and *Chlamydia trachomatis* are the most common isolated pathogens (77.4%). Polymicrobial salpingitis is an often identified phenomenon. The initiation of acute salpingitis is predominantly due to the ascending spread of sexually transmitted microorganisms. Bacterial vaginosis is a common concurrent disorder of women with acute salpingitis (52). Tubal interaction with the ovum (driven by the tubal secretion) and tubal function may be impaired or destroyed by acute salpingitis (9). How micropathogence is spread in an ascending pattern from the lower genital tract to the upper genital tract is not definitively established. Theories range from passive transport to active transport by either sperm or trichomonas (53).

Classification

Acute salpingitis is classified either by the type of microbial infection or by the clinical severity of infection:

A. *The microbial type* of salpingitis is categorized (54) as follows:
   1. Gonococcal salpingitis (some authorities also classify this as gonococcal/chlamydial salpingitis)
   2. Nongonococcal salpingitis (some authorities also classify this as nongonococcal/nonchlamydial salpingitis) can be caused by polymicrobial agents such as aerobic bacteria (*Escherichia coli*) or anaerobic bacteria, particularly bacteroides or peptostreptococci species. Rarely, *Mycoplasma hominis, Ureaplasma urealyticum,* tuberculosis, parasitic, or mycotic flora can cause acute salpingitis. Contrary to gonococcal/chlamydial salpingitis, the onset of acute salpingitis of nongonococcal/nonchlamydia is not associated with the commencement of the last menses (55).

Occasionally, acute salpingitis may occur in association with surgical procedures (up to 15%) such as abortion, dilatation and curettage, hysterosalpingography, or IUD insertion. Also, this condition may occur in about 1% of any intraabdominal bacterial infection, e.g., acute appendicitis.

Predisposing factors for acute salpingitis include the following:

1. Multiple sexual partners are a factor, especially in young women (<25 years).
2. Previous salpingitis causes mucosa damage, making a patient more susceptible to subsequent infection.
3. The use of an IUD is an independent risk factor for acute salpingitis and increases salpingitis and its sequelae by two- to fourfold. Shortly after IUD insertion, salpingitis may occur due to contamination of the endometrium with cervical microflora.

B. The severity of acute salpingitis is difficult to establish due to very broad clinical manifestations; it is generally classified as follows (56):
   1. Uncomplicated acute salpingitis (the absence of peritoneal inflammation signs or abscess formation)
   2. Complicated acute salpingitis (inflammatory complex or tuboovarian abscess formation), which occurs in approximately 30%

Diagnosis

To adopt very strict diagnostic criteria for acute salpingitis can lead to overlooking nontypically manifested disease. On the contrary, too liberal an interpretation of the clinical picture may lead to a false-positive clinical diagnosis.

Pertinent medical history associated with acute salpingitis may include the following:

1. *Sexually active*, nonpregnant, and menstruating women can be affected by this condition.

2. *The presence of abdominal-pelvic pain* may or may not be reported. Manifestation of pain can be presented in different degrees of severity, including as mild, moderate, and severe. Practical and easy clinical categorization of abdominal-pelvic pain can be established using the patient's ability to concentrate on daily tasks, daily functioning, and what remedies relieve pain. For instance, a mild form of lower abdominal and pelvic pain can be defined as pain that does not affect the patient's ability to concentrate and does not influence daily function nor requires pain medication (or requires only a weak painkiller). Conversely, when pain affects the ability to concentrate and daily functions (bedridden), and ordinary pain medication does not relieve pain sufficiently, a severe form of pain is present.
3. *Vaginal discharge* (leukorrhea) may be noted and reported by the patient.

Physical examination findings may range from no signs to tachycardia, warm skin, elevated core body temperature, abdominal-pelvic tenderness, and/or muscle guarding. In acute salpingitis, rebound tenderness can be elicited. The hill-draped test can be positive (elevating body on toes and draping on the hill may evoke or aggravate lower abdominal-pelvic pain).

Pelvic examination can disclose yellowish vaginal discharge; cervical motion can induce or can aggravate pelvic pain. Varied degrees of tenderness in the adnexal area unilaterally or bilaterally can be induced.

Laboratory tests are not specific; although, they may provide information leading to a clinical diagnosis. The following tests are routinely performed:

1. White count can be elevated (leucocytosis).
2. Erythrocyte sedimentation rate may be elevated.
3. Gram-stain may reveal the presence of pathogenic microbial flora.
4. Cervical culture may identify a specific micropathogen and its antibiotic sensitivity.

Less frequently, the following laboratory tests are also suggested:

1. Indirect immunoperoxidase test (Ipazyme kit) is offered for Chlamydial trachomatis.
2. Enzyme-linked immunosorbent assay (ELISA kit) can be ordered. (Neither of these first two tests are useful in an early state of salpingitis.)
3. C-reactive protein (C–RP) is a sensitive and nonspecific inflammatory marker that begins to rise 6 to 12 hours from commencement of inflammatory processes. Sequential C–RP determinations have greater diagnostic value and commonly reflect the clinical course. The clinical significance of C–RP in salpingitis is not fully defined. The test and its clinical interpretation should be analyzed in the context of the overall clinical picture (57).

4. CA-125 levels above 7.5 units may modestly improve the clinical diagnosis of salpingitis; however, limitations of the test (can be elevated in other condition such as neoplasia or endometriosis) make its clinical utilization less practical (58).
5. *Fallopian tube culture* can be obtained laparoscopically, and, recently, the hysteroscopic approach has been introduced. The specimen is obtained during hysteroscopy with a cytobrush (59). This approach has not yet been clinically validated.
6. *Laparoscopic confirmation* of acute salpingitis can be achieved in approximately 82.3% of cases (58), but requires significant experience in identifying infections through laparoscopy.

Differential Diagnosis

Differential diagnosis of acute salpingitis embraces several pelvic conditions, with the most frequent being the following:

1. Ectopic pregnancy and threatened early pregnancy abortion
2. Acute appendicitis, diverticulitis (left lower quadrant abdominal pain), and Crohn's disease
3. Pelvic inflammatory disease, endometriosis, and urinary tract infections
4. Adnexal torsion, isolated tubal torsion, lipoid or granulomatous salpingitis, ovarian cyst, and large paraovarian cyst
5. Degenerating uterine leiomyomata

Conventional Therapy

The Centers for Disease Control and Prevention recommends the following antibiotic modalities (56):

1. Uncomplicated acute salpingitis
   a. Cefotetan, 2 g IV every 12 hours
   b. Cefoxitin, 2 g IV every 6 hours
   c. Doxycycline, 100 mg IV or oral every 12 hours, in combination with a and b for 14 days

Also, uncomplicated acute salpingitis can be treated in an ambulatory setting:

a. A combination of Ceftriaxone, 250 mg IM with Doxycycline, 100 mg orally twice daily for 10 to 14 days
b. A combination of Cefoxitin, 2 g IM and Doxycycline, 100 mg orally twice daily for 10 to 14 days

A second line of ambulatory management includes the following:

a. Ofloxacin, 400 mg orally twice daily
b. Clindamycin, 450 mg orally four times daily
c. Metronidazole, 500 mg orally twice daily

It is important to offer an appropriate combination of antibiotics, which are active against gonococcal, chlamydial, enterobacteria, and anaerobes infection, since acute salpingitis is commonly caused by polymicrobial infection (60).

2. *Complicated acute salpingitis* will require a combination of broad-spectrum antibiotics:
   a. Clindamycin, 900 mg IV every 8 hours and Gentamicin, 2 mg/kg IV loading dose followed by 1.5 mg/kg IV every 8 hours
   b. Metronidazole, 500 mg IV every 8 hours and Gentamicin, 2 mg/kg IV loading dose followed by 1.5 mg/kg IV every 8 hours

Acute salpingitis sequelae can be treated as follows:

1. *Recurrent salpingitis* diagnosis can be reached with second-look laparoscopy followed by acute salpingitis. Recurrent salpingitis is estimated in 16% of cases. Therapy is based on culture and sensitivity, and the patient should be hospitalized for IV antibiotic therapy (61).
2. *Tuboovarian abscess (TOA)* formation as a complication of acute salpingitis is a well-documented sequel. Lower abdominal-pelvic pain and the presence of pelvic mass with elevated body core temperature and white blood cells raises the suspicion of TOA; although, fever and leucocytosis is not present in each case. The diagnosis can be confirmed either by imaging study, laparoscopy, or exploratory laparotomy. TAO can be present unilaterally or bilaterally. TOA is a polymicrobial infection with a preponderance of Gram-negative anaerobic pathogens, which are isolated in 63% to 100% (resistant *Bacteroids fragilis* and *Bacteroids bivius* are the most common microorganisms). Initially, unruptured TOA is treated with antimicrobial drugs for 48 to 72 hours; if the patient does not respond, surgical intervention is indicated. Ruptured TAO requires emergent surgical treatment with unilateral adnexectomy (62). If ruptured TAO is diagnosed bilaterally, total hysterectomy with bilateral salpingo-oophorectomy is executed. Laparoscopic drainage (63) and percutaneous drainage (64) are gaining clinical acceptance, but clinical data on safety and efficacy of these techniques are absent. Surgical preservation of tubes or adnexa is a possible option with the current combination of therapy with antimicrobial agents and conservative surgical intervention; however, fertility is significantly compromised and the use of assisted reproductive technology may help in the management of this aspect of TAO sequelae.
3. *Chronic salpingitis* is a residual form of acute salpingitis and may create multiple tuboovarian adhesions, resulting in occlusion of the distal tube. This persistent inflammatory process due to chronic infection can damage tubal folds, with scarring and plical disappearance. Such tubal destruction is beyond surgical reconstruction, since the function of the tube cannot be restored, even if successful restoration of tubal patency is accomplished. Pregnancy can be achieved with the use of *in vitro* fertilization.
4. *Tubal occlusion* with or without hydro- or pyosalpinx formation caused by acute salpingitis is a frequent clinical event. Bilateral tubal occlusion prevalence depends upon the severity of salpingitis and is present in approximately 9.5%, 20%, and 32.1% of mild, moderate, and severe cases, respectively (61). The mucosal plicae of the Fallopian tubes adhere to one another as a result of surface fibrin deposition and, in the final result, may completely obliterate the lumen of the oviduct. Surgical treatment for tubal occlusion is frequently performed; although, more and more cases are managed by *in vitro* fertilization. Distal tube occlusion with the presence of hydrosalpinx has a better outcome of pregnancy with *in vitro* fertilization than with surgical tubal reconstruction. Initial clinical observation indicates that salpingectomy for unilateral hydrosalpinx may improve *in vivo* fecundity without the need for *in vitro* fertilization (65). The use of microsurgical techniques and the application of magnification during surgery, either by operating microscope with magnification of ×4 to 16 or Loupes with magnification of ×2 to 4.5 (a nonsignificant reduction in outcome regardless of the form of magnification used) is the recommended approach. Overall, there is no significant difference when using CO_2 laser as compared to standard techniques for tubal reconstruction or adhesiolysis (66).

A multicenter prospective study of tubal mucosal lesions associated with hydrosalpinx documented that the most important factor in determining fertility outcomes from reconstructive surgery is the quality of tubal mucosa. At the time of performing salpingoneostomy for hydrosalpinx, the diameter and quality of the mucosa's appearance macroscopically (poor prognosis is associated with a thick wall of hydrosalpinx; the presence of peritubal adhesions or their extent does not influence the pregnancy rate) and microscopically (with an operating microscope) should be determined. The following clinical characteristics play a significant role in the surgical outcome:

- Mucosal abnormality of more than 50% will yield intrauterine pregnancy in about 7% of cases. Mucosal abnormality of less than 50% or 75% will result in intrauterine pregnancies in 50% and 69%, respectively.
- The small hydrosalpinx size of <1 cm presents a better prognosis than the medium size of 1 to 2 cm and the large size of >2 cm.
- Mucosal adhesions associated with hydrosalpinx decrease the intrauterine pregnancy rate postoperatively, to about 22%. The absence of mucosal adhesions significantly increases the intrauterine pregnancy, to approximately 58%. Also, the presence of mucosal adhesions increases the potential risk for tubal pregnancy (67).

5. *Pelvic adhesions*, especially peritubal and periovarian adhesions, may lead to a mechanical type of infertility and may require either laparoscopic or open microsurgical adhesiolysis. Pelvic adhesions strongly correlate with bilateral tubal occlusion and are estimated to occur after acute salpingitis episode in about 38.1% of cases (61). When comparing open adhesiolysis to no treatment, adhesiolysis provides significantly more pregnancies (66).

6. *Chronic pelvic pain* (history of pelvic pain lasting at least for 6 months) was noted in approximately 66.7% of cases (61). It is a very complex clinical entity, which requires a comprehensive approach, including consideration of multiple organ systems, and empiric treatment with nonsteroidal antiinflammatory agents, low-dose oral contraceptives, antimicrobial drugs, or antispasmodic medication should be considered. Diagnostic and/or operative laparoscopy is indicated; if pelvic pathology is identified, appropriate surgical intervention should be considered. The gynecological differential diagnosis may include endometriosis, endosalpingiosis, salpingitis, or adenomyosis; appropriate diagnostic and therapeutic measurements should be entertained (68).

7. *The Fitz-Hugh-Curtis* syndrome is a perihepatitis condition resulting from genital infection. *Chlamydia trachomatis* is the most common pathogen causing this syndrome. It can manifest with acute or recurrent right upper abdominal pain. The diagnosis can be suspected based upon the ELISA test; diagnostic laparoscopy is confirmatory. Intraabdominal fluid can be cultured on multimedia to identify specific microorganisms and their sensitivity to antimicrobial agents. The typical laparoscopic appearance of perihepatitis (glissonitis with pseudo-membranes) is the presence of inflamed peritoneum, and adhesions between the liver serosa and the abdominal wall peritoneum, with a small amount of fluid usually present (69). Initial experimental antibiotic therapy for chlamydia infection should be instituted in combination with other antimicrobial agents to address potential polymicrobial infection. Upon receiving culture results, therapy should be adjusted appropriately.

Complementary and alternative therapy is not addressed specifically for acute salpingitis; however, it is generally offered for pelvic inflammatory disease.

GENITAL TRACT TUBERCULOSIS
Tuberculous Salpingitis
Definition

Tuberculous salpingitis (tubal tuberculosis) is infection of the Fallopian tube caused by the *Mycobacterium tuberculosis* microorganism.

Incidence

In the United States, the prevalence of female genital tuberculosis was highest in 1956 at 5.5%. The prevalence declined in 1964 as a result of a nationwide antituberculosis campaign, falling to 0.27% in 1977 (70). Recently, the incidence of genital tuberculosis is rapidly rising not only in the United States (71) but also in other industrialized countries (72–74); although, the recent, actual incidence or prevalence of genital tuberculosis has not been established. The African continent and the Indian subcontinent are particularly affected, but European countries are also affected (75,76). In recent years, the incidence of genital tuberculosis has changed from being present primarily in patients aged 25 to 35 years old (66%) (70), to being present in a much larger proportion of patients over 40 years of age (to a prevalence of 3.7% of postmenopausal women) (77).

Etiology

Genital tract tuberculosis is caused by *Mycobacterium tuberculosis*, which is the main pathogen responsible for granulomatous salpingitis.

Classification

Genital tuberculosis can be classified as follows:

- *Primary genital tuberculosis* infection is considered to be extremely low. Primary direct transmission can occur from genitourinary tuberculosis of an infected sexual partner during coitus.
- *Secondary genital tuberculosis* infection is spread from the primary site of infection, which must be an organ other than the genital tract. The tuberculosis pathogen is the blood-borne organism. Dissemination to the genital tract is primarily from a primary pulmonary lesion, which may not be documented by x-ray.

Genital tract tuberculosis is usually presented according to the genital organ infection and the percentage of involvement of different organs of the genital tract varies (70):

- Fallopian tubes are infected in 100% of cases when genital tuberculosis is present; it is still unknown why tuberculosis preferentially infects tubes rather than other genital organs.
- Endometrium is affected in 79% of cases.
- Cervix in approximately 24%
- Ovaries 11%
- Vagina and vulva in about 0.07%
- Genital tuberculosis associated with tuberculous peritonitis is present in 0.01% of the outpatient population and 0.05% of hospitalized women (78).

Diagnosis

The diagnosis of genital tuberculosis is still a challenging process. The symptoms are not specific, and an asymptomatic clinical course has been reported (71).

Pertinent medical history includes the following:

- History of tuberculosis (significant number of patients will have negative history of tuberculosis)
- Travel history
- Infertility is the most common symptom and accounts for approximately 47.2% of cases (79) [primary infertility in 94% or secondary infertility 6% (69)].
- Pelvic pain in 32% is present (79).
- Abnormal endometrial bleeding occurs in about 11% (79).
- Habitual abortion is occasionally associated with endometrial tuberculosis (79).

Physical examination usually is normal.

Pelvic examination demonstrates the same form of pelvic pathology in approximately 68.4% of cases (79). An adnexal mass, unilateral or bilateral, can be present with or without symptoms (71).

A *clinical test* in the form of a skin test is performed with a purified protein derivative of tuberculin, which can produce positive findings.

Additional tests fall into several groups:

1. *Imaging studies* can assist in the detection of upper genital tract tuberculosis:
   a. *Hysterosalpingogram* may produce characteristic features such as beading, rigid patterning, and sacculation or sinus formation.
   b. *Chest x-ray* may document the evidence of healed pulmonary tuberculosis (80).
   c. *Ultrasound* may depict a large amount of loculated fluid containing debris (80).
   d. *MRI* can suggest the diagnosis (80).
2. *Menstrual effluence* can be collected either in a vaginal or cervical cup submitted for a culture. It has been postulated that culture is more reliable than biopsy (81).
3. *Histology examination* will confirm the diagnosis.
4. Acid-fast stain is also used; although, it demonstrates less sensitivity than histology or tuberculous culture.
5. CA-125 may disclose rising serum levels (71).

Differential Diagnosis

Differential diagnosis of tuberculosis includes the following:

- Other causes of infertility
- Other causes of pelvic pain
- Other causes of abnormal endometrial bleeding
- Another origin of a pelvic mass

Conventional Therapy

Conventional therapy falls into the following modalities:

- *Medical treatment* is the principal approach in the management of genital tract tuberculosis. The therapy consists of multiple, two or three, antituberculous medica-

tions and is administered for 18 to 24 months. Initially, Streptomycin, PAS, and Isoniazid were used, and later Rifampicin and Ethambutol were introduced (81). A combination of Rifampicin, Ethambutol, and Isoniazid has been successfully used in the treatment of genital tract tuberculosis (77).
- *Surgical treatment* following the failure of drug therapy is much higher in those women who had received short drug courses of therapy than in those who had received longer ones (82). Tubal reconstructive surgery for posttuberculosis tubal occlusion yields very poor outcomes (79).
- *In vitro fertilization* represents a useful treatment, with a rate of 28.6% of intrauterine pregnancies (83).

No specific recommendation is present in the form of complementary or alternative therapy for genital tract tuberculosis.

Other Causes of Salpingitis

Tubal Actinomycosis

Tubal actinomycosis is an inflammatory response to actinomycetes infection. It is a rare disease, and its pathogenesis is poorly understood. Actinomycetes are a natural habitant of the female genital tract. Due to this fact, identification of this microorganism in the vagina or cervix by means of Pap smear or culture, or a specific immunofluorescence technique cannot demonstrate pathology of the genital tract, nor does it have any predictive value for potential pelvic infection (84).

Some authorities divide actinomycotic infection, based upon clinical symptoms and therapeutic implications, into the following categories:

1. *Reactive infection*, which is associated with the use of an IUD and causes endocervicitis, endometriosis, pelvic infection, and tuboovarian abscess formation

The diagnosis is based on clinical symptoms such as vaginal discharge, abnormal endometrial bleeding, lower-abdominal-pelvic pain, and fever.

Physical examination may document elevated core body temperature, tachycardia, and lower abdominal tenderness with or without rebound tenderness.

Pelvic examination may reveal vaginal discharge, cervical and uterine tenderness to palpation and motion, tender adnexal areas, or the presence of an adnexal mass.

Laboratory tests can assist in establishing the diagnosis of genital tract actinomycosis, including the following:

a. A culture with anaerobic media and technique is often confirmatory.
b. Gram stain is suggestive.
c. Specific actinomycocyte immunofluorescence test can be suggestive.
d. Pap smear can be suggestive.

e. Histological examination with a special silver stain will reveal sulfur-granules.

Conventional therapy of reactive actinomycosis of the female genital tract is with antimicrobial drugs such as Penicillin, Tetracycline, Clindamycin, or Chloramphenicol, and IUD removal. Ordinarily, Penicillin is administered parentally in high dose for a 6-week course. Doxycycline is frequently added at the time of initial therapy. Medically conservative therapy appears to be quite effective even in shrinkage of the tubo-ovarian abscess; although, TOA often requires surgical intervention either by performing adnexectomy or TOA drainage, which is usually combined with antibiotics. IUD reinsertion can be offered to the patient following 4 to 8 weeks of an effective therapy (85).

2. *Nonreactive infection* or actinomycotic colonization is the asymptomatic colonization of the vagina, and it is considered natural vaginal flora; therefore, no therapy is required, nor is IUD removal (84,85). The consequences and management of asymptomatic Actinomyces-like organisms continues to be controversial and recent clinical data indicate that 294 Actinomyces-like organisms have been isolated (86). Whether or not coincidental findings of the presence of actinomyces on routine cervical cytologic smears should constitute an indication for IUD removal is an open question; some clinicians support removal (87), and others do not (84).

3. *Pseudoactinomycotic granules* are a condition identified histologically when PAS or Grocott-Kossa-staining is used; nevertheless, it is not a true infection, and no therapy or IUD removal should be offered (85).

Tubal Schistosomiasis

Schistosomiasis is a tubal granulomatous infection caused by helminthic ova of *Schistosoma haematobium* (most common) and *Schistosoma mansoni* eggs (88).

Travelers to endemic areas usually acquire schistosomiasis of the female genital tract in the United States and other industrialized countries. An early state of this parasitosis is asymptomatic or presents with hematuria and progresses to fever, dysuria and/or urinary frequency, neurological symptoms, and genital dysesthesias (89,90).

Laboratory tests include the following (91):

1. Detection of *Schistosoma haematobium* ova in urine
2. Detection of *Schistosoma haematobium* in vaginal lavage
3. Serum-circulating antigen
4. Histological verification

Initial clinical results indicate that Praziquantel, 40 mg/kg in a single dose, may be effective therapy (91); although, there is a lack of randomized controlled data to establish the safety and efficacy of this mode of therapy.

Sequelae of this infection fall into the following categories, particularly when there is a delay in diagnosis and treatment (92,93):

1. Tubal ectopic pregnancy
2. Infertility
3. Asherman's syndrome induced by schistosomiasis (tuberculosis can also cause the syndrome)

POSTTUBAL STERILIZATION SYNDROME

Posttubal sterilization syndrome is defined as the presence of emotional and physical symptomatology as the sequelae of tubal surgical sterilization.

The syndrome is characterized by:

1. Premenstrual physical and emotional distress
2. Menstrual dysfunction (prolonged and heavy menstrual bleeding)
3. Dysmenorrhea

Most well-designed, controlled studies have not determined significant changes to support the relationship between tubal sterilization and the occurrence of the syndrome, except in women who undergo tubal sterilization between 20 and 29 years of age (94). Therefore, the tubal sterilization procedure after the age of 30 has only a remote potential to produce the posttubal sterilization syndrome.

Conventional therapy is initial conservative treatment with nonsteroidal antiinflammatory drugs combined with oral contraceptive. If this management fails to relieve symptoms or symptoms are very severe, laparoscopic or laparotomy salpingectomy is recommended.

Recently, it has been reported that this syndrome has been more frequently observed in association with endometrial ablation and a history of tubal sterilization (95). However, there is no convincing data available in the literature to verify the validity of this observation.

BENIGN TUBAL NEOPLASIA

The prevalence of tubal benign masses is low and is scantly represented in the literature. Most of these masses are typically incidental findings observed during unrelated surgical intervention or at autopsy. The presence of tubal lesions may cause severe clinical consequences (tubal torsion, hematosalpinx or ectopic pregnancy, or heterotopic pregnancy); diagnostic processes and clinical management are not clearly established.

Tubal Endosalpinx Hyperplasia

Tubal endosalpinx hyperplasia (mucosal epithelial proliferation) is defined as overgrowth (proliferation) of the endosalpinx. The presence of this condition in the Fallopian tubes and its clinical significance have not yet been determined. This condition may cause total obliteration of the oviducts. The condition is observed in about 4.5% of the excised tube, when an examination is performed during a tubal ligation procedure of a healthy woman. Prevalence increases to 35% to 46% when associated with other benign or malignant lesions of the genital tract such as ectopic pregnancy, salpingitis, uterine leiomyomata, and other benign tubal disorders or gynecologic tumors. The diagnostic clinical process and clinical management have not yet been established. Hysterosalpingogram may determine occluded Fallopian tubes in an infertile patient. If reconstructive surgery is performed, histological examination may incidentally document the presence of endosalpinx hyperplasia (96).

Tubal Leiomyomata

Tubal leiomyoma of the oviduct arises from either smooth muscle of the tubal muscular layer or smooth muscle of blood vessels. The occurrence of this mass of the Fallopian tube is rare, and most are asymptomatic (97).

Symptoms are nonspecific and may manifest as abdominal-pelvic pain. On pelvic examination, an adnexal mass can be present and can be confirmed ultrasonographically as a solid mass located outside of the uterus. Intraoperative findings consist of the presence of a firm mass within the Fallopian tube. The tube can be twisted with edematous changes (98). The definitive diagnosis is established by histology.

It has been reported that the presence of tubal leiomyoma may predispose to tubal torsion, ectopic pregnancy, or heterotopic pregnancy (97–99).

Tubal Adenofibroma

The presence of benign glands and smooth muscle constitute an adenofibroma tumor of the Fallopian tube. It is a very rare, benign mass and can affect one or both tubes. The diagnosis is reached by histological examination. Simple tumor excision with tubal preservation is recommended (100). Also, cystadenofibroma in nonpregnant and pregnant women has been reported (101). The tumor is benign and may affect fimbriated segments of the Fallopian tube (102).

OTHER TUBAL BENIGN NEOPLASIA

- *Tubal inclusion cyst* results from invigilation of the tubal serosa. It is a gross cyst or complex of cysts of 1 to 2 mm in diameter present on the surface of the tubal serosa. Usually, intraoperative findings are of no clinical significance (103).
- *Tubal idiopathic pigmentosus* causes infertility by complete tubal occlusion. Usually, the condition is diagnosed by histology; hysterosalpingogram demonstrates tubal blockage and laparoscopy may lead to establishing the diagnosis of this extremely rare condition (104).

- *Tubal hematosalpinx* has been reported to be associated with torsion of the Fallopian tube. The condition may occur with no identifiable predisposing factors and at a young age (105).
- *Tubal polyps*, or epithelial papillomas, occur infrequently. They are often associated with an inflammatory process within the tube and may cause infertility by obstructing the lumen of the Fallopian tube (106).
- *Tubal benign cystic teratoma* as a primary lesion of the Fallopian tube is extremely uncommon and can be observed in reproductive age women. The size of the mass varies from 1 to 2 cm to 10 to 20 cm, which often fills the tubal lumen (107). A well-differentiated tumor comprises mesodermal, ectodermal, and endodermal rudiments and may be associated with subfertility (108) or ectopic tubal pregnancy (107) or intrauterine pregnancy (110), or may not be associated with pregnancy.

When small, tubal mature teratoma remains asymptomatic, but may cause infertility by tubal obstruction. A larger tumor may cause pelvic pain, and pelvic examination may reveal a pelvic mass. Ultrasonographic examination and laparoscopic evaluation usually leads to the diagnosis of a tubal mass. The definitive diagnosis is established by histology.

Conventional therapy is conservative surgical intervention.

MALIGNANT TUBAL NEOPLASIA

Primary Fallopian Tube Carcinoma

Definition

Fallopian tube malignancy is defined as a transformation of the oviduct tissue to malignant neoplastic lesion.

Incidence

The prevalence of primary Fallopian tube carcinoma is estimated at 0.3% (range, 0.1% to 0.5%) of all gynecological malignant neoplasia. Most commonly, tubal cancer is observed in the sixth decade, but it has been reported to occur between ages of 18 to 80. The Fallopian tube is a common site of metastatic disease and accounts for approximately 80% to 90% of tubal malignant neoplasia (109).

Etiology

The etiology of Fallopian tube carcinoma is unknown. It is a rare, biologically aggressive tumor. It has been postulated that its aggressiveness correlates with TP53 gen mutation and p53 immunopassivityAQ[10]. It shows a relationship with short-term survival in primary Fallopian tube cancer. Also, it is hypothesized that TP53 gen mutation may play a role in the risk of malignant transformation in various forms of tubal hyperplasia (110).

The occurrence of posthysterectomy Fallopian tube carcinoma has also been reported (111).

Classification

General classification of the Fallopian tube carcinoma proceeds as follows:

- Primary tubal carcinoma
- Secondary or metastatic carcinoma tubal carcinoma

Additionally, malignant tubal carcinoma is classified based upon its histological origin and falls into the following categories by the World Health Organization:

I. Epithelial malignant tumors
   A. Serous carcinoma
   B. Mucinous carcinoma
   C. Endometrioid carcinoma
   D. Clear cell carcinoma
   E. Transitional cell carcinoma
   F. Squamous cell carcinoma
   G. Undifferentiated and other
II. Mixed epithelial-mesenchymal tumors
   A. Mesodermal (Müllerian) mixed tumor
      1. Homologous (carcinosarcoma)
      2. Heterologous
III. Mesenchymal tumors
   A. Leiomyosarcoma
   B. Others

Diagnosis

Pertinent medical history is quite consistent but not specific, and a patient may report the following:

- Watery vaginal discharge, often bloody
- Intermittent lower abdominal-pelvic pain of a colicky type
- Vaginal bleeding that is usually noticed in advanced disease (111)
- Hydrops tubae profluens or an occasional release of watery, tinted discharge from hydrosalpinx

Physical examination is usually within normal limits in the early stage of malignancy; nevertheless, ascites and abdominal mass can be appreciated in the advanced stage.

Pelvic examination may identify firm adnexal mass.

Imaging studies such as ultrasonography, CT, or MRI may document the presence of an adnexal or isolated tubal mass.

Cytology may suggest the presence of adenocarcinoma; even though, it is not a reliable tool for screening tubal malignancy (111).

Culdocentesis material may document the presence of tubal malignancy.

Laparoscopic or culdoscopic evaluation may assist in reaching the diagnosis.

Histology of the tissue will provide definitive diagnosis of tubal carcinoma.

The *staging system* of tubal carcinoma is similar to ovarian staging, due to the remarkable similarity in biological characteristics. Also, management for tubal carcinoma is based on malignant ovarian neoplasia. In 1992, the International Federation of Gynecology and Obstetrics (FIGO) proposed a staging system for tubal carcinoma (Table 21.1) (112).

To differentiate between primary and secondary tubal carcinoma, the following criteria have to be met (113):

1. The core of the tumor must be within the tube by gross evaluation.
2. Tubal mucosa must be primarily involved, with a papillary pattern on microscopic examination.
3. The transition between benign and malignant tubal epithelium should be present, when the tubal wall is involved extensively.

TABLE 21.1. FIGO FALLOPIAN TUBE STAGING

Stage	Description
0	Carcinoma *in situ* (limited to tubal mucosa).
I	Growth limited to the Fallopian tubes.
IA	Growth limited to tube with extension into submucosa and/or muscularis but not penetrating serosal surface; no ascites.
IB	Growth limited to both tubes with extension into submucosa and/or muscularis but not penetrating serosal surface; no ascites.
IC	Tumor either stage IA or IB with extension through or onto tubal serosa or with ascites containing malignant cells or with peritoneal washings.
II	Growth involving one or both Fallopian tubes with pelvic extension.
IIA	Extension and/or metastases to the uterus and/or ovaries.
IIB	Extension to other pelvic tissue.
IIC	Tumor either stage IIA or IIB with ascites containing malignant cells or with peritoneal washings.
III	Tumor involving one or both tubes with peritoneal implants outside pelvis and/or positive retroperitoneal or inguinal nodes. Superficial liver metastasis equals stage III. Tumor appears limited to true pelvis but with histologically proved malignant extension to small bowel or omentum.
IIIA	Tumor grossly limited to true pelvis with negative nodes but with histologically confirmed microscopic seeding of abdominal peritoneal surface.
IIIB	Tumor involving one or both tubes with histologically confirmed implants of abdominal peritoneal surface, none exceeding 2 cm in diameter. Lymph nodes are negative.
IIIC	Abdominal implants >2 cm in diameter and/or positive retroperitoneal or inguinal nodes.
IV	Growth involving one or both Fallopian tubes with distant metastases. If pleural effusion is present, cytological fluid must be present for malignant cells to be stage IV. Parenchymal liver metastases equals stage IV.

Differential Diagnosis

Differential diagnosis of Fallopian tube carcinoma includes the following:

- Ovarian tumor
- Uterine tumor
- Another pelvic mass

Conventional Therapy

Conventional initial therapy is surgery. Upon entering the abdominal cavity, the following steps should be undertaken:

1. Abdominal fluid, if present, should be aspirated for cytology evaluation.
2. Washing material for cytologic examination should be obtained from left and right colonic gathers, the hepatic and spleen flexure, and the posterior cul-de-sac of Douglas.
3. Abdominal content should be inspected by visual examination and by palpation, with biopsy of any lesion.
4. Diaphragmatic inspection with biopsy of any abnormality should be performed (a laparoscope can be used to enhance visualization).
5. Omental inspection and biopsy, when indicated should be performed.
6. In the classic approach, a total hysterectomy with bilateral salpingo-oophorectomy is usually executed. Tubal carcinoma infiltration to the endocervix or upper vagina will require radical hysterectomy with omentectomy and pelvic/paraaortic lymphadenectomy.

The importance of lymph node metastasis and its influence on the overall survival rate is not well understood, and there are only a few, conflicting results in the literature. Appropriate staging of tubal carcinoma can be established only on the basis of pelvic/paraaortic lymphadenectomy; therefore, performing radical hysterectomy, bilateral salpingo-oophorectomy, omentectomy, and pelvic/para-aortic lymph node dissection is recommended at the present time (114).

External irradiation has been used and reported, yet the positive therapeutic outcome of this modality is not well documented.

Intraperitoneal installation of ^{32}P (phosphorus 32) following surgery is advocated to control peritoneal dissemination, although limited clinical evidence supports this therapeutic modality (115).

Chemotherapy with multiple agents may cause regression of advanced disease (116); however, clinical validation of such claim is absent. Second-look laparotomy may provide useful prognostic information in patients with tubal cancer; approximately 80% of patients who have a negative second-look following platin-based chemotherapy will remain disease-free (117).

In general, the prognosis in Fallopian tube carcinoma is poor. Early diagnosis followed by surgical treatment provides optimal results. The overall 5-year survival rate is estimated to about 38% (118). It has been postulated that poor prognosis in tubal carcinoma correlates with early lymphatic metastasis. Therefore, radical lymphadenectomy is suggested to improve the survival rate (119).

OTHER TUBAL CARCINOMA

- *Gestational choriocarcinoma* of the Fallopian tube has been reported following ectopic tubal pregnancy. The conventional chemotherapy regimen with Methotrexate is recommended and provides satisfactory results (120).
- *Primary tubal transitional cell carcinoma* (urothelial carcinoma) arising from tubal epithelium is extremely uncommon. Surgical intervention (total abdominal hysterectomy, bilateral salpingo-oophorectomy, pelvic/paraaortic lymphadenectomy, and omentectomy), followed by cisplatin-based adjuvant chemotherapy is suggested. This form of primary tubal carcinoma has good prognosis (121,122).
- *Primary tubal leiomyosarcoma* is a very rare and aggressive malignant neoplasm. Clinical manifestations of Fallopian tube sarcomas are usually nonspecific and comprise lower abdominal-pelvic pain and pelvic pressure. A median age of diagnosis is 47 years (range, 21 to 70 years). Conventional therapy is surgery, and chemotherapy or radiation can be of some benefit. In general, prognosis is poor; nevertheless, long-term survival has been reported (123).
- *Tubal malignant mixed Müllerian tumors* occur least commonly in the Fallopian tube. The median age at diagnosis is 59 years. Lower abdominal-pelvic pain often is present, but it is not a specific symptom. Pelvic or abdominal tumor is present in approximately 75% of cases. Diagnosis is usually made at the time of exploratory surgery, and histology provides verification of the type of excised tumor. Conventional therapy is surgery with postoperative radiation and/or chemotherapy. Platin-based chemotherapy may improve the outcome, although only limited clinical data are available (124).

In general, complementary or alternative treatment for tubal carcinoma has not been offered.

TUBAL ECTOPIC PREGNANCY

Tubal ectopic pregnancy is a subject that is customarily analyzed in abnormal obstetrics under the broader scope of ectopic pregnancy. Since the Fallopian tubes are the most common site of ectopic pregnancy location, a summary of this condition is presented here. For more detailed information on this subject, please consult obstetrical textbooks.

Tubal pregnancy is a part of ectopic pregnancy that can be defined as a product of conception implants that occurs elsewhere than within the endometrium.

The *incidence* of ectopic pregnancy is estimated at 19.7 occurrences per 1,000 pregnancies in North America, with a 98.3% location in the Fallopian tube, distributed as 79.6% ampulla, 12.3% isthmus, 6.2% fimbriae, and 1.9% interstitial area (location in the abdominal cavity occurs in approximately 1.4%, and in 0.15% at the ovarian and cervical location) (125). Ectopic pregnancy is a leading cause of maternal mortality in the first trimester and is estimated in 0.4 per 1,000 ectopic pregnancies (126).

The *etiology* of ectopic pregnancy is unknown. Altered tubal function may compromise a fertilized ovum migration through the tubal lumen. Clinically identified predisposing factors fall into the following categories (127,128):

- Tubal reconstructive operations may increase predisposition for ectopic pregnancy 21-fold.
- Prior ectopic pregnancy causes a six- to eight-fold increase of ectopic pregnancy.
- Tubal infection (particularly chlamydia or gonorrhea) and its sequelae increase the ectopic pregnancy prevalence 3.5-fold.
- Salpingitis isthmica nodosa
- *In utero*–exposed diethylstilbestrol increases the possibility of ectopic pregnancy fivefold.
- IUD
- Vaginal douching minimally increases the risk for ectopic pregnancy.
- Cigarette smoking slightly increases the risk of ectopic pregnancy.

Classification of ectopic pregnancy is based on the site of location and is categorized as follows:

1. Tubal pregnancy
2. Abdominal cavity pregnancy
3. Ovarian pregnancy
4. Cervical location
5. Heterotopic pregnancy, defined as the simultaneous presence of an intrauterine and extrauterine pregnancy

Diagnosis of early ectopic pregnancy has significantly increased due to better recognition and knowledge of potential risk factors, heightened awareness of patients, increased index of suspicion by clinicians, improved sensitivity of biochemical markers such as serum quantitative beta-human chorionic gonadotropin (beta-hCG) immunoassay, and improved ultrasonography technology.

Symptoms of ectopic pregnancy are frequently reported as the presence of oligomenorrhea or, exceedingly rarely, amenorrhea, abnormal uterine bleeding, and lower abdominal-pelvic unilateral or (less often bilateral) pain. An asymptomatic course is frequently present, particularly at the early stages of extrauterine pregnancy. When shoulder pain is reported, with or without syncope, a ruptured ectopic pregnancy with hemoperitoneum can be suspected. Occasionally, a patient can be seen in hemodynamic shock due to excessive bleeding.

Signs of abdominal tenderness and, to a lesser extent, rebound tenderness can be identified. Pelvic examination is nonspecific, but may reveal spotting or uterine bleeding, cervical tenderness to motion, fullness, the presence of a unilateral adnexal mass, and tenderness.

The diagnosis of ectopic pregnancy can be summarized as follows:

- Serum beta-hCG levels of >1,500 mIU/mL and the absence of an intrauterine gestational sac documented by transvaginal ultrasonography (TVS) raise suspicion for ectopic pregnancy. Multiple pregnancies may have higher serum beta-hCG levels. Serum beta-hCG levels and TVS should be repeated 3 days later, and an increasing serum beta-hCG level with the absence of an intrauterine pregnancy on TVS highly suggests ectopic pregnancy. Such results and the presence of an adnexal mass increase the possibility of an ectopic pregnancy.
- Serum beta-hCG levels of <1,500 mIU/mL and no intrauterine pregnancy present by TVS examination warrant the repetition of these examinations twice per week (beta-hCG levels are expected to double within 48 hours during the initial 6 to 7 weeks of pregnancy). Nondoubling beta-hCG levels within that time period may suggest an ectopic pregnancy or an abnormal intrauterine pregnancy.
- Serum progesterone levels of <5 ng/mL (15.9 nmol/L) suggest a nonviable pregnancy and warrant uterine evacuation to exclude spontaneous abortion (the absence of chorionic villi is suggestive of ectopic pregnancy). Levels of >25 ng/mL (79.5 nmol/L) indicate intrauterine pregnancy in about 97.5%.

In selective cases, culdocentesis (needle aspiration of the posterior cul-de-sac content) is performed; if unclotted blood is retrieved, one should consider the diagnosis of ectopic pregnancy.

Conventional therapy presents various types of treatment:

1. Expectant management is usually recommended for asymptomatic patients with serum beta-hCG levels of <1,000 mIU/mL and with a trend of decreasing levels. It is appropriate to closely observe and wait.
2. *Medical treatment* can be considered for hemodynamically stable patients with an unruptured tubal pregnancy, when the TVS measurement of the gestational sac does not exceed 4 cm, and when there is no fetal heart beat present, and when serum beta-hCG levels are <5,000 mIU/mL. The following laboratory tests should be performed before the initial dose of Methotrexate is administered:

- Complete blood count
- Blood type and Rh with titer
- Liver and renal function tests
- Serum quantitative beta-hCG
- TVS

Before treatment is initiated, it is important for the patient to do the following:

- Discontinue folic acid if taken for supplementation.
- Refrain from sexual intercourse.
- Reduce vigorous exercise.
- RhoGAM, 300 microgram single dose, should also be administered intramuscularly when indicated for the Rh-negative patient without titer elevation

A single dose treatment is offered as follows (129):

- *Methotrexate,* 50 mg/m^2 intramuscularly, is administered (low-dose). The serum beta-hCG level is determined on day 4 following the initial injection. On day 7, the serum beta-hCG level and TVS are obtained. If the quantitative beta-hCG levels drop to <25% of preinjection levels, a second identical dose is injected. Weekly serum quantitative beta-hCG levels are determined until the level drops to <10 mIU/mL. Also, weekly TVS is recommended. If TVS demonstrates intraperitoneal fluid of >100 mL or severe or acute abdominal pain is present, either laparoscopic or laparotomy intervention is indicated.
- Methotrexate, 1 mg/kg (high-dose), is recommended, but extreme caution should be exercised when treating interstitial gestations with single dose Methotrexate (130).

Multiple doses seem to be more reliable and are administered as follows:

- *Methotrexate,* 1 mg per kilogram body weight intramuscularly, is administered on alternated days: 1, 3, 5, and 7 days. To reduce Methotrexate's toxic effects following high-dose therapy, Leucovorin calcium, 0.1 mg/kg intramuscularly, is added on the alternate days 2, 4, 6, and 8. Follow-up with serum quantitative beta-hCG levels on a weekly basis until levels drop to >10 mIU/mL and with TVS is performed to determine intraabdominal fluid levels; when fluid levels are >100 mL or when severe or acute abdominal pain occurs, either laparoscopic or laparotomy intervention is indicated.

3. Surgical treatment is divided into the following:

   a. Conservative surgery or tubal preservation operation presents an outcome similar to radical surgery; nevertheless, the recurrence rate is higher with the conservative approach. The following conservative surgery for tubal pregnancy is generally accepted:

- *Fimbrial expression* requires unruptured tubal pregnancy located within the fimbriated end of the tube.
- *Linear salpingectomy* (a 1- to 1.5-cm longitudinal incision is made on the distended antimesosalpinx surface of the Fallopian tube) is designated for unruptured tubal pregnancy located in the ampulla. The procedure should be avoided when uncontrollable bleeding is present, when there is a recurrent pregnancy in the same tube, or pregnancy exceeds 5 cm, when a severely damaged tube is

identified, or when reproductive capacity is not a concern.

- *Tubal segmental resection* is usually performed when the pregnancy is located in the isthmus.

b. *Radical surgery* for ectopic pregnancy is salpingectomy with contralateral tubal preservation. Total hysterectomy is often performed in the interstitial or cervical location. A conservative procedure can be offered even through the laparoscopic approach, although it requires considerable laparoscopic skill and experience (31). In light of the current ability to reach diagnosis in an early stage and the available conservative medical therapies, there is very little room for total hysterectomy.

Today, early diagnosis and the laparoscopic approach almost eliminate laparotomy from the surgical armamentarium. A meta-analysis of randomized studies documented that laparoscopic intervention, for conservative surgical management of tubal extrauterine pregnancy, offers compatibility with laparotomy long-term outcome (tubal patency and future fertility). Yet, it is significantly less effective in the short-term; as primary treatment success, persistent tubal ectopic pregnancy, and re-intervention for clinical symptoms or persistent ectopic tubal pregnancy (132).

REFERENCES

1. Association of Professors of Gynecology and Obstetrics (APGO). *Medical student educational objectives,* 7th ed. Washington, DC: APGO, 1997.
2. Council on Resident Education in Obstetrics and Gynecology (CREOG). *Educational objectives core curriculum for residents in obstetrics and gynecology,* 5th ed. Washington, DC: CREOG, 1996.
3. American College of Obstetricians and Gynecologists (ACOG). *Technical bulletin no. 183.* Washington, DC: ACOG, 1996.
4. Bransilver BR, Franczy A, Richart RM. Female genital tract remnants. An ultrastructural comparison of hydatid of Morgagni and mesonephric ducts and tubules. *Arch Pathol* 1973;96:255–261.
5. Crosby EC, Humphrey T, Lauer EW. *Corrective anatomy of the nervous system.* New York: Macmillan, 1962.
6. Jansen RPS. Cyclic changes in the human fallopian tube isthmus and their functional importance. *Am J Obstet Gynecol* 1980;136:292–308.
7. Jansen RPS. Endocrine response in the fallopian tube. *Endocr Rev* 1984;5:525–542.
8. Surrey ES. Falloposcopy. *Obstet Gynecol Clin North Am* 1999;26:53–62.
9. Mastroianni L Jr. The fallopian tube and reproductive health. *J Pediatr Adolesc Gynecol* 1999;12:121–126.
10. Knab DR, Blanco LJ. Müllerian duct agenesis with a unilateral functioning segment of the rudimentary uterine horn. *Am J Obstet Gynecol* 1978;132:222–224.
11. Faber M, Mitchell GW Jr. Bicornuate uterus and partial atresia of the fallopian tube. *Am J Obstet Gynecol* 1979;134:881–884.
12. Zaitoon MM, Florentin H. Crossed renal ectopia with unilateral agenesis of fallopian tube and ovary. *J Urol* 1982;128:111–113.
13. Tulusan AH. Complete absence of the muscular layer of the

ampullary part of the fallopian tubes. *Arch Gynecol* 1984;234: 279–281.

14. Silverman AY, Greenberg EI. Absence of the proximal portion of the tube. *Obstet Gynecol* 1983;62:90S–91S.

15. Beyth Y, Kopolovic J. Accessory tubes: a possible contributing factor in infertility. *Fertil Steril* 1982;38:382–383.

16. DeCherney AH, Cholst I, Naftolin F. Structure and function of the fallopian tubes following exposure to diethylstilbestrol (DES) during gestation. *Fertil Steril* 1981;36:741–745.

17. Daw E. Duplication of the uterine tube. *Obstet Gynecol* 1973;442:137–138.

18. Bernardus RE, Van der Slikke JW, Roex AJM, et al. Torsion of the fallopian tube: Some consideration on its etiology. *Obstet Gynecol*1984;64:675–678.

19. Krissi H, Orvieto R, Dicker D, et al. Torsion of a fallopian tube following Pomeroy tubal ligation: a rare case report and review of the literature. *Eur J Obstet Gynecol Reprod Biol* 1997;72: 107–109.

20. Raziel A, Mardechai E, Friedler S, et al. Isolated recurrent torsion of the Fallopian tube: case report. *Hum Reprod* 1999;14: 3000–3001.

21. Barisic D, Bagovic D. Bilateral tubal torsion treated by laparoscopy: a case report. *Eur J Obstet Gynecol Reprod Biol* 1999;86:99–100.

22. Jaluvka V, Entezami M, Becker R, et al. Acute torsion of hydrosalpinx. Two cases after laparoscopic sterilization. *Ultraschall Med* 1995;16:33–35.

23. Bayer AI, Wiskind AK. Adnexal torsion: can the adnexa be saved? *Am J Obstet Gynecol* 1994;171:1506–1510.

24. Kurzbart E, Mares AJ, Cohen Z, et al. Isolated torsion of the fallopian tube in premenarcheal girls. *J Pediatr Surg* 1994;29: 1384-1385.

25. Jamieson MA, Sobolewski D. Isolated tubal torsion at menarche—a case report. *J Pediatr Adolesc Gynecol* 2000;13:93–94.

26. Ferrera PC, Kass LE, Verdile VP. Torsion of the fallopian tube. *Am J Emerg Med* 1995;13:312–314.

27. Thonell SH, Kam A, Resnick G. Torsion of accessory fallopian tube: ultrasound findings in two premenarchal girls. *Australas Radiol* 1993;37:393–395.

28. Filtenborg TA, Hertz JB. Torsion of the fallopian tube. *Eur J Obstet Gynecol Reprod Biol* 1981;12:177–181.

29. Case Record of the Massachusetts General Hospital (Case 9-1971). *N Engl J Med* 1971;248:491–496.

30. Ramin SM, Ramin KD, Hemsell DL. Fallopian tube prolapse after hysterectomy. *South Med J* 1999;92:963–966.

31. Wolfendale M. Exfoliative cytology in a case of prolapsed fallopian tube. *Acta Cytol* 1980;24:545–548.

32. Schmid J, Schreiner WE, Sauberi H, et al. Prolapse of the small bowel through the vaginal vault following hysterectomy. *Geburtshilfe Frauenheilkd* 1983;43:515–516.

33. Wheelock JB, Schneider V, Goplerud DR. Prolapsed fallopian tube masquerading as adenocarcinoma of the vagina in a postmenopausal woman. *Gynecol Oncol* 1985;21:369–375.

34. Letterie GS, Byron J, Salminen ER, et al. Laparoscopic management of fallopian tube prolapse. *Obstet Gynecol* 1988; 72:508-510.

35. Adams BE. Intussusception of a fallopian tube. *Am J Surg* 1969; 118:591–592.

36. Kuzela DC, Speers WC. Heterotopic endometrium of the fallopian tube. *Fertil Steril* 1985;44:552–553.

37. Outwater EK, Siegelman ES, Chiowanich P, et al. Dilated fallopian tubes: MR imaging characteristics. *Radiology* 1998; 208:463–469.

38. Clausen I. Peritoneal endosalpingiosis. *Zentralbl Gynakol* 1991;113:329–332.

39. Santeusanio G, Ventura L, Partenzi A, et al. Omental endosal-pingiosis with endometrial-type stroma in a woman with extensive hemorrhagic pelvic endometriosis. *Am J Clin Pathol* 1999;111:248–251.

40. La Borgne J, Nomballais MF, Lehur PA, et al. Intestinal endosalpingiosis. Apropos of 2 cases. *Ann Chir* 1995;49:73–75.

41. Laufer MR, Heerema AE, Parsons KE, et al. Endosalpingiosis: clinical presentation and follow-up. *Gynecol Obstet Invest* 1998;46:195–198.

42. DeHoop TA, Mira J, Thomas MA. Endosalpingiosis and chronic pelvic pain. *J Reprod Med* 1997;42:613–616.

43. Keltz MD, Kliman HJ, Arici AM, et al. Endosalpingiosis found at laparoscopy for chronic pelvic pain. *Fertil Steril* 1995;64:482–485.

44. Wiedelmann R, Sterzik K, Gombish V, et al. Beyond recanalizatizing proximal tube occlusion: the argument for further diagnosis and classification. *Hum Reprod* 1996;11:986–991.

45. Jenkins CS, Williams SR, Schmidt GE. Salpingitis isthmica nodosa: a review of the literature, discussion of clinical significance, and consideration of patient management. *Fertil Steril* 1993;60:599–607.

46. Wrork DH, Broders AC. Adenomyosis of the Fallopian tube. *Am J Obstet Gynecol* 1942;44:412–432.

47. Beenjamin CL, Beaver DC. Pathogenesis of salpingitis isthmica nodosa. *Am J Clin Pathol* 1951;21:212–222.

48. Honore LH. Salpingitis isthmica nodosa in female infertility and ectopic pregnancy. *Fertil Steril* 1978;29:164–168.

49. Confino E, Tur-Kaspa I, DeCherney A, et al. Transcervical balloon tuboplasty. A multicenter study. *JAMA* 1990;246: 2079–2082.

50. Thurmond AS, Burry KA, Novy MJ. Salpingitis isthmica nodosa: results of transcervical fluoroscopic catheter recanalization. *Fertil Steril* 1995;63:715–722.

51. Houston JG, Machan LS. Salpingitis isthmica nodosa: technical success and outcome of fluoroscopic transcervical fallopian tube recanalization. *Cardiovasc Intervent Radiol* 1998;21:31–35.

52. Soper DE, Brockwell NJ, Dalton HP, et al. Observations concerning the microbial etiology of acute salpingitis. *Am J Obstet Gynecol* 1994;170:1008–1014.

53. Keith LG, Berger GS, Edelman DA, et al. On the causation of pelvic inflammatory disease. *Am J Obstet Gynecol* 1984;149: 215–224.

54. Bjartling C, Osser S, Persson K. The frequency of salpingitis and ectopic pregnancy as epidemiologic markers of *Chlamydia tracomatis. Acta Obstet Gynecol Scand* 2000;79:123–128.

55. Sweet RL, Blankfort-Doyle M, Robbie MO, et al. The occurrence of chlamydia and gonococcal salpingitis during the menstrual cycle. *JAMA* 1986;255:2062–2064.

56. Centers for Disease Control. Sexually transmitted disease guidelines. *MMWR* 1993;42:1–102.

57. Hansen JG, Dahler-Eriksen BS. C-reactive protein and infections in general practice. *Ugesker Laeger* 2000;162:2457–2460.

58. Moore E, Soper DE. Clinical utility of CA 125 levels in predicting laparoscopically confirmed salpingitis in patients with clinically diagnosed pelvic inflammatory disease. *Infect Dis Obstet Gynecol* 1998;6:182–185.

59. Haeusler G, Tempfer C, Lehner R, et al. Fallopian tissue sampling with a cytobrush during hysteroscopy: a new approach for detecting tubal infection. *Fertil Steril* 1997;67:580–582.

60. Judlin PG, Koebele A. Acute salpingitis: current antibiotic protocols. *Contracept Fertil Sex* 1997;25:572–575.

61. Gerber B, Krause A. A study of second-look laparoscopy after acute salpingitis. *Arch Gynecol Obstet* 1996;258:193–200.

62. Landers DV, Sweet RL. Current trends in the diagnosis and treatment of tuboovarian abscess. *Am J Obstet Gynecol* 1985; 151:1098–1110.

63. Henry-Suchet J, Soler A, Loffredo V. Laparoscopic treatment of tuboovarian abscesses. *J Reprod Med* 1984;29:579–582.

64. Wiesenfeld HC, Sweet RL. Progress in the management of tuboovarian abscesses. *Clin Obstet Gynecol* 1993;36:433–444.

65. Choe J, Check JH. Salpingectomy for unilateral hydrosalpinx may improve *in vivo* fecundity. *Gynecol Obstet Invest* 1999;48: 285–287.

66. Watson A, Vandekerekhove P, Liford R. Technique for pelvic surgery in subinfertility. *Cochrane Database Syst Rev* 2000;2: CD000221.

67. Vasquez G, Boeckx W, Brosens I. Prospective study of tubal mucosal lesions and fertility in hydrosalpinges. *Hum Reprod* 1995;10:1075–1078.

68. Scialli AR, from the Pelvic Pain Expert Working Group. A consensus of recommendation. *J Reprod Med* 1999;44:945–952.

69. Garcia Compean D, Blane P, d'Abrigeon G, et al. Fitz-Hugh and Curtis syndrome. *Presse Med* 1995;24:1348–1351.

70. Nogales-Ortiz F, Tarancon I, Nogales FF. The pathology of female genital tuberculosis. A 31-year study of 1436 cases. *Obstet Gyenecol* 1979;53:422–428.

71. Miranda P, Jacobs AJ, Roseff L. Pelvic tuberculosis presenting as an asymptomatic pelvic mass with rising serum CA-125 levels. A case report. *J Reprod Med* 1996;41:273–275.

72. Lueken RP, Bormann C, Scotland V. Genital tuberculosis—increased incidence or coincidence. *Zentralbl Gynecol* 1997;119: 39–41.

73. Mizuno K. Tuberculosis in the field of gynecology. *Nippon Rinsho* 1998;56:3153–3156.

74. Seufert R, Casper F, Bauer H. Genital tuberculosis in the women—only of interest in medical history. *Geburtshilfe Frauenhilkd* 1992;52:56–58.

75. Valentini AL, Summaria V, Marano P. Diagnostic imaging of genitourinary tuberculosis. *Rays* 1998;23:126–143.

76. Parikh FR, Nadkarni SG, Kamat SA, et al. Genital tuberculosis—a major pelvic factor causing infertility in Indian women. *Fertil Steril* 1997;67:497–500.

77. Sutherland AM. Postmenopausal tuberculosi of the female genital tract. *Obstet Gynecol* 1982;59:54S–57S.

78. Weerakiet S, Rojanasakul A, Rochanawutanon M. Female genital tuberculosis: clinical features and trends. *J Med Assoc Thai* 1999;82:27–32.

79. Saracoglu OF, Mungan T, Tanzer F. Pelvic tuberculosis. *Int J Gynaecol Obstet* 1992;37:115–120.

80. Crowley JJ, Ramji FG, Amundson GM. Genital tract tuberculosis with peritoneal involvement: MR appearance. *Abdom Imaging* 1997;22:445–447.

81. Oosthuizen AP, Wessels PH, Hefer JN. Tuberculosis of the female genital tract in patients attending an infertility clinic. *S Afr Med J* 1990;77:562–564.

82. Sutherland AM. The changing pattern of tuberculosis of the female genital tract. A thirty-year survey. *Arch Gynecol* 1983;234:95–101.

83. Soussis I, Trew G, Matalliotakis I, et al. *In vitro* fertilization treatment in genital tuberculosis. *J Assist Reprod Genet* 1998; 15:378–380.

84. Lippes J. Pelvic actinomycosis: a review and preliminary look at prevalence. *Am J Obstet Gynecol* 1999;180:265–269.

85. Horn LC, Bilek K. Reactive and areactive actinomycosis infection of the female genitals and differentiation of pseudoactinomycosis. *Zentralbl Gyneakol* 1995;117:466–471.

86. Sabbe LJ, Van De Merwe D, Schoules L, et al. Clinical spectrum of infections due to the newly described Actinomyces species *A. turicensis, A. radingae, and A. europaeus. J Clin Microbiol* 1999;37:8–13.

87. Dehal SA, Kaplan MA, Brown R, et al. Clinically in apparent tuboovarian abscess in a women with an IUD. A case report. *J Reprod Med* 1998;43:595–597.

88. Feldmeier H, Daccal RC, Martins MJ, et al. Genital manifesta-

89. Crump JA, Murdouch DR, Chambers ST, et al. Female genital schistosomiasis. *J Travel Med* 2000;7:30–32.

90. Laven JS, Vleugels MP, Dofferhoff AS, et al. Schistosomiasis haematobium as a case of vulvar hypertrophy. *Eur J Obstet Gynecol Reprod Biol* 1998;79:213–216.

91. Richter J, Poggensee G, Kjetland EF, et al. Reversibility of lower reproductive tract abnormalities in women with Schistosoma haematobium infection after treatment with praziquantel—an interim report. *Acta Trop* 1996;62:289–301.

92. Nouhou H, Seve B, Idi N, et al. Schistosomiasis of the female genital tract: anatomoclinical and histopathological aspects. Apropos of 26 cases. *Bull Soc Pathol Exot* 1998;91:221–223.

93. Krolikowski A, Janowski K, Larsen JV. Asherman syndrome caused by schistosomiasis. *Obstet Gynecol* 1995;85:898–899.

94. Gentile GP, Kaufman SC, Helbig DW. Is there any evidence for a post-tubal sterilization syndrome? *Fertil Steril* 1998;69: 179–186.

95. Townsend DE, McCausland V, McCausland A, et al. Post-ablation-tubal sterilization syndrome. *Obstet Gynecol* 1993;82: 422–424.

96. Yanai-Inbar I, Silverberg SG. Mucosal epithelial proliferation of the fallopian tube: prevalence, clinical associations, and optimal strategy for histopathologic assessment. *Int J Gynecol Pathol* 2000;19:139–144.

97. Mroueh J, Margono F, Feinkind L. Tubal pregnancy associated with ampullary tubal leiomyoma. *Obstet Gynecol* 1993;81: 880–882.

98. Misao R, Niwa K, Iwagaki S, et al. Leiomyoma of the fallopian tube. *Gynecol Obstet Invest* 2000;49:279–280.

99. schust D, Stovall DW. Leiomyomas of the fallopian tube. A case report. *J Reprod Med* 1993;38:741–742.

100. Chen KT. Bilateral papillary adenofibroma of the fallopian tube. *Am J Clin Pathol* 1981;75:229–231.

101. Valerdiz Casasola S, Pardo Mindan J. Cystadenofibroma of fallopian tube. *Appl Pathol* 1989;7:256–259.

102. Alvarado-Cabrero I, Navani SS, Young RH, et al. Tumors of the fimbriated end of the fallopian tube: a clinicopathologic analysis of 29 cases, including nine carcinomas. *Int J Gynecol Pathol* 1997;16:189–196.

103. Wheeler JE. Disease of the Fallopian tubes. In: Kurman RJ, ed. *Blaustein's pathology of the female genital tract,* 4th ed. New York: Springer-Verlag, 1994:529–561.

104. Bolaji II, Meehan FP. Idiopathic pigmentosis tubae. *Int J Fertil Menopausal Stud* 1994;39:86–89.

105. Furui T, Imai A, Yokoyama Y, et al. Hematosalpinx and torsion of the fallopian tube in a virgin girl. *Gynecol Obstet Invest* 1993; 35:123–125.

106. Gisser SD. Obstructing fallopian tube papilloma. *Int J Gynecol Pathol* 1986;5:179–182.

107. Mazzarella P, Okagaki T, Richart RM. Teratoma of the uterine tube. *Obstet Gynecol* 1972;39:381–388.

108. Lai SF, Lim-Tan SK. Benign teratoma of the fallopian tube: a case report. *Singapore Med J* 1993;34:274–275.

109. Kutteh WH, Albert T. Mature cystic teratoma of the fallopian tube associated with an ectopic pregnancy. *Obstet Gynecol* 1991;78:984–986.

110. Hseih CS, Cheng GF, Liu YG, et al. Benign cystic teratoma on unilateral fallopian tube associated with intrauterine pregnancy: a case report. *Chung Hua I Hsueh Tsa Chih (Taipei)* 1998; 61:239–242.

111. Warshal DP, Burgelson ER, Aikins JK, et al. Post-hysterectomy fallopian tube carcinoma with a positive Papanicolaou smear. *Obstet Gynecol* 1999;94:834–836.

112. Creasman WT. Revision in classification by International Fed-

eration of Gynecology and Obstetrics. *Am J Obstet Gynecol* 1992;167:857–858.

113. Hu CY, Taymor ML, Hertig AT. Primary carcinoma of the fallopian tube. *Am J Obstet Gynecol* 1950;59:58–61.

114. Rosen AC, Klein M, Hafner E, et al. Management and prognosis of primary fallopian tube carcinoma. Austrian Cooperative Study Group for Fallopian Tube Carcinoma. *Gynecol Obstet Invest* 1999;47:45–51.

115. Benedet JL, White GW, Fairey RN, et al. Adenocarcinoma of the fallopian tube. *Obstet Gynecol* 1977;50:654–657.

116. Podczaski E, Herbst AL. Cancer of the vagina and fallopian tube. In: Knapp RC, Berkowitz RS, eds. *Gynecologic oncology.* New York: Macmillan, 1993.

117. Barakat RR, Rubin SC, Saigo PE, et al. Second-look laparotomy in carcinoma of the fallopian tube. *Obstet Gynecol* 1993; 82:748–751.

118. Sedlis A. Carcinoma of the fallopian tube. *Surg Clin North Am* 1978;58:121–129.

119. Klein M, Rosen AC, Lahousen M, et al. Lymphadenectomy in primary carcinoma of the Fallopian tube. *Cancer Lett* 1999; 147:63–66.

120. Logani KB, Sharama S, Kohli TP, et al. Gestational choriocarcinoma of the fallopian tube—a case report. *Indian J Cancer* 1995;32:183–185.

121. Rabczynski J, Kochman A, Hudziec P. Primary urothelial carcinoma of the fallopian tube. *Przeg Lek* 1998;55:572–575.

122. Takeuchi S, Hirano H, Ichio T, et al. A case report: rare case of primary transitional cell carcinoma of the fallopian tube. *J Obstet Gyneaecol Res* 1999;25:29–32.

123. Jacoby AF, Fuller AF, Thor AD, et al. Primary leiomyosarcoma of the fallopian tube. *Gynecol Oncol* 1993;51:404–407.

124. Weber AM, Hewett WF, Gajewski WH, et al. Malignant mixed müllerian tumors of the fallopian tube. *Gynecol Oncol* 1993;50: 239–243.

125. Breen JL. A 21-year survey of 654 ectopic pregnancies. *Am J Obstet Gynecol* 1970;106:1004–1019.

126. Tenore JL. Ectopic pregnancy. *Am Fam Physician* 2000;61: 1080–1088.

127. Ankum WM, Mol BWJ, Van der Veen F, et al. Risk factors for ectopic pregnancy; a meta-analysis. *JAMA* 1996;65:1093–1099.

128. Carr RJ, Evans P. Ectopic pregnancy. *Prim Care* 2000;27: 169–183.

129. Carson SA, Buster JE. Ectopic pregnancy. *N Engl J Med* 1993; 329:1174–1181.

130. Gherman RB, Stitely M, Larrimore C, et al. Low-dose methotrexate treatment for interstitial pregnancy. A case report. *J Reprod Med* 2000;45:142–144.

131. Ostrzenski A. A new laparoscopic technique for interstitial pregnancy resection. *J Reprod Med* 1997;42:363–366.

132. Hajenius PJ, Mol BW, Bossuyt PM, et al. Interventions for tubal ectopic pregnancy. *Cochrane Database Syst Rev* 2000;2: CD000324.

22

BENIGN OVARIAN DISORDERS

EDUCATIONAL OBJECTIVES

Medical Students (1)	*Residents in Obstetrics/Gynecology (2)*	*Practitioners (3)*
APGO Objective No. 59	*CREOG Objective*	*ACOG Recommendation*
Ovarian neoplasia	No specific recommendation	No specific recommendation
Patient evaluation with an		
adnexal mass		
Characteristics of:		
Functional cyst		
Benign neoplasms		

OVARIAN EMBRYOLOGY

Genetically predetermined by 46,XX chromosomes at the time of conception, the product of conception will develop ovaries (see Chapter 4). Ovarian embryonic development commences at 4 weeks of postconceptional life. Medially to the mesonephric ridge, the genital ridge initiates its development. Initially, the genital ridge has two components of embryonic tissues: the inner core of mesenchyme and the thick outer layer of coelomic tissue. The mesenchymal cell condensation creates the primitive sex cord. In addition to the mesenchymal and coelomic epithelium, the primordial germ cells are necessary to complete ovarian development.

The mesenchymal epithelium will create the ovarian stroma and the ovarian theca. The ovarian stroma is additionally divided into the cortex (the follicles are scattered irregularly throughout the superficial cortex) and the medulla. In the outer-superficial cortex, condensation of fibrotic tissue is typically more accentuated than elsewhere; this portion is termed the "tunica albuginea." Within the ovarian stroma, a variety of other cells can be found such as enzymatically active stromal cells, endometrial stroma-type cells, or smooth muscle cells. The ovarian stroma becomes functionally mature and able to respond to gonadotropin stimulation with steroidogenesis.

The coelomic epithelium will create the granulosa cells and the surface ovarian epithelium.

The primordial germ cells will eventually progress to differentiate into primordial follicles (approximately 400,000 are present at birth), which comprise oocytes (40 to 70 micromillimeters and surrounded by granulosa cells).

The undifferentiated gonad begins differentiating into the female gonad at about 12 weeks of embryonic life. Insertion of the coelomic epithelium into the ovarian mesenchymal epithelium creates the secondary sex cords (the cortical sex cords). The primordial follicles are generated when primordial germ cells invade the secondary sex cords and became oogonia. Oogonia undergo mitosis that pauses and eventually transforms from oogonia to primary oocytes. Primary oocytes enter the first meiotic division in the prophase stage and remain in this stage until puberty. From then on, they can be recruited for the maturation and ovulation process. Granulosa cells originate from the secondary sex cords and surround the primary oocyte. The primordial follicles are formed from granulosa cells and oocytes. Fetal ovaries are not hormonally active. Differentiation from primordial follicle to mature ovarian follicle is depicted in Fig. 22.1.

Ovarian follicular function and ovulation are presented in Chapter 11.

OVARIAN ANATOMY

The mature ovary is an ovoid, pair organ, which is on average 3.0 to 5.0 cm in length, 1.5 to 3.0 cm in width, and 0.6 to 1.5 cm in thickness. It weighs 5 to 8 g. The normal anatomical location of the ovaries is on either side of the

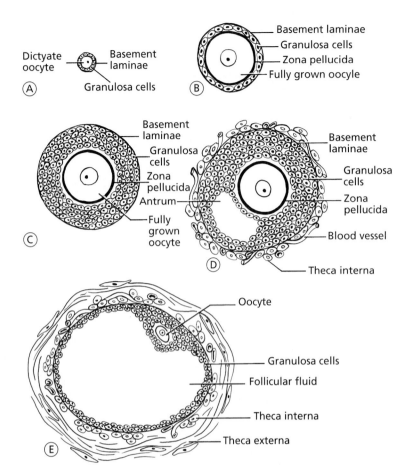

FIG. 22.1. Ovarian follicle development. **A:** Primordial follicle. **B:** Primary follicle. **C:** Primary follicle. **D:** Secondary follicle. **E:** Mature ovarian follicle (ripe Grafian follicle).

uterus, behind the broad ligament, and anteriorly to the rectum. Ovarian suspension is provided by the following structures (Fig. 22.2):

1. *The mesovarium* is a double fold of the peritoneum, which attaches the anterior margin of the ovary to the posterior surface of the broad ligament. The anterior ovarian margin is also termed the "ovarian hilus," through which blood vessels and nerves enter the ovary.
2. *The utero-ovarian ligament* (the ovarian ligament) is the fibromuscular structure, which suspends the ovarian medial inferior pole to the cornual segment of the uterus.
3. *The infundibulopelvic ligament* (the suspensory ligament) suspends the ovarian superior pole from the lateral pelvic wall.

The ovarian artery and the branches of the ascending *uterine artery* supply ovarian blood. The ovarian arteries are direct branches from the aorta and take off just below the renal artery bilaterally. They traverse obliquely downward and laterally over the psoas major muscle and the ureter, and enter the infundibulopelvic ligament. Upon reaching the infundibulopelvic ligament, they give off small arterial branches to the Fallopian tube. The main branch of the ovar-

ian artery reaches the ovary through the ovarian hilus. Within the ovary, the ovarian artery divides two separate medullary arteries. One branch supplies each opposing ovarian pole. Also, the main artery anatomizes with the ascending branch of the uterine artery to create approximately 10 arterial arcade branches, which penetrate the ovarian hilus. The arteries in the medullary part of the ovarian stoma are the coiled type of arteries, which become straight arterioles in the ovarian cortex and run in a radial arrangement. Arterioles create vascular arcades, from which a small but dense network is created to supply blood to the ovarian follicles.

Blood return is drained from the ovarian cortex to the medulla, where veins became large and tortuous. They connect together in the ovarian hilus, developing the plexus, which conducts vein blood from the ovary to the ovarian veins. The ovarian vein runs within the mesovarium and traverses along the infundibulopelvic ligament. The right ovarian vein returns blood directly to the inferior vena cava, and the left ovarian vein drains to the left renal vein.

Ovarian lymphatic channels initiate in the theca layer of the follicle and then traverse through the ovarian stroma and connect with larger in diameter lymphatics in the ovarian hilus. Upon parting from the ovary, lymphatics join the

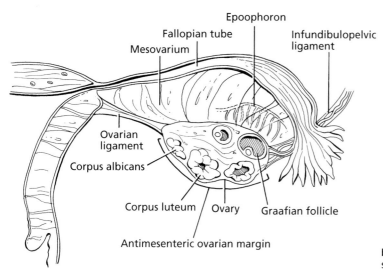

FIG. 22.2. The ovary, ovarian suspension, and adjacent structures.

Fallopian tube, and the uterine corpus branches. The major lymphatic ovarian drainage is in the cephalic aortic nodes. Accessory channels also are present and can be identified in the internal and external iliac lymph nodes and even in the inguinal lymph nodes.

Ovarian innervention comprises of the aortic and renal sympathetic plexuses. Also, the celiac and mesenteric ganglia supply nerves to the ovary.

OVARIAN FUNCTION AND ITS DISORDERS

Ovarian function and its disorders as well as genetic ovarian disorders are presented in Chapters 2, 3, 4, 8, and 11.

BENIGN OVARIAN DISORDERS

Ovarian Nonneoplastic Ovarian Cysts (Functional)

Benign nonneoplastic ovarian disorders can be categorized as follows:

- Follicular ovarian cysts
- Corpus lutein cysts
- Theca-lutein cysts

Follicular Ovarian Cyst

Failure of the follicle to regress and continue to grow is considered a follicular ovarian cyst. Current literature supports the hypothesis that angiogenesis participates in various (polycystic ovary, ovarian stimulation syndrome and other benign and malignant neoplasms) ovarian pathologic processes, including follicular cyst formation (4). It is a general clinical consensus that ovarian dysfunction with anovulation will result in follicle enlargement and eventually will form a cyst. Follicular ovarian cyst is a frequent clinical occurrence and can be identified in any age from birth to the postmenopausal period. Shortly after the postneonatal period, a follicular cyst can be present and is related to maternal estrogen stimulation during pregnancy. Also, prenatal follicular cyst can be diagnosed during obstetrical ultrasonography of a mother (5). These cysts usually spontaneously regress shortly after delivery. Clinical features of follicular ovarian cyst are different in the prepubertal period than in puberty. Before the age of 7 years, girls may display precocious pseudo-puberty with low pituitary gonadotropin levels associated with the presence of follicular cysts (5) or central precocious puberty with the presence of a follicular cyst as a result of gonadotropin elevation and stimulation (6). After the age of 10 years, abnormal menses, acute abdominal pain, and pelvic mass are dominant clinical characteristics (5). In healthy adolescent girls, follicular ovarian cyst formation is observed in approximately 12.2%, and all of them will spontaneously regress within the first 3-month period (7).

The potential risk of follicular ovarian cyst development in association with tamoxifen therapy for breast cancer in postmenopausal women has been also reported. The possible mechanism of tamoxifen induction of follicular cyst is direct stimulation of the granulosa cells within the follicle (8).

The diagnosis of follicular ovarian cyst is based upon different clinical features in the different age groups. *Before the age of 7* years, precocious puberty is the chief reported symptom. *After the age of 10* years, abnormal menses and abdominal-pelvic pain are leading symptoms. *Adolescent* and *reproductive age* women will report symptoms of menstrual cycle irregularity and abdominal-pelvic pain. Nevertheless, an asymptomatic course of follicular ovarian cyst is also observed. Acute abdominal pain with nausea and vomiting can be present in association with ovarian torsion.

Physical examination may disclose the presence of an abdominal mass when a cyst reaches the pelvic rim. Muscle guarding and rebound tenderness can be present when ovarian or adnexal torsion has developed.

Pelvic examination may reveal an adnexal cystic mass with various degrees of tenderness.

Ultrasonography will document a solitary (unilocular) thin-walled cyst filled with clear fluid. The cyst is usually under 5 cm in diameter, but it may attain a size of 8 to 9 cm or even greater (clinically, a follicular cyst is defined as a size of >2.5 cm).

Magnetic resonance imaging (MRI) will provide not only the characteristics of the follicular cyst but also distinct features of the ovarian stroma (9).

Histological verification will provide definitive diagnosis.

Differential diagnosis. includes other ovarian cystic masses; particular attention should be given to a complex cystic ovarian mass when cystic and solid components are present. A cystic complex mass may represent a potential for harboring malignancy.

Conventional therapy. of a follicular ovarian cyst falls into the following approaches:

1. *Ovarian cystectomy or oophorectomy* is indicated when torsion of the ovary or adnexa occurs (5) in precocious pseudopuberty (autonomous follicular ovarian cyst with no pituitary gonadotropin elevation), before the age of 7 years. Such an approach is advised to iradicate symptoms and signs of precocious puberty (5,10). Attention should be given to exclude central precocious puberty (pituitary gonadotropin elevation), since pelvic surgical intervention by means of cystectomy or oophorectomy will be inappropriate (6). In girls over the age of 10, management will fall into general management modality for an ovarian cyst.
2. *Close clinical observation,* including ultrasonography for 1 to 3 months, is the first line of management in the majority of cases, since spontaneous resolution may occur, particularly when a cyst is small (<5.5 cm) (5,10,11).
3. *Conservative medical management* with a low dose of oral contraceptive and oral pain medication, as indicated, for 3 months may be of help. Close clinical follow-up with appropriate patient education is necessary, so the early symptoms of ovarian torsion will not be overlooked. Such an approach is recommended for women in their reproductive period, but it is inappropriate for pediatric patients and postmenopausal women.
4. *Surgical management* is occasionally necessary when spontaneous rupture of the cyst with intraperitoneal bleeding, a cyst persisting for over three months (malignant tumors must be excluded), and severe symptoms are present. There is a potential risk of ovarian torsion, which can occur in about 17.8% in girls and young women (12), or of malignancy, when the cyst is of a large size. The principal approach for surgical intervention for ovarian cyst is laparotomy exploration. Minilaparotomy can be considered as an initial step, since it presents the option of extending the minilaparotomy to a full-size laparotomy, if necessary, for potential oncologic exploration. Also, minilaparotomy can be performed in an outpatient (ambulatory) setting, is safe, is a quick procedure for the management of ovarian cysts, and avoids intraperitoneal spill and potential seeding of malignant cells (13). Laparoscopic ovarian cystectomy or ovariectomy can be executed; however, it should be discouraged when an ovarian mass is present, due to the potential risk of peritoneal dissemination of the malignant content of an ovarian cyst (14,15). Laparoscopic control of ovarian bleeding following rupture of follicular cysts is recommended. Also, transcutaneous ovarian cyst aspiration with ultrasonographic guide or laparoscopic cyst aspiration is not recommended, not only for the obvious oncological reason but also because of the high recurrence rate following aspiration (16).
5. *Ovarian hyperstimulation* caused by infertility drugs with large and multiple follicular cyst formation may occur. The therapy requires medical conservative, supportive treatment in most of the cases (17) (see Chapter 11).

Corpus Luteum Cyst

Corpus luteum cyst is a functional cyst that may occur during the female reproductive period, including both the periods of pregnancy (18), and that of puerperium (19).

The symptomatology and clinical characteristics are very similar to those of the follicular ovarian cyst, including the sonographic appearance and the natural clinical course (spontaneous regression occurs within 1 to 2 months). Corpus luteum cyst may require ovarian cystectomy for hemorrhagic rupture associated with bleeding or torsion. Conservative medical management does not depart from that for the follicular ovarian cyst. Corpus luteum cyst histologically presents as luteinized granulosa and theca internal cells, and these features distinguish it from follicular ovarian cyst, in which the inner layer of the cyst is composed from granulosa cells and the outer layer comprises theca internal cells. In the physiological event, during the menstrual cycle, the corpus luteum is spontaneously converted to the corpus albicans, which rarely becomes a cyst.

Theca-Lutein Cyst

Theca-lutein cyst is a functional cyst and represents the least common occurrence among functional ovarian cysts. Theca-lutein cysts frequently accompany in conditions, in which beta-human chorionic gonadotropin (beta-hCG) secretion is elevated. Clinical behavior does not depend entirely on changes in beta-hCG levels, for it has been shown that these cysts can persist for as long as 15 to 18 weeks after beta-hCG regression. In postmolar trophoblastic disease, bilateral theca-lutein cysts occur frequently. Hydatidiform mole, choriocarcinoma, and pregnancy, particularly multiple pregnancies, are often associated with this condition. The mean cyst size is 7.3 cm (range, 3 to 20 cm); the size itself does not correlate with postmolar trophoblastic disease. The characteristic histologic feature of the cyst wall is the presence of theca cells, with or without luteinization. Infrequently, theca-lutein cysts can be associated with "hyperreactio luteinalis," a condition that can mimic ovarian malignancy. A wedge ovarian biopsy and frozen section, to avoid unnecessary extirpative surgical intervention, will establish the definitive diagnosis. Clinical sequelae of theca-lutein cysts are not serious and sooner or later will spontaneously resolve after the underlying cause is eradicated and sometimes after beta-hCG has ceased. Clinically, serial sonograms and beta-hCG levels provide necessary information for safety management (20–23).

All ovarian functional cysts may frequently present as "chocolate cysts," which can develop from ovarian follicles. At any time when bleeding within a functional cyst occurs, chocolate cysts can develop. Grossly, such cysts resemble endometriotic chocolate cysts, so clinical misdiagnosis of endometriosis may happen. Serial transvaginal ultrasonography or biochemical analysis of the cyst's fluid may assist in reaching the differential diagnosis between functional chocolate cyst and endometriotic cyst (24,25).

Complementary and alternative therapies can be considered in the management of functional cysts, since cyst formation results frequently from anovulation. Relevant clinical suggestions are presented in Chapters 3 and 11.

Benign Neoplastic Ovarian Tumors

Germ Cell Tumors

- Mature cystic teratomas
- Stroma ovarii
- Mature solid teratomas

Mature Cystic Teratomas
Definition. Mature teratoma (dermoid cyst) is a benign cystic neoplasia that consists of ectodermal, mesodermal, and endodermal layers of germ cells.

Incidence. In general, the overall incidence of dermoid cyst is unknown. It is a common ovarian tumor in childhood and in young women (26). Those tumors account for 25% to 40% of all ovarian masses, with only a 15% prevalence in the postmenopausal period; malignancy within tumors occurs in approximately 19% (27). Also, the occurrence of mature teratoma has been reported as late as in the eighth decade of life (28).

Etiology. A totipotential (the single cell potential to develop in any direction) single germ cell development in benign ecto-, meso-, or endo-dermal tissue may occur. The tumor can be present unilaterally or bilaterally (10.8%), with the rate of malignant transformation being approximately 0.17%. Larger tumors undergo torsion approximately 3.5% more than the cases involving smaller tumors (29). Malignant transformation to squamous cell carcinoma and adenocarcinoma (30) occurs, although occasionally other forms such as spindle-cell sarcoma or trabecular carcinoid will occur (31).

Classification. In general, teratomas are divided into the following categories:

- Mature cystic teratoma (benign ovarian neoplasia)
- Immature teratoma (malignant ovarian neoplasia)

Diagnosis. Most mature teratomas, up to approximately 60% of them, are asymptomatic (29). Pertinent medical history is lower abdominal-pelvic pain in the remaining patients. When ovarian or adnexal torsion occurs, acute abdominal pain associated with nausea and vomiting can be reported (32–34). Sporadically, virilization can be associated with ovarian dermoid cyst; nevertheless, it is an infrequent occurrence (35).

Physical examination may establish the presence of a nontender abdominal mass. When torsion or rupture occurs, spillage of sebaceous material from the cyst may produce a chemical granulomatous peritonitis (36) and signs of acute abdominal pain may develop. A ruptured dermoid cyst may produce symptoms of peritonitis such as diffuse abdominal pelvic tenderness, abdominal muscles guarding, rebound tenderness, and decreased bowl sounds.

Pelvic examination will identify a nontender pelvic mass in most cases, with the mean tumor size 6.4 ± 3.5 cm (29). Frequently, the anterior cul-de-sac can be occupied by the tumor. When ovarian torsion takes place, the pelvic area, including the tumor, becomes very tender.

Imaging studies such as ultrasound present characteristic features of dermoid cyst, and plain abdominal radiography may document the presence of teeth or boney structures (32). Recently, transvaginal color Doppler ultrasonographic characterization of benign and malignant ovarian cystic teratomas has been postulated for differential diagnosis; although, it will require clinical validity (37).

Blood tests may document the presence of a hemolytic type of anemia, which usually resolves after removing the tumor (38,39).

Histological verification establishes definitive diagnosis. Rokitansky's protuberance (a nodule within the tumor, where different types of tissues are present) should be carefully examined, since it is a common site of malignancy occurrence. Grossly, within the tumor all three embryologic tissue components are represented in different proportions (ecto-, meso-, and endo-dermal tissues) and usually comprise the elements of skin, hair, fragments of extremities, bones, and teeth.

Differential Diagnosis. Differential diagnosis of dermoid ovarian cyst includes the following:

- Immature teratomas
- Omental dermoid cyst (40)
- Benign or malignant tubal tumors
- Other benign or malignant ovarian tumors
- Pedunculated uterine or intraligamentary leiomyomata

Conventional Therapy. Conventional therapy for benign ovarian mature teratomas is surgical intervention executed through classic laparotomy or laparoscopic approach. The following surgical treatments are recommended:

1. Ovarian cystectomy alone
2. Ovariectomy
3. Salpingo-oophorectomy
4. Hysterectomy with salpingo-oophorectomy

When laparoscopy is contemplated, the potential risk of teratoma containing malignancy and potential chemical peritonitis due to spillage of the cyst irritative content should be considered. The malignant component of the tumor can be ruled out by histologic verification only. Nevertheless, preoperatively the use of serum tumor markers combined with diagnostic imaging technology may provide diagnostic clinical featured indicating, to some degree, the benign character of a dermoid ovarian cyst (36); however, it is not absolutely convincing evidence to exclude the presence of mature teratoma containing a malignant element.

Although, the laparoscopic removal of dermoid ovarian cyst is associated with a high spillage rate, the prevalence of chemical peritonitis is low and is estimated to be 0.2% in retrospective observational studies (41). The absence of randomized controlled study results makes this procedure unproven in safety and efficacy.

Stroma Ovarii

Stroma ovarii is an infrequent ovarian teratoma comprised either entirely or in part of thyroid tissue. It may present as a cystic structure with or without a solid component (42, 43). The definitive diagnosis rests on the histological verification, although imaging technology, including MRI, can be helpful preoperatively (44).

Symptoms of hyperthyroidism such as nervousness, heart palpitation, emotional lability, insomnia, heat intolerance, frequent defecation, excessive perspiration, menstrual irregularity (oligomenorrhea or secondary amenorrhea), apathy, increased appetite, and diarrhea can be reported. Also, recurrent pelvic pain can be associated with struma ovarii.

Signs of hyperthyroidism may include warm, moist, velvet skin, the presence of Plummer's nails (fingernails separate from the nail bed), silky hairs, erythematous palms, and weight loss. A pelvic mass can be appreciated on pelvic examination. Infrequently, benign struma ovarii may produce acute pseudo-Meigs' syndrome with elevated serum CA-125 levels (45).

Laboratory tests of thyroid hormone (TSH, T3, and T4) imbalance, associated with adnexal mass, may strongly indicate this condition.

Conventional therapy is surgical extirpation of the tumor and has a very favorable outcome. Shortly after removing the tumor, complete resolution of symptoms and signs, including hydrothoraces and ascites, as well as of laboratory abnormalities are usually noticed (42–45).

Solid Mature Teratoma

Solid mature teratoma derives from the three germ cell layers and comprises only mature tissues. Due to the solid character of the tumor, the clinical impression is malignancy. Solid mature teratoma can be associated with gliomatosis peritonei, which introduces a further suggestion of malignant spread of the ovarian tumor to the peritoneum and/or omentum. Gliomatosis peritonei is a benign condition, in which multiple nodular implants of mature glial tissue on the visceral and parietal peritoneum and/or omentum occur. In light of the malignant clinical picture, extensive intraoperative sampling is essential to exclude the presence of immature teratoma, which will require not only more aggressive therapy but will also carry a poor prognosis.

The diagnosis is difficult due to lack of specific symptoms or signs. Most of the patients are asymptomatic until tumor-size–related symptomatology occurs (mainly lower abdomen-pelvic pain with various characterizations of pain).

Physical examination may identify the presence of a nontender abdominal mass when a tumor reaches the size to be palpable in the abdominal cavity.

Pelvic evaluation will determine a solid adnexal mass ranging in size from a small to a massive tumor. At the time of diagnosis, it is usually large. The tumor has a slow growing pace and is unilaterally located.

Imaging studies and laboratory tests are similar to those presented for mature cystic teratoma.

Histological verification of the mature nature of the tumor and peritoneal seedlings are necessary before the appropriate surgical intervention is selected.

Conventional therapy is surgical extirpation of the tumor; due to the large size at the time of diagnosis usually, oophorectomy or salpingo-oophorectomy is often necessary. Prognosis for cure of solid mature teratoma with or without gliomatosis peritonei is good, and conservative surgical management with reproductive capacity preservation is recommended, since it is a benign condition (46–49).

Epithelial Cell Neoplasia

Benign epithelial cell neoplasia can be classified as follows:
1. Serous tumors
   a. Serous cystadenomas

b. Cystadenofibromas (it is debatable whether or not this type should be classified as serous cystadenomas)
c. Serous adenofibromas
2. Mucinous tumors
    a. Mucinous cystadenomas
    b. Mucinous cystadenofibroma
    c. Mucinous adenofibromas
3. Endometrioid tumors
    a. Endometrioid benign cysts
    b. Adenoma
    c. Cystadenofibroma
    d. Adenofibroma
4. Brenner cell tumor

Serous Cystadenoma

Serous cystadenoma is a benign tumor arising from the ovarian epithelium. It is the most frequent ovarian mass among epithelial tumors—approximately 20% of all ovarian tumors in the reproductive period, yet pediatric and postmenopausal cases have been reported. Serous cyst adenoma is predominantly unilaterally located; nevertheless, in about 10% to 15% of cases, the tumor can be identified bilaterally. The tumor usually grows asymptomatically and reaches a large size before it is diagnosed.

The diagnosis is suggested by the presence of lower abdomen-pelvic discomfort, pelvic pressure, and increasing abdominal girth.

Imaging technology plays an essential role not only in establishing the diagnosis but also in differentiating clinically between a benign and malignant serous cystadenoma. Accuracy for the overall characterization of benign versus malignant tumors appears to be not significantly different between MRI and CT (86% with MRI and 92% with CT). The sensitivity of CT is significantly higher when compared with that of ultrasonography (50,51).

Often ultrasonography reveals a unilocular or multilocular ovarian cyst with smooth walls; although, projections from the cyst wall can be observed, particularly in cystadenofibroma.

Grossly, the serous cyst is a large structure with smooth walls (papillary projections can be present), filled with serous fluid. Histology demonstrates a single layer of cuboidal epithelium with a base location of the nuclei and the absence of mitosis.

Cystadenofibroma constitutes about half of all benign serous cysts; it is a rare, benign tumor, which is predominantly diagnosed in the fourth and fifth decades (at a mean age of 53 years) (52). The tumor has very little malignant potential, even when epithelial atypia is present (53).

Ultrasonography and macroscopic intraoperative appearance highly suggests a malignant process (54); therefore, frozen section examination should be obtained before selecting an aggressive surgical approach, especially in young patients (55).

Serous adenofibromas are benign solid tumors of epithelial origin, consisting of small gland-like shapes of various size, surrounded by the dense fibrotic-connective tissue of the ovarian stroma. It resembles an ovarian fibroma. The tumor is rarely seen in gynecologic practice.

Conventional therapy is conservative surgery—either ovarian cystectomy when the tumor is small or ovariectomy with contralateral preservation of the ovary when the tumor is large and the ovarian tissue is destroyed.

In postmenopausal women, total hysterectomy with bilateral salpingo-oophorectomy is performed not only because of the potential risk of future malignancy but also because of the risk of developing serous epithelial nonmalignant neoplasia in the remaining ovary.

Neither complementary nor alternative surgery is presently recommended for serous benign tumors.

Mucinous Cystadenomas

Mucinous cystadenoma is an ovarian epithelial benign cystic tumor that has the ability to produce mucin. Two types of tissues exist: that resembling the endocervical-type epithelium and the gastrointestinal-type epithelium responsible for mucin production. Either one of them or both can be represented in mucinous cystadenoma. The prevalence of this tumor has not been pinpointed, although it is estimated to occur in approximately 20% of all benign ovarian neoplasms. In young adult women, mucinous cystadenomas occur as frequently as 50%, among benign ovarian neoplasia; yet, they are most commonly observed between the ages of 30 and 50 years. In approximately 5% of cases, the ovaries are bilaterally affected.

On gross examination, such a cyst is 10 to 39 cm in size and multiloculated with a smooth wall; occasionally, papillary projections can be present. Histology comprises a single layer of tall columnar epithelium with mucin-containing cytoplasm with nucleus located at the base.

Cystadenofibromas and adenofibromas are extremely uncommon tumors.

Clinical diagnosis is based on findings similar to those presented above.

Conventional therapy is a surgically conservative approach analogous to that used in a serous-type tumor.

Pseudomyxoma peritonei (PMP) is defined as the presence of mucin-type (gelatinous material) peritoneal implants. Recently, a new concept in origin and nomenclature has been offered. Currently, PMP can be viewed as two pathologically and prognostically distinct disease processes. The following classification of pseudomyxoma peritonei is suggested (56):

1. *Disseminated peritoneal adenomucinosis* is characterized by the presence of copious mucinous peritoneal implants in the abdominal cavity, similar to ascites (the classical clinical syndrome of pseudomyxoma peritonei). The condition can be attributed to a ruptured appendical mucinous adenoma in the vast majority of cases. This

condition has an indolent course when treated surgically, but may recur over months or years.

2. *Peritoneal mucinous carcinomatosis* presents with mucinous tumors and has clinical manifestations similar to those of adenomucinosis. Histology demonstrates gastrointestinal mucinous adenocarcinoma characteristics. The prognosis is significantly worse than in adenomucinosis.

3. *Intermediate histologic features*, their clinical manifestation and clinical course, are very similar to cases of pure peritoneal carcinomatosis.

Frequently, women have concomitant ovarian mucinous tumors that suggest primary ovarian neoplasia. However, morphologic, molecular, and immunohistochemical data support the view that the ovarian tumors are secondary and that appendiceal adenomucinosis is a primary tumor (56). Occasionally, pseudomyxoma peritonei can also be associated with a malignant tumor of the ovary or colon (57).

The clinical diagnosis is based on diffused abdominal pain and gastrointestinal symptoms. Ultrasonography and CT will suggest the diagnosis of PMP, and histological examination provides the definitive diagnosis (56,57).

Conventional therapy is either exploratory laparotomy with debulking of implants or peritoneal lavage for removal of the gelatinous implants (58).

Endometrioid Tumors

A benign ovarian endometrioid tumor looks like neoplasia of endometrial origin (endometrial-like glandular tissue) with epithelial and/or stromal components. It is an extremely rare tumor, and this fact is reflected in scarce data present in the literature (mainly, only case reports are present).

Cystadenofibroma is primarily located unilaterally; although, bilateral occurrence has also been reported (59). It occurs most commonly in the fourth to fifth decades, with a median age of 57 years; although, the tumor has been reported in patients as young as 17 years old. Grossly, the tumor is on average 10 cm in diameter and has a smooth wall. The interior structure of the mass resembles a honeycomb, and there is a polypoid nodule within the cyst. The long-term malignant potential of the endometrioid cystadenofibroma has not yet been established, even in cases linked with proliferating atypia (59–61).

Endometrioid adenofibroma of the ovary is an equally rare tumor. This tumor is characterized by proliferation of endometrial-type glands without atypical cells within the dense and thick stroma (62).

Conventional therapy for endometrioid tumors is cystectomy or ovariectomy. When the tumor is not removed completely, growth of the mass may continue.

Brenner Tumors

A benign solid Brenner's ovarian tumor arises from the ovarian epithelium and, through a metaplastic process, trans-

forms into urothelial-like epithelium. Among ovarian tumors, the prevalence of the tumor is approximately 0.23% (63). It occurs in the late premenopausal and postmenopausal periods (the tumor has been reported even in the eighth decade of life) and usually is unilateral, but it may be present bilaterally as well, as seen in about 5% of the cases.

Grossly, this solid tumor presents as white, whirled, and with a size of 2 to 20 cm in diameter. Histologic examination reveals cells that look like coffee beans with longitudinal grooves in the nucleus. Occasionally, cystic structures with solid components can be identified (63,64). The tumor is considered benign; nevertheless, malignant tumors of the ovary have been reported (63,65). Brenner tumors, therefore, can display benign, borderline, and malignant variations, but the vast majority of the tumors are benign (66). In about one-third of cases, Brenner tumors occur ipsilaterally. They can be associated with mucinous cystadenomas and cystic teratomas.

Histological verification establishes the definitive diagnosis. Preoperatively, MR and CT may document extensive amorphous calcification in a solid mass or a solid component in a multilocular cystic mass (67,68).

Conventional therapy for benign Brenner tumor is conservative surgical tumor extirpation with ovarian preservation. Ovariectomy is indicated when the tumor is large enough to destroy ovarian tissue. In postmenopausal women, total hysterectomy with bilateral salpingo-oophorectomy is indicated.

Benign Sex Cord–Stromal Ovarian Tumors

Ovarian Fibroma

Benign ovarian fibromas are gynecologic tumors with a prevalence of about 1% to 3% of all ovarian tumors (69). The tumor can grow at any age, including in premenarcheal girls, and during the reproductive and postmenopausal periods (but most commonly in postmenopausal women). It is predominantly unilaterally located (77% in the left ovary), but bilateral occurrence has been reported (70). On gross examination, the average size at diagnosis is about 9 cm; the tumor is white, smooth-surfaced, and solid, with a cystic area within the tumor (69). The tumor can be associated with a classic form of the Meigs' syndrome or abdominal ascites only (the pseudo-Meigs' syndrome). Meigs' syndrome is a rare clinical condition characterized by the presence of ovarian tumor, ascites, and hydrothorax (71). Usually, a patient presenting with Meigs' or pseudo-Meigs' syndrome and an adnexal mass raises the question of malignancy. Histological confirmation is mandatory to exclude malignant neoplasia.

Presumptive clinical diagnosis is based on the presence of a pelvic mass, since the condition is often asymptomatic (72).

Imaging technology, including plain radiographs, ultrasound, CT, and MRI, can document the presence of a pelvic mass (72,73).

Blood tests may document elevation of serum CA-125 levels, which additionally may suggest a malignant process (74).

Conventional therapy is guided by the benign nature of the lesion and consists of tumor extirpation. This course of action is taken because of the notion that there is a risk of recurring fibromas.

Thecomas

Thecomas are regarded as benign tumors of the sex cord–stroma origin. They are very similar to ovarian fibromas, and frequently it is difficult to differentiate those two.

The clinical diagnosis is based on the tumor's ability to secrete estrogens, which leads to abnormal postmenopausal endometrial bleeding or a variety of menstrual irregularities, including metrorrhagia, in the reproductive period (75). Lower abdominal-pelvic symptoms such as pain, pressure, and abdominal swelling are usually related to the presence of a pelvic mass (76).

Imaging studies will document the ovarian origin of the tumor. Radiography may reveal the presence of extensive calcification within adnexa, particularly in young women (77).

Laboratory tests will establish a hypoestrogenic state.

Conventional therapy is surgical extirpative conservative intervention with preservation of the reproductive capacity in young women.

Fibrothecomas

Ovarian fibrothecoma is composed of both thecal cells and fibroblasts of ovarian stromal origin. It is a benign ovarian tumor, and, regardless of having thecal cell components, fibrothecomas are hormonally inactive [thecoma tumors themselves are estrogen producing (75)].

The diagnosis is reached on the clinical presence of adnexal mass. Ultrasonographic findings, even though nonspecific, can provide a clinician with useful information preoperatively (78). MRI may display a relatively specific appearance (79).

Serum levels of Ca-125 tumor marker can be elevated over 200 UI/mL, suggesting ovarian malignancy; tumor markers will return to normal values shortly after tumor removal.

Conventional therapy is surgical removal of the tumor, oophorectomy, or total hysterectomy with bilateral salpingo-oophorectomy, depending upon the patient's age.

Mesenchymal Benign Ovarian Tumors

Ovarian Leiomyoma

Primary ovarian leiomyoma is a tumor probably originating from the smooth muscles of blood vessels within the ovary. The prevalence is very low (81). Usually it is unilateral, small, and concomitant with uterine leiomyomata. It ranges in size from only a few millimeters to being a massive tumor (82,83). The tumor has been diagnosed bilaterally (83,84). Primary ovarian leiomyoma, in most cases, are asymptomatic and can affect women between the second and eighth decade of life, though they are commonly diagnosed in the postmenopausal period (82,85,86).

Ovarian leiomyoma grossly presents itself as a solid, white tumor and may demonstrate degenerative processes identical to those of uterine leiomyomata (87).

The diagnosis can be made on pelvic examination if a tumor is large enough to be appreciated on pelvic bimanual examination. In most instances, ovarian leiomyoma are found incidentally.

Ultrasonography and/or MRI can be a useful tool in documenting the presence of an ovarian solid mass (81,87); definitive diagnosis is reached by histological confirmation.

Conventional therapy is surgical tumor extirpation or oophorectomy in young women. In postmenopausal women, total hysterectomy with bilateral salpingo-oophorectomy is recommended (88).

Neither complementary nor alternative therapy is suggested for this entity.

Ovarian Hemangioma

Ovarian hemangioma or ovarian angioma originates from ovarian vessels. This tumor is extremely rare, with size ranging from 3 mm to 10 cm (89,90). The reported ages of occurrence are from 30 to 80+ (90,91). A small sized tumor is asymptomatic; as the tumor increases in size, symptoms such as pelvic pain and pelvic pressure may occur (90). A routine workup for a pelvic mass is required preoperatively. Conventional therapy is tumor removal, adnexectomy, or total hysterectomy with bilateral salpingo-oophorectomy, depending on the patient's age.

Other Benign Ovarian Tumors

- *Germinal inclusion cyst* originates by invagination of the ovarian surface epithelium through the opening caused by ovum expulsion as the last step of the ovulation process. These cysts may occur at any age; they are not hormonally active or dependent. Germinal inclusion cyst does not fluctuate in size during the menstrual cycle and is not responsive to OC suppression. The persistent character of the cyst usually leads to surgical exploration. Definitive diagnosis is established by histology, which documents the flat or columnar, or cuboidal epithelium. The diagnosis of this pelvic mass is documented by the standard evaluation of adnexal mass. Due to the persistent natural behavior of the cyst, tumor markers are recommended. Simple cyst excision (cyst enucleation is difficult to achieve) is definitive therapy.
- *Endometrioma* is presented in Chapter 9.
- *Polycystic ovarian syndrome* is detailed in Chapter 8.
- *Ovarian hyperthecosis* is described in Chapter 8.

Adnexal Mass Evaluation

The essence of adnexal mass evaluation is to exclude malignant neoplasia. Although, the definitive diagnosis of any pelvic mass is histological confirmation, the preoperative workup may suggest benign versus malignant characteristics of a mass and may decrease the number of aggressive surgical interventions in nonneoplastic (functional) ovarian cyst.

The presence of a pelvic or adnexal mass is determined or confirmed by the following imaging technology:

1. *Ultrasonography* not only documents the presence of a pelvic mass but also will distinguish a solid tumor from a cyst or a complex mass (cystic and solid components within the same tumor). A transvaginal ultrasonographic transducer significantly improves the sensitivity and specificity of preoperative clinical diagnosis of a pelvic mass. Ultrasonographic evaluation may also provide information relating to the tumor and its effect on adjacent pelvic structures, and may demonstrate pelvic fluid collection. The evidence of negative predictive value of malignancy can be established with an accuracy of 95.6%. The positive predictive value evidence of malignancy can be reached in about 73% (92) of cases by depicting suspicious features for malignancy within an adnexal mass such as a complex ovarian mass, multiloculated cyst, or irregular protrusion from the surface wall. In current practice, sonography is an indispensable technology for the evaluation of a pelvic mass in women, including masses of the ureter and kidney.
2. *Magnetic Resonance Imaging* is an exceptional technology, particularly in soft tissue evaluation, and provides more specific information. Recently, preoperative evaluation with MRI has become more frequently used in adnexal mass evaluation.
3. *Computed Tomography* can assist, particularly in pelvic and periaortic nodes evaluation. CT for an adnexal mass evaluation is not often used.
4. *Radiographic intravenous pyelogram* is a useful modality in evaluating the urinary tract in relation to a pelvic mass and its effect on the ureter and the kidney.
5. *Plain radiographs* are frequently used, particularly when mature ovarian teratoma are clinically suspected.

Laboratory tests include the following:

1. Routine tests such as CBC with differential, ESR, SMA-20, platelets, PT, and PTT should be done. The presence of hypercalcemia may indicate a malignant neoplasia (93).
2. Tumor markers play an important role in the preoperative workup for an adnexal mass. The sensitivity and specificity of tumor markers are not sufficient enough to exclude or include malignancy with certainty (e.g., Ca-125 can be elevated above 35 mIU/mL in endometriosis, pelvic infections, and benign ovarian cyst). Tumor markers can enlighten the existing potential risk of

TABLE 22.1. OVARIAN TUMOR MARKERS

Serum Tumor Marker	Ovarian Tumor
AFP (alpha-fetoprotein)	Endodermal sinus tumors Embryonal carcinoma Mixed germ tumors (immature teratoma) Polyembryoma
CEA (carcinoembryonic antigen)	Not specific for ovarian cancer
CA-125	All types of nonmucinous epithelial tumors Immature teratoma
CA-19-9	Mucinous epithelial ovarian carcinoma
hCG (human chorionic gonadotrophin)	Choriocarcinoma Embryonal carcinoma Mixed germ tumors Polyembryoma
LDH (lactate dehydrogenase)	Dysgerminoma Mixed germ cell tumor
Estradiol	Granulosa cell tumor Thecomas
Testosterone	Sertoli's cell tumor Leydig's cell tumor

malignancy preoperatively and also may play a significant role in evaluating a therapeutic progress in selective malignant neoplasia. Table 22.1 presents the usefulness of tumor markers in ovarian tumors.

Diagnostic laparoscopy—is used to determine the origin of the pelvic mass (adnexa v/s uterus or other pelvic mass origin), to aspirate pelvic free fluid (not ovarian cyst content) for a cytology and abdominal cavity content for a microbiology study, or to perform peritoneal lesion biopsy, which is a procedure of choice.

Laparoscopic surgical intervention in an ovarian mass is a highly controversial issue. As long as the malignant process of an ovarian tumor (cystic or solid) cannot be excluded preoperatively beyond clinical doubt, the laparoscopic approach is not recommended. It has been observed that intraoperative rupture of malignant epithelial neoplasms may worsen the prognosis of patients with stage I ovarian cancer by upstaging it (94). On the other hand, it is estimated that ovarian masses, including those classified as tumors suspicious for malignancy, are approximately 80% benign (95). Future progress in laparoscopic technique and technological advancement are needed to make laparoscopic approaches safe and effective in oncologic cases.

REFERENCES

1. Association of Professors of Gynecology and Obstetrics (APGO). *Medical student educational objectives,* 7th ed. Washington, DC: APGO, 1997.

2. Council on Resident Education in Obstetrics and Gynecology (CREOG). *Educational objectives core curriculum for residents in obstetrics and gynecology,* 5th ed. Washington, DC: CREOG, 1996.

3. American College of Obstetricians and Gynecologists (ACOG). *Technical bulletin no. 183.* Washington, DC: ACOG, 1996.

4. Abulafia O, Sherer DM. Angiogenesis of the ovary. *Am J Obstet Gynecol* 2000;182:240–246.

5. Liapi C, Evain-Brion D. Diagnosis of ovarian follicular cysts from birth to puberty: a report of twenty cases. *Acta Paediatr Scand* 1987;76:91–96.

6. Arisaca O, Shimura N, Nakayama Y, et al. Ovarian cysts in precocious puberty. *Clin Pediatr (Phila)* 1989;28:44–47.

7. Poreu E, Venturoli S, Dal Prato L, et al. Frequency and treatment of ovarian cyst in adolescence. *Arch Gynecol Obstet* 1994; 225:69–72.

8. Terada S, Uchide K, Susuki N, et al. A follicular cyst during tamoxifen therapy in a premenopausal breast cancer woman. *Gynecol Obstet Invest* 1993;35:62–64.

9. Outwater EK, Mitchell DG. Normal ovaries and functional cysts: MR appearance. *Radiology* 1996;198:397–402.

10. Fakhry J, Khoury A, Kotval PS, et al. Sonography of autonomous follicular ovarian cyst in precocious pseudopuberty. *J Ultrasound Med* 1988;7:597–603.

11. Gerber B, Muller H, Kulz T, et al. Simple ovarian cysts in premenopausal patients. *Int J Gynaecol Obstet* 1997;57:49–55.

12. Templeman C, Fallat ME, Blinchevsky A, et al. Noninflammatory ovarian masses in girls and young women. *Obstet Gynecol* 2000;96:229–233.

13. Flynn MK, Niloff JM. Outpatient minilaparotomy for ovarian cysts. *J Reprod Med* 1999;44:399–404.

14. Aubriot FX, Dubuisson JB, Pasteur Y. Is it necessary to operate on every ovarian cyst. *Contracept Fertil Sex* 1993;21:49–52.

15. Hopkins MP, von Gruenigen V, Gaich S. Laparoscopic port site implantation with ovarian cancers. *Am J Obstet Gynecol* 2000; 182:735–736.

16. Trimbos JB, Hacker NF. The case against aspiration ovarian cyst. *Cancer* 1993;72:828–831.

17. Jacobs HS, Agrawal R. Complication of ovarian stimulation. *Baillieres Clin Obstet Gynaecol* 1998;12:565–579.

18. Haddad A, Mulvany N, Billson V, et al. Solitary luteinized follicle cyst of pregnancy. Report of a case with cytologic findings. *Acta Cytol* 2000;44:454–458.

19. Pezzica E, Buzzi A, Sonozogni A, et al. Large size solitary luteinizing follicular cyst in peerperium. *Minerva Ginecol* 1992;44: 201–204.

20. Montz FJ, Schlaerth JB, Morrow CP. The natural history of theca lutein cysts. *Obstet Gynecol* 1988;72:247–251.

21. Lupien C, Wagner H, Sauerbrei EE. Delayed regression of huge theca lutein cysts monitored by serial sonogram and beta-HCG levels. *J Can Assoc Radiol* 1984;35:70–72.

22. Esposito JM. An unusual theca lutein cyst. Report of a case. *Obstet Gynecol* 1967;30:260–263.

23. Schnorr JA Jr, Miller H, Davis JR, et al. Hyperreaction luteinalis associated with pregnancy and review of the literature. *Am J Perinatol* 1996;13:95–97.

24. Jain S, Dalton ME. Chocolate cysts from ovarian follicles. *Fertil Steril* 1999;72:852–856.

25. Christensen B, Schindler AE. The so-called "chocolate cyst"—frequently interpreted as ovarian endometriosis. *Geburtshilfe Frauenheilkd* 1996;56:482–484.

26. Bezuidenhout J, Schneider JW, Hugo F, et al. Teratomas in infancy and childhood at Tygerberg Hospital, South Africa, 1973 to 1992. *Arch Pathol Lab Med* 1997;121:499–502.

27. Gordon A, Rossenshein N, Parmley T, et al. Benign cystic teratomas in postmenopausal women. *Am J Obstet Gynecol* 1980; 138:1120–1123.

28. Takahashi K, Shinno T, Watanabe Y, et al. Benign teratoma in an 85-year-old women. *Arch Gynecol Obstet* 2000;263:188–190.

29. Comerei JT Jr, Lieciardi F, Bergh PA, et al. Mature cystic teratoma: a clinicopathological evaluation of 517 cases and review of the literature. *Obstet Gynecol* 1994;84:22–28.

30. Zorulu CG, Kuseu E, Soysal ME, et al. Malignant degeneration of mature cystic teratomas. *Aust NZ J Obstet Gynaecol* 1996;36: 221–222.

31. Richardson G, Robertson DI, O'Connor ME, et al. Malignant transformation occurring in mature cystic teratomas of the ovary. *Can J Surg* 1990;33:499–503.

32. Mahour GH, Wooley MM, Landing BH. Ovarian teratomas in children. A thirty-three year experience. *Am J Surg* 1976;132: 587–589.

33. Portuondo JA, Gimenez B, Rivera JM, et al. Clinical and pathologic evaluation of 342 benign ovarian tumors. *Int J Gynaecol Obstet* 1884;22:263–267.

34. Ahmed S. Enlargement and maturation in benign cystic ovarian teratoma. *Pediatr Surg Int* 1999;15:435–436.

35. Lopez-Beltran A, Calanas AS, Jimena P, et al. Virilizing mature ovarian cystic teratomas. *Virchows Arch* 1997;431:149–151.

36. Waxman M, Boyce JG. Intraperitoneal rupture of benign cystic ovarian teratoma. *Obstet Gynecol* 1976;48:9S–13S.

37. Emoto M, Obama H, Horiuchi S, et al. Transvaginal color Doppler ultrasonic characterization of benign and malignant ovarian cystic teratomas and comparison with serum squamous cell carcinoma antigen. *Cancer* 2000;88:2298–2304.

38. Payne D, Muss HB, Homesley HD, et al. Autoimmune hemolytic anemia and ovarian dermoid cysts: case report and review of the literature. *Cancer* 1981;48:721–724.

39. Cobo F, Pereira A, Nomdedeu B, et al. Ovarian dermoid cyst-associated autoimmune hemolytic anemia: a case report with emphasis on pathogenic mechanism. *Am J Clin Pathol* 1996; 105:567–571.

40. Smith R, Deppe G. Selvaggi S, et al. Benign teratoma of the omentum and ovary coexistent with an ovarian neoplasm. *Gynecol Oncol* 1990;39:204–207.

41. Nazhat CR, Kalyconcu S, Nezhat CH, et al. Laparoscopic management of ovarian dermoid cyst: ten years of experience. *JSLS* 999;3:179–164.

42. Okada S, Ohaki Y, Kawamura T, et al. Cystic struma ovarii; imaging findings. *J Comput Assist Tomogr* 2000;24:413–415.

43. Schutz R, Bauermeister U, Fiedler B, et al. Struma ovarii—a case report. *Geburtshilfe Frauenheilkd* 1996;56:154–155.

44. Matsuki M, Kaji Y, Matsuo M, et al. Struma ovarii: MRI findings. *Br J Radiol* 2000;73:87–90.

45. Bethune M, Quinn M, Rome R. Struma ovarii presenting as acute pseudo-Meigs syndrome with an elevated CA 125 level. *Aust NZ J Obstet Gynaecol* 1996;36:372–373.

46. Nada S, Kalra B, Arora B, et al. Massive mature solid teratoma of the ovary with giomatosi peritonei. *Aust NZ J Obstet Gynaecol* 1998;38:329–331.

47. Hamada Y, Tanano A, Sato M, et al. Ovarian teratoma with gliomatosis peritonei: report of two cases. *Surg Today* 1998;28: 223–226.

48. Nielsen SN, Scheithauer BW, Gaffey TA. Gliomatosis peritonei. *Cancer* 1985;56:2499–2503.

49. Robboy SJ, Scully RE. Ovarian teratoma with glial implants on the peritoneum. An analysis of 12 cases. *Hum Pathol* 1970;1(4): 643–653.

50. Ghossain MA, Buy JN, Ligeneres C, et al. Epithelial tumors of the ovary: comparison of MR and CT findings. *Radiology* 1991; 181:863–870.

51. Buy JN, Ghossain MA, Sciot C, et al. Epithelial tumors of the ovary: CT findings and correlation with US. *Radiology* 1991; 178:811–818.

52. Randrianjafisamindrakotroka NS, Gasser B, Philippe E. The malignant potential of adenofibroma and cystadenofibroma of the ovary and mesovarium. 118 cases including 13 proliferative and 5 carcinoma. *J Gynecol Obstet Biol Reprod (Paris)* 1993;22:33–38.

53. Kao GF, Norris HJ. Cystadenofibromas of the ovary with epithelial atypia. *Am J Surg Pathol* 1978;2:357–363.

54. Groutz A, Wolman I, Wolf Y, et al. Cystadenofibroma of the ovary in young women. *Eur J Obstet Gynecol Reprod Biol* 1994;54:137–138.

55. Puls L, Heidtman E, Hunter JE, et al. The accuracy of frozen section by tumor weight for ovarian epithelial neoplasms. *Gynecol Oncol* 1997;67:16–19.

56. Ronnett BM, Shmookler MB, Sugarbaker PH, et al. Pseudomyxoma peritonei: new concepts in diagnosis, origin, nomenclature, and relationship to mucinous borderline (low malignant potential) tumors of the ovary. *Anat Pathol* 1997;2:197–226.

57. Yasar A, De Keulenaer B, Opdenakker G, et al. Pseudomyxoma peritonei in association with primary malignant tumor of the ovary and colon. *J Belge Radiol* 1997;80:233–234.

58. Piver MS, Lele SB, Patsner B. Pseudomyxoma peritonei: possible prevention of mucinous ascites by peritoneal lavage. *Obstet Gynecol* 1984;64:95S–96S.

59. Eichhorn JH, Scully RE. Endometrioid ciliated-cell tumors of the ovary: a report of five cases. *Int J Gynecol Pathol* 1996;15:248–256.

60. Nasca D. Proliferative endometrioid cystadenofibroma of the ovary. Report of a case in teenager. *Diagn Gynecol Obstet* 1982;4:317–324.

61. Kao GF, Norris HJ. Unusual cystadenofibroma: endometrioid, mucinous and clear cell types. *Obstet Gynecol* 1979;54:729–736.

62. Chebrou DM, Provendier B, Chebrou C, et al. Endometrioid adenofibroma of the ovary. An anatomoclinical case report. *J Gynecol Obstet Biol Reprod (Paris)* 1993;22:254–256.

63. Kanajet D, Pirkic A. Branner's tumor of the ovary. *Jugosl Ginekol Perinatol* 1990;30:54–56.

64. Woodruff JD, Dietrich D, Genadry R, et al. Proliferative and malignant Brenner tumors. Review of 47 cases. *Am J Obstet Gynecol* 1981;141:118–125.

65. Austin RM, Norris HJ. Malignant Brenner tumor and transitional cell carcinoma of the ovary: a comparison. *Int J Gynecol Pathol* 1987;6:29–39.

66. Hermanns B, Faridi A, Rath W, et al. Differential diagnosis, prognostic factors, and clinical treatment of proliferative Brenner tumor of the ovary. *Ultrastruct Pathol* 2000;24:191–196.

67. Outwater EK, Siegelman ES, Kim B, et al. Ovarian Brenner tumors: MR imaging characteristics. *Magn Reson Imaging* 1998;16:1147–1153.

68. Moon WJ, Koh BH, Kim SK, et al. Brenner tumor of the ovary: CT an MR findings. *J Comput Assist Tomogr* 2000;24:72–76.

69. Silvanesaratnam V, Dutta R, Jayalakshmi P. Ovarian fibromas—clinical and histopathological characteristics. *Int J Gynaecol Obstet* 1990;33:243–247.

70. Howell CG Jr, Rogers DA, Gable DS, et al. Bilateral ovarian fibromas in children. *J Pediatr Surg* 1990;25:690–691.

71. Santangelo M, Battaglia M, Vescio G, et al. Meigs's syndrome: its clinical picture and treatment. *Ann Ital Chir* 2000;71:115–119.

72. Laufer L, Barki Y, Mordechai Y, et al. Ovarian fibromas in a prepubertal girl. *Pediatr Radiol* 1996;26:40–42.

73. Schwartz RK, Levine D, Hatabu H, et al. Ovarian fibromas: findings by contrast-enhanced MRI. *Abdom Imaging* 1997;22:535–537.

74. Spinelli C, Gadducci A, Bonadio AG, et al. Benign ovarian fibromas associated with free peritoneal fluid and elevated serum CA 125 levels. *Minerva Ginecol* 1999;51:403–407.

75. Robert HG, Dutranoy G, Vu J, et al. Thecal tumors of the ovary. *Nouv Presse Med* 1976;6:1459–1462.

76. Barrenetxea G, Schneider J, Centeno MM, et al. Pure theca cell tumor. A clinicopathologic study of 29 cases. *Eur J Gynaecol Oncol* 1990;11:429–432.

77. Young RH, Clement PB, Scully RE. Calcified thecomas in young women. A report of four cases. *Int J Gynecol Pathol* 1988;7:343–350.

78. Conte M, Guriglia L, Benedetti Panici P, et al. Ovarian fibrothecoma: sonographic and histologic findings. *Gynecol Obstet Invest* 1991;32:51–54.

79. Troiano RN, Lazzarini KM, Scoutt LM, et al. Fibroma and fibrothecoma of the ovary: MR imagining findings. *Radiology* 1997;204:795–798.

80. Le Bouedec G, Glowaczowaer E, de Latuour M, et al. Demons-Meigs' syndrome. A case of thecoma and ovarian fibroma. *J Gynecol Obstet Biol Reprod (Paris)* 1992;21:651–654.

81. Kabayashi Y, Murakami R, Sugizaki K, et al. Primary leiomyoma of the ovary: a case report. *Eur Radiol* 1998;8:1444–1446.

82. Danihel L, Losch A, Kainz C, et al. Bilateral primary leiomyoma of the ovary. *Wien Klin Wochenschr* 1995;107:436–438.

83. Kandalaft PL, Esteban JM. Bilateral ovarian leiomyoma in a young woman: a case report with review of the literature. *Mod Pathol* 1992;5:586–589.

84. Seinera P, Raspollini M, Privitera S, et al. Bilateral ovarian leiomyoma. *Acta Obstet Gynecol Scand* 1997;76:488–489.

85. San Marco L, Londero F, Stefanutti V, et al. Ovarian leiomyoma. Case report. *Clin Exp Obstet Gynecol* 1991;18:145–148.

86. Gut R, Wozniak F, Listos T. A rare case of ovarian leiomyoma. A case report with review of literature. *Ginekol Pol* 1997;68:567–571.

87. Kohno A, Yoshikawa W, Yunoki M, et al. MR findings in degenerated ovarian leiomyoma. *Br J Radiol* 1999;72:1213–1215.

88. Sato Y, Tanaka T. An ovarian leiomyoma; a case report. *J Obstet Gynaecol Res* 1998;24:349–354.

89. Rivasi F, Philippe E, Walter P, et al. Ovarian angioma. Report of 3 asymptomatic cases. *Ann Pathol* 1996;16:439–441.

90. Loverro G, Cormino G, Perlino E, et al. Transforming growth factor–beta 1 in hemangioma of the ovary. *Gynecol Obstet Invest* 1998;46:210–213.

91. Rodriguez MA. Hemangioma of the ovary in 81-year-old woman. *South Med J* 1979;72:503–504.

92. Hermann UJ Jr, Locher GW, Goldhirsh A. Sonographic patterns of ovarian tumors: prediction of malignancy. *Obstet Gynecol* 1987;69:777–781.

93. Holtz G. Paraneoplastic hypercalcemia in gynecologic malignancy. *Obstet Gynecol Surv* 1980;35:129–136.

94. Sainz de la Cuesta R, Goff BA, Fuller AF Jr, et al. Prognostic importance of intraoperative rupture of malignant ovarian epithelial neoplasms. *Obstet Gynecol* 1994;84:1–7.

95. Canis M, Botchorishvili R, Manhes H, et al. Management of adnexal masses: role and risk of laparoscopy. *Semin Surg Oncol* 2000;19:28–35.

23

MALIGNANT OVARIAN DISORDERS

EDUCATIONAL OBJECTIVES

Medical Students (1)
APGO Objective No. 59

Characteristics of
  carcinomas
Evaluation and management of
  ovarian carcinomas:
  Symptoms and physical findings
  Risk factors
  Histologic classification
Impact of staging on management
  and prognosis

Residents in Obstetrics/Gynecology (2)
CREOG Objectives

Ovarian carcinoma
  History
  Physical examination
  Diagnostic studies
  Diagnosis
  Management
  Follow-up

Practitioners (3)
ACOG Recommendations

Ovarian cancer
  Screening
  Diagnosis
  Diagnostic workup
  Management
  Adjunctive therapy
  Factors affecting survival
Ovarian tumors in children
  and teenagers
Ovarian tumors in pregnancy

DEFINITION

Ovarian cancer is diversified ovarian tissues transformed to biologically divergent express neoplasia.

INCIDENCE

The incidence of ovarian cancer in the United States remains relatively unchanged at approximately 14.3/100,000 in recent decades. The mortality rate is 7.8/100.000 women per year. Ovarian cancer is uncommon before the age of 40 and sharply increases thereafter, with a peak at ages 65 to 75 (4). The incidence of ovarian cancer fluctuates in frequency among geographic regions and ethnic groups. The highest rate is in northern Europe (Scandinavia), intermediate rates appear in western Europe and North America, and low rates appear in Japan and in the developing countries (5). In the United States, the incidence rate distribution of ovarian cancer is highest among white and Hawaiian women, intermediate among African-American, Hispanic, and Asian-American women, and lowest among Native American women (6).

The majority of ovarian cancer is sporadic, and 5% to 10% is regarded as hereditary (7,8). Ovarian cancer is recognized as the fourth leading cause of cancer death among women in the United States (7), and a comparison of ovarian cancer with other genital tract cancers with respect to incidence and mortality in the United States is presented in Table 23.1.

TABLE 23.1. OVARIAN AND OTHER GYNECOLOGICAL CANCER

	Ovary	Endometrium	Cervix	Other
Incidence	32.5%	41.4%	19.1%	6.9%
Mortality	55.0%	22.3%	18.2%	4.5%

Data from Parker SL, Tong T, Bolden S, et al. Cancer statistics. *CA Cancer J Clin* 1996;46:5–27.

ETIOLOGY

Ovarian cancer etiology is poorly understood. One of the hypotheses of ovarian cancer development is incessant ovulation (lifetime number of ovulation expresses the index of relative ovarian cancer).

Another hypothesis focuses on the retrograde transport from the lower genital tract through the Fallopian tubes of carcinogens. Recognizable factors have been identified that influence the potential risk, prevention, and prognostic factors.

Risk Factors for Ovarian Cancer

The following risk factors can be identified:

■ A *family history* is considered the strongest risk factor for ovarian cancer development (4). Progress in molecular genetics supports this clinical view. Mutations or overexpression in the BRCA 1 and BRCA 2 tumor suppressor genes are accountable for the vast majority of familial occurrence of ovarian cancer; these are inherited by autosomal dominant factor (7,8,10,11) BRCA 1 and BRCA 2 genes located on chromosomes 17 and 13, respectively. The mutation of these genes is considered the hereditary ovarian–breast cancer syndrome. Women with BRCA 1 mutation have a 85% and 60% chance of developing breast and ovarian cancer by the age of 70, respectively. Most commonly, ovarian epithelial adenocarcinoma occurs from transmitting the germ-line of the BRCA 1 mutation; women with the BRCA 2 gene mutations have a lesser chance of developing ovarian cancer (12).

■ *Advanced age, early menarche, late menopause, and nulliparity* represent an increased risk of developing ovarian cancer (4,13).

■ *Refractory infertility* alone is an independent risk factor for ovarian cancer development. A combination of refractory infertility and nulliparity may present an even higher risk than either of these factors independently (14). In spite of these two factors, the use of fertility drugs independently may pose a potential risk for predominantly epithelial ovarian cancer development (between 1982 and 1977, at least 43 cases have been linked to the user of fertility drugs, and 25 out of 43 cases [58.1%] were epithelial tumors). Anovulation that requires induction of ovulation with fertility drugs among infertile women is approximately 33%. In 1998 alone, over 2 million women in the United States used medical induction of ovulation with various drugs (15). The possible association of epithelial ovarian cancer with ovulation induction has been postulated for some time; nevertheless, the causation of fertility drugs in ovarian cancer has not yet been established (14). Cancer in women previously treated with fertility drugs occurs in a younger population (mean age, 30.3 years) than does cancer in women not receiving these medications) (15).

■ *Race,* the incidence and mortality rate among different ethnic groups probably relates to genetic makeup (cancer predisposing genes) and epidemiological risk factors (4,6,16).

■ *History of endometrial or breast cancer* is considered an increased risk factor associated with epithelial ovarian tumor (4).

The literature concerning hormonal replacement therapy *(HRT)* and epithelial ovarian risk is inconsistent; although, most of the results indicate either a weak or no influence present (5).

■ *Contributing factors* such as excessive ovarian stimulation with *gonadotropins and androgens* may play a role predisposing for ovarian cancer development (8).

■ *Cosmetic talc exposure* is considered to be associated with an increase in ovarian cancer when talcum powder is applied to the perineum over an extended period of time (6).

Preventive Factors for Ovarian Cancer

The following factors help prevent the development of ovarian cancer, to various degrees (4,5):

■ *One or more full-term pregnancies* (increasing parity) consistently give strong protection against epithelial ovarian cancer; interruption of pregnancy before reaching full-term, for any reason, provides a lesser degree of protection (4,5).

■ *A history of breast-feeding* provides some protective value in ovarian cancer, but less protection than a full-term pregnancy (4,5).

■ *Users of oral contraceptive (OC)* receive protection, with a greater degree of protection following a longer duration of OC use; such use may lower a woman's risk up to 30% no matter when OC was used. A reduced risk up to 50% is possible after 5 years of OC use; this protection may last for 10 years after cessation of OC use (5).

■ *Tubal ligation and hysterectomy* provides protection against epithelial ovarian cancer by two mechanisms:

1. Suppression of ovarian hormone production (ovarian steroidal hormones influence the development of ovarian cancer) (5);
2. Elimination of the path of ascent for carcinogens [e.g., cosmetic talc (6)] to reach ovaries by obliterating the connection between the lower genital tract and the upper genital tract (17).

Prognostic Factors in Ovarian Cancer

These are the prognostic factors in ovarian cancer (8):

1. Stage of disease at the time of diagnosis
2. Maximum residual disease following cytoreductive surgery
3. Performance status

CLASSIFICATION

A comprehensive classification for malignant ovarian tumors is based upon the diversified origins of ovarian cells, according to the World Health Organization (WHO) (18). In general, malignant ovarian tumors are categorized as follows:

1. *Primary ovarian malignancy,* which includes the following origins:

a. Epithelial tumors account for 70% of all ovarian neoplasia.
b. Germ cell tumors account for approximately 15% to 20% of all ovarian neoplasia.
c. Sex cord–stromal tumors represent 5% to 10% of all ovarian neoplasia.
d. Other ovarian tumors
2. *Secondary (metastatic) tumors* are present in about 5% of cases, most commonly metastasizing from breast or colon cancer.

DIAGNOSIS

Pertinent medical history in the early stage of this disease, contrary to popular clinical conviction, is present; menstrual irregularity is one of the most common symptoms that cause a patient to seek professional help. Late ovarian cancer symptomatology is usually related to an enlarging tumor and falls into the following categories:

- Abdominal swelling is the most commonly reported complaint.
- Pelvic discomfort, urinary frequency, and constipation may result from tumor compression of adjacent anatomical structures.
- Abdominal discomfort or even acute abdominal pain may be reported when torsion or rupture (with leaking content) of the tumor takes place.
- Gastrointestinal symptoms such as nausea, vomiting, heartburn, abdominal bloating, anorexia, and weight loss usually demonstrate the metastasis of ovarian cancer to the upper abdomen and/or ascites.
- Abnormal, irregular endometrial bleeding is frequently present.

- Shortness of breath is commonly linked to the Meigs' syndrome (the presence of an ovarian mass, ascites, and hydrothorax).
- A triad of ovarian cancer symptoms—abdominal swelling, fatigue, and abdominal pain—is the most frequent clinical manifestation, regardless of the stage of disease (19).

Physical examination may demonstrate the following:

- A breast mass and enlargement of the axillary lymphatic nodes.
- Abdominal examination may determine the presence of ascites and/or an abdominal tumor.
- Percussion and auscultation of the lungs can determine pleural effusions.
- Evaluation of the lower extremities may establish a warm, tender, and red cord-like structure, suggesting vein thrombosis.

Pelvic examination may reveal the following abnormalities:

- The cervix can be displaced from its natural location by a tumor.
- The uterus can be fused with an ovarian mass presenting as one enlarged structure, it can be a separate organ, or it can be displaced by a mass.
- Adnexa can be enlarged, or only the ovary may be enlarged (on average, the normal ovary size for premenopausal women is $3 \times 2 \times 2$ cm and for postmenopausal women is $2 \times 1 \times 0.5$ cm).
- The posterior cul-de-sac nodules can be palpated on recto-vaginal examination.

Detailed pelvic mass evaluation is presented in Chapter 22. The differences in benign and malignant characteristics of an adnexal mass are presented in Table 23.2.

TABLE 23.2. CLINICALLY SUSPECTED BENIGN VERSUS MALIGNANT ADNEXAL MASS

	Benign (Follow-up Within 4–6 Weeks)	Malignant (Surgical Intervention)
Age	Reproductive	1. Perimenarcheal 2. Postmenopausal
Initial size	<8 cm	>8 cm
Changing size	Decreasing in size	1. Persistence through 2–3 menses 2. Increase in size
Symptoms	Asymptomatic	Symptomatic
Location	Unilateral	Bilateral
Tumor mobility	Mobile	Fixed
Tumor characteristics	Cystic and smooth	Solid and irregular
Ultrasonography	Simple cyst	1. Complex mass 2. Multiloculated cyst 3. Irregular surface
Ascites	Absence	Presence

Data from Young RC, Perez CA, Hoskins WJ. Cancer of the ovary. In: DeVita VT, Hellman S, Rosenberg SA, eds. *Cancer: principles and practice of oncology,* 4th ed. Philadelphia: JB Lippincott, 1993:1226–1263.

Ovarian Cancer Staging

Ovarian cancer staging is surgical and is applied regardless of the origin of the ovarian cells. The process of staging incorporates clinical, surgical, histological, and cytological findings. The International Federation of Gynecology and Obstetrics (FIGO) classification is formally recommended in the United States (21). The staging process commences with an adequate abdominal incision. Upon entering the abdominal cavity, fluid, if present, is aspirated for cytology evaluation.

Thorough and methodological inspection of the entire peritoneal cavity should begin with any suspicious peritoneal and/or diaphragmatic lesion; a biopsy should be obtained and submitted as a frozen section (intraoperative pathological consultation). Tumor resection or unilateral salpingo-oophorectomy is performed if conservative surgical treatment is applicable. Total hysterectomy with bilateral salpingo-oophorectomy is performed when definitive extirpative surgery is indicated. Surgical specimens are submitted for frozen-section histological evaluation. The accuracy of frozen-section is very high in regard to the sensitivity and specificity of ovarian tumors, with the exception of borderline tumors. Frozen-section has profound implication not only on the type of tumor, but also the extent of surgery to be executed at the initial surgical intervention (22). Following these steps, paraaortic and pelvic node sampling and subtotal omentectomy are recommended. An appendectomy is performed when a mucinous type of ovarian cancer is present. Ovarian carcinoma staging is presented in Table 23.3.

It is estimated that approximately 75% of women with ovarian cancer will be diagnosed with a stage of II or greater at the time of initial surgery. Staging itself is an independent prognostic factor; although, some studies indicate histologic grade (grade 1 or grade 2, etc.) of the tumor is the leading prognostic indicator, followed by stage and histologic origin (23). Contrary to these suggestions, it has been postulated that the single most important factor that significantly influences survival rate is residual disease (cutoff point of residual disease, <0.5 cm) (24).

Ovarian Cancer Grading System

FIGO (25) and WHO (26) are the most common histologic grading systems of epithelial ovarian carcinoma. For practical purposes, the following ovarian tumor grading system is useful:

- Grade 1 stands for well-differentiated cells.
- Grade 2 is moderately (intermediate) differentiated cells.
- Grade 3 is poorly differentiated or undifferentiated cells (the biologically most aggressive tumors).

The absence of a universal, simple grading system for ovarian cancer makes it difficult to establish the prognostic significance of histologic grade. Recently, however, a prog-

TABLE 23.3. FIGO OVARIAN CANCER STAGING

Stage	Description
I	Growth is limited to the ovaries.
IA	Growth is limited to one ovary; no ascites present containing malignant cells. There is no tumor on external surface; capsule is intact.
IB	Growth is limited to both ovaries; no ascites present containing malignant cells. There is no tumor on external surface; capsule is intact.
IC	Tumor is classified as either stage IA or IB but with tumor on the surface of one or both ovaries; or with ruptured capsules; or with ascites containing malignant cells present or with positive peritoneal washings.
II	Growth involves one or both ovaries, with pelvic extension.
IIA	There is extension and/or metastases to the uterus and/or tubes.
IIB	There is extension to other pelvic tissue.
IIC	Tumor is either stage IIA or IIB but with tumor on the surface of one or both ovaries; or with capsules ruptured; or with ascites containing malignant cells present or with positive peritoneal washing.
III	Tumor involves one or both ovaries with peritoneal implants outside the pelvis and/or positive retroperitoneal or inguinal nodes. Superficial liver metastasis equals stage III. Tumor is limited to the true pelvis but with histologically proven malignant extension to small bowel or omentum.
IIIA	Tumor is grossly limited to the trough pelvis with negative nodes but with histologically confirmed microscopic seeding of abdominal peritoneal surfaces.
IIIB	Tumor involves one or both ovaries with histologically confirmed implants of abdominal peritoneal surfaces, none exceeding 2 cm in diameter; nodes are negative.
IIIC	There are abdominal implants greater than 2 cm in diameter and/or positive retroperitoneal or inguinal nodes.
IV	Growth involves one or both ovaries, with distant metastases. If pleural effusion is present, there must be positive cytologic findings to assign a case to stage IV. Parenchymal liver metastasis equals stage IV.

Data from International Federation of Gynecology and Obstetrics (FIGO). *Annual report on the results of treatment in gynecological cancer,* 22nd ed. Stockholm: FIGO, 1994.

nostically relevant, universal histological grading system for invasive ovarian carcinoma has been proposed (27).

When the type and grade of a tumor are combined, the result may give, to some degree, favorable versus unfavorable treatment outcome. The tumor type offers less prognostically relevant information than the stage or grade of the disease (28). The histological type of tumor best determines the predictive value of the tumor responsiveness to a specific chemotherapeutic agent; therefore, the most appropriate chemotherapy can be selected based upon the histologic type of the tumor. The histologic grade of the tumor will not influence the responsiveness of the tumor to chemotherapy, but the histology grade will significantly affect the duration of a progression-free period (29).

DIFFERENTIAL DIAGNOSIS

Differential diagnosis of ovarian cancer, for practical purposes, is divided into the following categories:

1. Nongynecologic disorders comprise these conditions:
   a. Primary malignancy such as intestinal tumors, lymphoma, retroperitoneal tumors, and mesothelial tumors should be excluded.
   b. Benign disorders such as appendiceal abscess, Crohn's disease, and diverticulitis can mimic ovarian cancer.
   c. Pelvic kidney may present as a pelvic mass and can be ruled out either by intravenous pyelogram or cystoscopy and retrograde pyelography.
2. Gynecologic disorders embrace these conditions:
   a. Ectopic pregnancy should be considered in the reproductive period.
   b. Other gynecologic malignancies such as of the Fallopian tube or the uterus should be excluded
   c. Benign tumor of the upper genital tract, particular pedunculated uterine leiomyomata, should be taken into clinical consideration.
   d. Tuboovarian abscess as sequelae of pelvic inflammatory disease or salpingitis, or oophoritis may suggest the presence of ovarian cancer.

CONVENTIONAL THERAPY

In general, conventional therapy for ovarian cancer falls into the categories of surgical therapy, chemotherapy, and radiotherapy.

Surgical intervention depends upon the stage and type of disease and is categorized as follows:

1. *Conservative treatment* should be given special consideration in the following clinical scenarios (3):
   a. A patient requests preservation of childbearing capacity after full disclosure of potential clinical consequences of such a decision.
   b. The ovarian cancer is unilateral, is unruptured, is intracystic, is not adherent, and has a negative washing cytology (stage IA).
   c. The ovarian cancer is a borderline or well-differentiated epithelial cell type tumor.
   d. Germ cell tumors such as dysgerminoma, immature teratoma, endodermal sinus, embryonal carcinoma, and choriocarcinoma are frequently unilaterally located and can be considered for conservative surgical intervention in a stage IA tumor.

   e. Sex cord–stromal origin ovarian cancer can be managed by unilateral salpingo-oophorectomy in an early stage of the tumor.
2. *Primary cytoreductive* or debulking surgery involves extirpating tumor and metastatic masses as much as possible. The surgical procedure consists of total hysterectomy with bilateral salpingo-oophorectomy, total omentectomy, and resection metastatic lesions. Occasionally, intestinal resection is necessary. When residual tumor is >1.5 cm in diameter, it should be considered a suboptimal resection; although, some researchers adopt a standard diameter of 1 cm of the largest residual tumor node as an optimal cytoreduction (30,31). A retrospective study has documented that the probability of achieving optimal cytoreduction (1 cm residual nodule) in stage III ovarian cancer with preoperative CA-125 levels higher than 500 U/mL is possible in one out of five patients (31).
3. *Interval cytoreductive surgery* or interval debulking surgery is designed for patients in whom appropriate debulking at the initial surgery could not be executed (22). Randomized controlled clinical results support the view that interval debulking surgery significantly lengthened progression-free and overall survival rate (33).
4. *Second-look laparotomy* plays an essential role in clinical assessment and documentation of ovarian cancer responsiveness to chemotherapy.
5. *Palliative surgery* is usually performed for resection or bypass surgery. Most commonly, this operation is performed for intestinal obstruction related to advanced ovarian cancer. The serious complications of the surgery may reach 49%, with a mortality rate reaching 30%. For 4 to 6 months following surgery, the ability to eat can be improved with this surgery, but no benefit in survival can be expected.

Chemotherapy can benefit most ovarian cancer patients; 57% to 80% will respond to chemotherapy. The most favorable response to chemotherapy is observed among women with optimal debulking before primary chemotherapy.

1. *Primary chemotherapy* can be commenced at the time of the initial debulking surgery by intraperitoneal chemotherapy instillation, particularly when the residual lesion is less than 1 cm in diameter and limited to the peritoneal cavity. When a larger residual tumor (>1 cm) is present, systemic chemotherapy should be administered.
2. *Salvage chemotherapy* is provided to those patients who develop resistance to chemotherapy before their ovarian cancer is completely eradicated.

Radiation therapy demonstrates beneficial effects in the early-stage or microscopic residual of ovarian cancer. Also, this mode of therapy can be applied as a form of palliative therapy.

In general, *overall 5-year survival rates*, when considering aggressive cytoreductive surgical interventions in combination with chemotherapy, are as follows (8):

- Stage I, approximately 93%
- Stage II, 70%
- Stage III, 37%
- Stage IV, 25%

Complementary and alternative therapies do not provide any specific treatment for ovarian cancer.

OVARIAN TUMORS IDENTIFIABLE BY HISTOLOGY

Diversified ovarian cells give rise to different histological types of malignant ovarian tumor such as epithelial (from the coelomic epithelial cells, which is the outer lining of the ovarian layer), sex cord–stromal (from the mesenchymal tissue), and germ cell (from the germinal epithelium).

Epithelial Malignant Ovarian Tumors

WHO's modified classification of malignant epithelial ovarian tumors can be identified as follows (18):

1. *Serous malignant tumors*
   a. Borderline malignancy (carcinoma of low malignant potential)
   b. Adenocarcinoma (papillary adenocarcinoma and papillary adenocarcinoma and papillary cystadenocarcinoma)
   c. Surface papillary carcinoma
   d. Malignant adenofibroma or cystadenofibroma
2. *Mucinous malignant tumor*
   a. Borderline malignancy (carcinoma of low malignant potential)
   b. Adenocarcinoma
   c. Malignant adenofibroma or cystadenofibroma
3. *Endometrioid malignant tumors*
   a. Borderline malignancy (carcinoma of low malignant potential)
   b. Adenocarcinoma
   c. Adenoacanthoma
   d. Adenosquamous carcinoma
   e. Malignant adenofibroma or cystadenofibroma
4. *Epithelial stroma and stromal tumors*
   a. Adenosarcoma
   b. Stromal sarcoma
   c. Mesodermal (Müllerian) mixed tumor, homologous and heterologous
5. *Clear cell (mesonephroid) tumors*
   a. Borderline malignancy (carcinoma of low malignant potential)
   b. Adenocarcinoma (carcinoma)

6. *Transitional cell malignant tumors*
   a. Borderline malignancy (carcinoma of low malignant potential)
   b. Malignant Brenner's tumor
7. *Mixed epithelial malignant tumors*
   a. Borderline malignancy (carcinoma of low malignant potential)
   b. Malignant mixed epithelial tumors
8. *Undifferentiated carcinoma*
9. *Unclassified epithelial malignant tumors*

Borderline Malignant Tumors

A borderline malignant tumor, of low malignant potential, is a biologically and histologically well defined epithelial ovarian tumor with prevalence estimated at 4% to 14% among female tract malignant neoplasm (34,35). Here, it has been purposely included in Chapter 23, on ovarian malignancy, since it clinically requires staging and treatment according to an oncologic management schema. It can be analyzed from a benign proliferative gynecologic condition with an oncological therapeutic approach. Epithelial tumors of low malignant potential are not an intermediate or premalignant stage between benign and malignant tumors.

The diagnosis is similar to that in a case of adnexal mass; surgical staging follows the FIGO staging for carcinoma of the ovary. The age of diagnosis is younger and an earlier stage of the disease can be determined when compared with other epithelial ovarian cancers.

Conventional therapy is surgery and can be offered in a conservative form with unilateral oophorectomy, preserving the contralateral ovary and the uterus in stage IA, when a patient desires the preservation of her reproductive capacity. If the stage of the disease is greater than stage IA or a future pregnancy is not an issue, peritoneal washing, tumor debulking, total abdominal hysterectomy, bilateral salpingo-oophorectomy, and pelvic and paraaortic lymphadenectomy is recommended.

In general, these tumors have a very favorable prognosis, though about 10% to 20% exhibit a progressively worsening clinical course with widespread peritoneal implants and death of patients within 5 years. It has been suggested that the prediction of the poor clinical outcome, among patients in this group, can be determined by DNA cytophotometry. The presence of aneuploidy can be regarded as an indicator of biologically aggressive behavior (36).

The survival rate in stage I is 99%, and 92% in stage II at a mean 7-year follow-up (34,35).

Epithelial Malignant Tumors

Despite improved overall surgical techniques and adjuvant therapies for early stage high-risk ovarian cancer, approximately 20% of women with the disease will experience a

TABLE 23.4. THERAPY FOR EPITHELIAL OVARIAN CANCER

Cancer Progression	Clinical Findings	Surgical Cytoreduction		Therapy
		Optimal	Suboptimal	
Early, low risk	1. Stage IA 2. Grade 1	—	—	1. Unilateral salpingectomy and full surgical staging 2. TAH and BSO 3. No postoperative therapy
Early, high risk	1. Stage IA, IB, IC, Stage IIA, IIB, IIC 2. Grade 1 and 2	No residual cancer	—	1. TAH and BSO 2. Platinum-based chemotherapy 3. Alternative: whole-abdomen radiation
Advanced	1. Stage II 2. Stage III and IV		Residual cancer >1 cm Residual cancer <1 cm	1. Maximal surgical cytoreduction 2. TAH and BSO 3. Full staging 4. Chemotherapy with platinum and paclitaxel 5. Second look Alternative: whole abdominal radiotherapy
		No gross residual cancer	Residual cancer >1 cm	1. Same as above 2. Chemotherapy with cisplatin and paclitaxel 3. No alternative therapy 4. Second look
Persistent or recurrent	—	—	—	1. Chemotherapy, including investigational treatment 2. Palliative surgery as indicated

TAH, total abdominal hysterectomy; BSO, bilateral salpingo-oophorectomy.
Data from American College of Obstetricians and Gynecologists (ACOG). *Educational bulletin 141*. Washington, DC: ACOG, 1990; and Young RC, Walton LA, Ellenberg SS, et al. Adjuvent therapy in stage I and stage II epithelial ovarian cancer: results of two prospective randomized trials. *N Engl J Med* 1990;322(15):1021–1027.

relapse. It has been demonstrated, in a randomized study with long-term (10 years) follow-up, that neither whole-abdominal radiotherapy (2,250 rads in 10 fractions), nor Melphalan (8 mg/m²/day for 4 weeks with a total of 18 courses), nor intraperitoneal chromic phosphate (10 to 20 mCi) present statistically significant differences. Therefore, surveillance for life is required, since second primary malignancies can be expected in approximately 35% of epithelial malignant tumors (38).

Among epithelial cancers, a serous type is the most common and has a less favorable prognosis than mucinous and endometrioid types. Clear cell carcinoma clinical behavior is controversial, and some authorities categorize it as a highly aggressive form of cancer; other clinicians believe that clear cell carcinoma has a relatively favorable course.

Management of epithelial tumors is diversified; therapeutic modalities are summarized in Table 23.4.

Follow-up of patients with an early stage of epithelial ovarian cancer includes gynecological examination with serum CA-125 for serous or CA-19-9 for mucinous epithelial ovarian cancer every 3 months for the first year. If no persistence or recurrence is noticed, follow-up should continue every 4 months for the second year and every 6

months for the next 3 years. Following 5 years of disease-free survival, only an annual examination and Pap smear are suggested.

In advanced ovarian cancer, clinical surveillance is via second-look laparotomy to evaluate chemotherapy effects and also includes follow-up. Pelvic examination and serum CA-125 or CA-19-9 levels every 3 months for the first 2 years and every 6 months thereafter for 3 years should be executed. If a patient has not been subjected to second-look laparotomy or laparoscopy, either CT or MRI can be utilized as needed.

In Table 23.5, the most commonly used tumor markers in epithelial cell malignant tumors are presented.

TABLE 23.5. TUMOR MARKERS IN EPITHELIAL CELL TUMORS

Marker	Type of Tumor
CA-125	All types of nonmucinous epithelial tumors Immature teratoma
CA-19-9	Mucinous epithelial ovarian carcinoma

OVARIAN GERM CELL MALIGNANT TUMORS

The WHO classification of ovarian tumors of germ cell origins falls into the following categories (18):

I. Dysgerminoma
  A. Variant:
    1. With syncytiotrophoblast cells
II. Yolk sac tumor (endodermal sinus tumor)
  A. Variants:
    1. Polyvesicular vitelline tumor
    2. Hepatoid
    3. Glandular
      a. Variant: "Endometrioid"
III. Embryonal carcinoma
IV. Polyembryoma
V. Choriocarcinoma
VI. Immature teratomas
  A. Solid
  B. Cystic with secondary tumor formation (specify type)
  C. Fet–form (homunculus)
  D. Monodramal and highly specialized
    1. Carcinoid
    2. Insular
    3. Trabecular
  E. Stromal carcinoid
  F. Mucinous carcinoid
  G. Neuroectodermal tumors
  H. Sebaceous tumors
  I. Other
  J. Mixed (specify types)
VII. Mixed (specify types)

Germ cell tumors can affect prepubertal girls, reproductive aged women, and postmenopausal women. These tumors are predominantly observed in the second and third decades of life. The following malignant germ cell tumors are commonly seen in gynecologic practice:

1. *Dysgerminoma* is the most common tumor among all germ cell tumors and is estimated to occur in about 35% to 45% of all germ cell tumors. The tumor can be present bilaterally in approximately 10% to 15%. On gross examination, dysgerminoma is a solid, lobulated, and smooth surface tumor (39). LDH is a tumor marker that is utilized in dysgerminoma. Dysgerminoma can be associated with pure XY gonadal dysgenesis (40) and can also be seen in patients with 45,X/46,XY mosaic karyotype. Also, dysgerminoma can arise from gonadal dysgenesis associated with the pure Turner syndrome (45,X) (41). Gonadoblastoma and its association with the chromosome Y are described in Chapter 4.

2. *Endodermal sinus tumor* is categorized as a yolk sac tumor and is considered a biologically aggressive malignancy, with a survival rate in the early stage between 60% and 100%, and in stage III and IV approximately 50% to 75% when appropriate therapy is implemented (42). The AFP tumor marker is used to evaluate therapeutic progress or recurrence (43).

3. *Immature teratomas* account for approximately 4.0% to 20% of all malignant germ cell tumors and 2.1% of all ovarian neoplasms. Diagnosis is reached predominantly in stage I, grade 1, and the tumor is normally unilateral (44). Overall incidence is not established. Immature teratomas infrequently may be associated with elevation of serum AFP, LDH, and CA-125 levels of tumor markers.

4. *Embryonal carcinoma* is a rare ovarian cancer. It has been associated with high levels of AFP and/or hCG (45); however, pure embryonal carcinoma does not demonstrate an elevation of ATP and hCG. The tumor is unilateral normally; very infrequently is it present bilaterally (46).

5. *Choriocarcinoma* of germ cell origin is an uncommon and biologically aggressive ovarian malignancy that is categorized as follows (47):

- *Nongestational primary choriocarcinoma* arises from germ cells and occurs in a pure or mixed form. The mixed type is more frequently observed in clinical practice than the pure type.
- *Gestational primary ovarian choriocarcinoma* arises from ovarian ectopic pregnancy.
- *Secondary ovarian choriocarcinoma* (metastatic) originates from other organs—for the most part, from the uterus.

Nongestational, gestational, and metastatic choriocarcinoma consists of cytotrophoblastic and syncytiotrophoblastic cells with large mononucleated intermediated cells (47–49). This form of ovarian cancer may occur in pediatric patients, young women of reproductive age, and postmenopausal women (47–52). In prepubertal girls, choriocarcinoma may induce isosexual precocity in about 50% of cases. Serum hCG can be used as a tumor marker to evaluate treatment outcome and tumor persistence or recurrence. Pregnancy, including ectopic pregnancy, must be taken into account if there is hCG elevation, since ovarian choriocarcinoma may coexist with an otherwise uncomplicated pregnancy (53). Large theca lutein cysts can be present in both ovaries or unilaterally.

6. *Polyembryoma* is an exceedingly rare germ cell tumor, which is composed of embryoid bodies in different stages of development. Embryoid bodies are tissues that usually correspond to early stage embryonal development (15- to 16-day embryonal life is able to produce AFP and hCG). Tumor markers such as AFP and hCG can be elevated. Polyembryoma may be present in mixed germ cell tumors as one of the tumor components. Due to serum hCG elevation, the tumor may cause precocious puberty in prepubertal girls (54).

7. *Ovarian mixed germ cell tumor* is defined by the presence of more than one histologic variety of tissue within the tumor. These types of tumors affect girls and adolescents

predominantly, with a median age of 16 years; they are estimated at 10% to 15% of all germ cell tumors (55,56). There are different components of tissues within the tumor. The following illustrates such arrangements: dysgerminoma combined with choriocarcinoma (56), polyembryoma mixed with mature and immature teratomas (57), polyembryoma and immature teratoma (58), polyembryoma and choriocarcinoma (59), or ovarian gonadoblastoma in women with 46,XX associated with mixed germ cell tumor consisting of choriocarcinoma, embryonal carcinoma, and dysgerminoma (60). The most common symptom is abdominal pain, which occurs in approximately 90% of cases (55).

In the pediatric population, germ cell tumors are uncommon, and they are estimated at 3% of all childhood malignancies (in the United States, the incidence is about 4 per million individuals under the ages of 15). Germ cell tumors can occur in both gonadal and extragonadal sites (extragonadal occurrence is common under 3 years of age; a gonadal location is observed frequently at puberty and after). Extragonadal tumors are believed to develop from abnormal migration of primordial germ cells (55). Primary gonadal tumor location presents a more favorable prognosis than an extragonadal location, and gonadal germ cell tumors offer more prognostic value than histology (56).

The diagnosis, surgical staging, and histological verification with grading are reached in a fashion similar to that presented for pelvic mass evaluation in Chapter 22, in the discussion of benign ovarian disorders, and above, in the discussion of epithelial cell tumors. Germ cell tumors can occur in any age, with frequent occurrence in the pediatric and adolescent group; although, postmenopausal women also can be affected (55,57). Tumor metastasis is divided into two categories: pulmonary versus nonpulmonary visceral metastasis (liver, bone, and central nervous system). CT or MRI is required for clinical metastatic investigation.

At laparotomy, a germ cell tumor frequently presents as a large necrotic mass and, often, a large theca lutein cyst associated with choriocarcinoma (51).

Preoperative diagnosis of germ cell tumors is difficult, particularly to distinguish gestational from nongestational choriocarcinoma in reproductive age women (51,52).

Conventional therapy is fertility sparing management in young patients whenever clinically achievable. The malignant process in germ cell tumors does not commonly affect the contralateral ovary, even in advanced disease. This natural behavior of these tumors favors conservative approach.

Surgery is the primary mode of therapy, which includes complete surgical resection and staging with histological grading, followed by selective use of platin-based chemotherapy (55).

Patients with early stages of the disease (stage I or II), regardless of histologic type, can be safely treated with conservative surgery such as unilateral salpingo-oophorectomy, appropriate staging, and tumor grading, followed by, if indicated, three to four courses of cisplatin-based chemotherapy. Even in advanced stages of the endodermal sinus tumor, conservative surgery can be considered (58,59).

In general, surgical intervention consists of total abdominal hysterectomy, bilateral salpingo-oophorectomy, and extensive surgical staging in those patients who do not desire to preserve reproductive capacity. Recently, unilateral adnexectomy, with or without comprehensive surgical staging in stage I of the disease, has been recommended. Overall, the 5-year survival rate is estimated to be approximately 93% (60). In patients with persistent serum marker elevation during and after chemotherapy, salvage surgery is recommended even in patients with visceral metastasis. Postchemotherapeutic residual tumor resection (salvage surgery) offers over 50% long-term success. Therefore, even patients with visceral metastasis will benefit from salvage surgery (61). Second-look laparotomy should be included when indicated.

In the pediatric group, management consists of surgical resection for localized disease, chemotherapy for residual or metastatic disease, and neoadjuvant chemotherapy with delayed surgical excision for nonresectable lesions. Current survival for early-stage (stage I or II) gonadal sites is almost 100%, and for advanced stages, III and IV, is approximately 95%. The survival rate for extragonadal germ cell tumor location in the early stage is about 95%, and for stages III and IV is approximately 75% (62–70).

Follow-up of germ cell tumors distinguishes itself by the presence of serum tumor markers, which are indispensable in the evaluation of the extent of tumor resection and in tumor persistence or recurrent monitoring. Normalizing levels of a tumor marker during chemotherapy indicate tumor regression or complete reemission. Rising levels of serum marker correspond closely with progression of the tumor. The disappearance of tumor markers during chemotherapy is a very encouraging sign; yet, it does not always indicate complete destruction of the tumor. Table 23.6 presents the tumor markers most commonly associated with germ cell tumors. The follow-up schedule does not differ from that presented for the epithelial tumors.

TABLE 23.6. TUMOR MARKERS IN GERM CELL TUMORS

Serum Tumor Marker	Ovarian Tumor
AFP (alpha-fetoprotein)	Endodermal sinus tumors
	Embryonal carcinoma
	Mixed germ tumors (immature teratoma)
	Polyembryoma
hCG (human chorionic gonadotropin)	Choriocarcinoma
	Embryonal carcinoma
	Mixed germ tumors
	Polyembryoma
LDH (lactate dehydrogenase)	Dysgerminoma
	Mixed germ cell tumor

OVARIAN SEX CORD–STROMAL TUMORS

Sex cord–stromal tumors are gonadal cell type tumors derived from either the coelomic epithelium (sex cord) or mesenchymal cells of the embryonic gonads and incorporate granulosa cells, theca cells, Sertoli cells, and Leydig cells. Ovarian sex cord–stromal tumors represent approximately 5% to 8% of all ovarian masses. The most common tumor among them is granulosa-theca cells, followed by fibrothecomas, and Sertoli-Leydig cell tumors. Sex cord–stromal tumors exhibit hormonal activity by producing estrogens that may cause hyperestrogenism and its manifestations such as isosexual precocious puberty, abnormal endometrial bleeding in prepubertal girls (<5%) and in women in the reproductive and postmenopausal periods (>50%), and endometrial hyperplasia and/or cancer as high as 60%. Excessive androgen production by the tumor may lead to hyperandrogenism and its sequelae (hirsutism, oily skin, deep voice, and clitorimegaly). In addition to hormonal abnormality, sex cord–stromal tumors can be associated with: Peutz-Jeghers syndrome (an autosomal dominant disease, characterized by melanin spots on lips and buccal mucosa, and multiple gastrointestinal hamartomatous polyps), Maffucci's syndrome (its cardinal characteristics include the coexistence of enchondromatosis and vascular anomalies, particularly the presence of large hemangioma), or Ollier's disease (where the presence of enchondromatosis and the absence of vascular anomalies distinguish it from Maffucci's syndrome) (71,72).

According to the WHO classification, sex cord–stromal malignant ovarian tumors include the following (18):

I. Granulosa–stromal cell tumor
   A. Granulosa cell tumor
      1. Juvenile
      2. Adult
   B. Tumors in the thecoma-fibroma group
      1. Fibrosarcoma
II. Sertoli–stromal cell tumors; androblastomas
   A. Well differentiated
      1. Sertoli cell tumor; tabular androblastomas
      2. Sertoli-Leydig cell tumor
      3. (Leydig cell tumor)
   B. Of intermediate differentiation
      1. Variant: With heterologous elements (specify types)
   C. Poorly differentiated (sarcomatoid)
      1. Variant: With heterologous elements (specify types)
   D. Retiform
   E. Mixed
III. Sex cord tumor with annular tubules
IV. Gynandroblastoma
V. Steroid (lipid) cell tumors
   A. Stromal luteoma

   B. Leydig cell tumor; hilus cell tumor (a rare Leydig cell tumor that is nonhilar)
   C. Unclassified

Ovarian Granulosa Stromal Tumor

Granulosa cell tumors consist of granulosa cells or a combination of granulosa and the theca epithelium. These ovarian tumors are divided into the following categories:

- Juvenile granulosa cell tumors
- Adult granulosa cell tumors

Juvenile Granulosa Cell Tumors

Juvenile granulosa cell tumors (JGCT) occur at approximately 97% in the population under 30 years of age; although, the neoplastic malignant disease may affect a patient from newborn to postmenopausal periods, with the average age being 13 years (73). It has been postulated that the presence of chromosomal trisomy 12, an extra abnormal chromosome 12 (74,75) and chromosomal monosomy 22 may indicate a genetic predisposition to this form of malignancy. In the adult type of granulosa cell tumors, chromosomal trisomy 12 abnormality may or may not be present (76). Yet, monosomy 22 is suggested to be present in both types of granulosa cell tumors (74). These genetic findings will need validation before clinical acceptance.

The diagnosis of juvenile granulosa may be suggested by signs of isosexual pseudoprecocious puberty in children (not associated with ovulation) and is present in about 70% of ovarian tumors in the pediatric population (77). Abnormal endometrial bleeding in perimenarcheal girls is associated frequently with a pelvic mass and abdominal distention or acute abdomen. Infrequently, Ollier's disease and Maffucci's syndrome, or Peutz-Jeghers' syndrome, or painful enlargement of the breast can be manifested (72,73,78). In young women, abdominal pain or swelling, menstrual irregularity, or amenorrhea can be present. In postmenopausal women, abnormal endometrial bleeding is the main symptom (73).

Physical examination in children may demonstrate the premature presence of secondary sex characteristics (see Chapter 2), and a distended and enlarged abdomen. An abdominal mass may be palpable. In adult women, an abdominal tumor can be appreciated by palpation, and sequelae of hyperestrogenism can be identified (see Chapter 3).

Pelvic evaluation in children may reveal a mature occurrence of external genitalia, a developed cervix with copious mucous, uterine enlargement, and a pelvic mass. Adult women will demonstrate the presence of a pelvic tumor with hyperestrogenic characteristics.

Laboratory tests may document serum elevation of estrogen levels.

Imaging studies (ultrasonography, MRI, or CT) will confirm and document the presence of a unilateral or bilateral mass of ovarian origin (72,73).

At laparotomy, surgical staging is performed according to the FIGO ovarian staging discussed above. The majority of tumors are in FIGO stage I as established at the time of diagnosis (78–80).

A tumor usually is located unilaterally and occasionally may be present bilaterally in about 2% (73). On gross examination, an average size is approximately 12.5 cm (range, 3 to 32 cm). A tumor in both juvenile and adult subtypes appears similar to a solid/cystic mass in 49%, a solid mass in 37%, and a large, often multicystic mass in 14%, frequently filled with bloodstain fluid. Also, this can appear as a small solid tumor, yellow-gray in color, and often associated with necrosis and/or hemorrhage (73).

Histologic examination discloses a diffused and follicular pattern with luteinized granulosa cells; Call-Exner bodies are absent or rare in the juvenile type (73,81). Grading of the tumor should be established during microscopic examination, which follows the general ovarian grading system presented above.

Conventional therapy in the early stage of the disease is surgical resection of the affected site of the tumor or salpingo-oophorectomy in pediatric and reproductive aged patients who request fertility sparing. Adjuvant multidrug chemotherapy, including platin-based regiments, is recommended (78). In more advanced stages (FIGO II to IV), aggressive debulking, appropriate staging, salpingo-oophorectomy of the affected site with preservation of the uterus and contralateral adnexa, followed by Carboplatin and Etoposide chemotherapy (the clinical safety and effectiveness of which has not yet been fully determined) is recommended (79).

In women whose fertility is of no concern to them or in postmenopausal women, total abdominal hysterectomy, bilateral salpingo-oophorectomy, and appropriate staging, followed by multidrug platinum-based chemotherapy, is recommended.

The prognosis in juvenile granulosa cell tumors depends on the stage of the tumor at the time of diagnosis. The higher the stage of the disease, the less favorable a clinical outcome is expected. It has been reported that in stage IA the survival rate is over 95% (72,78,80), and then survival decreases about 10-fold with advanced Stage IV (72).

In relapse of the disease, the prognosis is poor and pregnancy does not modify the prognosis (82).

Follow-up of JGCT is not different than with other histological types of ovarian cancer. Estradiol can be used to monitor the disease. It is crucial to establish lifelong follow-up due to possible late recurrence of the tumor (83). Poor prognosis in recurrent disease opens the possibility of prophylactic oophorectomy of the remaining ovary upon completion of the patient's family.

Adult Granulosa Cell Tumor

Adult granulosa cell tumors are uncommon neoplasms characterized by a long natural history and a tendency to late, local recurrence following initial therapy. Recurrence of these tumors has a very poor prognosis associated with a low survival rate. Among granulosa cell tumors, the adult type is the most common one (95%). It occurs more frequently than the juvenile type in postmenopausal periods than it does in premenopausal periods, with the peak age being between 50 to 55 years old. The majority of tumors are hormonally active and secrete estrogens, leading to endometrial hyperplasia and/or cancer. These tumors demonstrate less malignantly aggressive behavior than most of the ovarian carcinomas and customarily are detected at an early stage (84). The principal symptoms in reproductive age are changes in the menstrual cycle pattern (most commonly abnormal endometrial bleeding as a result of estrogen stimulation), and in postmenopausal women, abnormal endometrial bleeding is reported. In both age groups, abdominal distension with pain is present (85,86).

The diagnosis is reached in process similar to that presented in juvenile granulosa cell tumors.

Conventional therapy is surgical. The extent of surgery depends upon age and fertility-sparing concerns. In the young population, conservative surgery alone with preservation of the contralateral ovary, the contralateral Fallopian tube, and the uterus, and appropriate staging are recommended in an early stage of the disease. In the early stage when intermediate or poor differentiation of the tumor occurs, adjuvant therapy is indicated. In the older group, where reproductive capacity is of no concern or in postmenopausal women or in advanced disease, total hysterectomy, bilateral salpingo-oophorectomy, and staging are offered and adjuvant combination chemotherapy (cis-platin/vinblastine/bleomycin) appear to provide the highest response rate. Individualized treatment for metastatic or recurrent disease is offered, and the general approach for advanced ovarian cancer treatment is utilized (87).

Clinical prognostic factors in adult granulosa cell tumor of the ovary can be categorized as follows (88):

1. Tumor stage is statistically the most significant prognostic factor.
2. Tumor size is also an important prognostic factor; although, to a lesser extent than tumor stage.

Significant pathologic prognosticators can be identified as follows (88):

1. The presence of the degree of atypia is a statistically significant prognostic factor and is often observed in patients with recurrent tumor.
2. The presence of a higher mitotic rate is also noticed more frequently in patients with recurrent tumor.
3. The presence of Call-Exner body occurs more frequently in tumors in those patients who remained disease free.

In general, higher degrees of atypia, higher mitotic rates, and fewer Call-Exner bodies will occur in early recurring tumors (88).

The overall 5- and 10-year survival rates are 90% and 77%, respectively (77,86,89); the 5-year survival rate in stage I is 100% and for stage II and IV is 33%(90). *Follow-up* procedures in both juvenile and adult granulosa cell tumor forms are the same; it is important to establish long-term follow-up due to indolent growth and the tendency toward late recurrence.

The clinical characteristics of juvenile and adult granulosa cell tumors are presented in Table 23.7.

Thecomas

Thecomas are very rare solid (grossly, yellow-orange masses) ovarian malignant tumors and are very difficult to differentiate from ovarian fibromas; they are often called "fibrothecomatous tumors of the ovary." Thecomas are most commonly diagnosed at a mean age of 59.5 years (91). Thecoma may produce estrogen and fibroma not, and clinical behavior may assist in making the diagnosis. Sequelae of hyperestrogenism can be present, including but not limited to abnormal endometrial bleeding, endometrial hyperplasia, and cancer in the postmenopausal period. Also, fibrothecoma may result in secondary amenorrhea and infertility due to inhibin-B–producing substance, which has the ability to suppress FSH (92). The definitive diagnosis of malignant fibrothecoma is established by histological confirmation, and the same criteria apply as in ovarian fibrosarcoma (93).

Conventional therapy is fertility sparing surgery that consists of tumor resection and staging. In postmenopausal women or when reproductive capacity is not of concern, total abdominal hysterectomy, bilateral salpingo-oophorectomy, and appropriate staging are recommended.

Ovarian Sertoli's Tumors

Ovarian Sertoli's tumors arise from sex cord–stromal tissue that differentiated in the male (testicular) direction. These tumors have the ability to secrete hormones (estrogen, androgen, and progesterone) or to be inactive as well. It is estimated that the occurrence of this ovarian tumor is less than 1% of all ovarian masses.

Pure Sertoli cell tumor may cause isosexual precocious puberty, hyperestrogenism and its clinical sequelae, virilization, or a combination of virilizing and estrinizing signs (94); although, lack of clinical hormonal activity can also be observed (95). In extreme cases, there are markedly elevated serum estrogen and progesterone levels, at the same time that the endometrium exhibits pronounced decidualization and mimics a gestation state with no actual pregnancy (96). Occasionally, Sertoli's cell tumor of the ovary can be associated with the Peutz-Jeghers syndrome (97).

The diagnoses are difficult due to a wide variety of hormonal activities or lack of them; therefore, symptomatology will depend upon the types of hormones being produced. The symptoms of isosexual precocious puberty, hyperestrogenism symptoms, virilization or a combination of both, secondary amenorrhea, and even galactorrhea can be present. Tumor-related symptoms such as pelvic pain, abdominal enlargement, or swelling can be present (94–97).

Physical examination will also depend on the type of hormone secretion by the tumor and will range from no signs to virilization or hyperestrogenism signs (for more details, see Chapters 2, 8 and 11). An abdominal mass can be present.

Pelvic evaluation of the lower genital tract will reflect hormonal activities ranging from hyperestrogenic to hyperandrogenic or a combination of the two. An adnexal mass is customarily palpable.

TABLE 23.7. JUVENILE AND ADULT GRANULOSA CELL TUMORS

	Juvenile Form	Adult Form
Age	Infrequently after 30 years	Frequently between 50 and 55 years
Trisomy 12	Consistently present	Customarily present
Pubertal occurrence	Up to 50%	<1%
Occurrence	Infrequently among sex cord stromal	Frequent (95%)
Recurrence	Early	Often very late, rarely early
Aggressiveness	More aggressive in advanced stage	Less aggressive
Histology:		
a. Call-Exner bodies	a. Often absent	a. Commonly present
b. Follicles	b. Irregular with mucin	b. Regular without mucin
c. Nuclei	c. Dark, occasionally grooved	c. Pale, often grooved
d. Luteinization	d. Frequently present	d. Infrequently present

Data from Young RH, Dickersin GR, Scully RE. Juvenile granulosa cell tumor of the ovary. A clinicopathological analysis of 125 cases. *Am J Surg Pathol* 1984;8:575–596; Lindgren V, Wagginer S, Rotmensch J. Monosomy 22 in two ovarian granulosa cell tumors. *Cancer Genet Cytogenet* 1996;89:93–97; Tanyi J, Rigo J Jr, Csapo Z, et al. Trisomy 12 in juvenile granulosa cell tumor of the ovary during pregnancy. A report of two cases. *J Reprod Med* 1999;44:826–832; and Fletcher JA, Gibas Z, Donovan K, et al. Ovarian granulosa-stromal cell tumors are characterized by trisomy 12. *Am J Pathol* 1991;138:515–520.

Imaging studies can confirm and document the presence of a complex ovarian mass (solid and cystic structures).

Laboratory tests may reveal serum elevation of estrogen and/or progesterone or testosterone. Also, an ovarian selective venous percutaneous catheterization can be performed for hormonal studies, when the diagnosis is in question.

Surgical staging of the tumor falls into the general ovarian staging system. Grading of the tumor is part of the histological evaluation.

The definitive diagnosis is established by histology, which determines, among several criteria [well dedifferentiated with solid neoplastic cells and tubular formation (94,98)], the presence of characteristics of Charcot-Bottcher filaments that unequivocally identify Sertoli differentiation (94,95). Histologically, endometrium can demonstrate pronounced decidualization, but an actual gestational sac is not present (96).

At laparotomy, the tumor is gray to brown, and generally solid with a cystic area and can be large (95,98).

Conventional therapy is similar to that previously described for this group of tumors, with fertility-sparing surgery appropriate for the early stage of the disease.

Recurrent tumor may involve multiple intraabdominal sites, and individualized therapy is recommended.

Follow-up does not differ from the generally established recommendation of observing serum levels of estradiol and/or progesterone or testosterone as tumor markers.

Sertoli-Leydig Cell Tumors

A Sertoli-Leydig cell tumor consists of both Sertoli's and Leydig's cells; contrary to Sertoli's cell tumors, which tend to secrete estrogens, Sertoli-Leydig cell tumors tend to be an androgenic type of tumor (approximately 40% of the cases) (99). These tumors occur as less than 0.5% of all ovarian tumors, and they are usually located unilaterally, with 58% being solid/cystic, 38% solid, and 4% cystic. These tumors mainly affect young women of age 30 or younger (75%); approximately 10% of women in the postmenopausal period are affected (range, 2 to 75 years of age; average, 25 years of age).

Signs and symptoms of hyperandrogenism (see Chapter 8), abdominal swelling or abdominal pain, and abdominal-pelvic mass (ranges from millimeters to 51 cm in diameter; average of 13.5 cm) are the most common clinical findings (100). Elevated serum peripheral testosterone levels are usually found at >200 ng/dL (101). Imaging examination (ultrasonography, CT scan, and/or MRI scan) will confirm the presence of the tumor. Histological verification determines the presence of Sertoli-Leydig tumors and grading (approximately 54% is intermediate differentiation, 22% is poorly differentiated, and 11% well differentiated tumors). Infrequently, well-differentiated Sertoli-Leydig cells tumor of the ovary may exhibit calcification/ossification (102).

Stage I of the tumor is present in 97.5% at the time of diagnosis (stage II in about 1.5% and stage III in the remaining 1%); the tumor can be identified bilaterally in 1.5% (100).

Conventional therapy is conservative surgery and does not depart from the general approach in this group of tumors. In follow-up, serum testosterone levels are utilized.

Prognosis correlates most significantly with the stage of the disease and the degree of differentiation of the tumor at the time of initial diagnosis (100).

Sex Cord Tumor with Annular Tubules

Sex cord tumor with annular tubules is predominantly a benign ovarian tumor, but a malignant degeneration of this disease has been reported (103). The Peutz-Jeghers syndrome frequently is associated with a benign type of these tumors, which are typically located bilaterally, small in size, and calcified. Unilateral location is not associated with the Peutz-Jeghers syndrome; this tumor is solid and yellowish, with varying degrees of cystic degeneration, is large, and it produces estrogen (in up to 50% of cases, which may cause sexual precocity, menstrual irregularity, and postmenopausal bleeding). Those symptoms can be associated with a malignant tumor (104). A sex cord tumor with annular tubules may produce both estrogen and progesterone, which may be responsible for menorrhagia followed by amenorrhea (105).

The clinical diagnosis is reached by detecting an adnexal mass, if the tumor is palpable, associated with symptoms (not specific), and confirmed by imaging examination.

Laboratory tests in some cases may document elevated levels of serum estrogen and occasionally progesterone.

Histological confirmation is necessary to verify the type and grade of the tumor. Microscopic examination shows simple or complex annular tubules; many tumor cells may show lipids in cytoplasm and Sertoli cell differentiation with Charcot-Bottcher filaments (106).

Conventional therapy is conservative surgery with staging, and in more advanced disease, total abdominal hysterectomy and bilateral ovarian-oophorectomy with staging is recommended. Radiotherapy is suggested for recurrent or metastatic disease (105).

Leydig Cell Tumor

Leydig (hilus) cell tumors arise from hilar cells, which are homologous with Leydig cells in the testis. Less frequently they may arise from ovarian stromal cells. Due to tumor location in the ovarian hilar area, they are in the vicinity of the mesovarium vessels and are predominantly unilateral. The tumors are small, usually less than 5 mm in diameter, and the color ranges from light brown to dark brown; they are well-circumscribed (107).

These tumors usually affect women in their 50s (mean age, 50 years) and cause hirsutism and/or virilization; they are almost never malignant (see Chapter 8).

When peripheral blood tests and imaging examinations (ultrasonography, CT scan, and/or MRI scan) fail to identify an ovarian source of hyperandrogenism, percutaneous selective ovarian vein catheterization may assist in establishing a diagnosis.

Conventional therapy for management is presented in Chapter 8.

OVARIAN METASTATIC TUMORS

Ovarian metastatic tumors can be divided into the following categories:

1. Metastasis from the genital tract, which includes the following:
   a. Tubal carcinoma
   b. Endometrial carcinoma
   c. Uterine sarcomas
   d. Vaginal and vulvar carcinomas
   e. Gestational and nongestational trophoblastic genital tumors
2. Metastasis from other organs
   a. Breast carcinoma
   b. Stomach carcinoma, including the Krukenberg tumor
   c. Intestinal carcinoma
   d. Tumor of the appendix
   e. Carcinoid tumors
   f. Lung tumors
   g. Pancreatic tumors
   h. Liver and gallbladder tumors
   i. Urinary tract tumors (renal, ureteral, bladder, and urethra)
   j. Adrenal gland tumor
   k. Malignant melanoma

REFERENCES

1. Association of Professors of Gynecology and Obstetrics (APGO). *Medical student educational objectives,* 7th ed. Washington, DC: APGO, 1997.
2. Council on Resident Education in Obstetrics and Gynecology (CREOG). *Educational objectives core curriculum for residents in obstetrics and gynecology,* 5th ed. Washington, DC: CREOG, 1996.
3. American College of Obstetricians and Gynecologists (ACOG). *Educational bulletin no. 141.* Washington, DC: ACOG, 1990.
4. Tortolo-Luna G, Mitchell MF. The epidemiology of ovarian cancer. *J Cell Biochem Suppl* 1995;23:200–207.
5. Riman T, Persson I, Nilsson S. Hormonal aspect of epithelia ovarian cancer; review of epidemiologic evidence. *Clin Endocrinol (Oxf)* 1998;49:695–707.
6. Daly M, Obrams GI. Epidemiology and risk assessment for ovarian cancer. *Semin Oncol* 1998;25:255–264.
7. Berchuck A, Schildkraut JM, Marks JR, et al. Managing hereditary ovarian cancer risk. *Cancer* 1999;86:2517–2524.
8. Holschneider CH, Berek JS. Ovarian cancer: epidemiology, biology, and prognostic factors. *Semin Surg Oncol* 2000;19:3–10.
9. Parker SL, Tong T, Bolden S, et al. Cancer statistics. *CA Cancer J Clin* 1996;46:5–27.
10. Zweemer RP, Verheijen RH, Menko FH, et al. Differences between hereditary and sporadic ovarian cancer. *Eur J Obstet Gynecol Reprod Biol* 1999;82:151–153.
11. Aunoble B, Sanches R, Didier E, et al. Major oncogenes and tumor suppressor genes involved in epithelial ovarian cancer. *Int J Oncol* 2000;16:567–576.
12. Farghaly SA. Current status of management of hereditary ovarian-breast cancer syndrome. *Obstet Gynecol* 2000;95:S51.
13. Thompson SD. Ovarian cancer screening: a primary care guide. *Lippincott Prim Care Pract* 1998;2:244–250.
14. Bristow RE, Karlan BY. Ovulation induction, infertility, and ovarian cancer. *Fertil Steril* 1996;66:499–507.
15. Franco C, Coppola S, Prosperi Porta R, et al. Ovulation induction and the risk of ovarian tumors. *Minerva Ginecol* 2000;52:103–109.
16. Neuhausen SL. Ethnic differences in cancer risk resulting from genetic variation. *Cancer* 1999;86:2575–2582.
17. Westhoff C. Ovarian cancer. *Annu Rev Public Health* 1996;17:85–96.
18. The World Health Organization (WHO). *Histological typing of ovarian tumors.* Geneva: WHO, 1973.
19. Smith EM, Anderson B. The effects of symptoms and delay in seeking diagnosis on stage of disease at diagnosis, among women with cancer of the ovary. *Cancer* 1985;56:2727–2732.
20. Young RC, Perez CA, Hoskins WJ. Cancer of the ovary. In: DeVita VT, Hellman S, Rosenberg SA, eds. *Cancer: principles and practice of oncology,* 4th ed. Philadelphia: JB Lippincott, 1993.
21. The International Federation of Gynecology and Obstetrics (FIGO). *Annual report on the results of treatment in gynecological cancer,* 22nd ed. Stockholm: FIGO, 1994.
22. Rose PG, Rubin RB, Nelson BE, et al. Accuracy of frozen-section (intraoperative consultation) diagnosis of ovarian tumors. *Am J Obstet Gynecol* 1994;171:823–826.
23. Sorbe B, Frankendal B, Veress B. Importance of histologic grading in the prognosis of epithelial ovarian carcinoma. *Obstet Gynecol* 1982;59:576–582.
24. Vaccarello L, Rubin SC, Vlamis V, et al. Cytoreductive surgery in ovarian carcinoma patients with a documented previously complete surgical response. *Gynecol Oncol* 1995;75:61–65.
25. The International Federation of Gynecology and Obstetrics (FIGO). Classification and staging of malignant tumors in the female pelvis. *Acta Obstet Gynecol Scand* 1971;50:1–7.
26. Serov SF, Scully RE, Sobin LK, eds. Histological classification of tumors. In: *International histological classification of tumors. No. 9.* Geneva: WHO, 1973:17–54.
27. Silverberg SG. Histologic grading of ovarian carcinoma: a review and proposal. *Int J Gynecol Pathol* 2000;19:7–15.
28. Silverberg SG. Prognostic significance of pathologic features of ovarian cancer. *Curr Top Pathol* 1989;78:85–109.
29. Shimizu Y, Kamoi S, Amada S. The grade and the type should be friends: a study of comparative value of histologic grading and typing of ovarian epithelial carcinoma [Abstract]. *Mod Pathol* 1998;11:115A.
30. Soper JT, Couchman G, Berchuck A, et al. The role of partial sigmoid colectomy for debulking epithelial ovarian carcinoma. *Gynecol Oncol* 1991;41:239–244.

31. Chi DS, Venkatraman ES, Masson V, et al. The ability of pre-operative serum CA-125 to predict optimal primary tumor cytoreduction in stage III epithelial ovarian carcinoma. *Gynecol Oncol* 2000;77:227–231.

32. Dauplat J, Le Bouedec G, Pomel C, et al. Cytoreductive surgery for advanced stages of ovarian cancer. *Semin Surg Oncol* 2000; 19:42–48.

33. van der Burg ME, van Lent M, Buyse M, et al. The effect of debulking surgery after induction chemotherapy on the prognosis in advanced epithelial ovarian cancer. Gynecological Cancer Cooperative Group of the European Organization for Research and Treatment of Cancer. *N Engl J Med* 1995;332: 629–634.

34. Trimble CL, Trimble EL. Management of epithelial ovarian tumors of low malignant potential. *Gynecol Oncol* 1994;55: S52–S61.

35. Barakat RR. Borderline tumors of the ovary. *Obstet Gynecol Clin North Am* 1994;21:93–105.

36. Dietel M, Hauptmann S. Serous tumors of low malignant potential of the ovary. 1. Diagnostic pathology. *Virchows Arch* 2000;436:403–412.

37. Young RC, Wlton LA, Ellenberg SS, et al. Adjuvant therapy in stage I and stage II epithelial ovarian cancer: results of two prospective randomized trials. *N Engl J Med* 1990;322: 1021–1027.

38. Dent SF, Klaassen D, Pater JL, et al. Second primary malignancies following the treatment of early stage ovarian cancer: update of a study by the National Cancer Institute of Canada–Clinical Trials Group (NCIC-CTG). *Ann Oncol* 2000; 11:65–68.

39. Gordon A, Lipton D, Woodruff JD. Dysgerminoma: a review 158 cases from the Emil Novak Ovarian Tumor registry. *Obstet Gynecol* 1981;58:497–504.

40. Helpap B, Schwinger E, Spiertz K. Dysgerminoma in pure gonadal dysgenesis. *Geburtsilfe Frauenheilkd* 1980;40:381–384.

41. Pierga JY, Giacchetti S, Vilain E, et al. Dysgerminoma in a pure 45,X Turner syndrome: report of a case and review of the literature. *Gynecol Oncol* 1994;55:459–464.

42. Gerhenson DM, Del Junco G, Herson J, et al. Endometrial sinus tumor of the ovary: the M.D. Anderson's experience. *Obstet Gynecol* 1983;61:194–202.

43. Talerman A, Haije WG, Baggerman L. Serum alpha-fetoprotein (AFP) in patients with germ cell tumors of the gonads and extragonadal sites: correlation between endodermal sinus (yolk sac) tumor and raised serum AFP. *Cancer* 1980;46:380–385.

44. Ayhan A, Aksu T, Selcuk Tuncer Z, et al. Immature teratoma of the ovary. *Eur J Gynecol Oncol* 1993;14(3):205–207.

45. Ueda G, Abe Y, Yoshida M, et al. Embryonal carcinoma of the ovary: a six-year survival. *Int J Gynaecol Obstet* 1990;31(3): 287–292.

46. Hulewicz G, Golfier F, Chatte G, et al. Pure embryonal carcinoma of the ovary. A review of the literature apropos of a case. *Bull Cancer* 1996;83:718–724.

47. Axe SR, Klein VR, Woodruff JD. Choriocarcinoma of the ovary. *Obstet Gynecol* 1985;66:111–114.

48. Rivoire M, Treilleux I, Kaemmerlen P, et al. Salvage liver surgery of a chemorefractory ovarian choriocarcinoma. *Gynecol Oncol* 1997;65:185–187.

49. Jacobs AJ, Newland JR, Green RK. Pure choriocarcinoma of the ovary. *Obstet Gynecol Surv* 1982;37:603–609.

50. Trigueros Velazquez M, Sereno Colo JA, Villagran Urive J. Pure form of primary ovarian choriocarcinoma. Report of a case. *Ginecol Obstet Mex* 1995;63:341–345.

51. Wheeler CA, Davis S, Degefu S, et al. Ovarian choriocarcinoma: a difficult diagnosis on unusual tumor and review of the hook effect. *Obstet Gynecol* 1990;75:547–549.

52. Babu MK, Kini U. Choriocarcinoma of the ovary in a postmenopausal woman. *Indian J Cancer* 1996;33:111–115.

53. Cunanan RG Jr, Lippes J, Tancinco PA. Choriocarcinoma of the ovary with coexisting normal pregnancy. *Obstet Gynecol* 1980;55:669–672.

54. Takada A, Ishizuka T, Goto T, et al. Polyembryoma of ovary producing alpha-fetoprotein and HCG: immunoperoxidase and electron microscopic study. *Cancer* 1982;49:1878–1889.

55. Gershenson DM, Del Junco G, Copeland LJ, et al. Gershenson cell tumors of the ovary. *Obstet Gynecol* 1984;64(2):200–206.

56. Fanning J, Walker RL, Shah NR. Mixed germ cell tumor of the ovary with pure choriocarcinoma metastasis. *Obstet Gynecol* 1986;68:84S–85S.

57. King ME, Hubbell MJ, Talerman A. Mixed germ cell tumor of the ovary with a prominent polyembryoma component. *Int J Gynecol Pathol* 1991;10:88–95.

58. Takemori M, Nishimura R, Yamasaki M, et al. Ovarian mixed germ cell tumor composed of polyembryoma and immature teratoma. *Gynecol Oncol* 1998;69:260–263.

59. Nishida T, Oda T, Sugiyama T, et al. Ovarian mixed germ cell tumor comprising polyembryoma and choriocarcinoma. *Eur J Obstet Gynecol Reprod Biol* 1998;78:95–97.

60. Zhao S, Kato N, Enoh Y, et al. Ovarian gonadoblastoma with mixed germ cell tumor in a women 46,XX karyotype and successful pregnancies. *Pathol Int* 2000;50:332–335.

61. Rescorla FJ, Breitfeld PP. Pediatric germ cells tumors. *Curr Probl Cancer* 1999;23:257–303.

62. Bethel CA, Mutabagani K, Hammond S, et al. Nonteratomatous germ cell tumors in children. *J Pediatr Surg* 1998;33(7): 1122–1126.

63. Doss BJ, Jacques SM, Qureshi F, et al. Immature teratomas of the genital tract in older women. *Gynecol Oncol* 1999;73: 433–438.

64. Linasmita V, Srisupundit S, Wilailak S, et al. Recent management of malignant ovarian germ cell tumors: a study of 34 cases. *J Obstet Gynaecol Res* 1999;25(5):315–320.

65. Chang FH, Lai CH, Chu KK, et al. Treatment of malignant germ cell tumors of the ovary. *J Formos Med Assoc* 1994;93: 411–416.

66. Tewari K, Cappuccini F, Disaia PJ, et al. Malignant germ cell tumors of the ovary. *Obstet Gynecol* 2000;95:128–133.

67. Albers P, Ganz A, Hannig E, et al. Salvage surgery of chemorefractory germ cell tumors with elevated tumor markers. *J Urol* 2000;164:381–384.

68. Rescorla FJ. Pediatric germ cell tumors. *Semin Surg Oncol* 1999; 16:144–158.

69. Gobel U, Calaminus G, Harms D. Germ cell tumors in children and adolescents. *Schweiz Rundsch Med Prax* 1995;84: 1063–1067.

70. Gobel U, Schneider DT, Calaminus G, et al. Germ-cell tumors in childhood and adolescence. GPOH MAEI and MAHO study groups. *Ann Oncol* 2000;11:263–271.

71. Gell JS, Stannard MW, Ramnani DM, et al. Juvenile granulosa cell tumor in a 13-year-old girl with enchondromatosis (Ollier's disease): a case report. *J Pediatr Adolesc Gynecol* 1998;11: 147–150.

72. Outwater EK, Wagner BJ, Mannion C, et al. Sex cord–stromal and steroid cell tumors of the ovary. *Radiographics* 1998;18: 1523–1546.

73. Young RH, Dickersin GR, Scully RE. Juvenile granulosa cell tumor of the ovary. A clinicopathological analysis of 125 cases. *Am J Surg Pathol* 1984;8:575–596.

74. Lindgren V, Wagginer S, Rotmensch J. Monosomy 22 in two ovarian granulosa cell tumors. *Cancer Genet Cytogenet* 1996;89: 93–97.

75. Tanyi J, Rigo J Jr, Csapo Z, et al. Trisomy 12 in juvenile gran-

ulosa cell tumor of the ovary during pregnancy. A report of two cases. *J Reprod Med* 1999;44:826–832.

76. Fletcher JA, Gibas Z, Donovan K, et al. Ovarian granulosa–stromal cell tumors are characterized by trisomy 12. *Am J Pathol* 1991;138:515–520.

77. Cronje HS, Niemand I, Bam RH, et al. Granulosa and theca cell tumors in children: a report of 17 cases and literature review. *Obstet Gynecol Surv* 1998;53:240–247.

78. Calaminus G, Wessalowski R, Harms D, et al. Juvenile granulosa cell tumors of the ovary in children and adolescents: results from 33 patients registered in a prospective cooperative study. *Gynecol Oncol* 1997;65:447–452.

79. Powell JL, Otis CN. Management of advanced juvenile granulosa cell tumor of the ovary. *Gynecol Oncol* 1997;64:282–284.

80. Powell JL, Johnson NA, Bailey CL, et al. Management of advanced juvenile granulosa cell tumor of the ovary. *Gynecol Oncol* 1993;48:119–123.

81. Bouffet E, Basset T, Chetail N, et al. Juvenile granulosa cell tumor of the ovary in infants: a clinicopathologic study of three cases and review of the literature. *J Pediatr Surg* 1997;32:762–765.

82. Leveque J, Meunier B, Berger D, et al. Juvenile ovarian granulosa tumor associated with pregnancy. A case report. Review of the literature. *J Gynecol Obstet Biol Reprod (Paris)* 1994;23:283–287.

83. Hines JF, Khalifa MA, Moore JL, et al. Recurrent granulosa cell tumor of the ovary 37 years after initial diagnosis: a case report and review of the literature. *Gynecol Oncol* 1996;60:484–488.

84. Evans AT III, Gaffey TA, Malkasian GD Jr, et al. Clinico-pathologic review of 118 granulosa and 82 theca cell tumors. *Obstet Gynecol* 1980;55:231–238.

85. Schweppe KW, Beller FK. Clinical data of granulosa cell tumor. *J Cancer Res Clin Oncol* 1982;104:161–169.

86. Ayhan A, Tuncer ZS, Tuncer R, et al. Granulosa cell tumor of the ovary. A clinicopathological evaluation of 60 cases. *Eur J Gynaecol Oncol* 1994;15:320–324.

87. Segal R, DePetrill AD, Thomas G. Clinical review of adult granulosa cell tumors of the ovary. *Gynecol Oncol* 1995;56:338–344.

88. Miller BE, Barron BA, Wan JY, et al. Prognostic factors in adult granulosa cell tumor of the ovary. *Cancer* 1997;79:1951–1955.

89. Bartl W, Spernol R, Breitencker G. The significance of clinical and morphological parameters for the prognosis of granulosa cell tumors of the ovaries. *Geburtshilfe Frauenheilkd* 1984;44:295–299.

90. Piura B, Nemet D, Yanai-Inbar I, et al. Granulosa cell tumor of the ovary: a study of 18 cases. *J Surg Oncol* 1994;55:71–77.

91. Bjorkholm E, Silfversward C. Theca-cell tumors. Clinical features and prognosis. *Acta Radiol Oncol* 1980;19:241–244.

92. Meyer AC, Papadimitriou JC, Silverberg SG, et al. Secondary amenorrhea and infertility caused by inhibin-B–producing ovarian fibrothecoma. *Fertil Steril* 2000;73:258–260.

93. McCluggage WG, Sloan JM, Boyle DD, et al. Malignant fibrothecomatous tumor of the ovary: diagnostic value of anti-inhibin immunostaining. *J Clin Pathol* 1998;51:868–871.

94. Tavassoli FA, Norris HJ. Sertoli tumors of the ovary. A clinico-pathologic study of 28 cases with ultrastructural observations. *Cancer* 1980;46:2281–2297.

95. Harris M, Balgobin B. Pure Sertoli cell tumor of the ovary: report of a case with ultrastructural observation. *Histopathology* 1978;2:449–459.

96. Tracy SL, Askin FB, Reddick RL, et al. Progesterone secreting Sertoli cell tumor of the ovary. *Gynecol Oncol* 1985;22:85–96.

97. Ferry JA, Young RH, Engel G, et al. Oxyphilic Sertoli cell tumor of the ovary: a report of three cases, two in patients with the Peutz-Jeghers syndrome. *Int J Gynecol Pathol* 1994;13:259–266.

98. Ramzy I, Bos C. Sertoli cell tumors of ovary: light microscopic and ultrastructural study with histologic consideration. *Cancer* 1976;38:2447–2456.

99. Young RH. Sertoli-Leydig cell tumors of the ovary: review with emphasis on historical aspects and unusual variants. *Int J Gynecol Pathol* 1993;12:141–147.

100. Young RH, Scully RE. Ovarian Sertoli-Leydig cell tumor. A clinicopathological analysis of 207 cases. *Am J Surg Pathol* 1985;9:543–569.

101. Arai M, Jobo T, Iwaya H, et al. Androgen-producing ovarian tumors: a clinicopathological study of 3 cases. *J Obstet Gynecol Res* 1999;25:411–418.

102. Mooney EE, Vaidya KP, Tavassoli FA. Ossifying well-differentiated Sertoli-Leydig cell tumor of the ovary. *Ann Diagn Pathol* 2000;4:34–38.

103. Lele SM, Sawh RN, Zaharopoulos P, et al. Malignant ovarian sex cord tumor with annular tubules in a patient with Peutz-Jeghers syndrome: a case report. *Mod Pathol* 2000;13:466–470.

104. Young RH, Welch WR, Dickersin GR, et al. Ovarian sex cord tumor with annular tubules: review of 74 cases including 27 with Peutz-Jeghers syndrome and four with adenoma malignum of the cervix. *Cancer* 1982;50:1384–1402.

105. Shen K, Wu PC, Lang JH, et al. Ovarian sex cord tumor with annular tubules: a report of six cases. *Gynecol Oncol* 1993;48:180–184.

106. Ahn GH, Chi JG, Lee SK. Ovarian sex cord tumor with annular tubules. *Cancer* 1986;57:1066–1073.

107. Moore A, Permezel M, Mulvany N, et al. Hillus cell tumor of the ovary in a virilized, postmenopausal women. Case report and review of hyperandrogenism of ovarian origin. *Aust NZ J Obstet Gynaecol* 1999;39:75–78.

24

PELVIC SUPPORT AND SUSPENSION DYSFUNCTION

EDUCATIONAL OBJECTIVES

Medical Students (1)
APGO Objective No. 48

Predisposing risk factors for pelvic
  organ prolapse and incontinence
Anatomic changes, fascial defects,
  and neuromuscular pathophysiology
Signs and symptoms of pelvic
  organ prolapse
Physical exam
  Cystocele
  Rectocele
  Enterocele
  Vaginal vault or uterine prolapse
Nonsurgical and surgical treatments
  including the following:
    Pessary
    Medications
    Reconstructive surgery

Residents in Obstetrics/Gynecology (2)
CREOG Objectives

History
Physical examination
Diagnostic studies
  Tenaculum traction
  Valsalva maneuver
  Anatomic assessment while
    patient is standing
Diagnosis
  Uterine prolapse and procidentia
  Cystocele and Cystourethrocele
  Enterocele
  Rectocele
  Healed vaginal and perineal obstetric laceration
Management
  Possible interventions
  Factors influencing decisions regarding intervention
Potential complications of intervention
Potential complications of intervention
Potential complications of nonintervention
Follow-up

Practitioners (3)
ACOG Recommendations

Pelvic organ prolapse
Contributing factors
Pelvic support system
Signs and symptoms
Evaluation
Management
  Nonsurgical
  Surgical
Follow-up

The clinical management of pelvic support and suspension dysfunction is challenging, even for a practitioner specializing in these aspects. The functional complexity of maintaining female internal genitalia in place and the mechanism of pelvic relaxation are not fully understood. They can cause controversy in diagnosis and management. Additionally, most of the essential supporting and suspending structures are located retroperitoneally, deep within the pelvis, and require three-dimensional appreciation. Understanding the pelvic anatomy and its accurate function are essential for establishing defects in the underlying anatomical structure. Pelvic support structures in the erect posture of human females, as opposed to the plantigrade (or quadruped) postures of other mammals, must balance the forces of gravity and intra-abdominal pressure, which are the main contributors to pelvic relaxation.

PELVIC FLOOR FUNCTIONAL ANATOMY

Female pelvic bone and structures underwent unique evolutionary changes preparing women to cope effectively with the challenges imposed by nature. Accordingly, pelvis bones adopted changes to match the demands of erect posture as follows:

■ Alternation of lumbosacral angulations (which effectively disperse intraabdominal pressure directing it to the abdominal wall, the pubic symphysis, the iliac bones, and the widened sacrum hollow)

- Broadening of the hollowed sacrum
- Horizontal positioning of the pubic symphysis

With evolutionary changes of the pelvis bone, changes in pelvic floor structures occurred:

- Relocation and reduction of tail-moving muscles that partially fill the pelvis
- Horizontal closing of the low pelvis space by the urogenital diaphragm (a characteristic structure for human being)
- Forward (towards the pubis symphysis) movement of the hiatus upon the levator ani muscle (5)

The pelvic floor, which is created by the pelvis bones, plays multiple roles in the human female:
1. Secures the outlet of the pelvis
2. Prevents the prolapse of abdominal-pelvic organs
3. Permits conception
4. Assists in maintaining the pregnant uterus in the pelvic-abdominal location
5. Allows childbirth
6. Controls urine as well as stores and evacuates fecal material

The vagina fuses in several points, ranging from the perineum though the cervix to the pelvic floor structures. The pelvic outlet determines *the perineum* boundaries, with the following diamond-shaped anatomical formations:

- The pubic symphysis establishes the anterior aspect.
- The ischiopubic rami define the anterolateral boundaries.
- The ischial tuberosities determine lateral position.
- The sacrotuberous ligaments delineate posterolateral borders.
- The coccyx demarcates the posterior margins.

Drawing an imaginary line between the two ischial tuberosities, the diamond-shaped perineum will be composed of two anterior and posterior triangles. The anterior triangle (also called the "urogenital triangle") can be identified between the inferior fascia of the urogenital diaphragm and the superficial perineal fascia.

I. *The urogenital triangle* (anterior triangle) is divided into two compartments:
  A. *Superficial perineal area*, which harbors the following structures:
    1. *The superficial transverse perineal muscle* inserts from one side to the ischial tuberosity, and the other end fuses with the perineal body. It functions to stabilize the perineal body. The perineal branch of the pudendal nerve provides innervations.
    2. *The ischiocavernous muscle* is attached to the ischiopubic ramus and the inner surface aspect of the ischial tuberosity, and inserts into the corpus

cavernosum (the crus of the clitoris). The perineal branch of the pudendal nerve provides innervations. The function of this muscle is to retard the venous return by compressing the crus and the deep dorsal clitoral vein.
    3. *The bulbocavernosus muscle* (the bulbospongiosus muscle) arises from the central perineal tendon and inserts to the clitoral corpus spongiosum. The perineal branch of the pudendal nerve provides innervation. It functions to contract the vaginal introitus and squeeze the vestibular bulb.
    4. *The vestibular bulb* is covered by the bulbocavernosus muscle.
    5. *Bartholin's gland*, or the greater vestibular gland, is located behind the vestibular bulb. It produces and secretes mucus that lubricates the vagina during sexual intercourse. The Bartholin's gland duct orifice is located between the labium minora and the hymen.
    6. *The central tendon* of the perineum (the perineal body or the central point of the perineum) contains fibromuscular tissues located in the midline between the anal canal and the vagina. It is a place of fusion for the following:
      a. The superficial transverse perineal muscles
      b. The deep transverse perineal muscles
      c. The fibers of the levator ani muscle
      d. The bulbocavernous muscles
      e. The external sphincter muscles

The perineal body functions to provide a major support for the posterior vagina, which rests on this structure.
    7. *The superficial perineal fascia* (Colles' fascia) establishes the lower margin of the superficial perineal space, providing the deep membranous layer to this structure.
    8. *The inferior fascia* of the urogenital diaphragm or the perineal membrane plays dual roles:
      a. The superior edge of the superficial space
      b. The inferior margin of the deep space
  B. *Deep perineal space* is located between the superior and inferior fascias and encapsulates the urogenital diaphragm, which is composed of the following:
    1. *The deep transverse perineal muscle* is attached to the inner plane of the ischial ramus and inserts to the wall of the vagina and the perineal body. The perineal branch of the pudendal nerve provides innervations. It functions to support the vagina and to stabilize the perineal body.
    2. *Sphincter urethral muscle* surrounds the urethra and is attached to the inferior pubic ramus and inserts into the perineal body and anterolateral wall of the vagina. The perineal branch of the pudendal nerve provides innervations.
    3. *The superior and inferior fascia* invests the urogenital diaphragm

4. Bulbourethral glands or Cowper's glands, which are located on the posterolateral urethra
5. Branches of the internal vessels
6. Pudendal nerve

II. *Posterior anal triangle* is delineated as follows:

- Anteriorly, the superficial and deep transverse perineal muscles create the boundaries.
- Posteriorly, the sacrotuberous ligaments and the gluteus maximus muscles represent the borders.
- Laterally, the obturator muscle and fascia form the boundary.
- Medially, the external anal sphincter and the levator ani muscle form the boundary.

The anal triangle contains the following:

- *Ischiorectal fossa* incorporates the internal pudendal vessels, the pudendal nerve, and a perineal branch of the posterior femoral cutaneous nerve.
- The *Levator ani muscle* is partially connected with the posterior anal triangle. This muscle has multiple points of attachments such as the pubic bones, the arcus tendineus of levator ani, and the ischial spine. It inserts into the coccyx and anococcygeal raphe. The levator ani muscle is divided into the three branches according to the points of origin and in analogy with its phylogenetic derivation: the puborectalis, pubococcygeus, and iliococcygeus. These branches of the levator ani muscle form a firm muscle plate that is called the "levator plate," which is located between the coccyx and the anus. Also, the levator ani muscle forms two crura that delineate the boundaries of the levator hiatus laterally. The third and fourth sacral nerves and the perineal branch of the pudendal nerve provide the innervations to the muscles. The function of the levator ani is to form the pelvic floor with the coccygeus muscle, which is the main supporting structure of the pelvis viscera by continuous tonic contraction of the striated muscle (6). Such tonic contractions of the muscle will change in response to fluctuating intraabdominal pressure. The puborectalis and the pubococcygeus of the levator ani directly surround the levator ani hiatus, and their contractions will not only reduce the anterior-posterior detentions of the levator hiatus but also will close the visceral organ canals that pierce the levator hiatus (the rectum, the vagina, the urethra). In addition to the closure of the pelvis aperture, the levator ani muscle coordinates the intraabdominal pressure distribution between the abdominal wall muscles and the pelvic diaphragm.
- *Coccygeous muscle* attaches to the ischial spine and the sacrospinous ligament, and inserts into the coccyx and the lower segment of the sacrum. This muscle is innervated by the third and fourth sacral nerves. Functionally, the coccygeus muscle together with the levator ani muscle creates the pelvic floor and, as part of this structure, supports and raises the pelvic floor.

- *Obturator internus muscle* is inserted to the inner surface of the obturator membrane, and its tendon is attached to the greater trochanter of the femur. The obturator internus nerve provides innervation. The function of this muscle is to laterally rotate the thigh.
- *External anal sphincter muscle* fuses with the tip of the coccyx and anococcygeal ligament, and inserts into the perineal body. The inferior rectal nerve provides the innervations and functionally is responsible for anal closure.

The anterior and posterior triangles constitute the lowest segment of the pelvic outlet viscera supporting structures. In this segment of pelvic floor support, the *paracolpium* (the portion of the fascia that fuses with the vagina) and *parametrium* (the portion of the fascia that combine to the uterus) are also important structures that play a role in supporting the pelvic viscera. The next level of pelvic floor support is the urogenital diaphragm.

The urogenital diaphragm is a strong musculomembranous structure that spreads out between the ischiopubic rami and supports the anterior half of the pelvic outlet. The superior and inferior fascia encapsulates the deep transverse perineal muscle, the striated sphincter urethral muscles, the pudendal vessels, and pudendal nerves are part of this anatomical structure. The vagina and the urethra pierce the urogenital diaphragm in a different angle, apart from the levator ani hiatus. Such an unaligned configuration between these two structures efficiently enhances the pelvic floor.

The endopelvic fascia is a structure that forms a connective tissue envelope, encapsulating all the pelvic supportive structure. It also forms ligaments such as the cardinal ligaments (which attach to the posterolateral aspect of the cervix and the vagina bilaterally, and insert into the pelvis wall), and the uterosacral ligaments (which run from the posterior cervix bilaterally to the sacrum) which suspend the pelvic viscera. The Douglas pouch is situated between the uterosacral ligaments. The pubocervical fascia stretches anteriorly from the pubic bone and incorporates the vagina, from the vesicovaginal septum, and the urethra enhancing their support in the pelvis. Posteriorly, it provides the support between the posterior wall of the vagina and the anterior wall of the rectum (the rectovaginal septum).

Vaginal Support and Suspension

The uterovaginal fascia (endopelvic fascia) encompasses the vaginal walls, providing connective tissue for merging with supportive and suspensory structures. The introitus or vestibule of the vagina posteriorly in the midline fuses with the perineal body and laterally with the bulbocavernous muscles. Between the bulbocavernous muscle and the inferior fascia of the urogenital diaphragm, the vestibular bulb is located adjacent to the lateral wall of the vagina. Laterally, the inferior and posterior fascia of the urogenital diaphragm and the deep transverse perineal muscle support the vagina bilaterally. Just above this vicinity, the vagina is attached to the crura of the levator ani. The upper part of the vagina is suspended from the Mackenrodt's ligament (the cardinal ligaments). There are four vaginal fornices: anterior, posterior, and two laterals. Among them the posterior vaginal fornix is the deepest one and is considered a reservoir for semen after ejaculation. The vaginal fornices fuse around the cervix. The arcus tendineus fascia pelvis or white line (stretches between the pubic bone and ischial spine and superiorly rests on the pelvic diaphragm) merges with the vaginal lateral-superior pubocervical fascia (the vaginal superior-lateral sulci) and supports a middle part of the vagina (7).

The vagina and terminal rectum lie parallel to the levator plate within the pelvis. At rest, the vagina is bent, creating an angle of approximately 130 degrees between the parallel course to the rectum and the part that lies on the perineal body.

The pudendal nerve supplies innervations to the vagina with low numbers of sensory nerve endings.

Uterine Support and Suspension

The major source of uterine support is the pelvic diaphragm, more specifically the levator plate (part of the pelvic diaphragm which is not a separate anatomical or functional organ), over which the uterus rests. When intraabdominal pressure increases (during straining, coughing, loafing, sneezing, defecating, or urinating), this triggers pelvic diaphragm contractions, which manifest by increasing the tension (strength) of this structure. Such increased tension effectively resists abdominal pressure. The continuous resting tone of the levator ani not only closes the urethral, vaginal, and rectal lumen (obliterating the pelvic floor aperture, thereby preventing pelvic viscera from descending), but also places the uterus over the levator plate (with the cervix located at the posterior aspect of the levator plate, close to the coccyx). Such uterine placement shifts the uterus away from the levator hiatus, preventing prolapse. It is essential that all the levator ani muscle attachments in the pelvis, innervations, contractions, and functions remain intact. When one or more of these parameters are impaired, resistance can be ineffective, predisposing to pelvic floor relaxation. Therefore, increased intraabdominal pressure with adequate pelvic diaphragm contractions result in resistance, so that the pelvic viscera will remain above the pelvic diaphragm, behind and away from the levator hiatus (the urogenital hiatus), aligned backward, downward, and against the levator plate. To stabilize the uterus, appropriate interaction between the pelvic floor and uterine ligaments is essential.

The broad ligament of the uterus is a double reflection of the parietal peritoneum that stretches from the lateral superior aspect of the uterine isthmus bilaterally and attaches to the inner pelvic walls. The bladder and the rectal peritoneum merge with the broad ligaments. The ligament invests the round ligaments and inserts to the anterior inferior surface of the Fallopian tube. The broad ligament between the Fallopian tubes and ovaries is called the "mesosalpinx," or "tubal mesentery," which contains small-caliber vessels. Together with the uterus, the broad ligament establishes the anterior and posterior sections of the pelvis. This structure encompasses areolar tissue, blood vessels, and nerves.

The cardinal ligaments, also known as the transverse cervical ligaments or Mackenrodt's ligaments, are situated at the inferior base of the broad ligament and the lateral isthmic-cervical areas. They fuse the anterior cervical and the upper part of the endopelvic fascia. The lateral-posterior aspect of the ligament, together with the uterosacral ligaments, create the cardinal complex. Laterally, the cardinal ligaments merge with the fascia of the obturator and pelvis floor muscles. The function of the cardinal complex is to directly support, suspend, and stabilize the cervix and the upper vagina. This mechanism also indirectly supports, suspends, and stabilizes the uterus in the midline. These ligaments effectively assist the pelvic diaphragm in preventing the pelvic viscera from descending or prolapsing.

The uterosacral ligaments attach to the posterior aspect of the cervix at the level projecting to the internal cervical os and insert to the second and third sacral vertebrae. This strong connective tissue is mainly responsible for maintaining the following:
1. The corpus of the uterus in normal anteverted position
2. The cervix at the right angle to the vagina

By this mechanism, the uterine body axis is unaligned with the vaginal longitudinal axis, providing effective protection for the pelvis viscera descent or prolapse.

The round ligaments arise from the anterior corneal area of the uterine corpus bilaterally, then pass retroperitoneally, traverse the inguinal canals, and insert to the labia majora. The round ligaments have little, if any, effect on uterine support or stabilization.

The uteroovarian ligaments or ovarian suspensory ligaments arise between the Fallopian tubes and the round ligaments, and insert to the inferior edge of the ovary and the mesovarium (the extended part of the broad ligament). Their function is to stabilize the ovaries; although, they do not participate in support of the pelvic floor diaphragm.

The posterior cul-de-sac or the pouch of Douglas (the rectovaginal pouch) stretches between the uterosacral ligaments. The peritoneum covers the posterior uterine cervix, then descends over the posterior vaginal fornix and the small upper part of the vagina, and over the anterior rectal ampulla fascia. The mean depth of the rectovaginal pouch is about 5.3 cm, and the mean length of rectovaginal septum is about 2.1 cm (8).

The Denonvilliers' fascia is also known as the rectovaginal septum; it stretches from the perineal body to the pouch of

Douglas. The fascia arises from the perineal body, extends under the posterior vaginal wall, traverses along the anterior margin of the rectovaginal space, and inserts into the posterior cul-de-sac of Douglas.

The pelvic bones are the fundamental structures to which, directly or indirectly, all the genital supportive and suspensory anatomical elements are ultimately fused.

GENITAL SUPPORT DYSFUNCTION AND DEFECTS

Retrodisplacement of the Uterus

Definition

The posterior cul-de-sac or the Douglas' pouch sometimes opens so wide that the uterine body moves inside it.

Incidence

In the general female population, uterine retrodisplacement prevalence is approximately 20% to 30% (9,10).

Pathophysiology

The uterine body may fill the posterior cul-de-sac when the space between the uterosacral ligaments is greater than the uterine corpus itself. Such a wide opening of the pouch of Douglas may result from weakening of the uterosacral ligaments, particularly the retroperitoneal part of the ligaments. The retroperitoneal part of the cardinal complex appears to be stronger than the extraperitoneal segment of the uterosacral ligaments, which is the weak peritoneum. The uterosacral ligament is one unit anatomically; nevertheless, two functional layers of these ligaments have been distinguished in the literature (the superficial layer or peritoneal structure, and the deep layer made of connective tissue) (11).

In nonpregnant women, the round ligament may have little, if any, role in maintaining the uterus in anteversion (9). Therefore, placating the round ligaments for uterine suspension merely transitionally elevates the uterus.

Classification

The uterine retrodisplacement is divided into the following (12) the classifications:

1. Uterine *retroversion* is defined by the angle between the cervix and the vagina.
2. Uterine *retroflexion* is determined by the angle between the long axis of the uterine corpus and the cervix.
3. *Retrocession* is where both the corpus and cervix are in the backward (towards the sacrum) position.

These variations of uterine displacement, in the most cases, may coexist, although either may exist independently (9,13).

Diagnosis

Essentially, the diagnosis of symptomatic uterine retrodisplacement is based upon a clinical picture and the absence of pelvic pathology. Therefore, the diagnosis of exclusion of other gynecological entities is recommended.

Pertinent medical history is characterized by the presence of the following:

- Deep dyspareunia
- Dysmenorrhea
- Pressure in the bladder with frequent urination
- Pressure in the rectum
- Backaches
- Pelvic pressure and pain
- Bearing-down sensation
- Pregnancy loss due to pregnant uterine fixation or sacculation
- Constipation

General physical examination reveals no identifiable abnormality.

Pelvic examination will determine uterine retroversion, retroflexion, or retrocession. Occasionally, an incarcerated uterus (uterine wedging into the pelvis) can be identified.

Differential Diagnosis

The differential diagnosis includes the following:

- Allen-Masters' syndrome includes the broad ligament or the uterosacral ligament laceration, the universal join of the cervix (cervical hypermobility in all directions), and uterine enlargement/engorgement (14). In the majority of cases of Allen-Masters' syndrome, uterine retroversion is present.
- Pelvic congestion syndrome is considered a vascular congestion manifested by dysmenorrhea, menorrhagia, dyspareunia, diffused suprapubic pain, postmenstrual low-back pain, and, in about 35% of patients, uterine retrodisplacement. On pelvic examination, the uterus can be retroverted, enlarged, soft, and congestive, and adnexal tenderness can be present (15).

Conventional Therapy

Initially, a patient with symptomatic uterine retroflexion should be *treated conservatively* with the following regimes (16):

1. Combined medical therapy of a low-dose oral contraceptive and nonsteroidal antiinflammatory drugs for at least 6 months.

2. Bimanual replacement of the retrodisplaced uterus followed up by vaginal Smith-Hage insertion. A pessary may not only provide transitional therapeutic benefit but also may predict the outcome of the surgical correction, if surgery is contemplated.

If both medical approaches fail, the surgical approach is recommended.

When the pregnant uterus is incarcerated in the posterior cul-de-sac, an attempt can be made to displace the uterus. With a patient in the knee-chest position, finger pressure is applied through the rectum to the wedged uterus in the pelvis. Upon a successful attempt, a Smith-Hage pessary is inserted and kept in place until the end of the first trimester. The most common side effect of an intravaginal pessary is occasional local irritation and vaginal discharge. It can be overcome with ease by periodically applying a vaginal cream such as Sultrin.

Surgical therapy, historically, is executed on the extraperitoneal anatomical suspensory structures by shortening or plication of the round ligaments [either by Gilliam's technique (17) or its modification (18)] or of the uterosacral ligaments [the peritoneal, superficial layer of the uterosacral ligaments (9)]. Some pelvic surgeons also do peritoneal reconstruction of the posterior cul-de-sac, either by Moschcowitz's (19) or Halban's technique (20).

The idea that placation of the round ligament can convert uterine retrodisplacement to anteversion, as well as its durability, has been questioned for several decades (21,22). In this procedure, by elevating the uterus, the posterior cul-de-sac and the rectovaginal space are exposed to fluctuating intraabdominal pressure, which creates a predisposition to enterocele formation. Shortening of the peritoneal part of uterosacral ligament (9) does not reconstruct the defective retroperitoneal part of the uterosacral ligament. Therefore, retroperitoneal structures of the uterosacral ligaments stronger than peritoneal composition appear more suitable for durable surgical outcome. The retroperitoneal reconstructive technique utilizes the deep layer of the uterosacral ligaments, rectal fascia, and vaginal-uterine fascia for durable reconstruction; initial promising results have been discussed in the literature. The retroperitoneal hysteropexy can be executed via laparotomy or from the laparoscopic approach (16).

It is important to stress that not all women with uterine retrodisplacement (20% to 30% in general population) will require surgery for this condition. Those women who have not responded to conservative management and in whom symptoms are interfering with daily activity are candidates for surgical treatment. It is crucial to select the type of operation that will correct the cause of symptomatic uterine retroflexion (16).

Occasionally, symptomatic *anteroflexion* can occur. Dysmenorrhea and bladder pressure with frequent urination may be present. In the lithotomy position without anesthesia or analgesia, a gentle reposition with synchronized bimanual transvaginal pressure can be applied. The internal finger identifies and firmly supports the angle between the uterine corpus and the cervix, while the external hand pushes the uterine corpus against the internal hand. Such gentle uterine reposition is helpful in both symptomatic retroflexion and anteroflexion. To decrease endometrium bleeding during menses and menstrual pain, oral contraceptive and nonsteroidal antiinflammatory drugs can be administered.

Complementary-Alternative Therapy

There is no data available for a specific therapy for symptomatic uterine retroflexion. Selective therapies offered for dysmenorrhea and dyspareunia can be theoretically applied in this medical entity. However, scientific clinical data to support such an approach are not present.

Pelvic Viscera Descent or Prolapse
Central Compartment

Pelvic organ descent or prolapse may occur in different locations of anatomic support and/or suspension; affecting pelvic organs anatomically related to these structures. Gross and functional anatomy and a clinical picture of a particular case should be analyzed intensely. For pragmatic purposes, the pelvic structures can be compartmentalized:

I. *Central compartment defect* is the result of compromising the effectiveness of the cardinal-uterosacral ligament complex associated with congenital weakness, injury, or an iatrogenic cause such as pelvic surgery. The following clinical abnormality can be identified in the central compartment defects:
   A. Enterocele
   B. Vaginal eversion or prolapse
   C. Uterine prolapse
II. *Anterior compartment defects*
   A. Urethrocele
   B. Cystocele
      1. Vaginal wall defect(s)
      2. Anterior paravaginal defects
III. *Posterior compartment defects*
   A. Rectocele
   B. Perineal deficiency
   C. Perineal descent

Pelvic organ prolapse and pelvic floor dysfunction have been standardized by a site-specific system that provides a tool for staging pelvic support disorders. Such a system eases both clinical and scientific communication in reference to an individual patient or research (23).

The following site-specific staging is offered (23):

- Stage 0 (no prolapse)
- Stage I (the presenting part is >1 cm above the hymen)

- Stage II (the presenting part is >1 cm above or below the hymen)
- Stage III (the presenting part is >1 cm beyond the hymen but <1 cm from the total vaginal length)
- Stage IV (complete eversion)

For quantification of pelvic organ prolapse, the following nine-point profile is used:

- The six vaginal reference points are used (two anterior, two posterior, and two at the apex). Their relationship from the hymen (the hymen is considered as the cutoff point, or the 0 point) to the presenting part is determined, and the distance above the hymen is expressed as minus (e.g., −3 cm meaning that the presenting part of the descending organ is 3 cm above the hymen). The distance below the hymen is expressed as plus.
- The genital hiatus, the perineal body, and the total vaginal length make additional three points. In general, from a clinical point of view, the genital hiatus (measurement from the middle of the external urethral meatus to the inferior hymeneal ring), the vaginal length (measurement from the hymeneal ring to the vaginal apex), and the perineal body (measurement from the inferior hymeneal ring to the middle of the anal orifice) should be quantitatively evaluated.

Such prolapse quantification seems to be sufficient for an individual presentation of a patient; even though, this system is ineffective when group comparisons are needed.

Enterocele

Definition. Enterocele is a detachment of the retroperitoneal anterior rectal fascia and the posterior vaginal-uterine musculofascial structures (the rectovaginal septum), with or without abdominopelvic organs present in the hernia sac (the small intestine, omentum or ovary) (24).

Incidence. The prevalence of enterocele is estimated to be approximately 0.1% to 16% in women undergoing gynecological procedures (25).

Pathophysiology. Enterocele, from the clinical point of view, meets all the criteria to satisfy the true definition of hernia and is, therefore, considered by some to be a misnomer (26). "Entero-" refers to the intestine, which is not a diseased organ and merely is entrapped in the hernia sac. There is no other hernia in the human body that is termed according to the organ trapped inside a hernia sac.

- Enteroceles involve anatomic defects of the retroperitoneal anterior rectal fascia and the posterior vaginal fascia (the rectovaginal septum).

Classification. Enteroceles are generally divided into these four categories (27):

1. *Congenital enterocele* sac is located between the posterior vaginal wall and anterior rectal wall, and results from the failure of fusion of the peritoneum.
2. *Pulsion enterocele* sac has the same location as the congenital enterocele, but, additionally, vaginal wall eversion is present. Mechanics of this defect are associated with forces generating from pushing by intraabdominal pressure. Some authorities call this form of enterocele a *true enterocele* (the hernia sac is distended by intraabdominal pressure, with intestine filling the sac).
3. *Traction enterocele* sac is located similarly to the congenital enterocele, with lower vaginal vault eversion caused by the pulling forces of cysto- and rectocele; it is not filled by intestine.
4. *Iatrogenic enterocele* is considered a postsurgical (a vesicourethral pin-up procedure such as Marshall-Marchetti-Krantz procedure, Burch operation, or ventral suspension) complication that changes the vaginal axis. It can occur anteriorly or posteriorly to the vagina.

Diagnosis. *Pertinent medical history* reveals the following (24):

- Bearing down sensation
- Pressure or feeling fullness in the rectum
- Falling-out sensation
- Sensation of a bulging mass in the vagina pool
- Pelvic pressure
- Pelvic and/or low back pain (absent on arising from bed in the morning, occurring during daily activities, and getting better with resting in the lying down position) are together highly suggestive of genital organ prolapse. Pain that presents at the time of arising from a bed and gets better during the day suggests an orthopedic origin.
- Deep dyspareunia or difficulty during sexual intercourse
- Dyschesia

These symptoms are nonspecific for enterocele and can be present in other pelvic relaxation conditions as well.

General physical examination is performed with particular attention to the presence of abdominal skin striae. If striae are present, their width should be assessed (the presence of numerous, wide abdominal striae may suggest an elastic tissue defect, and the wider the striae the greater the chance of pelvic relaxation disorder).

On *pelvic examination*, positive findings may include any of the following:

- Vulvar atrophy
- Anterior and posterior perineal triangles should be evaluated.
- Site-specific abnormality should be noticed, and staging in dorsolithotomy at rest and with strain should be performed,
- The damage assessment of primary enterocele is initially performed with the anterior blade of the speculum gently inserted in the anterior vaginal fornix. Two cotton-

tipped swabs should be centrally applied to the leading enterocele part. Gentle pressure is applied until the enterocele is reduced. The upper blade of the speculum is released, and the relationship of the anterior and posterior vaginal walls and their defects are evaluated.

■ Bowel sounds may be appreciated on sac enterocele auscultation.
■ Upon rectovaginal examination with the patient in the standing position and straining, an examiner may appreciate a sliding movement of the intestine into the herniated sac.

Some authorities suggest performing defecography and/or electromyography of the pelvic floor muscles in the case of enterocele (28). However, these approaches have not met wide clinical acceptance.

Differential Diagnosis

■ High located rectocele
■ Communicating rectocele with the pouch of Douglas

Conventional Therapy. Taking into consideration the anatomic defect location associated with symptomatic enterocele, it is obvious that retroperitoneal, and not peritoneal, reconstruction should be executed (24). There are several techniques that have been developed and applied transabdominally (19,20), laparoscopically (24) or transvaginally (29,30).

A surgical therapy that corrects the specific-site retroperitoneal damage—reconstruction with an option to approach via laparotomy, vaginally or laparoscopically—has been developed (24). Surgical techniques and the differences in anatomical structures are presented in Table 24.1.

Complementary-Alternative Therapy. Since enterocele is an anatomical defect, conservative medical approach can only be used to cope with general symptoms; however, definitive therapy is surgical reconstruction. No complementary or alternative specific treatment has been reported.

Partial or Total Vaginal Prolapse
Definition. Sliding down the vaginal wall from its supportive and suspensory structure is considered a vaginal descent. The extreme stage is complete vaginal wall migration beyond the hymen, which is called a "total vaginal prolapse."

Incidence. The prevalence of posthysterectomy vaginal vault prolapse is unknown; however, it is suspected to be in the range of 900 to 1,200 cases per year in the United States (31).

TABLE 24.1. DIFFERENCES AMONG SURGICAL THERAPIES FOR ENTEROCELE

Study	Surgical Technique	Anatomic Structure Used for Reconstruction	Comments
Moschowitz (19)	To obliterate the posterior cul-de-sac with multiple, concentric purse-string nonabsorbable sutures	Peritoneum and sigmoid colon serosa and peritoneal portion (superficial layer) of the uterosacral ligaments	1. Endopelvic or rectal fascia, or paravaginal fascia is not incorporated into reconstruction. 2. Deep layer (retroperitoneal) of the uterosacral ligaments is not used.
Halban (20)	To obliterate the posterior cul-de-sac with multiple, saggittal nonabsorbable sutures	Peritoneum, sigmoid colon serosa, and posterior uterine erosa	1. Endopelvic or rectal fascia, or paravaginal fascia is not incorporated into reconstruction 2. Deep layer (retroperitoneal) of the uterosacral ligaments is not used.
Torpin (29)	To narrow the cul-de-sac and vaginal apex by vaginal and posterior cul-de-sac wedge excision	Peritoneal portion (superficial layer) of the uterosacral ligament, cul-de-sac peritoneum, and posterior vaginal wall	1. Endopelvic or rectal fascia, or paravaginal fascia is not incorporated into reconstruction. 2. Deep layer (retroperitoneal) of the uterosacral ligaments is not used.
McCall (30)	To narrow the cul-de-sac by placating the uterosacral ligaments and suspending the vaginal apex from the stumps of the uterosacral ligaments	Peritoneum, peritoneum portion (superficial layer) of the uterosacral ligaments, and the vaginal apex in the midline	1. Endopelvic or rectal fascia, or paravaginal fascia is not incorporated into reconstruction. 2. Deep layer (retroperitoneal) of the uterosacral ligaments is not used.
Ostrzenski (24)	Retroperitoneally, to reconstruct the cul-de-sac and the rectovaginal septum	Retroperitoneal deep layer of the uterosacral ligaments connective tissue, rectal fascia, and uterovaginal fascia	1. Retroperitoneal concept of surgery. 2. Retroperitoneal reconstruction. 3. Retroperitoneal connective tissue (and not peritoneum) is utilized for the cul-de-sac and rectovaginal septum reconstruction. 4. Neither vaginal length nor width is compromised.

Pathophysiology. Damage to any of the supportive or suspensory structures may lead to vaginal eversion or total prolapse. The following structures may play a role to different degrees in eversion and/or total vaginal prolapse.

- The uterovaginal fascia (endopelvic fascia)
- The perineal
- The urogenital diaphragm
- The crura of the levator ani
- The Mackenrodt's ligament (the cardinal ligaments)
- The vaginal fornices: anterior, posterior and two laterals fuse around the cervix.
- The arcus tendineus fascia pelvis or white line
- Pelvic diaphragm with the levator plate

Upon removing the uterus, the vaginal apex loses 70% of its support, and a posthysterectomy event is the leading cause of vaginal vault eversion or prolapse. Race also plays a role (i.e., the Caucasian population is more affected than the African-American population).

Classification

1. Partial vaginal eversion (descent) without cystocele and rectocele present
2. Partial vaginal eversion with cystocele, rectocele, and enterocele present
3. Total vaginal prolapse

Diagnosis. *Pertinent medical history* includes the following:

- The vagina protruding from the hymen
- Pelvic fullness and pressure
- Bearing down
- Backaches that eases in the laying down position and gets worse during physical activities
- Sexual vaginal intercourse difficulty
- In some cases, difficulty with defecation that requires manual assistance
- Pelvic pressure and discomfort
- Feeling that something is dropping down
- Occasionally, urinary incontinence is present.

General physical examination may uncover wide and numerous abdominal striae.

Pelvic examination is performed in the dorsolithotomy position at rest with straining (a Valsalva maneuver). Then with the patient in standing position with and without a Valsalva maneuver, the examination is continued to determine the stage of vaginal descent or prolapse by utilizing site-specific staging (23). It is important to determine the site of primary damage, which usually appears first at the vulva and will require particular attention during reconstruction.

Differential Diagnosis

- Enterocele
- Cystocele
- Rectocele

Conventional Therapy for Vaginal Prolapse. The therapy of this condition falls into the following categories:

I. *Nonsurgical treatment may include the following:*
  A. Oral estrogen replacement therapy or local vaginal application of estrogen (initially, 2 g of equivalent or conjugated estrogens at bedtime, 3 times weekly for 2 to 4 weeks; and then after that, 1 g at bedtime once per week) is recommended if hypoestrogenism is present (see Chapter 12).
  B. A long-term perineal resistance exercise or Kegel's exercise (15 strong voluntary pelvic and perineal muscle contraction, each lasting for 3 seconds, and six times daily).
  C. An effective size of intravaginal pessary may be helpful in the following (32):
    1. Anterior compartment disorders—a plastic ring or a Smith/Hodge pessary
    2. Central compartment disorders—a plastic ring or a Gellhorn/flex pessary
    3. Posterior compartment disorder—a Donut or Risser pessary
    4. Total prolapse (procidentia)—Gellhorn/flex or Donut pessary

Other pessaries such as an inflatable pessary can be used at the physician's discretion.

A patient should not feel a properly fitted pessary; nevertheless, to retain a pessary intravaginally, some strength in the perineal body and the pelvic diaphragm must be preserved. A trained person should clean the pessary at the first month and then quarterly as indicated until after the patient becomes proficient at doing it.

In general, a pessary may assist in patient management in the following clinical scenario (33):

- A patient refuses surgery.
- Surgery is contraindicated.
- A patient is awaiting surgery

A pessary may provide very valuable information as to the potential outcome of surgery. It is a general clinical conviction that a pessary will reduce symptoms associated with pelvic organ prolapse; although, how a pessary affects the progress of pelvis relaxation and influences site-specific supportive structures remains an open question.

Complications resulting from the use of a vaginal pessary are as follows:

- Vaginal wall ulceration or vaginal irritation (34)
- Bowel herniation (35)
- Vaginal fistula formation (36)

To minimize such complications, the following measures may be helpful:

- Avoiding excessive tension or stretching of the vaginal walls
- Establishing appropriate follow-up (at the first month and every 3 months thereafter)
- Treatment of any hypoestrogenism before pessary insertion
- Vaginal application of an antibacterial cream
- Concomitant pelvic-perineal muscle exercises

Controlling chronic constipation, adequate treatment of chronic respiratory disease, cardiac disease, diabetes, or arthritis, and weight control should be incorporated into a management program.

II. *Surgical treatment*

Recently, *a new surgical technique for vaginal vault suspension (colpopexy)* has been introduced (37). In this reconstructive operation, the vagina is reattached to the following:

A. The uterosacral ligaments posteriorly
B. The cardinal ligaments lateral-posterior aspect of the vaginal apex
C. The pubocervical fascia anteriorly
D. The tendinous arch, obturator fascia, and the pubo-coccygeus muscle fascia in the middle part of the vagina when traversing through the pelvic floor area [the lateral superior vaginal sulci are attached to these structures (37)]
E. Retroperitoneal reconstruction of cul-de-sac endopelvic fascia [by performing retroperitoneal culdoplasty (24)]
F. Reconstruction of the perineum and the perineal body with reattachment of the lower vagina to the Denonvilliers' fascia and perineal body.
G. When cyst- and/or recto-cele, and enterocele, or perineal, or other defect(s) defects are present, all of them must be corrected with an appropriately selected procedure.

Commonly, extragenital structures such as the sacrospinous ligament [transvaginal sacrospinous colpopexy (9)] or the sacrum [abdominal sacral colpopexy (38) or sacrotuberous fixation (39)], or the Cooper's ligament (40) are used for vaginal vault suspension. The fascia lata (41) or other materials are also utilized for the treatment of total vaginal prolapse.

Occasionally, complete vaginal obliteration by *LeFort operation* is suggested; even though, the procedure eliminates the potential for vaginal sexual intercourse and access to the cervix for Pap smears or other diagnostic and/or therapeutic procedures (9).

In a clinical setting, a life-threatening condition such as small intestinal eventration through the necrotized vaginal wall may develop in an unattended patient (42). Therefore, education about the potential sequelae of untreated vaginal prolapse, of a large enterocele, or of pessary therapy should occur, and the importance of compliance with the management plan should be emphatically stressed.

Complementary-Alternative Therapy. Complementary therapeutic approaches of lifestyle changes to decrease intra-abdominal pressure and a weight reduction program will assist in management. However, there is no clinical experience in the application of these complementary-alternative modalities.

Partial or Total Uterine Prolapse

Partial or total uterine prolapse is one of the central or apical support-suspensory defects that may occur when one or more of these structures compromise functional or anatomical strength. A defect of the following supportive structure may affect the uterine stability in the pelvis:

- *The pelvic diaphragm* with the levator plate (the part of the pelvic diaphragm not separate anatomical or functional organ)
- The cardinal ligaments
- The uterosacral ligaments
- All other supportive pelvic viscera structures may also affect uterine position stability.

Symptoms and the diagnostic approach are very similar to the ones presented for vaginal prolapse.

Conservative management does not deviate from the approaches presented for vaginal prolapse above.

Surgical management consists of total vaginal hysterectomy with posterior culdoplasty and vaginal vault suspension; repair of the existing supportive-suspensory structures appears to be a major trend in the clinical management of this condition. Prophylactic (at the time of hysterectomy) and therapeutic posterior retroperitoneal culdoplasty with vaginal vault suspension is best executed by incorporating retroperitoneal structures, but not peritoneal components (43,44).

In some cases associated with cervical elongation, the Manchester's operation that involves cervical amputation with reattachment of the cardinal ligaments to the anterior surface of the cervix is recommended (9).

There is a psychological aspect to hysterectomy because of issues surrounding the preservation of childbearing capacity for many women. Removing the healthy uterus in women who desire to preserve their childbearing capacity should not be taken lightly. There is a way to preserve the uterus from extirpation. The uterus can be saved when multiple points of suspension of the uterus are created by narrowing the pelvic hiatus. The uterine and vaginal reconstruction techniques, posterior culdoplasty, and anterior-posterior colpomyoperineorrhaphy have been presented above. Nevertheless, additional clinical study is needed to determine the safety and effectiveness of such complex multipelvic supportive-suspensory organ reconstructive procedures.

Complementary Therapy. Kegel's exercise is recommended to tone the pelvic floor and perineal muscles. Also, a vaginal pessary is suggested in selective cases. There is no scientific data to support the notion that perineal resistance exercises can improve or cure total uterine or vaginal vault prolapse.

Alternative Therapy. *Patient Education.* Patient education is recommended to familiarize affected women with the nature of pelvic relaxation, available conventional-complementary-alternative therapies, and their success rates. Lifestyle changes and compliance with the established management program should be explored with patients. The risks, benefits, complications, and expected success rates of various surgical procedures should be presented, as well as the potential consequences that may result from no treatment.

Diet. Diet recommendations include the following:
- Approximately 75% of the diet should consist of raw fruits and vegetables, as well as whole grains such as brown rice and millet
- Drinking 8 to 10 full glasses of water daily

Nutritional Supplements
  Minerals
- Calcium, 1,500 mg daily
- Magnesium, 1,000 mg daily
- Zink, 50 mg daily

  Vitamins
- Vitamin B complex
- Vitamin C, 3,000 to 5,000 mg daily
- Multivitamin

  Nutrients
- L-Carnitine, 500 mg, BID
- L-Glycine, 500 mg, BID
- Amino acid complex
- Fiber supplement daily

Herbal Medicine. Natural hormonal therapy is recommended if hypoestrogenism is present. Moreover, natural products containing phytoestrogens are recommended (see Chapter 12).

    Aletris is recommended in the form of powdered root (about 6 g daily, as a liquid extract [1:1 of 45% ethanol water] or infusions [1.5 g is added to 100 mL of water], is recommended). No side effects have been reported in these doses (45).

Homeopathic Therapy. Alteris (Alteris farinose) is a plant regiment also known as Blackroot, Bitter grass, Culver's physic or root, Devil's bit, Colic root, Blazing starts, or Star-Grass. The active ingredients of the remedy increase motility and serve as a tonic. The dose used is 5 to 10 drops, 1 tablet, 5 to 10 globules, or 1 mL in an intramuscular injection.

    Traditional and anecdotal data support such a clinical approach, but a well-designed control study is needed to validate it. This form of management is also suggested for vaginal descent or prolapse (45).

Anterior Compartment Defect

Urethrocele
Urethrocele (sagging of the urethra) is considered by some a misnomer, since no urethral walls displace, distend, or overstretch. Cystourethrocele is the concurrent occurrence of urethrocele and cystocele. Urethrocele itself will not cause urinary incontinence.

Definition. Urethrocele is the descent of the anterior distal (about 4 cm) vaginal wall from its normal position.

Incidence. The incidence is unknown.

Classification
- Congenital urethrocele is the result of inherited weakness of the endopelvic fascia or fascia of the pelvic floor muscles (46).
- Acquired urethrocele (47)

Pathophysiology. A weakening of the pubocervical fascia may cause urethral posterior rotation and descent from its fusion with the pubic bone. Straining with a Valsalva maneuver will cause the changes that are clinically observed in association with urethrocele.

    Compression and traction of a fetal head during its passage through the vaginal canal during delivery may result in urethrocele formation.

Diagnosis. *Pertinent medical history* is reported as vaginal pressure, protruding anterior vaginal wall, recurrent infection, or chronic inflammation and dyspareunia.

    On *general physical examination*, no abnormality is identified.

    Pelvic examination identifies bulging of the anterior distal (4 cm) vaginal wall.

    Clinical verification is best established with ultrasonographic study and cystourethrography (46).

    Laboratory tests include urine analysis and culture, urethroscopy, and ultrasonography.

Differential Diagnosis
- Anterior cystocele
- Urethral diverticulum
- Enterocele of the anterior cul-de-sac

Conventional Therapy for Urethrocele. Conventional therapy is surgery, which can be executed either endoscopically or via classic excision (urethroplasty) (46–48). Surgery is indicated when symptoms are present or recurrent infection caused by urethrocele is documented. The most common surgical complication is a high recurrent rate, postoperative fistula formation, and stenosis (48).

Complementary-Alternative Therapy. There are no available data for urethrocele treatment.

Cystocele

Definition. Cystocele is herniation of the bladder to the vaginal pool through the anterior vaginal wall.

Incidence. The incidence is unknown.

Classification

- *Distention cystocele* is overstretching of the vaginal wall associated with damage of the deep transverse perineal and pubococcygeus muscles
- *Displacement cystocele* is bladder displacement associated with vaginal vault prolapse; urethral kinking may prevent of stress incontinence, replacement of the prolapse vagina and cystocele may result in stress incontinence
- *Anterior cystocele* or psuodocystocele is bladder herniation to the distal half of the vagina
- *Posterior cystocele* or distention cystocele is bladder herniation to the distal half of the anterior vaginal wall. Anterior and posterior cystoceles often coexist. Isolated posterior cystocele is not associated with stress incontinence; however, large posterior cystoceles may create a problem in emptying the bladder, which may require digital reduction to assist in complete emptying.

Pathophysiology

- *Anterior vaginal* wall defects are associated with damage (stretching, tearing) or atrophy of support structures such as the bladder neck, urethrovesical junction, and the proximal urethra. This form of cystocele is associated with stress incontinence.
- *Anterior paravaginal* defects are partial or complete detachment of the lateral superior vaginal sulci from the arcus tendineus and of the pubourethral ligament.

Diagnosis. *Pertinent medical history* includes the following:

- Sensation of incomplete bladder emptying after urination
- In some cases, a digital reduction of the cystocele to void
- Pressure in the vagina
- Falling out of the vagina
- Increased urinary frequency
- In some cases, the presence of stress urinary incontinence

On *general physical examination*, no abnormality is identified.

Pelvic examination will reveal, with straining (a Valsalva maneuver, or coughing), an increase in the bulging size of the vaginal wall and descent of the anterior vaginal wall. A soft, reducible bulging mass into the vaginal pool is appreciated.

A lateral paravaginal defect

A lateral paravaginal defect is suspected, when, upon squeezing of the pelvic-perineal muscle, the anterior vaginal wall is not elevated from the resting position (*elevation test*).

The lateral vaginal sulci reflections are shallow, absent, or everted, but anterior vaginal wall rugae are present (displacement cystocele). Elevating the vaginal sulci with sponge forceps or Baden's vaginal defect analyzer may completely reduce the cystocele, if it is a pure case of cystocele caused by lateral defect. If there is another cause of the cystocele such as transverse or central fascia damage or combination of both, the elevation test will not completely reduce the cystocele.

Laboratory tests include the following:

- Urine analysis and culture
- Urethrocystoscopy
- Ultrasonography with or without contrast (49,50)

Differential Diagnosis

- Urethrocele
- Urethral diverticulum
- Enterocele of the anterior cul-de-sac

Conventional Therapy for Cystocele

- Cystocele associated with detrusor instability, incontinence will not require corrective surgery for cystocele.
- Symptomatic cystocele will not qualify a patient for hysterectomy.
- Symptomatic cystocele will necessitate reconstructive surgery.
- Symptomatic cystocele without stress incontinence can be treated with anterior colpomyorrhaphy.
- *Paravaginal colpopexy* or paravaginal reconstruction is indicated when paravaginal defect is established clinically and documented by ultrasonography with or without contrast. To reconstruct the damage between arcus tendineus fascia pelvis, the lateral superior vaginal sulci is recommended. The procedure can be executed from the transvaginal approach (51), from the transabdominal approach (52), or from a laparoscopic approach (53).

Complementary-Alternative Therapy. There are no available data for cystocele treatment.

Posterior Compartment Defects

Rectocele

Definition. Rectocele is herniation of the rectum to the vaginal pool through the posterior rectovaginal fascia.

Incidence. The incidence is unknown, although a small asymptomatic rectocele can be identified in a majority of multiparous women.

Pathophysiology

- Trauma of parturition
- Congenital weakness of connective tissue

- Predisposing factors such as long-term constipation

Diagnosis. *Pertinent medical history:*

- Small rectocele is asymptomatic
- Rectal fullness
- Difficult defecation in some cases manual reduction or immobilization of rectocele is necessary to evacuate feces
- Digital evacuation of firm feces
- Incomplete evacuation
- Vaginal pressure
- Frequent enemas and/or disproportionate laxatives used
- Occasionally, rectal bleeding may be reported and is due to hemorrhoidal bleeding most commonly.

On *general physical examination,* no abnormality is identified.

Pelvic examination is best performed with the index finger in the vagina and the middle finger in the rectum (determining the size of the sack) simultaneously. Valsalva maneuver or coughing demonstrates the posterior vaginal wall with a soft, reducible mass bulging into the vaginal pool, an old perineal laceration, and a flat perineal body. The rectovaginal septum is thin and bulging into the vagina. Palpation of the perineal body (between the middle finger in the rectum and the thumb on the perineum) may reveal the skin and the intestinal wall, and the absence of a perineal body.

Colonoscopy is recommended to rule out concomitant colonic lesions, when rectal bleeding is present.

Differential Diagnosis

- Enterocele (bowel sound may be appreciated on auscultation)
- Tumor of the rectovaginal septum

Conventional Therapy for Rectocele

I. *Conservative medical management* is recommended until after completion of childbearing. Such management includes the following:
   A. Eight glasses of fluid intake per day
   B. Avoiding a diet that causes constipation
   C. Oral stool softeners and/or laxatives
   D. Glycerin suppositories
   E. Intravaginal pessary (an inflatable doughnut or a rubber ring pessary); usually a large size is required.
2. *Surgical management* is indicated when a symptomatic rectocele is present, or other central and/or anterior compartments defects are concomitantly present.

Posterior colpomyoperineorrhaphy is recommended and is quite successful when executed correctly, and if any concomitant pelvic relaxation condition is not overlooked and appropriately treated (9).

Postoperative management includes the following:

- Patient education
- Lifestyle changes with appropriate diet recommendations (increased fluid intake to control constipation, avoidance of straining physical activity, etc.)
- Using stool softeners and/or laxative, and/or lubricating suppositories
- Immediate medical attention given to respiratory tract infections to minimize coughing, which increases intra-abdominal pressure.
- Subsequent vaginal delivery discouraged

Complementary-Alternative Therapy. There are no data available for rectocele treatment.

Perineal Disorders
Classification And Definition

1. *Perineal deficiency* is separation of the perineum from pelvic diaphragm muscles (obstetrical trauma during parturition).
2. *Perineal descending or perineal prolapse syndrome* is sagging of the perineum due to an anatomical defect of the pelvic diaphragm.

Incidence. The incidence is unknown.

Pathophysiology:

- *Perineal deficiency* is the result of obstetrical trauma that leads to separation and retraction of the bulbocavernosus and superficial transverse muscles with one end detached from the perineal body. Such a mechanism will cause not only urogenital dysfunction but also may cause anal sphincter muscle dysfunction.
- *Perineal descending syndrome* results from chronic straining during bowel evacuation (54).

Diagnosis. *Pertinent medical history*

I. Perineal deficiency symptoms are related to the extent of the disorder and its association with other forms of pelvic relaxation.
II. Perineal descending syndrome
   A. Initially can be asymptomatic
   B. Difficulties on evacuation
   C. Diminishing stool diameters (a pencil size stool)
   D. Constipation and/or fecal impaction can be present, leading to evacuation difficulties.

On *general physical examination,* no abnormality is identified.
   Pelvic examination

I. Perineal deficiency determination on physical examination is similar to what was described for rectoceles above.
II. Perineal descending syndrome:
   A. The anus is the most dependent portion intergluteally

B. The perineum bulges and widens, and descends below the pelvic bones during straining

Laboratory tests

I. Perineal deficiency testing will depend upon associated clinical symptoms and signs of other forms of pelvic relaxation; described above.

II. Perineal descending syndrome
   A. Clinical measurement of perineal descent is a simple noninvasive method that assesses the location of perineum in reference to the ischial tuberosities. The perineum being below the tuberosities at rest or >2.5 cm during straining may assist in making the diagnosis (54).
   B. Perineometry is not as reliable a method as defecography (55).
   C. Defecography is a functional anatomy evaluation by means of radiographic examining technique of the rectum and anal canal in a sitting down position at rest and during straining (56).

Differential Diagnosis

I. Perineal deficiency
   A. Posterior compartment disorders
   B. Perineal descending syndrome
II. Perineal descending syndrome
   A. Anorectal prolapse
   B. Perineal deficiency

Conventional Therapy for Perineal Defects

I. Perineal deficiency
   A. Conservative symptomatic management
   B. Surgical management is usually effective with an adequate perineoplasty performed. It is imperative to reconstruct all associated pelvic supportive disorders (9).
II. Perineal descending syndrome delays diagnosis, and untimely surgical reconstructive treatment may lead to permanent nerve damage in the levator ani and the external anus sphincter muscles. Such inadvertent denervation will result in fecal incontinence.

Management falls into the following categories:

I. Conservative management includes:
   A. Avoiding straining at defecation
   B. Defecating through a 3-inch (a 7.6-cm) diameter hole to create support around the anus
   C. Administering stool softener and/or laxative
   D. High-fiber diet to prevent constipation
   E. Perineal muscles exercise
II. Surgical treatment is based on the retrorectal levatoroplasty, which involves placing the patient in a jackknife position. A skin incision is made between the anus and the coccyx, the levator plate is identified and bisected,

and dissection is continued until the retrorectal space is reached. On the posterior surface of the rectum, plication stitches 1 cm apart are placed (usually three to four stitches) and tied. Each stitch is attached to the sacral periosteum in the pelvic hollow individually. The levator plate is reconstructed in the middle with single sutures and approximation of the pubococcygei muscle in the midline. If necessary, the pubococcygeus muscle can be shortened by utilizing a Z-shaped type of suture (9).

Complementary-Alternative Therapy. There are no available data for Perineal Disorders treatment.

REFERENCES

1. Association of Professors of Gynecology and Obstetrics (APGO). *Medical student educational objectives,* 7th ed. Washington, DC: APGO, 1997.
2. Council on Resident Education in Obstetrics and Gynecology (CREOG). *Educational objectives core curriculum for residents in obstetrics and gynecology,* 5th ed. Washington, DC: CREOG, 1996.
3. American College of Obstetricians and Gynecologists (ACOG). *Technical bulletin no. 214.* Washington, DC: ACOG, 1995.
4. American College of Obstetrician and Gynecologists (ACOG). *Technical bulletin no. 213.* Washington, DC: ACOG, 1995.
5. Berglas B, Rubin IC. Study of the supportive structures of the uterus by levator myography. *Surg Gynecol Obstet* 1953;97:677–692.
6. Parks AG, Porter NH, Melzak J. Experimental study of the reflex mechanism controlling muscles of the pelvic floor. *Dis Colon Rectum* 1962;5:407–411.
7. DeLancey JOL. Anatomic aspect of vaginal eversion after hysterectomy. *Am J Obstet Gynecol* 1992;166:1717–1728.
8. Kuhn RJP, Hollyock VE. Observations on the anatomy of the rectovaginal pouch and septum. *Obstet Gynecol* 1982;59:445–447.
9. Thompson JD. Retrodisplacement of the uterus. In: Rock JA, Thompson JD, eds. *Te Linde's operative gynecology,* 8th ed. Philadelphia: Lippincott Williams & Wilkins, 1997.
10. Barr SJ, Barr KJ. Retroversion and infertility. *Am J Obstet Gynecol* 1983;146:990–991.
11. Okabayashi H. Radical abdominal hysterectomy for cancer of the cervix uteri. *Surg Gynecol Obstet* 1929;23:335–341.
12. Beckmann CRB, Ling FW, Herbert WNP, et al., eds. *Obstetrics and gynecology,* 3rd ed. Baltimore: Williams & Wilkins, 1998.
13. Mann WJ, Stenger VG. Uterine suspension through the laparoscope. *Obstet Gynecol* 1978;51:563–566.
14. Chatman DL. Pelvic peritoneal defects and endometriosis: Allen-Masters syndrome revisit. *Fertil Steril* 1981;36:751–756.
15. Taylor HC Jr. Vascular congestion and hyperemia: their effect on function and structure in the female reproductive organs. III. Etiology and therapy. *Am J Obstet Gynecol* 1949;57:654–663.
16. Ostrzenski A. Laparoscopic retroperitoneal hysteropexy. A randomized trial. *J Reprod Med* 1998;43:361–366.
17. Gilliam DT. Round ligament ventrosuspension of the uterus: a new method. *Am J Obstet Gynecol* 1900;41:299–303.
18. Candy JW. Modified Gilliam uterine suspension using laparoscopic visualization. *Am J Obstet Gynecol* 1976;47:242–243.
19. Moschowitz AV. The pathogenesis, anatomy and cure of the perirectum. *Surg Gynecol Obstet* 1912:15:7–11.

20. Halban J. *Gynekologische opertionslehere*. Berlin: Urban and Schwarzenberg, 1932.
21. Fluhmann CF. The rise and fall of suspension operation for uterine displacement. *Bull Johns Hopkins Hosp* 1955;96:59–70.
22. Ostrzenski A. Carter-Thomason uterine suspension and positioning by ligament investment, fixation and truncation. *J Reprod Med* 2000;45:79–82.
23. Bump RC, Mattiasson A, Bo K, et al. The standardization of terminology of female pelvic organ prolapse and pelvic floor dysfunction. *Am J Obstet Gynecol* 1996;175:10–17.
24. Ostrzenski A. A new laparoscopic retroperitoneal posterior culdoplasty technique. *J Reprod Med* 1999;44:504–510.
25. Holley RL. Enterocele: a review. *Obstet Gynecol* 1994;49:284–287.
26. Ostrzenski A. Endoscopic pelvic herniorrhaphy with CO_2 laser. *Gynecol Endoscopy* 1992;1:95–98.
27. Nichols DH. Types of enterocele and principles underlying the choice of operation for repair. *Obstet Gynecol* 1972;40:257–263.
28. Smith LE, ed. *Practical guide to anorectal testing*. New York: Igaku-Shoin, 1995.
29. Torpin R. Excision of the cul-de-sac of Douglas, for the surgical care of hernias through the female caudal wall, including prolapse of the uterus. *J Int Coll Surg* 1955;24:322–330.
30. McCall ML. Posterior culdoplasty: surgical correction of enterocele during vaginal hysterectomy. A preliminary report. *Obstet Gynecol* 1957;10:595–602.
31. Dunton JD, Mikuta J. Posthysterectomy vaginal vault prolapse. *Postgrad Obstet Gynecol* 1988;8:1–4.
32. Cundiff GW, Addison WA. Management of pelvic organ prolapse. *Obstet Gynecol Clin North Am* 1998;25:907–921.
33. Sulak PJ, Kuehl TJ, Shall BL. Vaginal pessaries and their use in pelvic relaxation. *J Reprod Med* 1993;38:919–923.
34. Muram D, Summitt RL, Feldment N. Vaginal dilators for intermittent pelvic support: a case report. *J Reprode Med* 1990;35:303–304.
35. Ott R, Richter H, Behr J, et al. Small bowel prolapse and incarceration cause by a vaginal ring pessary. *Br J Surg* 1993;80:1157–1159.
36. Goldstien I, Wise GJ, Tancer ML. A vesicovaginal fistula and intravesical foreign body: a rare case of neglected pessary. *Am J Obstet Gynecol* 1990;163:589–591.
37. Ostrzenski A. Laparoscopic colposuspension for total vaginal prolapse. *Int J Gynecol Obstet* 1996;55:147–152.
38. Backer MH. Success with sacrospinous suspension of the prolapsed vaginal vault. *Surg Gynecol Obstet* 1992;175:419–424.
39. Zweifel P. *Voresungen uber Klinische Gynekologie*. Berlin: Hirschwald, 1982.
40. Langmade CF. Cooper ligament repair of vaginal vault prolapse. *Am J Obstet Gynecol* 1965;92:601–604.
41. Beecham CT, Beecham JB. Correction of prolapsed vagina or enterocele with fascia lata. *Obstet Gynecol* 1973;42(4):42–47.
42. Poreba R, Pozowski J, Ciszek V. Spontaneous small intestine prolapse through the vaginal wall. *Ginekol Pol* 1987;58:128–131.
43. Ostrzenski A. A new, simplified posterior culdoplasty and vaginal vault suspension during abdominal hysterectomy. *Int J Gynecol Obstet* 1995;49:25–34.
44. Ostrzenski A. New retroperitoneal culdoplasty and colpopexy at the time of laparoscopic total abdominal hysterectomy. *Acta Obstet Gynecol Scand* 1998;77:1017–1021.
45. Hansel R, Keller K, Rimpler H, et al. *Hagers handbuch der pharmazeutischen praxis, 5. Aufl., Bde 4-6 (Dorgen)*. Berlin: Springer-Verlag, 1992.
46. Amrani A, Elquessar A, M'Bida R, et al. Congenital Urethrocele in children. A case report. *Ann Urol (Paris)* 1999;33:97–99.
47. Sachot JL, Ratajczak A. Female urethrocele. Difficult diagnosis and therapy. *Ann Urol (Paris)* 1989;23:156–157.
48. Ronzoni G, DeVecchis M, Raschi R. Urethroplasty of recurrent urethrocele: study of 41 cases. *Acta Urol Bel* 1992;60:1–8.
49. Ostrzenski A, Osborne NG, Ostrzenska MK. Method for diagnosing paravaginal defects using contrast ultrasonographic technique. *J Ultrasound Med* 1997;16:673–677.
50. Ostrzenski A, Osborne NG. Ultrasonography as a screening tool for paravaginal defects in women with stress incontinence: a pilot study. *Int Urogynecol J* 1988;9:195–199.
51. White GR. Cystocele. A radical cure by suturing lateral sulci of vagina to white line of pelvic fascia. *JAMA* 1909;53:1707–1713.
52. Richardson AC, Edmonds PB, Williams NL. Treatment of stress urinary incontinence due to paravaginal fascia defect. *Obstet Gynecol* 1981;57:357–362.
53. Ostrzenski A. Genuine stress in women. New laparoscopic paravaginal reconstruction. *J Reprod Med* 1998;43:477–482.
54. Ambrose S, Keighley MR. Outpatient measurement of perineal descent. *Ann R Coll Surg Engl* 1985;67:306–308.
55. Oettle GJ, Roe AM, Bartolo DC, et al. What is the best way of measuring perineal descent? A comparison of radiographic and clinical methods. *Br J Surg* 1985;72:999–1001.
56. Berkelmans I, Heresbach D, Leroi AM, et al. Perineal descent at defecography in women with straining at stool: a lack of predictive value for future anal incontinence. *Eur J Gastroenterol Hepatol* 1995;7:75–79.

25

UROGYNECOLOGY

EDUCATIONAL OBJECTIVES

Medical Students (1) *APGO Objective No. 48*	*Residents in Obstetrics/Gynecology (2)* *CREOG Objectives*	*Practitioners (3)* *ACOG Recommendations*
Urinary incontinence	History	Urinary incontinence
Methods of diagnosis:	Physical examination	Etiology
Urine culture	Diagnostic studies	Stress incontinence
Postvoid residual volume	Valsalva maneuver	Urge incontinence
Cystoscopy	Anatomic assessment while patient	Other conditions causing
Urodynamic testing	is standing	incontinence
Nonsurgical and surgical	Diagnosis	Diagnosis of incontinence:
treatments including:	Management	History
Pessary	Possible interventions	Voiding diary
Medications	Factors influencing decisions	Physical examination
Reconstructive surgery	regarding intervention	Urine culture
	Potential complications of intervention	Stress test
	Potential complications of intervention	Pad test
	Potential complications of nonintervention	Cystometry
	Follow-up	Cystourethroscopy
		Treatment
		Follow-up

MICTURITION AND CONTINENCE IN WOMEN

Urine collection, storage, continence, and micturition involve a complex synchronized interaction between the nervous system, pelvic floor, and lower urinary tract muscles. Micturition and continence in women require intact coordination between the following neurologic factors.

The *neuroanatomy* integrates the central nervous system (4) (brain, spinal cord, and central nerve bodies) and both the somatic (controlling voluntary activity of pelvic floor viscera and smooth muscles) and autonomic (both sympathetic and parasympathetic) peripheral nervous systems. The somatic parasympathetic efferent fibers, which are located in the proximal urethra, innervate the urethral sphincter. The pudendal nerve (S2–4) supplies innervations to the distal urethral sphincters (5). Thus, the pudendal nerve plays a major role in maintaining the integrity of storage and continence. Damage during childbirth or extensive vaginal dissection during pelvic reconstruction may result in incontinence (6).

The peripheral nervous system, essentially via the parasympathetic afferent pathway (the pelvic plexus and pelvic nerve), with sympathetic and somatic feedback, controls urinary collection (bladder filling) and storage reflexes. The bladder pressure receptors, located in the bladder wall, stimulate parasympathetic afferent input in the following spinal voiding reflexes (7,8):

- *Somatic* pathway—the pudendal nerve increases urethral resistance by stimulating muscle contraction.
- *Sympathetic* pathway—the hypogastric plexus stimulates alpha-mediated contraction of the bladder base and urethral smooth muscles, while at the same time inducing beta-mediated relaxation of the detrusor muscle.
- *Efferent* pathway— the pelvic plexus induces parasympathetic inhibition to the detrusor muscle of the bladder.
- *Afferent* pathway includes the pelvic plexus and the pelvic nerves.

The neurophysiology of storage, continence, and micturition presents the complexity of a neuromuscular interaction. The bladder's dual role in urine collection and evacuation depends on activation or inactivation of a switch-type mechanism, with simultaneous increase or decrease of urethral and pelvic floor resistance. The bladder's muscle contraction may commence with an intravesicular pressure of greater than 20 cm H_2O [threshold intravesicular pressure is between 15 and 20 cm H_2O [9]], where the impulse is conducted to the pontine micturition center via the sacral spinal cord.

The pontine micturition center is located in the brainstem (the dorsomedial pons of the central nervous system). The micturition center is responsible for coordination of a loss of cortical voiding parasympathetic inhibition (provokes detrusor contraction) and sympathetic pathway stimulation or inhibition of the external urethral sphincter. Such a mechanism leads to opening of the bladder neck (10). Upon entering the urethra, urine activates the urethrovesicular reflex, which in turn triggers involuntary detrusor contraction (the probable mechanism of stress and urge incontinence in some cases) (11). Initiation of micturition depends on simultaneous bladder muscle contraction and its outlet-reducing resistance.

Bladder Storage Compliance

The dorsal pons micturition center as the supraspinal center controls the bladder's storage compliance (10). The following parameters, under the control of the neurologic system, contribute to bladder compliance of urine filling and storage:

- Normal range of maximum urethral closure pressure
- Low detrusor pressure
- Absence of involuntary detrusor contractions
- Bladder's stretching ability
- Smooth muscle electromechanical properties
- Sacral neural input
- Parasympathetic efferents
- Sympathetic efferents
- Somatic efferents
- Visceral–visceral reflex (vagina, uterine cervix, and rectum) stimulation increases urethral resistance (12). This reflex is used in the treatment of detrusor instability with rectal or vaginal electrostimulation (13) or with biofeedback methods (14).
- Somatovisceral reflex, cutaneous stimulation inhibits micturition contractions. Through this mechanism acupuncture treatments may work in a selective group of patients (15).

When the quantity of urine exceeds the bladder's compliance threshold, a signal is sent via the pelvic nerve to the dorsal horn of the sacral spinal cord, which triggers the frontal cerebral cortex to relax the external urethral sphincter and the pelvic diaphragm by decreasing urethral resistance. External sphincter relaxation occurs 1 to 3 seconds before detrusor contraction in a normal female voiding

process, which is controlled by the pontine micturition center (10). Thus, any brain lesion that affects the pons may clinically manifest as detrusor instability, also known as detrusor hyperreflexia (16).

The neuropharmacology of micturition reflects neuroeffector junction and ganglionic transmission functions. Neurotransmitters of the lower urinary tract, the bladder and urethra, are divided into the adrenergic receptors and the cholinergic receptors (12).

Among *the adrenergic receptors*, alpha-receptors are primarily found in the bladder neck and smooth muscles of the urethra and are responsible for mediating contraction of the bladder base and urethral smooth muscles. Alpha-receptors are sensitive to the high levels of norepinephrine that trigger contraction of the smooth muscles. Through sympathetic pathway stimulation, the bladder storage capacity increases.

Beta-receptors are disseminated throughout the smooth muscle of the detrusor and participate in relaxation of this muscle by lowering norepinephrine levels.

Among *cholinergic receptors*, acetylcholine is the major neurotransmitter in the parasympathetic and somatic systems (12).

Lower Urinary Tract Functional Anatomy

The bladder requires a unique and complex infrastructure to perform its opposing dual tasks of storage and evacuation. The ureteral orifices divide the bladder into two compartments: the bladder dome, which is situated above the ureteral orifices, and the bladder base below. The transitional epithelium (urothelium) is furnished with connective tissue and covers the inner surface of the bladder.

The bladder base has three layers of detrusor muscle:

- Outer layer, with longitudinal muscle fibers
- Middle layer, with circumferential muscle fibers
- Inner layer, with longitudinal muscle fibers

The bladder base musculature plays a major role in urine storage and its evacuation. *The bladder dome* is not composed of the same three layers as the bladder base, but has a plexiform configuration. This part of the bladder assists the bladder base in storage and evacuation.

The bladder neck is the area where the detrusor creates two U-shaped loops that encompass the proximal urethra from opposing directions, with the proximal urethra centrally located between them.

The trigone is the area that stretches from the ureteral orifices to the internal urethral meatus and is composed of an expansion of the longitudinal muscle fibers of the ureter (12,17).

The female urethra is a tube (approximately 4 cm in length) that is composed of multiple layers of muscle, with the inner layer covered by the squamous epithelium mucosa. The squamous epithelium becomes the transitional epithelium upon approaching the bladder base. The urethral tube is connected to the bladder base and opens freely. It is attached to the lower third of the anterior vaginal wall and runs into the retropubic space. The urethra's function is to conduct urine from the bladder, to participate in the opening process of the bladder neck by relaxing muscles, and to enhance the closure mechanism. This complexity of the opening and closing mechanism requires that the anatomic, neurologic, and physiologic integrity of the urethra is intact. The urethra is composed of three layers:

- Outer layer, with circumferential smooth muscle fibers. This layer is considered the internal urethral sphincter.
- Inner layer, with longitudinal smooth muscle fibers
- The circumferential striated muscle sheath encompasses the outer and inner layers of the urethra and forms the external urethral sphincter. This skeletal muscle is distributed in two thirds of the proximal urethra and supports the circumferential pattern of the urethral closure mechanism. The distal one third of the urethral external sphincter ends with the urethrovaginal sphincter, which arises from the anterior vaginal wall, and the urethral compressor, which originates from the ischiopubic ramus (18).

Continence Mechanism

The functional complexity of the female continence mechanism depends not only on the lower urinary tract but also on the pelvic diaphragm and vagina. The specific mechanism of micturition and continence is not yet known. There are several commonly suggested theories.

The proximal urethral compression theory asserts that intraabdominal pressure is used to close off the urethral mechanism. At stress (sneezing, coughing, and etc.), intraabdominal pressure increases, transmitting pressure to the urethra, which causes the lumen to close (19).

The integral theory of female urinary micturition and continence is based on interaction of the closing–opening functional structures of the lower urinary tract with the pelvic floor muscles (levator plate, anterior segment of the pubococcygeus muscle), vagina, and longitudinal muscles of the anus. The mechanism is based on vaginal attachment to the pubourethral ligament and the vagina's ability to move forward at this point. Pubococcygeus muscle contraction induces this forward vaginal movement, closing off the urethra (20–23). This theory discounts the view that the lumen is closed by compression caused by increased intraabdominal pressure.

The common sphincter theory postulates that the harmonious contraction and relaxation of the puborectalis and external urethral sphincter muscles play a major role in micturition and continence processes. During micturition the common sphincter relaxes (24).

The hammock hypothesis suggests that the combination of the fascia and the anterior vaginal wall have a hammock-like construction, in which the bladder neck and proximal urethra lie. The fascia in this unit serves as a connecting, passive element that attaches the vagina to the pelvic floor muscles. The pelvic floor muscles (mainly the levator ani muscle) are considered an active part of this mechanism. Tonic pelvic diaphragm contractions elevate the bladder neck, and the proximal urethra closes off the urine outlet (25).

URINARY INCONTINENCE

Definition

The International Continence Society defines urinary incontinence as "involuntary loss of urine that is objectively demonstrable and a social or hygienic problem" (26), and the U.S. Urinary Guideline Panel characterizes urinary incontinence as "involuntary loss of urine, which is sufficient to be a problem" (27).

Incidence

The prevalence of female urinary incontinence is estimated to range from 10% to 25% among the population 15 to 64 years of age (28) and 17% to 45% among those 35 to 79 years of age (29).

Etiology

The pathophysiology of urinary incontinence is multifactorial and in brief can be categorized by the acronym DIAPPERS, which stands for reversible causes of stress incontinence:

- Delirium
- Infection
- Atrophic vaginitis
- Pharmacologic agents
- Endocrine disorders
- Restricted mobility
- Stool impaction

Classification

- *Stress urinary incontinence* (SUI) is involuntary urine leakage (intravesicular pressure surpasses the maximum urethral pressure) without detrusor contraction (27).
- *Detrusor instability*, or overactive bladder, is involuntary urine leakage associated with an abrupt and strong desire to void (urgency) (27).
- *Mixed incontinence* is coexisting SUI and detrusor instability.
- *Overflow incontinence* is involuntary urine leakage associated with overdistension of the bladder (30).
- *Functional incontinence*, or transient incontinence, is the inability to reach the toilet with an intact lower urinary tract (31).
- *Bypass of the anatomic continence mechanism* is a constant urine leakage due to an anatomic abnormality, such as fistulas, ectopic ureters, or epispadias (31).

■ *Urinary retention* is the result of obstruction of the urethra. A dynamic form of urinary retention is associated with pelvic visceral prolapse (32).

Clinical Evaluation of Stress Urinary Incontinence

Step I

Medical history is an important factor in reaching the diagnosis, but it is insufficient to initiate therapy for urinary incontinence. The *urogynecologic pertinent history* should include the following elements:

■ Onset of urine leakage (gradual onset may indicate a hypoestrogenic state; abrupt onset may indicate an allergic or infectious condition).
■ Duration of urinary incontinence.
■ Severity can be estimated by determining urinary leakage in the supine position with a comparatively empty bladder or the inability to voluntarily cease voiding (only in severe cases); how much urine is leaking (continuous perineal pad protection vs. other intermittent); and how often an incontinence episode occurs.
■ Related specific symptoms:
  Urgency in the context of urologic evaluation has two components: a strong desire to void and fear of leakage or pain, or both.
  Frequency is considered as abnormal when voiding occurs more than seven times per day or within 2 hours of the last void.
  Nocturia is defined as voiding two or more times per night.
  Nocturnal enuresis (bed wetting) is urine incontinence during sleep.
■ Circumstances that trigger urine leakage such as laughing, sneezing, coughing, strenuous physical activity, and changing position may indicate SUI. However, detrusor instability occasionally induces incontinence.
■ Medical history of diabetes mellitus, thyroid disease, multiple sclerosis, cerebrovascular accident, and neurologic illness should be explored (urinary incontinence may present without an underlying urologic abnormality).
■ Parity and mode of deliveries.
■ Urogynecologic or other pelvic surgery potentially affecting the lower genital tract anatomy or function.
■ Medication potentially affecting urine continence:
  Decreasing urethral smooth or skeletal muscle tone (diazepam, phenothiazine, prazosin, and alpha-methyldopa).
  Antihistamine or anticholinergic agents can cause urine retention.
■ *Psychiatric disorders* (urinary incontinence may be present without underlying urologic abnormality).
■ Herbal medicine affecting urinary incontinence:

Micturition disturbances include henbane, mandrake, and scopolia (display atropine and scopolamine properties).
Urinary urgency may be caused by stavesacre in compounds of diterpene alkaloids and may cause urinary and stool urgency.

■ A urolog, or voiding record, is a 24-hour record (can be conducted for 1 day to 2 weeks) of fluid intake, urine output, and incontinence episode(s) and its relationship to physical activities, and related symptoms. The record should be kept for 24 hours and evaluated at the time of clinical interview.
■ A practitioner should address questions in reference to established criteria that fill the DIAPPERS symptomatology.

Step II

General Physical Examination
Routine general examination is performed with particular emphasis on the following:

■ Nutritional status, including body mass index
■ Mental status
■ Mobility
■ Manual dexterity
■ Presence of hernia (abdominal, inguinal, or femoral)
■ Neurologic examination

Particular attention should be directed to the annual wink reflex or bulbocavernosus reflex which evaluates the integrity of the sacral cord reflexes L5 to S5, as well as the pudendal nerve. *The pudendal nerve* arises from S2 through S4 and supplies the following (33):

■ Levator ani muscle
■ Inferior hemorrhoidal (rectal) nerve
■ External anal sphincter
■ Striated urethral sphincter muscle

The wink test is performed with light stroking or tapping of the perineum or clitoris with an alcohol wipe (cold sensitivity test) and pinprick. The anus will normally respond with a "wink" (visible contraction of the external anal sphincter muscle). The test will determine the area of numbness or paresthesia (abnormal sensation), providing information about pudendal neuropathy. The absence of the anal wink reflex to stimulation may be a result from either damage to the pudendal nerve or sacral cord segment. Paresthesias may indicate the presence of a cord lesion, which may be associated with detrusor hyperreflexia or areflexia, depending on the level of the lesion location (34).
Deep tendon reflexes test may indicate the upper and lower motor neurons. Hyperreflexia indicates the presence of an upper motor lesion, and the absence of tendon reflexes indicates a lower motor lesion.

The Babinski sign shows the state of the corticospinal tract's integrity.

Muscle strength evaluation establishes either muscular neuropathy or weakness. Ascertaining lower extremity muscle strength shows the state of the lower sacral segment nerves.

The following testing is usually conducted:

- Visual inspection for symmetry and smooth contraction.
- Unequal muscle strength in both extremities suggests a central nervous system disorder.
- Plantar flexion integrity is controlled by the sacral segment of S1 to S2.
- Hip flexion is controlled by the motor S2 and S3 segments.
- Gait evaluation provides information on cerebellum integrity (lesion or stroke may affect the test).

Pelvic Examination

Pelvic examination should be performed routinely with cervical cytology. Initial inspection and examination is performed with the patient in a supine dorsolithotomy position with forceful straining and coughing; then in a semi-upright position (the position is reached by adjusting the examining table) with vigorous straining and coughing; and finally in the standing position with powerful straining and coughing. Particular attention should be directed to the following:

- Anterior urogenital and posterior anal triangles and anatomic structures within these configurations should be examined.
- Examination of the vaginal mucosa may reveal such changes as:
    - Hypoestrogenic atrophy (thin, smooth, and friable mucosa with decreasing vaginal rugae).
    - Vaginal fistula.
    - Urethral caruncle.
    - Partial vaginal fornix obliteration.
- Strength and symmetry of vaginal and anal sphincter muscle contractions should be evaluated.
- Genital hiatus (measurement from the middle of the external urethral meatus to the inferior hymenal ring), vaginal length (measurement from the hymenal ring to the vaginal apex), and the perineal body (measurement from the inferior hymenal ring to the middle of the anal orifice) should be evaluated.
- Pelvic organ descent or prolapse (see Chapter 24) in the central, anterior, and posterior compartments should be determined with appropriate staging; however, pelvic organ descent or prolapse may not cause urinary incontinence.
- Organ prolapse or a large cystocele must be reduced and urinary incontinence evaluation performed (prolapsed pelvic organ may kink the urethra, preventing urinary incontinence).
- Vaginal introitus, anterior, posterior walls, and apex should be inspected for any abnormality.

- Anterior vaginal defects

In paravaginal lateral superior defect evaluation, two ring forceps are introduced into the lateral aspects of the vaginal pool along the pelvic sidewall and gently elevated. If the cystocele is reduced and does not recur when a patient strains, a paravaginal defect may be present. However, a good correlation between this examination and intraoperative findings has not been achieved (35).

A midline (central and transverse) cystocele should be examined. A midline defect is established with a closed ring forceps placed and elevated in the midline. Reduction of the cystocele during straining suggests midline damage.

Other areas that should be addressed during the pelvic examination are as follows:

- Apical vaginal support evaluation should be conducted (see Chapter 24).
- Posterior vaginal wall abnormalities should be noted.
- The anal sphincter and rectovaginal septum should be examined (rectovaginal digital examination is performed with pelvic-perineal muscle contraction).
- Perineal sensation and the perineal body should be assessed.
- Elicit urethral discharge or tenderness should be noticed, which may suggest the presence of urethral diverticulum.
- Hypermobility of the urethra and the bladder neck is assessed by surveillance of the proximal urethra and bladder neck posterior rotational descent while the patient strains or coughs and with a posterior speculum blade retracting the posterior vaginal wall.
- Urethra and urethral meatus should be evaluated.

Step III

Additional Testing

A primary care physician may establish a clinically precise urinary incontinence diagnosis in about 80% of cases. To reach such a diagnosis, the following testing can be performed in the office setting:

- Urinalysis

Hematuria (may suggest infection, stone, or cancer), elevated white blood cell count (leukocytosis) may indicate infection and calls for urine culture; bacteriuria may indicate symptomatic or asymptomatic urinary tract infection (UTI), which warrants urine culture; glycosuria, and proteinuria must be ruled out.

- Urine culture as indicated.
- Serum creatinine or blood urea nitrogen levels should be determined.
- Urine cytology is indicated when malignancy is suspected.

Among the simple urodynamic tests performed during the bladder filling and storage phases (as well as during voiding) is the *1-hour pad test*, which is designed to objectively demonstrate and document urinary incontinence. After 1 hour of a series of physical activities, a weighted absorbable pad is reweighed and the difference noted (pyridium at a dose of 100–200 mg 30 minutes before ambulating can be used).

The cotton-tipped swab test is applied with the patient lying supine. The urethral meatus is prepared with povidone iodine. The cotton tip is then saturated with anesthetic jelly or cream and inserted into the bladder pool, then gently retracted to the position where some resistance is felt. With the patient straining or coughing, if the horizontal angle of swab reaches more than 30 degrees (measurement can be done with an orthopedic goniometer), it indicates compromised support to the urethrovesicular junction and bladder base (urethrovesicular junction hypermobility) (36). The test is nonspecific, and a positive test result does not usually indicate the presence of stress incontinence (37). Healthy and continent women commonly exhibit positive cotton swab test results (38).

Positive test results (a change of >30 degrees) are helpful because most of the patients with the stress incontinence have positive findings (90% sensitivity) (36,38). Negative test results (a change of <30 degrees) calls genuine stress incontinence into question, and a more sophisticated test may be required to reach the stress incontinence diagnosis (38).

The provocative stress test is performed under direct visualization. A patient in the dorsolithotomy or standing position with full bladder is asked to strain or cough. A pad can be used to substantiate the presence of leak. A synchronized urine leak with strain or cough suggests SUI. Delayed or persistent leak suggests detrusor instability (detrusor overactivity).

Postvoid residual (PVR) volume is determined shortly after a patient's voluntary void, and measurement is attained via the following methods:

- Catheter
- Transvaginal ultrasonography (39)
- Abdominal palpation and percussion, or bimanual pelvic examination

Results of the test are interpreted as follows:

- There is no maximum or minimum PVR urine volume to be considered as normal or abnormal.
- PVR volume of less than 50 mL is a sign of sufficient bladder evacuation, PVR volume of greater than 50 mL suggests an emptying phase dysfunction, and PVR volume of greater than or equal to 200 mL is a sign of insufficient bladder emptying.
- A PVR volume of 50 to 199 mL should be interpreted with regard to other parameters; although, this level suggests a bladder emptying phase dysfunction (owing to detrusor instability or obstruction), and further testing is necessary.

The uroflowmetry test determines the emptying phase of micturition through the urine flow rate. The test itself does not assist in establishing the type of incontinence (40). Nevertheless, the test identifies an abnormal voiding pattern. The time of bladder emptying phase is measured visually, electronically, or with a disposable unit from the beginning to the end of emptying. A urine volume of less than 100 mL is not an adequate volume for interpretation. The normal expected flow rate is 15 mL per second.

The cystometry test provides information on the following bladder characteristics:

- Sensation (sense of bladder filling)
- Capacity
- Filling phase function
- Storage function
- Voluntary and involuntary detrusor contractions

The test can be used to differentiate detrusor instability from urine outlet dysfunction. Cystometry is performed with the patient standing, with periodic straining or coughing [with the patient lying supine without provocation, approximately 30% of cases of detrusor instability would be missed (41)].

Simple cystometry or single-channel cystometry is performed in the office setting, and the test measures bladder pressure only. The bladder is filled with sterile saline or water using a catheter, and the cystometry machine records involuntary detrusor contractions. If a cystometry machine is not available, a fetal cardiotocographic monitor can be used to measure bladder pressure with filling (42). Because the test is executed without a rectal or vaginal catheter to record intraabdominal pressure, the analysis of results and the diagnostic conclusion should be undertaken with caution (43):

- Expected *first sensation* of bladder filling is at about 150 mL.
- *Bladder fullness* usually is reported at 200 to 300 mL.
- *Maximal bladder capacity* (patient cannot delay voiding) is reached at 400 to 700 mL.

Complex cystometrography or urethrocystometry is designed to evaluate several urodynamic parameters simultaneously:

- Subtracting detrusor pressure is the difference between intraabdominal pressure and intravesicular pressure. Intraabdominal pressure is obtained through either the vagina or rectum.
- Intravesicular pressure.
- Intraurethral pressure (urethral closure pressure is established by subtracting intravesicular pressure from urethral pressure).

Complex cystometry can establish the following information about the bladder:

- *Functional bladder capacity*, which also may be obtained via a voiding record (urolog).
- *Bladder compliance* is increasing when the bladder volume increased intravesicular pressure by 1 cm of water.

Bladder compliance of less than or equal to 60 mL/cm H_2O may indicate detrusor instability (44). Therefore, bladder compliance can help differentiate between stress incontinence and detrusor instability.

■ *Bladder sensation* (first filling sensation at about 150 mL; bladder fullness at 200– 300 mL; maximal bladder capacity at 400–700 mL).

The International Continence Society suggests that the following information be incorporated when results are reported due to differences in technique and technology of complex cystometry (45):

■ Access route (transurethral or percutaneous)
■ Filling medium (liquid or gas) and its temperature
■ Patient position during examination
■ Filling method (orthograde or retrograde, or continuous or incremental)
■ Retrograde filling rate
    Slow (<10 mL/min)
    Medium (10–100 mL/min)
    Rapid (>100 mL/min)
■ Technique
    Fluid-filled catheter (number of catheters, number of lumens, size, type, and manufacturer)
    Microtip transducers (number of catheters, size, and type)
    Measuring equipment description

Urethral pressure profilometry generates a urethral pressure curve by measuring pressure (with microtip pressure transducer catheters or a fluid-filled catheter) along the length of functional urethra. From the urethral pressure curve, functional urethral length, maximal urethral closure pressure (MUCP), and a pressure transmitted ratio (PTR is pressure equalization between the bladder and urethra without detrusor contractions) can be extrapolated. Urethral pressure profilometry identifies a patient with stress incontinence due to intrinsic sphincter deficiency (ISD). The test provides the following practical information:

■ Type III incontinence, such as ISD, which occurs when MUCP is less than 20 cm H_2O (46).
■ PTR of less than 90% establishes the definitive diagnosis of SUI due to urethral hypermobility (47).

Abdominal leak point pressure or Valsalva leak point pressure reflects the urethra's resistance to increasing intraabdominal pressure. The test assists in identifying stress incontinence due to ISD. At a bladder volume of 150 mL using a 10 French urethral catheter, a Valsalva leak point pressure of less than 60 cm H_2O strongly correlates with intrinsic urethral sphincter deficiency and is a highly reproducible technique (48).

A pressure flow study of micturition is designed to establish voiding dysfunction. It is usually performed as a complementary study to a simple uroflowmetry test. The test measures flow times and rates as well as premicturition pressure, opening pressure, maximal pressure, bladder pressure at maximal flow, and detrusor contraction pressure. Test results can be clinically interpreted as follows:

■ Poor flow and normal detrusor contraction suggest bladder outlet obstruction.
■ Detrusor external urethral sphincter dyssynergia is present.
■ Detrusor and urethral smooth muscle dyssynergia is present.

Video-urodynamic studies incorporate a radiographic contrast medium and fluoroscopy during cystometry. A fluoroscopic imaging study of the urethra or bladder and a urodynamic study may be combined as a functional test that can be recorded on videotape and viewed as needed.

Neurophysiologic testing is applied in the forms of *electromyography* (EMG) and *nerve conduction studies*. EMG is used to determine neuromuscular dysfunction in urinary incontinence, pelvic support disorders (descent or prolapse), and anal incontinence. The test can be applied to external urethral and anal sphincters, pubococcygeus muscles, and puborectalis muscles. EMG may provide information related to denervation of these muscles and may be a useful test in urinary and fecal incontinence cases.

A nerve conduction study provides information about different types of nerve dysfunction, such as demyelination of nerve sheathes or axonal degeneration.

A voiding cystourethrogram is recommended in bladder prolapse cases. It can help rule out other mechanical tribulations. When testing for stress incontinence, a patient is asked to strain either by coughing or by Valsalva maneuvers that will reproduce an incontinence episode. When testing for urge incontinence, filling the bladder with sterile water increases intravesicular pressure, which provokes detrusor involuntary contractions and urine leakage.

Differential Diagnosis

■ Excessive sweating
■ Vaginal discharge

STRESS INCONTINENCE

Definition

Stress incontinence is an objectively demonstrable urine leak associated with increased intraabdominal pressure induced either by Valsalva maneuver or a cough test.

Classification

Genuine stress incontinence includes anatomic (genuine) stress incontinence and ISD.

Incidence

■ Anatomic stress incontinence prevalence is unknown.
■ ISD prevalence is unknown.

Diagnosis

Medical pertinent history, physical examination, and specific urodynamic study should be performed. It is important to emphasize that genuine stress incontinence cannot be reliably diagnosed from only a urologic history, even when rigorous selection criteria are used, including a urinary diary. Cystometry is mandatory for ruling out detrusor instability (49). A urodynamic study should include the following elements:

- 1-hour pad test (objectively demonstrates urine loss)
- Cough test, when positive, is about 77% sensitive and 100% specific for genuine stress incontinence in women and with cough (during multichannel cystometrography, sensitivity is about 91% with a specificity of 100%) (50).
- Cotton swab test determines urethral hypermobility (angle changes over 30 degrees from rest to maximum urethral horizontal elevation with a Valsalva maneuver or cough) (51).
- PVR volume.
- Single-channel cystometry measures simple bladder filling. When a stress urine leak is demonstrated, SUI is probably and detrusor instability is ruled out (52).

For mixed urinary incontinence symptoms and for patients who have undergone anti-incontinence procedures for stress incontinence, a multichannel urodynamic test is recommended to rule out intrinsic urethral sphincter deficiency.

Differential Diagnosis

Before therapy is instituted for SUI, the definitive diagnosis must be established and the following differential diagnoses should be considered:

- Detrusor instability
- Reflex incontinence (detrusor hyperreflexia, involuntary urethral relaxation)
- Overflow incontinence
- Extraurethral incontinence (fistulas, ectopic ureter)

Conventional Therapy

Conservative Management

Alpha-adrenergic stimulating agents may provide improvement in the degree of stress incontinence. The following oral drugs are also commonly used for mild to moderate stress incontinence (53):

- Pseudoephedrine (30–60 mg orally, three or four times daily)
- Phenylpropanolamine (15–30 mg orally, two to four times daily)
- Imipramine (10–25 mg three times daily, up to 150 mg daily; it is particularly useful in mixed stress incontinence)

- Ornade spansules (contains phenylpropanolamine and chlorpheniramine; one tablet twice daily)
- Entex (contains phenylpropanolamine and quifenesin; one tablet twice daily)

Over-the-counter medications are available that contain phenylpropanolamine. Caffeine is often a component of such over-the-counter drugs, and should be avoided.

Estrogens exhibit properties that may improve alpha-adrenergic bladder and urethra receptor sensitivity. The best therapeutic effect is achieved when estrogen replacement therapy (see Chapter 12) is combined with alpha-adrenergic agents. A Combination of estriol and phenylpropanolamine provides significant improvement in mild to moderate cases of stress incontinence. A comparison of each drug alone did not yield the same results (54).

Estrogen vaginal cream (1–2 g applied locally three times per week for 6–12 weeks) may improve mild to moderate incontinence in up to 70% of hypoestrogenic women. This form of therapy improves the ureoepithelium, suburethral elastic tissue, and submucosal vascularity.

Vaginal pessaries, such as a fitted ring or Smith-Hodge type of pessary, may improve continence in about 75% of women affected by stress incontinence. The indications for pessary insertion as an alternative to surgery are as follows:

- Older women with genital prolapse and incontinence
- Poor surgical candidates
- Stress incontinence associated only with vigorous exercise

Other conservative measures include the use of *contraceptive diaphragms*, *vaginal tampons*, *Perineal resistant exercise* or Kegel's exercises (also known as pelvic floor rehabilitation), and *functional electrical stimulation*.

In general, conservative approaches are safe with minimum undesirable side effects, but they must be considered temporary improvements for stress incontinence. Such therapeutic modalities cannot restore permanent continence or reconstruct anatomic dysfunction or defects. On the other hand, surgical correction may relieve incontinence symptoms, reconstruct anatomy, and restore continence function.

A new field of tissue engineering and gene therapy has developed. The potential use of myoblasts to improve and expand the treatment of SUI is under clinical investigation. This area of study involves the use of myogenic or muscle-derived cells for tissue engineering and cell-mediated gene therapy (55).

Surgical Management

Surgical management of genuine stress incontinence falls into two categories: procedures for urethral hypermobility and those for intrinsic sphincter deficiency.

Urethral Hypermobility

Anterior vaginal repair or anterior colporrhaphy (Kelly plication or Kelly-Kennedy modification) is applicable for stress incontinence when anatomic support of the proximal urethra and urethrovesicular junction is impaired. The prerequisites for a successful outcome from this operation are a hypermobile urethra and intact function of the intrinsic urethral sphincter. The overall long-term success rate (≥5 years) is 37% (56), with complication rates of 1% to 3% and postoperative detrusor instability rates of about 2% to 6% (57).

Retropubic suspension or retropubic urethropexy is a surgical approach that can be undertaken via a variety of procedures.

Marshall-Marchetti-Krantz (MMK) urethropexy, the periurethral tissue is sutured to the periosteum of the pubic symphysis and has an initial success rate compatible with Burch colposuspension (58). The complication rate is high, with postoperative voiding dysfunction observed in approximately 28% and osteitis pubis in about 5% (59).

Burch's colposuspension is a modification of the MMK operation. The periurethral tissue is suspended to the Cooper ligament instead of to the periosteum. The initial success rate of the operation is approximately 82%. The long-term success rates are 71% after 5 years (56), 69% at 10–12-years (59), and 54% at 18 years (60). The most common complications associated with Burch colposuspension are enterocele formation (5%–17%) (61), detrusor instability (5%–18%), and voiding difficulties (8%–22%) (59). Older age (>65 year) had no significant impact on long-term outcome (59,61).

Burch colposuspension and MMK urethropexy can be executed via laparotomy or laparoscopy (62,63). Laparoscopic bladder injury is reported to be the most common complication, occurring in about 3.7%–8.3% of the procedures (62). However, laparoscopic Burch colposuspension has a statistically higher failure rate when compared with the laparotomy Burch procedure at 1-year follow-up (64).

Paravaginal defect reconstruction was originally designed to correct cystourethrocele due to lateral superior paravaginal defects. Later, this procedure was a part of the complex operation that included Burch colposuspension. In this combination, the initial success rate was approximately 97% (65). Paravaginal reconstruction for urinary stress incontinence yielded a 93% cure rate in short-term follow-up (56). These initial results were confirmed independently, with a cure rate of 79% (66). A new surgical technique for paravaginal defects has been presented, adding an extra fixation point to the anterior aspect of the ischial periosteum, with a similar success rate (66,67). The clinical diagnostic approach for paravaginal defects is presented in Chapter 24.

Needle bladder neck suspension originally was described in 1959, and is known as the Pereyra procedure (68). Since that time, various modifications of Pereyra's operation have been presented for stress incontinence, and have gained wider acceptance than others [Stamey operation (69), Raz modified Pereyra procedure (70), Muzsnai et al. procedure (71), and Gittes and Loughlin procedure (72)]. All of these procedures are transvaginal approaches to the retropubic space with a small, stub skin suprapubic incision. The suspending permanent suture anchors the periurethral and bladder neck tissues.

Complication rates are estimated at 2% to 60% and include urinary retention of longer than 3 weeks, vaginal granuloma, sepsis, vesicocutaneous fistula, hematoma, detrusor instability, suprapubic pain, and wound infection. The success rate of needle suspension at 48 months is about 67% and compares favorably with that of anterior colporrhaphy (61%) (73). In the absence of urethral hypermobility and documented low urethral pressure, any retropubic surgical corrective procedure for SUI is contraindicated (74).

Intrinsic Sphincter Deficiency

Surgery for intrinsic sphincter deficiency focuses on compensation for the inadequate function of the intrinsic urethral sphincter. *Periurethral bulk injection* is a minimally invasive procedure and has been used for ISD with an encouraging initial subjective cure range of 20% to 30%, with 50% to 60% showing a marked improvement (73, 75). Another study showed that long-term success rates vary (30%–70%) due to different injectable material being used (76). Medical collagen devices for the treatment of stress incontinence such as Contigen, Bard, and Collagen Implant, have been approved by the U.S. Food and Drug Administration (FDA). A 4-week skin test should be executed to rule out an allergic reaction to the cross-linked bovine collagen. It is estimated that 3% of individuals have a potential allergic response to the skin test, and the 4-week period is necessary to exclude late sensitivity reaction of a potential recipient.

The following guidelines are used to qualify a patient for periurethral bulking injections (73):

- Absence of urethral hypermobility
- Bladder capacity of greater than 250 mL
- PVR of less than 100 mL
- Valsalva leak point pressure of less than 100 cm H_2O
- Negative urine culture (sterile urine)
- Negative skin test to a collagen

The following injectable materials are available:

- Glutaraldehyde cross-linked bovine collagen (Contigen), most commonly used in the United States.
- Polytetrafluoroethylene (not approved by the FDA).
- Autologous fat injections are less effective than collagen injections, with success rates of 13% and 24%, respectively (75). Another study reported initial success rates of 23% to 65% (76).
- Silicone microimplants (still in developmental stage).

Periurethral injection or *transurethral injection* can deliver material. The periurethral injection technique is an office procedure and requires the application of local anesthetic at the lateral aspect of the urethral meatus close to the orifice of the Skene duct bilaterally. Under urethroscopic guidance, a spinal needle is advanced parallel to the urethra until it reaches the bladder neck, where submucosal injection of local anesthetic is applied (a mixture of indigo carmine with anesthetic may help to identify the area for collagen injections). Collagen is injected under direct visualization at the 3 and 9 o'clock positions until the urethrovesicular junction occludes. Usually 7.5 to 10 mL of collagen are needed. Clinical experience has shown that a patient will require initial catheterization; therefore, training beforehand is advised so those patients may perform self-catheterization (77).

The transurethral injection technique involves instilling approximately 5 mL of collagen material (Contigen) at the 3 and 5 o'clock positions under local anesthesia. A cystoscope with an oblique sheath with 0 degree or 12 degree lenses and transurethral injection needle may be inserted through a standard operating channel approximately 2 cm distal to the bladder neck, and the needle is advanced to 1 cm from the bladder neck. Anesthetic agent is injected under the urethral mucosa followed by collagen injection and is stopped until after the urethrovesical closes.

The following complications have been reported:

- Allergic reactions (77)
- Suburethral abscess formation (79)
- De novo urinary urgency in about 12.6% (80)
- Hematuria in about 5% (80)
- Urinary retention in about 1.9% (80)
- Delayed reaction at the skin test side associated with arthralgia in about 0.9% (80)
- Periurethral pseudocyst formation (81)
- Osteitis pubis (82)
- Urethral prolapse (83)

It also has been documented that coexisting urethral hypermobility should not preclude the use of collagen injection in women with SUI (84).

The sling procedure is recommended for ISD that is determined by low Valsalva leak point pressures or urethral closure pressure. This procedure is most commonly used under the following circumstances:

- ISD with hypermobility (may result from multiple surgeries causing urethral scarring)
- Recurrent stress incontinence due to failure of previous anti-incontinence procedures or due to chronic cough, or physical activity that significantly increases intraabdominal pressure
- Primary sling procedure for genuine stress incontinence

The surgical concept for all sling procedures is the same and involves the placement of a synthetic or tissue graft sling under the bladder neck (urethrovesicular junction) and anchoring a sling to the retropubic or abdominal structures. Inserted into the bladder lumen, a Foley catheter

helps determine the location of the bladder neck, over which the anterior vaginal wall is dissected (dissection should be performed at a 45 degree angle away from the urethra and bladder neck). The abdominal incision is made until the rectus fascia is perforated for a passage of instruments from the abdominal wall through the space of Retzius to the vaginal site. From the vaginal site, both ends of a sling are carried to the abdominal anchor site, either to the rectus fascia, the Cooper ligament, or the pubic bone. The bladder neck is attached to the sling with fine sutures. The elevation tension is established at the surgeon's discretion, but the sling should not be too tight or too loose (a cotton swab in the urethra with positive deflection should be observed after anchoring a sling). Upon completion of the operation, cystourethroscopy should be performed routinely to ensure urethral integrity and patency as well as bladder neck integrity.

Various materials may be used, such as autologous fascia lata from the lateral aspect of the thigh, fascia from a cadaver, and many synthetic materials. The cure rate ranges from 85% to 90% with similar long-term results. Patients who do not achieve cure with a suburethral sling are good candidates for periurethral or transurethral collagen injection (73).

The following complications have been observed with the suburethral sling procedure (73):

- Urine retention
- High residual volume
- Voiding dysfunction
- Urge incontinence
- Intraoperative bleeding
- Wound infection
- Urine leakage during sexual intercourse
- Early or delayed synthetic graft rejection
- Sling material erosion into the bladder or urethra

The artificial urinary sphincter procedure is executed via abdominal and transvaginal approaches, where a device is implanted. A patient activates the device for voiding. Complications include fluid leak, loose cuff, erosion, tubing occlusion, and infections (27,85).

Complementary Therapies for Stress Urinary Incontinence

Diet

Women with urinary incontinence may benefit from avoiding the following foods, which are considered to be bladder irritants, leading to urinary frequency and urgency:

- Acid food (citrus fruits and tomatoes)
- Spicy foods and spices
- Caffeine
- Chocolate
- NutraSweet

Acupuncture

Electroacupuncture, with the acupuncture needle placed into the skin of the lower legs and lower abdomen, has been shown to significantly increase urethral closure pressure as determined by cystourethrometry (86). Electroacupuncture therefore may be used in the treatment of stress incontinence, but additional study is needed.

Exercise

Kegel exercises, with or without weighted vaginal cones (20–100 g) or a perineometer, improve stress incontinence in 40% to 75% of women. The exercise is designed to increase tone of the pelvic floor, perineal muscle (particularly the pubococcygeus muscle), and voluntary external urethral muscle, and is designed to recruit new muscle fibers. At least 40 perineal-pelvic floor muscle contractions daily are needed for noticeable results. Contractions should last 3 seconds followed by 3 seconds relaxation for a total 5 minutes per exercise, five or six times per day. Reviewing pelvic floor randomized clinical trials based on levels-of-evidence criteria, evidence supports the assertion that pelvic floor muscle exercises effectively reduce the symptoms of SUI. There are limited data to determine the efficacy of a low-intensity versus high-intensity schedule of exercise. Also, there is no evidence that pelvic floor exercises with biofeedback are more effective than pelvic floor exercises alone (87).

Interrupting urine flow exercises, as many times as possible, during voiding are suggested for urinary stress incontinence. Scientific data are lacking to support any claims of improvement of symptoms.

Weighted vaginal cone exercises involve holding a vaginal cone (20–100 g) for 15 minutes twice daily. Such exercises are based on a reflex contraction of the pelvic floor muscles, which prevents the cone from impending slippage from the vaginal pool. Approximately 90% of women find this method acceptable, with 70% claiming improvement of symptoms. A highly significant correlation between decreased urine loss and increase in retaining cone weight has been determined (88). A set of five tampon-shape vaginal cones (Femina) is available. This exercise also appears to be a good teaching tool in the initial learning process for pelvic resistance exercise.

Perineometer exercises provide increased vaginal pressure, forcing the pelvic floor muscles to contract. Intraabdominal pressure may interfere with this type of exercise. Limited data are available for clinical recommendation.

Biofeedback

Biofeedback is a "mind over the body" relaxation technique, and is used as a therapeutic method for pelvic floor rehabilitation, conducted with visual or auditory displays. Physiologic changes are recorded either with electronic or mechanical instruments. A surface electrode, which is applied to the vaginal wall, gathers EMG information, and a manometric catheter placed in the rectum indicates pelvic, abdominal, and detrusor muscle activity. Biofeedback may play an important role in the treatment of female stress incontinence. However, a quantitative statistical analysis of the literature yielded different conclusions (89). At 2 years' follow-up, 27% of patients were (objectively) cured and 47% improved, but only 58% of patients accepted this form of treatment on a daily basis (90).

Functional Electrostimulation

Electrostimulation can be used to deliver electrical impulses to the pelvic viscera, pelvic muscle, or the nerve supplies of these anatomic structures. External (non-implantable) and internal (implantable) electrodes may be used for long-term, chronic, continuous, or short-term stimulation of the sacral nerve root. Duration, voltage amplitude, and frequencies vary (20–50 Hz) between studies; therefore, these differences should be considered when comparing results. Success rates for electrostimulation in the treatment of stress incontinence have been 30% to 50% in short- and long-term follow-up reports. When compared with pelvic floor exercises, electrostimulation has not demonstrated its superiority. A combination of pelvic floor exercises and electrostimulation yielded better results than either therapy alone (91). Such a therapeutic approach requires a minimum of 14 weeks of pelvic floor stimulation before significant objective improvements can be documented (92). Results from a placebo-controlled clinical trial showed that 62% of patients experienced significant improvement; although, only 20% of patients were continent. These findings were documented objectively by a provocative pad test (93). Pelvic muscle contraction can be achieved using the intravaginal electrical stimulation system (Innova system).

Absorbent Pad

Absorbent products are beneficial under the following circumstances:

- Immobilized patients, yet to be diagnosed
- Patients awaiting incontinence therapy
- Therapy failure

Absorbent products such as Serenity provide a good barrier, separating the skin from absorbed urine, offer good hygiene results, and prevent infection.

Continuous Urine Drainage

A bedridden, immobilized patient who is not able to perform self-catheterization requires the placement of a Foley catheter for gravity drainage. Such an approach is associated with a high rate of infection and urethral erosion, necessitating close follow-up.

Natural Alternative Therapy

Similar recommendations for pelvic relaxation disorders and urinary incontinence are offered, discussed in further detail in Chapter 24.

Herbal Medicine

Skullcap (94,95) (also known as helmet flower and hoodwort) capsules of 425 or 429 mg or liquid extract 1 and 2 ounces. *Side effects* include confusion, stupor, twitching, seizures, and giddiness. Large doses can be toxic, particularly to the liver. *Drug interactions* have been observed between Skullcap and Antabuse, as well as between Skullcap and immunosuppressive drugs such as Imuran, Prograf, and Sandimmune.

Follow-up should incorporate periodic liver function testing.

Homeopathic Therapy

Sweet sumac (also known as sweet fragrant sumac, sumach, smooth, and polecat-bush) is an herbal remedy that can be used in the form of a tincture of five drops, one tablet, or one globule one to three times daily.

Side effects have not been observed with the above doses (96, 96a).

DETRUSOR INSTABILITY AND URGE INCONTINENCE

Definition

Detrusor instability is involuntary detrusor contractions that may or may not produce incontinence.

Etiology

The etiology of detrusor instability and urge incontinence is unknown; however, it is often associated with stress incontinence, bladder outlet obstruction, and aging.

Classification

- Detrusor instability
- Detrusor hyperreflexia (secondary to an upper motor lesion such as in multiple sclerosis)
- Idiopathic low bladder capacity (considered by some clinicians to be a medical condition separate from detrusor instability)
- Urge incontinence

Incidence

Detrusor instability occurs in 8% to 50% of individuals, depending on age distribution, and reaches 80% in institutionalized women.

Diagnosis

Pertinent medical history includes the following:

- Urge incontinence (short period between urge to void and urine leakage)
- Increased frequency of urination
- Nocturia
- Enuresis
- Urine leakage associated with orgasm (particularly in younger population)
- SUI often present

General physical examination often identifies no abnormality.

Pelvic examination may or may not be associated with pelvic relaxation.

Laboratory study should include urinalysis and urine culture.

Clinical testing should include the following (97):

- Cystometry is diagnostic when during the filling phase either wavelike contraction is recorded or intravesicular pressure increases by at least 15 cm H_2O.
- Coughing may evoke detrusor contraction (shortly after coughing not simultaneously with cough), as may a patient changing position.
- Low bladder compliance may trigger involuntary detrusor contraction and may result from recurrent UTI, interstitial cystitis (IC), radical pelvic surgery, and radiotherapy.

Differential Diagnosis

- SUI
- Mixed incontinence
- Overflow incontinence
- Functional incontinence
- Bypass incontinence

Conventional Therapy

Conservative Management

Psychotherapy is implemented based on documented data that patients with detrusor instability and urge incontinence have high anxiety levels. Psychotherapy used alone demonstrates significant improvement in symptoms such as urgency, incontinence, and nocturia (98).

Behavioral modification plays a significant role in the management of detrusor instability and urge incontinence. Patient education, timed voiding, and positive reinforcement are essential aspects of this approach. Such behavioral modification may establish a patient's ability to control the urinary urge sensation and to urinate on a preplanned schedule.

Bladder retraining or bladder drill is designed to exercise the bladder-emptying reflex by resisting the urge sensation and to delay voiding according to a pre-established schedule. Increasing bladder volume by postponing voiding (increasing the step-up increment time between 15 and 30 minutes for each month until the ultimate desirable voiding interval of 2–3 hours is reached) and adjusting fluid intake; may provide an additional therapeutic benefit (six to eight glasses of fluid prevent bladder irritation caused by excessive concentrated urine) (99).

About 12% of patients who use *biofeedback* become continent, and approximately 75% experience improvement (100). A pressure catheter is inserted into the bladder and connected to a visual or auditory signal, which is activated when intravesicular pressure increases. Upon receiving a signal, a patient relaxes her muscles.

The U.S. Urinary Incontinence Guidelines Panel suggests *pharmacologic therapy* either as a primary or supplemental treatment to behavioral modification. The following pharmacologic agents are recommended:

- *Oxybutynin* (Ditropan tablet, 2.5–5.0 mg three or four times daily; Ditropan syrup, 5 mg) is considered the preferred anticholinergic agent. Oxybutynin exhibits properties such as strong antispasmodic (muscle relaxant), local anesthetic, and moderate antihistaminic as well as anticholinergic effects. The drug can reduce urinary incontinence frequency by 15% to 56%. The side effects often (76%) include dry mouth and eyes, abdominal distention, nausea, diarrhea, constipation, dysphagia, stomal ulcers, headaches, dizziness, blurred vision, and drowsiness (53).
- *Propantheline* (Pro-Banthine) is an anticholinergic agent recommended as second-line therapy at a dosage of 15 to 30 mg four times daily. Blurry vision, drowsiness, tachycardia, nausea, and constipation may occur. It decreases the frequency of urinary incontinence by 13% to 17%, which is statistically significant over the placebo (101).
- *Dicyclomine* (Bentyl) is an anticholinergic medication that exhibits smooth muscle relaxant properties. An oral dosage of 20 mg four times daily is recommended (53).
- *Hyoscyamine* is an anticholinergic agent used at a dose of 0.125 to 0.250 mg orally (53).
- *Tolterodine* (Detrol tablet 1–2 mg twice daily) is a relatively new competitive muscarinic antagonist. It displays a compatible effect with oxybutynin, with significantly fewer side effects (102).
- *Imipramine* (tricyclic antidepressants) at a dosage of 10 to 25 mg three times daily is recommended for detrusor instability and urge incontinence due to its direct spasmolytic, local anesthetic, and anticholinergic properties. The medication should be used with caution in older women and may cause side effects such as sedation, confusion, and drowsiness. A prospective, randomized, controlled study to verify safety and effectiveness has not been undertaken (53).
- *Terodiline* (calcium channel blockers) at the dosage of 25 mg twice daily is effective in approximately 70% of women in reducing urge incontinence and appears to be safe (103).

- *Estrogen replacement therapy (ERT)* in a hypoestrogenic state is recommended for women who do not have a history of breast and uterine cancer in their immediate family, and who are regularly screened for malignancy (Papanicolaou smear, mammography, colonoscopy as indicated). Because the bladder contains estrogen receptors, it may lead to a hypoestrogenic-related predisposition to tissue atrophy, decreased tissue blood flow, and infections. Such changes may lead to detrusor instability or urge incontinence.

The most commonly used pharmacologic agents for detrusor instability and urge incontinence are as follows:

- Antispasmodic agents (oxybutynin, probantine, and imipramine) cause bladder muscle relaxation.
- Sympathomimetics (phenylpropanolamine) stimulate the alpha-receptors in the bladder neck and urethra, in turn increasing the tone of the sphincter mechanism (caution should be exercised in patients with elevated blood pressure and cardiac conditions).
- Combination of psychotherapy and medical therapy.
- Electrical stimulation.

Surgical Management

Surgical management of urge incontinence is considered when conservative approaches fail. Several surgical procedures may be considered:

- Denervation
- Bladder transection
- Ileocystoplasty (bladder augmentation)
- Cystectomy with neobladder construction
- Urinary diversion

Bladder augmentation and bladder denervation are the most commonly selected operations for bladder instability; but not for detrusor dyssynergia. The cure rate is reported to be in the range of 77.2%, and improvement can be expected in approximately 80% (97).

Complementary Therapies

Patient Education

Because a success rate of detrusor instability or urge incontinence therapy depends on the patient's motivation and compliance, education is an important part of management. A patient should be familiarized with potential reversible causes of urinary incontinence (DIAPPERS), the diagnostic process, and the patient's role in reaching the diagnosis. Identifying therapeutic options and their success rates, and establishing patient cooperation, commitment, and compliance are essential factors in reaching a successful outcome. When surgery is contemplated, a second opinion should be advised to verify the indication for surgery and to verify a surgical procedure match (there are over 200 surgical operations for stress incontinence). Both the practitioner and patient should familiarize themselves with surgical procedure options to avoid merely choosing a surgical technique familiar to the surgeon rather than the most effective surgical technique that specifically addresses the patient's needs. When vaginal devices are recommended, the patient's must become educated about appropriate hygiene and early signs of possible complications.

The patient should understand the mechanics of perineal resistance exercise and its intensity, frequency, and continuity. When medications are selected, their undesirable side effects should be clearly presented to the patient.

Behavioral modification is not only a very demanding process in terms of time needed, but the patient must be properly motivated if such an approach can work.

Diet, nutritional supplements, and herbal medicines are not specifically designated for detrusor instability or urge incontinence, but the same approaches may be used. However, only anecdotal, traditional suggestions for such approaches have been made.

Acupuncture

Available data suggest that acupuncture is useful in the management of detrusor instability and urge incontinence. Acupuncture has been shown to significantly increase maximum bladder capacity and bladder compliance (104).

Two to eight acupuncture sessions are needed to achieve clinical improvement. Long-term (average 5.5-year) acupuncture at the Sp-6 point treatment follow-up has documented a transient effect, and repeated acupuncture has been necessary to maintain beneficial effects (105). A success rate of 77% has been reported by short-term follow-up of acupuncture therapy in objectively documented clinical and urodynamic studies (106).

Initial data are promising in using acupuncture for the treatment of detrusor hyperreflexia associated with chronic spinal cord injuries that lead to urinary incontinence (107).

Although, results in the treatment of detrusor instability and urge incontinence are promising, acupuncture remains insufficiently tested.

Exercise

Kegel exercises or perineal resistance exercises are recommended in stress incontinence and pelvic relaxation disorders, and some patients with detrusor instability or urge incontinence also benefit from this approach. Kegel exercises are discussed earlier in this chapter and in Chapter 24.

Electrostimulation

Results of electrostimulation for detrusor instability or urge incontinence are promising, but a long-term success rate has not been uniformly as good as preliminary data indicated. Reviewing various types of functional electrostimulation (including anogenital, long- and short-term maximal

stimulation, implantable stimulation, and transcutaneous stimulation), symptomatic improvement has reportedly occurred in 50% to 90% of women in uncontrolled studies (108). In contrast with stress incontinence, for which electrostimulation is implemented with high frequency and high amperage, detrusor instability is best managed with low frequency and moderate amperage (93). Before clinical implementation of electrostimulation can be widely recommended for the management of detrusor instability, additional well-designed and controlled studies need to be undertaken.

Hypnosis

Preliminary results suggest that hypnotherapy for detrusor instability or urge incontinence may be effective. An observational study was conducted for detrusor instability for a total of 12 sessions. Preliminary results showed that 58% of patients were symptom free, 28% demonstrated improvement, and 14% failed to respond to hypnosis (109).

New Technologies for Stress Urinary Incontinence

The FDA has approved the following products for SUI:

- *The Continence Guard* is a new design to support the bladder neck. It is made from hydroscopic material (polyurethane foam). It comes in three sizes and is inserted into the vaginal pool with an applicator. Upon insertion the device absorbs water and expands by approximately 30%.
- *The Extracorporeal Magnetic Innervation (ExMI)* system is a new device for stimulating nerve impulses through pulsing magnetic fields. In contrast to pelvic floor electrical stimulation, magnetic neuromodulation does not require electrodes to conduct electrical currents.
- *The Fem Soft Insert* is a disposable intraurethral device that provides catheter-like urethral occlusion.
- *The FemiScan system* is a product for biofeedback pelvic floor rehabilitation that provides an adjustable training device to meet the patient's needs at home.
- *A fitting set* provides individual sizing of an incontinence pessary. A set of six rings of different sizes helps to establish an optimum pessary size.
- *The Incontinent Dish* has dual uses: to support the bladder neck and the pelvic viscera (can be used in pelvic relaxation).

Natural Alternative Therapy

There is no specific reccomendation.

MIXED INCONTINENCE

Definition

Coexisting genuine stress incontinence and detrusor instability is referred to as mixed incontinence.

Incidence

The prevalence of SUI coexisting with urge incontinence (mixed incontinence) among community-dwelling women varies from 4% to 30% (110).

Pathophysiology

There are coexisting factors for SUI and detrusor instability. The degree of contribution of these factors varies, but one factor usually dominates.

Diagnosis

The diagnostic process incorporates genuine and urge incontinence clinical testing that is detailed elsewhere in this chapter. A patient's pertinent medical history usually includes the following elements (111):

- Urine leakage is larger in volume than either stress incontinence or detrusor instability alone.
- Incontinence episodes are more frequent than with either stress incontinence or detrusor instability alone.

Differential Diagnosis

- Genuine stress incontinence
- Urge incontinence
- Other forms of urinary incontinence

Conventional Therapy

A therapeutic approach is problematic for mixed incontinence, because an aggressive treatment of stress incontinence may or may not negatively affect urge incontinence. The dilemma is more accentuated when combined conservative management for stress incontinence and detrusor instability fails. Because performing surgery for the stress incontinence component alone may worsen mixed incontinence, a study was conducted to document the effects of such surgery (112). Results showed that when involuntary detrusor contractions were induced, surgical correction of stress incontinence was about 90% effective (if the intravesicular pressure was less than 25 cm H_2O). When the intravesicular pressure was greater than 25 cm H_2O, the success rate decreased to 50%.

The subject of surgery for mixed incontinence is widely debated among clinicians. On one side the claim is made that the degree of detrusor instability may affect the surgical outcome; the other side suggests that detrusor instability does not affect the outcome of stress incontinence surgery (113). Due to this clinical controversy the following conservative approach is recommended:

- Perineal resistance exercises with or without vaginal cones or electrostimulation as the first line of management.

- Pelvic floor exercises associated with bladder drilling and behavioral modification treatment.
- Combined pelvic floor exercises and pharmacologic agents for detrusor instability.
- Vaginal devices for stress incontinence with bladder drilling and behavioral modification therapy.
- Combining bladder drilling and anticholinergic drugs may lead to secondary urine retention, and the patient should be trained for self-catheterization.

Surgical therapy for stress incontinence may affect detrusor instability in the following ways:

- Worsening urge incontinence
- Improving urge incontinence
- No affect on detrusor instability

By and large, a practitioner should establish the dominant urinary incontinence type and focus the therapy on this condition. When ambiguous mixed incontinence is present, detrusor instability should be addressed first, and surgery should be offered only when the remaining stress incontinence is unbearable.

Complementary-Alternative Therapy

No data are available for the treatment of mixed incontinence, but individual therapies can be administered as described elsewhere in this chapter.

OVERFLOW INCONTINENCE AND URINARY RETENTION

Definition

Overflow incontinence is caused by a chronically full bladder leading to overdistension of the bladder wall.

Urethral obstruction or bladder outlet obstruction may result from the following (114):

- Pelvic organ prolapse
- Ovarian neoplasm
- Uterine retroflexion (either gravid or nongravid uterus); uterine leiomyomata
- Vaginal wall large mesonephric or paramesonephric cysts
- Postsurgical edema, large cystocele

Bladder atony or detrusor hyporeflexia may result from detrusor muscle dysfunction, which can be caused by the following (115):

- *Lesion in the lower motor neurons* (multiple sclerosis)
- *Peripheral neuropathy* (diabetic mellitus neuropathy, hypothyroidism, vitamin B^{12} deficiency), as well as peripheral pelvic nerve damage associated with radical surgery, AIDS, pelvic inflammation, psychogenic etiology, and iatrogenic origin
- *Central nervous system lesions* (stroke, spinal cord injury, damage, and cauda equina tumors)

- *Medication* such as alpha-adrenergic agonists, anticholinergic agents, beta-adrenergic agonists, and calcium channel blockers can be used (116)
- Large cystocele

Diagnosis

Pertinent medical history:

This medical condition manifests by unconscious small quantities of urine loss in association with changing position, standing, bending, or other physical activities through the day and night. The incontinence episodes occur with no urinary urge. The patient may have a history of urinary hesitancy, intermittent flow with decreased stream, dribbling, and prolonged urination. Manual suprapubic pressure or bending assists in evacuating the bladder.

Physical examination, including neurologic examination, may establish signs of underlying medical condition.

Pelvic examination may determine bladder location above the pubic symphysis, and the bladder may be tender to palpation. Evidence of pelvic pathology may be established.

Clinical testing should include the following:

- Measurement of PVR urine (>500 mL) either by catheterization or ultrasonographic determination.
- Cystometrography will demonstrate decreased bladder sensation and increased bladder capacity.
- Voiding study reveals high bladder pressure with low flow rate or low bladder pressure with low flow rate, which is associated with detrusor hyporeflexia.

Differential Diagnosis

Other forms of urinary incontinence

Conventional Therapy

The following management is recommended (117):

- Treatment of underlying causes (vaginal pessary, surgery as indicated, or medical therapy).
- Drainage (Foley catheter) for 24 to 48 hours if the cause is self-limited.
- Intermittent self-catheterization.
- Pharmacologic therapy is not usually successful.

Complementary and Alternative Therapies

No data are available for the use of complementary and alternative therapies, but a remedy may be administered to treat the underlying cause.

FUNCTIONAL INCONTINENCE

A patient who is not able to or is reluctant to reach a toilet and voids into garments is considered to have functional incontinence. Physical impairment (limited manual functions, inability to reach a toilet, multiple layers of underwear, etc.), mental impairment, and environmental factors (remote location or difficult accessibility, confusing surroundings, etc.) may contribute to functional incontinence. Treatments include correcting the environmental factors, patient education and encouragement to use a toilet, looser underwear that is easy to remove, and use of absorbent pads or a Foley catheter.

BYPASS OF ANATOMIC CONTINENCE MECHANISM

The presence of urine conduits circumventing a natural lower urinary path may be caused by a congenital or acquired abnormality. The following congenital causes may be observed:

- Epispadias results from the incomplete midline fusion. The absence of pubic hairs in the midline is also present.
- An ectopic ureter may open to the urethra (usually middle or distal urethra), the vagina, the cervix, or the uterine corpus.

The following acquired abnormalities also may be observed:

- Vesicovaginal, ureterovaginal, urethrovaginal, and vesicouterine fistulas may result from surgical injury, radiation therapy, or unfitted and the long presence of a vaginal pessary.
- Urethral diverticulum.

In the majority of cases, the clinical diagnosis is straightforward. A patient's medical history indicates continuous urine loss, and pelvic examination establishes the source of urine leakage. *Diagnosis of fistula*, when it is large, does not present a diagnostic dilemma; when it is small, an oral Pyridium Plus tablet (phenazopyridine hydrochloride; urinary dye) at a dose of 100 to 200 mg may help to identify the fistula orifice.

Urethrocystoscopy or radiographic contrast studies are indicated when simple tests cannot identify the fistula opening, multiple paths are suspected, or the fistula opens to the bladder neck or urethral sphincter.

Urethral diverticulum diagnosis is based on the classic history triad of dysuria, dyspareunia, and postvoid dribbling (urine builds up within the diverticulum during voiding and dribbles in a standing position). To confirm the clinical impression, ureteroscopy, voiding cystourethrography, urethral pressure profilometry, or a radiographic contrast study may be performed. Ultrasonography may be combined with double-balloon catheterization (one balloon obstructs the urethrovesicular junction and the other occludes the urethral meatus, forcefully placing contrast media into the diverticular compartment). Urethral diverticula are usually

1 to 3 cm in diameter and located in the distal or middle third of the urethra (118).

Conventional Therapy

Conventional therapy is usually surgical, because abnormalities are usually anatomic in nature.

Small fistulas may close spontaneously with time. Surgical treatment is successful when a *fistula* track is excised, the surrounding scar tissue is removed, and the appropriate reconstruction of structures has been undertaken. Approximation of the urethral structures must be performed without tension, and suprapubic catheterization should be an integral part of the procedure.

Diverticula, when symptomatic, require surgical therapy:

- Simple incision and drainage are performed when acute infection is present in the suburethral diverticulum (119).
- When subacute infection is present, the diverticular sac is excised with a margin of healthy tissue through a vaginal incision. Fine suturing material should be used, and no tension on the suture line is applied; suprapubic catheterization for several days is needed (120).
- Marsupialization is recommended when the diverticulum is present at the distal urethra (121). The operation itself is a simple incision carried from the external meatus of the diverticular sac, incorporating the vaginal mucosa and the urethral wall. The diverticular wall is excised, and the urethral mucosa is anchored to the vaginal mucosa, creating a new meatus. This procedure may lead to iatrogenic internal sphincter insufficiency.

Each surgical procedure may result in urethral stricture and fistula formation.

OTHER CONDITIONS OF UROGYNECOLOGY PRACTICE

Urinary Tract Infection (UTI)

Lower UTIs are the most common clinical entity encountered in a primary care practice. Timely diagnosis and appropriate management is essential to prevent severe sequelae such as acute pyelonephritis.

Definition

Microorganisms invade the lower urinary tract.

Incidence

Urinary tract infections occur at a rate of 2% to 5% in women 15 to 24 years of age, 10% after age 60, 20% after age 65, and 25% to 50% after age 80 (122).

Etiology

Pathogenesis of Urinary Tract Infections

Community-acquired infection is most commonly caused by *Escherichia coli* in about 80% of cases. The remaining 20% are caused by other bacterial flora, such as *Klebsiella* (approximately 5%) and *Enterobacter* and *Proteus* specious (about 2%) (123). *Staphylococcus saprophyticus* accounts for 10% of cases among young women (124), and *Staphylococcus epidermidis* is a common cause of nosocomial UTI (125). Other microorganisms, such as *Chlamydia trachomatis,* may be responsible for infection with negative urine culture (sterile infection).

Hospital-acquired infection is usually caused by *Serratia marcescens* and *Pseudomonas aeruginosa.*

Predisposing Factors to Urinary Tract Infections

- Hypoestrogenic state
- Diabetes mellitus
- Incomplete bladder evacuation
- Stones
- Cystic kidneys
- Diverticula
- Ureteric stumps

Classification

- Urethritis
- Cystitis
- Urethrocystitis

Diagnosis

Pertinent medical history is usually characterized by the following elements:

- *Frequency* of urination.
- *Urgency* of urination.
- *Dysuria* associated with UTI occurs by the end of urination, in contrast to the symptom of dysuria present at the beginning of urination, which is associated with periurethritis and vulvitis.
- *Suprapubic pain* or sensation of heaviness in this area may be reported.

Physical examination may reveal suprapubic tenderness. *Pelvic examination* usually elicits bladder tenderness.

Laboratory tests include: office urine microscopic examination of sediment displays numerous leukocytes (presence of white cells is termed pyuria) and bacteria. Pyuria itself is considered the best indicator of UTI. The absence of pyuria with a full clinical picture of UTI may suggest either papillary necrosis or the presence of stones.

An office urine dipstick test (positive for nitrites, which are metabolic products of bacteria) or other chemical markers are acceptable methods for UTI screening (as long as the screening method has a low false-negative rate).

Definitive diagnosis is reached by standard clean-catch, mid-stream urine sample culture (transurethral catheterization or suprapubic aspiration is indicated in selected cases), which not only identifies pathognomonic organisms, but also its spectrum of sensitivity to antibiotics (antibiogram). Any time that UTI is suspected, urine culture should be obtained. Bacterial colony counts of greater than or equal to 100,000/mL are indicative of the presence of significant bacteriuria (a significant infection).

Pyelonephritis, as a sequelae of cystitis or urethrocystitis, may occur with a characteristic clinical picture:

- Malaise, flank pain, dysuria, urinary frequency and urgency, and fever.
- Flank tenderness (unilateral or bilateral costovertebral tenderness).
- Microscopic examination of urinary sediment demonstrates an increased number of white blood cells, white blood cell casts, and red blood cells (gross hematuria).
- Blood test shows elevated white blood cells (leukocytosis), elevated erythrocyte sedimentation rate, and elevated C-reactive protein. When renal function is affected, elevated creatinine and blood urea nitrogen are present.
- Intravenous urography with renal enlargement, nonobstructive urinary collecting system dilatation, impaired contrast excretion, and ureteral striations may be seen. Contrast-enhanced CT is indicated when urography is not conclusive or pyelonephritis is retracted to a treatment.

Conventional Therapy

General measures include *rest* and *hydration*, which may dilute bacterial counts and break up some bacterial cell walls and may reduce bacterial adherence. Cranberry juice exhibits such a capacity (126).

Relieving the pain and burning associated with voiding is an important aspect. The urinary tract analgesic Pyridium (phenazopyridine hydrochloride) is particularly effective and does not interfere with antibacterial medication. A dosage of 100 to 200 mg three times daily for 2 to 3 days is recommended.

An antimicrobial agent should be selected by taking into account the following aspects:

- Effective for UTI treatment at a low serum concentration level (low serum levels will not change bacterial flora in another part of the body, such as the vagina, predisposing to development of fungal infection)
- Causing insignificant alteration in vaginal or fecal microorganisms
- Low adverse effects

The following medications are most commonly recommended for UTI and are usually prescribed after a urine sample is obtained to determine the spectrum of bacteria and the sensitivity to antimicrobial agents:

- *Nitrofurantoin* (one 50- to 100-mg tablet every 6-8 hours for 8 days) is very effective in the treatment of a community-acquired UTI. The side effect most commonly reported is gastrointestinal symptoms (nausea and vomiting). Overdose may lead to pneumonitis or peripheral neuropathy (127).
- *Septra DS or Bactrim DS (80 mg trimethoprim/400 mg sulfamethoxazole, or TMP-SMX)*, one tablet twice daily for 7 to 10 days, exhibits particular effectiveness against a wide range of uropathogens with rare bacterial resistance (128).
- *Norfloxacin (Noroxin)*, 400 mg every 12 hours, is a synthetic derivative of quinoline, has a wide spectrum, and is an effective agent either for gram-positive or gram-negative bacteria. Side effects, observed infrequently, are mainly gastrointestinal (129).
- *Ampicillin*, 250 to 500 mg every 6 hours for 7 to 10 days, has a predisposition to vaginal fungal infection in up to 25% of patients when administered for simple cystitis. Ampicillin is excreted undistorted with fecal material in about 70% of patients (130).
- *Tetracyclines*, 250 to 500 mg every 6 hours, predispose to vaginal candidal infection. Up to 80% is excreted unchanged with stool. It often causes gastrointestinal upset and skin rash, particularly when the skin is exposed to sunlight (131).

Acute pyelonephritis is an inflammatory process affecting the kidney. Management depends on clinical severity, with the knowledge that pyelonephritis is a potentially life-threatening condition. Mild symptoms *may not require hospitalization*, and TMP-SMX (one tablet every 12 hours for 14 days) can be effective (132). Urine culture and sensitivity must be obtained before commencing medication, and repeat urine culture and sensitivity should be performed 5 to 7 days from the time of initial therapy, and 4 to 6 weeks after discontinuation of therapy.

Severe illness *requires hospitalization* and administration of a parenteral antibiotic. An intravenous combination of ampicillin (1–2 g every 6 hours) and an aminoglycoside (e.g., gentamicin) is administered, when the serum creatinine is not elevated, at a loading dose of 1.5 mg/kg, followed by a maintenance dose of 1 mg/kg every 8 hours. The serum creatinine levels should be assessed every other day to monitor the patient for nephrotoxicity. After the third dose, serum gentamicin levels are determined 30 minutes before and 30 minutes after gentamicin administration.

If nephrotoxicity occurs or pathogenic bacteria are resistant to gentamicin, a third-generation cephalosporin is effective therapy. Initial urine culture and follow-up culture are recommended as described above. Appropriate hydration is recommended, usually with 3,000 mL normal, saline solution per day, with urine output monitored.

Pyelonephritis is *associated with hospitalization* or procedures such as catheterization or urogynecologic surgery. Similar parenteral therapy and follow-up as described above are recommended.

It has been estimated that relapse of pyelonephritis occurs in 10% to 30% of patients after 14 days of therapy. A second course of treatment, in accordance with antibiogram, for 14 days is a sensible approach. Some patients respond to this mode of treatment after 6 weeks of therapy (133).

Recurrent Urinary Tract Infection

After their initial UTI episode, 75% of patients have fewer that one recurrence per year; 25% have approximately three episodes per year (134). Recurrent UTIs usually are diagnosed by urine culture, and long-term management includes the following:

- A patient collects a urine sample for culture when UTI symptoms recur, and *self-administers* previously prescribed therapy with one of the antimicrobial agents for a consecutive 3-day period.
- Postcoital prophylaxis is an effective form of recurrent UTI management. Before or after vaginal intercourse, one dose of 100 mg nitrofurantoin or one tablet of TMP-SMX (or other antimicrobial agents) is sufficient for prevention of UTI (135).
- Continuous prophylaxis is usually initiated when urine is negative for bacterial flora following antimicrobial therapy. Usually nitrofurantoin, 100 mg or TMP-SMX one tablet (136), or cephalexin, 250 mg (137), is administered at bedtime.

Complementary Therapies

In randomized, controlled clinical trials, it has been documented that *acupuncture* is 85% effective in the treatment of recurrent UTI. When these results were compared with those of the sham acupuncture group, a statistically significant prophylaxis for recurrent lower UTIs was confirmed. Acupuncture is another option for the prevention of recurring lower UTIs in women (138).

Patient Education

Patient education includes hygiene, prophylaxis, and the diagnostic/therapeutic process. Understanding how to maintain personal genitalia hygiene is crucial. The patient must understand the anatomic relationship between the meatus and the anus, and the post defecation procedure for cleansing the perineal region from anterior to posterior is important to emphasize. Avoidance of irritating substances and local allergens also should be addressed.

Motivation and compliance of a patient can be greatly improved, when the pros and cons for diagnostic and therapeutic approaches are clearly presented. The risks and benefits of diagnostic procedures and therapeutic modes as well as the risks of unattended care for UTI should be conveyed to the patient. All available options, including conventional, complementary, and alternative therapies, their therapeutic success rates, current knowledge about them, and side effects associated with their use should be explained. Potential interaction between medications and alternative therapeutic remedies should be explored with the patient.

Diet

Coffee, tea, carbonated beverages, artificial sweeteners, and tomato-based foods should be avoided to improve the symptoms of UTI.

Nutritional Supplements

The following *minerals* may be beneficial for UTI:

- Calcium 1,500 mg daily (reduces bladder irritability)
- Magnesium 750 to 1,000 mg daily
- Zinc 50 mg daily
- Copper 3 mg daily
- Potassium 99 mg daily (replaces potassium lost as a result of frequent urination)

The following *vitamins* may be beneficial for UTI:

- Vitamin A 10,000 IU daily
- Vitamin B complex 50 to 100 mg twice daily with meals (used with antibiotics)
- Vitamin C 4,000 to 5,000 mg daily in divided doses (produces antibacterial effects
- Multivitamins

Natural Alternative Therapy

Herbal Medicine

Cranberry juice (pure, unsweetened juice, not commercial) has been tested in the laboratory, and results have confirmed that it inhibits bacterial adherence by 75% in over 60% of clinical isolates of *E. coli*. Cranberry juice also affects urine acidification and expresses bacteriostasis (139). It has been determined that *E. coli*, isolated from urine, adheres to urinary tract epithelial cells, and it has been established that cranberry juice exhibits anti-adherence activity against gram-negative rods isolated from urine (140). These experimental findings were clinically tested with *300 mL of cranberry juice cocktail daily* over the course of 6 months. This observational study suggests that consumption of cranberry juice is clinically useful and is more effective in treating than preventing bacteriuria and pyuria (140). A randomized, controlled clinical trial is needed to substantiate these observational findings.

Commercially available cranberry juice contains less than 30% pure cranberry juice and includes high-fructose corn syrup or other sweeteners. In this form, cranberry juice is not suitable as a remedy. When pure cranberry juice is not available, cranberry capsules can be used.

The active antimicrobial effect of *uva ursi* (*Arctostaphylos uva-ursi*) is associated with the aglycon hydroquinone that displays urine-sterilizing properties (141). Uva ursi has long been used for this purpose (142), but its safety and effectiveness have not been determined in a randomized, controlled study. The daily dose of powdered or finely sliced leaves of the plant is 10 g (equal to 400–800 mg of pure substance) or 0.4 g of the dry extract. Capsules are available in 150 mg, 455 mg, and 505 mg. Infusion is prepared with 3 g in 150 mL of sterile water (96,96a). A tea is prepared from 1 teaspoon of powdered drug (2.5 mg) placed into boiling water for 15 minutes.

Uva ursi should be avoided with medication or food that increases uric acid. The following side effects may be observed (95,96,96a):

- Bluish gray skin.
- Greenish urine.
- Nausea and vomiting.
- Large doses (>20 g) may cause ringing in the ears, vomiting, seizures, and blood vessel collapse.

Contraindications include pregnancy and periods of lactation (95,96,96a).

Crataeva decoction (varuna or three-leafed caper) displays antiinflammatory, bladder tonic, and antilithic properties. It is an ayurvedic herb and is used as a remedy of choice in urinary disorders. An uncontrolled, observational clinical study showed that up to 85% of patients with chronic UTIs became asymptomatic after 4 weeks of therapy on the daily dose of 15 to 25 g of the dried bark or root bark (143)

Birch leaves (*Betula* species) increase the amount of urine (diuretic) and are anecdotally recommended for inflammatory and bacterial diseases of the urinary tract. The daily dose is 2 to 3 g with more than 2 liters of fluid per day in three to four divided doses. Side effects include skin irritation or allergic reaction, and it is contraindicated during pregnancy or breast-feeding.

A *phytosynergistic* combination is designed to provide actions of four aspects of the treatment of UTI (144):

- Diuretic activity (*Agropyron repens,* also known as couch grass)
- Antiseptic properties (*Barosma betulina* or buchu)
- Immunostimulant properties that increase the body's resistant to both viral and bacterial infections (*Echinacea angustifolia* or Echinacea and *Glycyrrhiza globra* or licorice)
- Increasing resistance of the uroepithelium to bacterial penetration (licorice)
- Mucosa protection (licorice)

The following composition formula is recommended (145):

- *Agropyron repens* 1,500 mg
- *Barosma betulina* 500 mg
- *Echinacea angustifolia* 625 mg
- *Glycyrrhiza globra* 1,250 mg

This formula is contraindicated for patients with hypertension. No reported toxicity has been associated with this herbal composition. No randomized, controlled data are available to validate this clinical approach.

Other herbal remedies, such as marshmallow root, burdock root, juniper berries, kava kava (may cause drowsiness), and rose hips, are also anecdotally used as folk remedies for UTI.

Homeopathic Therapy

Uva ursi is taken at a dose of 5 to 10 drops of leaf extract, 1 tablet or 5 to 10 globules one to three times daily, or 1 mL injection solution twice weekly (96,96a).

Interstitial Cystitis

Definition

Chronic bladder mucosa inflammation produces significant urinary urgency, frequency, and bladder pain (midline suprapubic pain).

Incidence (IC)

The prevalence of IC in the United States is approximately 52 to 67 per 100,000 women and is more than 50% greater than originally reported. Caucasian women constitute about 95% of IC patients (146).

Etiology

The cause of IC is unknown. Several etiologic hypotheses have been suggested, such as infectious, lymphatic, immunologic, neurologic, or vascular abnormalities (147).

CLASSIFICATION

- Classic ulcer IC
- Nonulcer IC

Diagnosis

Pertinent medical history includes urinary complaints of frequency, urgency, and midline suprapubic pain. Duration of symptoms confirms chronic symptomatology (> 6 months' duration).

The *voiding diary* should be an integral part of the IC diagnosis. A 3-day voiding log usually is sufficient for analysis, which provides not only diagnostic information but also aids in planning a future treatment plan.

A voiding diary should include the following:

- Nocturia (more than two voiding episodes per night)
- Daytime frequency (fewer than eight voiding episodes per day)

- Urgency per day (mild form eight episodes and severe form >119)
- Pain and its characteristics (location, onset, radiation, duration, severity character, aggravation, and relief and severity) are important to evaluate.

A simple formula that helps to make the initial appraisal of pain severity is as follows:

- *Mild pain* does not interfere with concentration on a task.
- *Moderate pain* interferes with concentration; however, a physical or
- Mental task can be continued or completed.
- *Severe pain* causes loss of concentration and incapacitates a patient.

Physical examination is usually unremarkable or may demonstrate suprapubic tenderness.

Pelvic examination may reveal urethral tenderness or tenderness over the bladder base. Particular attention should be given to the presence of vulvovaginitis, vulvar vestibulitis, vulvodynia, urethral diverticulum, cervicitis, or posterior cul-de-sac tender lesions (may suggest endometriosis), because these abnormality are frequently associated with IC (148).

Laboratory testing should include the following (149, 150):

- *Urinalysis, culture* (must be negative in IC), and cytology (bladder malignant neoplasm may mimic IC) must be performed.
- *Cervical and urethral culture* (must be negative for gonorrhea and *Chlamydia trachomatis*) are indicated.
- *Vaginal secretion* wet preparation with normal saline and 10% KCl must be negative for fungus and trichomonas.
- *Cystometry* in IC has a characteristic picture, which includes sensory urgency, a small bladder capacity, and pain on bladder filling (the absence of an intense urge to void in the filling phase of the test rules out IC).
- *Cystoscopy with bladder hydrodistention* is the procedure that produces an intravesicular pressure of 80 to 100 cm H_2O and maintains it for 1 to 2 minutes. It is performed under general anesthesia. Cystoscopy with bladder hydrodistention may display not only characteristic (not diagnostic per se) changes of bladder mucosa such as diffused pinpoint petechial hemorrhages (glomerulations) or a mucosal red Hunner patch or ulcers, but also urethral or bladder abnormalities, tumors, and bladder stones (150). Glomerulations have only diagnostic value when symptoms of IC are present, because up to 45% of asymptomatic women display this clinical phenomenon, and the diagnosis of IC can be reached without the presence of glomerulation (151). An average bladder capacity is approximately 1,000 mL; in patients with IC, it is decreased to 650 mL (152).
- *The potassium sensitivity test* is a relatively new diagnostic tool and is designed to screen patients for defective blad-

der epithelial permeability. The test is initiated with 40 mL of water and then followed by 40 mL potassium chloride solution (40 mL of 40 mEq/100 mL). A patient with IC responds with urgency, and pain is recorded on a scale of 0 to 5 (5 represents maximum severity of urgency or pain, and 0 equals no urgency or pain). The test result is considered positive when the score is greater than or equal to 2. Intravesicular water installation does not provoke urgency or pain. The potassium solution produces a marked sensation of urge or pain in 75% of patients (153). An independent study has not validated the intravesicular potassium test and established a sensitivity of 69.5% and specificity of 50% (154). Therefore, the diagnosis of IC must depend more on the clinical presentation and endoscopic findings. The National Institute of Arthritis, Diabetes, Digestive, and Kidney Diseases (NIDDK) workshop on IC established research diagnostic criteria (155). Strict application of these criteria in clinical practice may comprise about 60% of the IC diagnosis (156).

NIDDK Diagnostic Criteria

At least one *symptom* must be present:

- Urgency to urinate (present in 91.7%) (157)
- Pain linked to bladder (present in 60%; pain location and its degree differ significantly between patients with a classic ulcer IC and nonulcers) (157)

At least one of the *cystoscopic* findings must be present:

- Diffuse glomerulations present in at least three bladder quadrants
- Hunner ulcer

The following criteria *exclude* IC:

- Age under 18
- Fewer than eight voids per day while awake
- Fewer than two voids during the night
- More than 350 mL maximum bladder capacity while awake
- No intense urge to void during cystometry with medium filling rate, with bladder filled to 100 mL of gas or 150 mL of water
- Involuntary bladder contractions on cystogram at medium filling rate
- Less than 9-month duration of persistent symptoms
- Symptoms relieved by antimicrobial, urinary antiseptic, anticholinergic or antispasmodic medications
- UTI in past 3 months
- Active genital herpes or vaginitis
- Urethral diverticulum present
- Bladder or lower urethral stones
- Uterine, cervical, vaginal, or urethral malignancy
- History of cystitis related to cyclophosphamide or similar chemicals, or radiation
- History of bladder tuberculosis
- History of benign or malignant tumors

Bladder biopsy should be performed after hydrodistention (may be predisposed to bladder rupture at the biopsy site); even though, the histologic examination is not diagnostic for IC (152), but will rule out other conditions such as malignant neoplasia.

Differential Diagnosis

- Voiding relieves or lessens IC pain in 73.6% (157)
- Constrictive clothing, sexual intercourse, and stress increase IC pain in about 50%
- Urethral syndrome
- Other causes of cystitis
- Other causes of chronic pelvic pain (gynecologic, urologic, or colorectal origin)
- Other causes of urinary frequency and urgency
- Pelvic infection, including tuberculosis
- Bladder or urethral stones
- Bladder malignancy

Conventional Therapy

Conservative Therapy

Oral pharmacologic therapy includes several drugs. *Elmiron (pentosan polysulfate sodium, or PPS)* is administered at a dose of 100 mg three times daily (can be increased to 400 to 600 mg/day as indicated). For uninterrupted administration, it is given for at least 3 to 6 months. Response to therapy is first seen until after 6 to 10 weeks but may take 6 to 9 months. PPS can be used for several years to control this condition. PPS is the only medication that has been approved by the FDA for the therapy of IC. PPS improves the uroepithelium mucus layer, creating a protective intravesicular barrier that prevents urine from reaching the cells. PPS decreases urinary frequency in 54%, bladder pain in 37%, and urgency in 28% of patients (158).

Antidepressant medication is a symptomatic adjunct therapy, and the following medications are often used:

- *Imipramine HCl*, starting dose of 10 to 25 mg 1 hour before bedtime; after 2 to 3 weeks the dose can be increased (initially the patient may be tired)
- *Elavil (amitriptyline)*, starting dose of 10 to 25 mg 1 hour before bedtime; after 2 to 3 weeks the dose can be increased (initially the patient may be tired)
- *Prozac (fluoxetine)*, initial dose of 20 mg per day; can be increased up to 40 mg daily
- *Zoloft (sertraline)*, starting dose of 50 mg; can be increased to 100 mg per day

Antihistamines in observational clinical trials demonstrated approximately 40% improvement with Atarax (hydroxyzine hydrochloride). *Atarax* or *Vstaril* is recommended at the dose 25 to 50 mg per day, administered for at least 2 to 3 months (160), particularly to patients with allergy and IC.

Antiinflammatory steroidal and nonsteroidal medications can be prescribed for IC. However, no data are available to substantiate their effectiveness.

Intravesicular pharmacologic therapy with dimethylsulfoxide (DMSO) has been approved by the FDA for the treatment of IC. DMSO intravesicular treatment offers 50% to 90% symptomatic improvement, although relapse (35%–50%) is often observed, and reinstating this mode of therapy results in relief of symptoms in 50% to 60% of patients (161).

Weekly, intravesicular installation of 50 mL DMSO is performed for a duration of 10 to 15 minutes, for a total of six to eight treatment sessions, and then can be continued every other week for 4 to 6 months (DMSO has been used successfully for several years without complications) (162). When DMSO causes symptoms to flare up (self-limited within 24 hours), 10 mL of 2% viscous xylocaine jelly for 15 minutes before DMSO instillation usually resolves this undesirable effect.

Other medications have been used for bladder distention, such as sodium oxychlorosene, heparin, hydrocortisone, and silver nitrate. Combinations of hydrocortisone, heparin, sodium bicarbonate, and local anesthetic also have been used (intravesicular cocktails).

Surgical Therapy

Occasionally, surgery for IC is performed (1%–5% among patients associated with IC). Surgery is indicated only when IC is refractory to conservative treatment and a severe form of IC persists (163). The following surgical procedures are presently used:

- *Hydrodistention* of the bladder under general anesthesia (162).
- *Electrocoagulation* in the classic subtype of IC is suggested as a mode of management (163).
- *Laser ablation* with the contact neodymium-YAG laser seams to be beneficial in the treatment of IC. Low complication rate and satisfactory initial results may assist in clinical management of this condition. The method needs to be validated before clinical recommendation (164).
- *Cystolysis, cysto-cystoplasty, and perivesicular denervation* are surgical procedures in which the main objective is to reduce bladder hypersensitivity through decreasing bladder innervation. One of these operations is performed when bladder capacity is within normal range (165). The outcome of surgery is unpredictable, and neurologic bladder with severe voiding pain is the most common complication of surgery (162).
- *Bladder augmentation* is a combination of cystectomy (resection of the detrusor can be performed supratrigonally, subtrigonally, or at the proximal urethra) and ileocystoplasty. The most common bladder resection is executed supratrigonally using the ileum for bladder

reconstruction (166). It has been postulated that supra-trigonal cystectomy with ileocystoplasty is an effective approach for a classic ulcerative IC subtype, and this technique seems to be unsuitable for a nonulcerative subtype of IC (167).

■ *Cystectomy and diversion* is a radical procedure. Before contemplating it, all conservative treatments must be tried and proven unsuccessful. It must be definitively established that the pelvic pain originates in the bladder (pain increases when a patient holds urine and pain subsides to some degree with voiding). Cystometrogram must prove that filling of the bladder causes the pain. It is estimated to be successful in 95% of patients (162).

Complementary Therapy

Acupuncture

Acupuncture has been tested in prospective, observational studies, and initial results indicate a limited effect on patients with IC. However, the small patient population is insufficient to establish evidence for clinical use (168).

Transcutaneous Electrical Nerve Stimulation

Transcutaneous electrical nerve stimulation (TENS) observational studies suggest that TENS is beneficial in the treatment of IC. The better outcome of this mode of therapy is observed when it is used in the classic subtype of IC (169).

Exercise and Behavioral Therapy

A combination of pelvic floor muscle exercise; behavioral modification such as timed voiding (bladder drilling); controlled fluid intake, and keeping a voiding diary may yield rates of up to 50% of symptoms markedly improved. 38% improvement was observed among patients refractory to conservative management. Such significant improvement is observed after a mean of 12 weeks of treatment (170). No studies have validated these findings either in short- or long-term observation.

Urethral Syndrome

Definition

Urethral syndrome is defined as symptoms mimicking a lower UTI in the absence of significant uropathogens.

Incidence

The true incidence of urethral syndrome is unknown. It is estimated to occur in approximately 20% to 30% of patients with urinary conditions (171).

Etiology

The cause of urethral syndrome is unknown.

Diagnosis

The diagnosis of urethral syndrome is reached by excluding other conditions manifesting similar symptoms.

Differential Diagnosis

The following conditions must be ruled out before the diagnosis of urethral syndrome can be entertained (172):

■ The absence of pyuria, bacteriuria, and urine pathogenic colony most likely eliminates bacterial infection of the lower urinary tract.

■ Hypoestrogenism (pale, atrophic urethral mucosa and bladder trigone). Therapy is usually with estrogens orally, locally, or both.

■ Urethral stenosis (Lyon ring or distal urethra constructive band must be disrupted under local infiltration with an anesthetic agent).

■ Urethral spasm [can be treated with a skeletal muscle (e.g., diazepam) or smooth muscle (alpha-blocker) relaxant].

■ Acute (dysuria, redness, exudative urethral mucosa, pyuria, and often a negative urine culture) or chronic urethritis (redness, exudates, polyp, granulation, and cyst in urethra and trigone). Therapy is recommended with antibiotics empirically before culture results are available.

■ Allergy (management includes eliminating the cause of allergy, and administering antihistamines or local steroids).

■ Trauma (reducing or excluding exposure to traumatic events).

■ Anatomic abnormality (management is usually surgery).

■ Neurologic disorders (treating the underlying neurologic cause).

■ Psychogenic (psychotherapy is required for management).

Conventional Therapy

Conservative management of urethral syndrome is based on a probable cause, and treatment is directed toward the dominant symptom.

A surgical procedure has been suggested, such as urethral dilatation, cryotherapy, and marsupialization or unroofing (Reiser operation). There are conflicting reports on outcomes over the short and long terms. Therefore, the surgical option should be approached with caution (171).

Complementary Therapy

A combination of acupuncture and moxibustion [cauterization by the burning of moxa (combustible substance) on the skin] intervention for urethral syndrome significantly improves symptoms in both the short and long terms by approximately 90.6% and 80.4%, respectively (172).

REFERENCES

1. Association of Professors of Gynecology and Obstetrics (APGO). *Medical student educational objectives,* 7th ed. Washington, DC: APGO, 1997.
2. Council on Resident Education in Obstetrics and Gynecology (CREOG). *Educational objectives core curriculum for residents in obstetrics and gynecology,* 5th ed. Washington, DC: CREOG, 1996.
3. American College of Obstetrician and Gynecologists (ACOG). *Technical bulletin no. 213.* Washington, DC: ACOG, 1995.
4. Weider AC, Versi E. Physiology of micturition. In: Ostergard DR, Bent AE, eds. *Urogynecology and urodynamics,* 4th ed. Baltimore, Williams & Wilkins, 1996:33–63.
5. deGroat WC. Neuroanatomy and neurophysiology: innervation of the lower urinary tract. In: Raz S, ed. *Female urology,* 2nd ed. Philadelphia, WB Saunders, 1996.
6. Allen RE, Hosker GL, Smith ARB, et al. Pelvic floor damage and childbirth: a neurophysiology study. *Br J Obstet Gynecol* 1990;97:770–779.
7. Benson JT, McClellan E. The effect of vaginal dissection on the pudendal nerve. *Obstet Gynecol* 1993;82:387–399.
8. Lalley PM, DeGroat WC, McLayn PL. Reflex firing on the hypogastric nerve (HGN) in response to stimulation of visceral afferent fibers. *Fed Proc* 1971;30:324–332.
9. DeGroat WC, Lalley PM. Reflex firing in the lumbar sympathetic outflow to activation of visceral afferent fibers. *J Physiol (London)* 1972;226:289–309.
10. Chai TC, Steers. Neurophysiology of micturition and continence in women. *Int Urogynecol J* 1997;8:85–97.
11. Kuru M. Nervous control of micturition. *Physiol Rev* 1965;45:425–494.
12. Grady M, Kozminski M, DeLencey J, et al. Stress incontinence and cystocele. *J Urol* 1991;145:1211–1213.
13. Wester C, Brubaker L. Normal pelvic floor physiology. *Obstet Gynecol Clin North Am* 1998;25:707–722.
14. Fall M. Does electrostimulation cure urinary incontinence? *J Urol* 1984;131:664–667.
15. Susset J, Galea G, Manbeck K, et al. A predictive score index for the outcome of associated biofeedback and vaginal electrostimulation in the treatment of female incontinence. *J Urol* 1995;153:1461–1466.
16. Sato A, Sato Y, Suzuki A. Mechanism of the relax inhibition of micturition contractions of the urinary bladder elicited by acupuncture-like stimulation in anesthetized rats. *Neurosci Res* 1992;15:189–198.
17. deGroat WC. Inhibition and excitation of sacral parasympathetic neurons by visceral and cutaneous stimuli in the cat. *Brain Res* 1971;33:499–503.
18. deGroat WC. Anatomy and physiology of the lower urinary tract. *Urol Clin North Am* 1993;20:383–401.
19. DeLencey JOL. Anatomy and physiology of lower urinary tract. In: Wall LL, Norton PA, DeLencey JOL, eds. *Practical urology.* Baltimore: Williams & Wilkins, 1993:6–40.
20. Enhorning G. Simultaneous recording of intravesicle and intraurethral pressure. *Acta Chir Scand* 1961;27(suppl):61–68.
21. Petros PE, Ulmsten U. An integral theory of female urinary incontinence. *Acta Obstet Gynecol Scand* 1990;69(suppl 153):1–79.
22. Petros PE, Ulmsten U. Role of the pelvic floor in the bladder neck opening and closure I: muscle forces. *Int Urogynecol J* 1997;8:74–80.
23. Petros PE, Ulmsten U. Role of the pelvic floor in the bladder neck opening and closure II: vagina. *Int Urogynecol J* 1997;8:69–73.
24. Shafik A. Micturition and urinary continence: new concept. *Int Urogynecol J* 1992;3:168–175.
25. DeLencey JOL. Structural support of the urethra as it relates to the stress incontinence: the hammock hypothesis. *Am J Obstet Gynecol* 1994;170:1713–1723.
26. International Continence Society Committee for the Standardization of Terminology of the Lower Urinary Tract Function. *Br J Obstet Gynecol* 1990;6(l):1–16.
27. Urinary Incontinence Guideline Panel. *Urinary incontinence in adults.* Rockville, MD: US Department of Health and Human Services. Agency for Health Care Policy and Research (AHCPR), 1992.
28. Thomas TM, Plymat KR, Blannin J, et al. Prevalence of urinary incontinence. *Br Med J* 1980;281:1243–1245.
29. Rekers H, Drogendijk AC, Valkenburg H, et al. Urinary incontinence in women from 35 to 79 years of age: prevalence and consequences. *Eur J Obstet Gynecol Reprod Biol* 1992;43: 229–234.
30. Koonings PP, Bergman A, Ballard CA. Low urethral pressure and stress urinary incontinence in women: risk factor for failed retropubic urethropexy. *Urology* 1990;36:245–248.
31. Weinberger MW. Differential diagnosis of urinary incontinence. In: Ostergard DR, Bent AE, eds. *Urogynecology and urodynamics. Theory and practice,* 4th ed. Baltimore: Williams & Wilkins, 1996.
32. Richardson DA, Bent AE, Ostergard DR. The effect of uterovaginal prolapse on urethrovesicle pressure dynamics. *Am J Obstet Gynecol* 1983;146:901–905.
33. Juenmann KP, Lue TF, Schmidt RA. clinical significance of sacral and pudendal nerve anatomy. *J Urol* 1988;139:74–80.
34. Bruskewitz R. Female incontinence: signs and symptoms. In: Raz S, ed. *Female urology.* Philadelphia: WB Saunders, 1983: 45–50.
35. Barber MD, Cundiff GW, Weidner AC, et al. Accuracy of clinical assessment of paravaginal defects in women with anterior vaginal wall prolapse. *Am J Obstet Gynecol* 1999;181:87–90.
36. Karram MM, Bhatia NN. The Q-tip test: standardization of the technique and its interpretation in women with urinary incontinence. *Obstet Gynecol* 1988;71:807–811.
37. Montz FJ, Stanton SL. Q-tip test in female urinary incontinence. *Obstet Gynecol* 1986;67:258–260.
38. Bergman A, McCarthy TA, Ballard CA, et al. Role of the Q-tip test in evaluating stress urinary incontinence. *J Reprod Med* 1987;32:273–275.
39. Hayen BT. Residual urine volumes in a normal female population: application of transvaginal ultrasound. *Br J Urol* 1989;64:347–349.
40. Fantl JA, Smith PJ, Schneider V, et al. Fluid weight uroflowmetry in women. *Am J Obstet Gynecol* 1983;145:1017–1024.
41. Godec GJ, Cass AS. Cystometric variations during postural changes. *J Urol* 1980;123:722–725.
42. Bergman A, Nguyen H, Koonings PP, et al. Use of fetal cardiotocographic monitor in the evaluation of urinary incontinence. *Isr J Med Soc* 1988;24:291–294.
43. Wall LL, Norton PA, Delancy JOL. Practical urodynamic. In: *Practical urogynecology.* Baltimore: Williams & Wilkins, 1993.
44. Harris RL, Cundiff GW, Theofrastous JP, et al. Bladder compliance in neurologically intact women. *Neurourol Urodyn* 1996;15:483–488.
45. Bottaccini MR, Gleason DM. Urodynamic norms in women. I. Normals versus stress incontinence. *J Urol* 1980;124:659–662.
46. McGuire EJ. Urodynamic findings in patients after failure of stress incontinence operations. *Prog Clin Biol Res* 1981;78:351–360.
47. Bump RC, Copeland WE, Hurt WG, et al. Dynamic urethral pressure/profilometry pressure transmission ratio determination

in stress-incontinent and stress-continent subjects. *Am J Obstet Gynecol* 1988;159:749–755.

48. McGuire EJ, Fitzpatric CC, Wan J, et al. Clinical assessment of urethral sphincter function. *J Urol* 1993;150:1452–1454.

49. James M, Jackson S, Shepherd A, et al. Pure stress leakage symptomatology: is it safe to discount detrusor instability? *Br J Obstet Gynecol* 1999;106:1255–1258.

50. Swift SE, Ostergard DR. Evaluation of current urodynamic testing methods in the diagnosis of genuine stress incontinence. *Obstet Gynecol* 1995;86:85–91.

51. Karram MM, Bhatia NN. The Q-tip test: Standardization of the technique and its interpretation in women with urinary incontinence. *Obstet Gynecol* 1988;71:807–811.

52. Summit RL, Stovall TG, Bent AE, et al. Urinary incontinence: correlation of history and brief office evaluation with multichannel urodynamic testing. *Am J Obstet Gynecol* 1992;166: 1835–1844.

53. Nygaard IE. Pharmacologic management of pelvic floor dysfunction. *Obstet Gynecol Clin North Am* 1998;25:867–882.

54. Kinn AC, Lindskog M. Estrogen and phenylpropanolamine in combination for stress urinary incontinence in postmenopausal women. *Urology* 1988;32:273–280.

55. Yokoyama T, Huard J, Chancellor MB. Myoblast therapy for stress urinary incontinence and bladder dysfunction. *World J Urol* 2000;18:56–61.

56. Bergman A, Elia G. Three surgical procedures for genuine stress incontinence: five-year follow-up of a prospective randomized study. *Am J Obstet Gynecol* 1995;173:66–71.

57. Beck RP, McCormick S, Nordstrom L. A 25-year experience with 519 anterior colporrhaphy procedures. *Obstet Gynecol* 1991;78:1011–1018.

58. Colombo M, Scalambrino S, Magginoni A, et al. Burch colposuspension versus modified Marshall-Marchetti-Krantz urethropexy for primary genuine stress urinary incontinence: a prospective, randomized clinical trial. *Am J Obstet Gynecol* 1994;171:1573–1579.

59. Alcalay M, Monga A, Stanton SL. Burch colposuspension: a 10–20 year follow-up. *Br J Obstet Gynecol* 1995;102:740–745.

60. Laursen H, Farlie R, Rasmussen KL, et al. Colposuspension Burch—an 18 year follow-up study. *Neurourol Urodyn* 1994;13:445.

61. Erikson BC, Hagen B, Eik-Nes SH, et al. Long-term effectiveness of the Burch colposuspension in female urinary stress incontinence. *Acta Obstet Gynecol Scand* 1990;69:45–50.

62. Polascik TJ, Moore RG, Rosenberg MT, et al. Comparison of laparoscopic and open urethropexy for treatment of stress incontinence. *Urology* 1995;45:647–652.

63. Vancaillie TG, Schuessler W. Laparoscopic bladder neck suspension. *J Laparoendosc Surg* 1991;1:169–173.

64. Burton G. A randomized comparison of laparoscopic and open colposuspension. *Neurourol Urodyn* 1994;13:497–498.

65. Shull BL, Baden WF. A six-year experience with paravaginal defect repair for stress urinary incontinence. *Am J Obstet Gynecol* 1989;160:1432–1440.

66. Bruce RG, El-Galley RE, Galloway NT. Paravaginal defect repair in the treatment of females stress urinary incontinence and cystocele. *Urology* 1999;54:647–651.

67. Scotti RJ, Garely AD, Greston WM, et al. Paravaginal repair of lateral vaginal wall defects by fixation to the ischial periosteum and obturator membrane. *Am J Obstet Gynecol* 1998;179: 1436–1445.

68. Pereyra AJ. A simplified surgical procedure for the correction of stress urinary incontinence in women. *West J Surg Obstet Gynecol* 1959;67:223–226.

69. Stamey TA. Endoscopic suspension of the vesicle neck for urinary incontinence. *Surg Gynecol Obstet* 1973;136:547–554.

70. Raz S. Modified bladder neck suspension for female stress incontinence. *Urology* 1981;17:82–85.

71. Muzsnai D, Carrillo E, Dubin C, et al. Retropubic vaginopexy for correction of urinary stress incontinence. *Obstet Gynecol* 1982;59:113–117.

72. Gittes RF, Loughlin KR. No-incision pubovaginal suspension for stress incontinence. *J Urol* 1987;138:568–570.

73. Bent AE, McLennan MT. Surgical management of urinary incontinence. *Obstet Gynecol Clin North Am* 1998;25:883–906.

74. Sand PK, Bowen LW, Panganiban R, et al. The pressure urethra as a factor in failed retropubic urethropexy. *Obstet Gynecol* 1987;69:390–402.

75. Haab F, Zimmern PE, Leach G. Urinary incontinence due to intrinsic sphincter deficiency: experience with fat and collagen injection periurethral injections. *J Urol* 1997;157:1283–1286.

76. Su TH, Hsu CY, Chen JC. Injection therapy for stress incontinence in women. *Int Urogynecol J Pelvic Floor Dysfunct* 1999;10:200–206.

77. Berg s. Polytef augmentation urethroplasty. *Arch Surg* 1973; 107:379–381.

78. Corcos J, Fournier C. Periurethral collagen injection for the treatment of female stress urinary incontinence: 4-year follow-up results. *Urology* 1999;54;815–818.

79. McLennan MT, Bent AE. Suburethral abscess: a complication of periurethral collagen injection therapy. *Obstet Gynecol* 1998;92:650–652.

80. Stothers L, Goldberg SL, Leone EF. Complications of periurethral collagen injection for stress urinary incontinence. *J Urol* 1998;159:806–807.

81. Wainstein MA, Klutke CG. Periurethral pseudocyst following cystoscopic collagen injection. *Urology* 1998;51:835–836.

82. Matthews K, Govier FE. Osteitis pubis after periurethral collagen injection. *Urology* 1997;49:237–238.

83. Harris RL, Cundiff GW, Coates KW, et al. Urethral prolapse after collagen injection. *Am J Obstet Gynecol* 1998;178: 614–615.

84. Steele AC, Kohli N, Karram MM. Periurethral collagen injection for stress incontinence with and without urethral hypermobility. *Obstet Gynecol* 2000;95:327–331.

85. Appell RA. Artificial urinary sphincter in the treatment of stress incontinence in females. In: Ostergard DR, Bent AE. *Urogynecology and urodynamics. Theory and practice,* 4th ed. Baltimore: Williams & Wilkins, 1996:581–590.

86. Kubisyta E, Altmann P, Kucera H, et al. Electro-acupuncture's influences on the closure mechanism of the female urethra in incontinence. *Am J Clin Med* 1976;4:177–181.

87. Berghmans LC, Hendriks HJ, Bo K, et al. Conservative treatment of stress urinary incontinence in women: a systemic review of randomized clinical trials. *Br J Urol* 1998;82: 181–191.

88. Peattie AB, Plevnic S, Stanton SL. Vaginal cones: a conservative method of treating genuine stress incontinence. *Br J Obstet Gynecol* 1988;95:1049–1053.

89. Weatherall M. Biofeedback or pelvic floor muscle exercises for female genuine stress incontinence: a meta-analysis of trials identified in a systemic review. *BJU Int* 1999;83:1015–1016.

90. Glavid K, Laursen B, Jaquet A. Efficacy of biofeedback in the treatment of urinary stress incontinence. *Int Urogynecol J Pelvic Floor Dysfunct* 1998;9:151–153.

91. Yasuda K, Yamanishi T. Critical evaluation of electro-stimulation for management of female urinary incontinence. *Curr Opin Obstet Gynecol* 1999;11:503–507.

92. Miller K, Richardson DA, Siegel SW, et al. *Int Urogynecol J Pelvic Floor Dysfunct* 1998;9:256–270.

93. Appell RA. Electrical stimulation for urinary incontinence. *Urology* 1998;51:24–26.

94. Chopra D, ed. *Alternative medicine. The definitive guide.* Tiburon, CA: Future Medicine Publishing, 1997:985.

95. Fetrow CW, Avila JR. *The complete guide to herbal medicines.* Springhouse, PA: Springhouse Corporation, 1999.

96. *PDR for herbal medicine.* Montvale, NJ: Medical Economics Company, 2000.

96a. Montella JM. Detrusor instability. In: Ostergard DR, Bent AE, eds. *Urogynecology and urodynamics. Theory and practice,* 4th ed. Baltimore: Williams & Wilkins, 1996:465–475.

97. Macaulay AJ, Stern RS, Holmes DM, et al. Micturition and the mind: psychological factors in the aetiology and treatment of urinary symptoms in women. *BMJ* 1987;294:540–543.

98. Frewen W. Role of bladder training in the treatment of the unstable bladder in the female. *Urol Clin North Am* 1979;6:273–277.

99. Fantl JA, Wymen JF, Harkins SW, et al. Efficacy of bladder training in older women with urinary incontinence. *JAMA* 1991;265:609–613.

100. Zarzitto ML, Jewett MAS, Fernie GR, et al. Effectiveness of propantheline bromide in the treatment of geriatric patients with detrusor instability. *Neurourol Urodyn* 1986;5:133–140.

101. Drutz HP, Appell RA, Gleason D, et al. Clinical efficacy and safety of tolteridine compared to oxybutynin and placebo in patients with overactive bladder. *Int Urogynecol J Pelvic Floor Dysfunct* 1999;10:283–289.

102. Norton P, Karram M, Wall LL, et al. Randomized double-blind trial of terodiline in the treatment of urge incontinence in women. *Obstet Gynecol* 1994;84:386–391.

103. Kitakoji H, Terasaki T, Honjo H, et al. Effect of acupuncture on the overactive bladder. *Nippon Hinyokika Gakkai Zasshi* 1995;86:1514–1519.

104. Chang PL, Wu CJ, Huang MH. Long-term outcome of acupuncture in women with frequency, urgency and dysuria. *Am J Chin Med* 1993;21:231–236.

105. Philip T, Shah PJ, Worth PH. Acupuncture in the treatment of bladder instability. *Br J Urol* 1988;61:490–493.

106. Honjo H, Kitakoji H, Kawakita K, et al. Acupuncture for urinary incontinence in patients with chronic spinal cord injury. A preliminary report. *Nippon Hinyokika Gakkai Zasshi* 1998; 89:665–669.

107. Okada N, Igawa Y, Nishizawa O. Functional electrical stimulation for detrusor instability. *Int Urogynecol J Pelvic Floor Dysfunct* 1999;10:329–335.

108. Freeman RM, Baxyby K. Hypnotherapy for incontinence caused by the unstable detrusor. *BMJ (Clin Res Ed)* 1982; 284:1831–1834.

109. Horzog AR, Fultz NH. Prevalence and incidence of urinary incontinence in community-dwelling populations. *J Am Geriatr Soc* 1990;38:273–280.

110. Fantl JA, Bump RC, McClish DK. Mixed urinary incontinence. *Urology* 1990;36(suppl):21–24.

111. Lockhart J. Vorstman B, Politano VA. Anti-incontinence surgery in females with detrusor instability. *Neurourol Urodyn* 1984;3:201–207.

112. Bowen LW, Sand PK, Ostergard DR, et al. Unsuccessful Burch urethropexy: a case-controlled urodynamic study. *Am J Obstet Gynecol* 1989;160:452–458.

113. Polsky MS, Agee RE, Berg SR, et al. Acute urinary retention in women. Brief discussion and unusual case report. *J Urol* 1973;110:541–543.

114. Herbaut AG. Neurologic urinary retention. *Int Urogynecol J* 1993;4:221–228.

115. Weinberger MW. Differential diagnosis of urinary incontinence. In: Ostergard DR, Bent AE. *Urogynecology and urodynamics. Theory and practice,* 4th ed. Baltimore: Williams & Wilkins, 1996:83–89.

116. Wheeler JS, Walter JS. Urinary retention in females: a review. *Int Urogynecol J* 1992;3:137–142.

117. Andersen MJF. The incidence of diverticula in the female urethra. *J Urol* 1967;98:96–98.

118. Ginsburg DS, Genadry R. Suburethral diverticulum in the female. *Obstet Gynecol Surv* 1984;39:1–7.

119. Kohoron EI, Glickman MG. Technical aids in investigating and management of urethral diverticula in the female. *Urology* 1992;40:322–325.

120. Spence H, Duckett J. Diverticulum of the female urethra: clinical aspects and presentation of simple operative technique for cure. *J Urol* 1970;104:432–437.

121. Mulholland SG. Controversies in the management of urinary tract infection. *Urology* 1986;27(suppl):3–8.

122. Cunha B. Urinary tract infections. I. Pathophysiology and diagnostic approach. *Postgrad Med* 1981;70:141–158.

123. Maskell R. Importance of coagulase-negative staphylococci as pathogens in the urinary tract. *Lancet* 1974;1:1155–1159.

124. Nicolle LE, Hoban SA, Harding GKM. Characterization of coagulase-negative staphylococci from urinary isolates. *J Clin Microbiol* 1983;17:267–271.

125. Sobota AE. Inhibition of bacterial adherence by cranberry juice: potential use for the treatment of urinary tract infections. *J Urol* 1984:131:1013–1016.

126. Parsons CL. Urinary tract infections in the female patient. *Urol Clin North Am* 1985;12:355–361.

127. Weinstein l, Madoff MA, Samet CM. The sulfonamides. *N Engl J Med* 1960;263:793–801.

128. Goldstein EJ, Alpert ML, Najem A. Norfloxacin in the treatment of complicated and uncomplicated urinary tract infections: a comparative multicenter trial. *AM J Med* 1987; 82:65–69.

129. Reed MD, Blumer JL. Urologic pharmacology in the office setting. *Urol Clin North Am* 1988;15:737–751.

130. Kunin CM, Finland M. Clinical pharmacology of the tetracycline antibiotics. *Clin Pharmacol Ther* 1961;2:51–56.

131. Ronald AR. Optimal duration of treatment for kidney infection. *Ann Intern Med* 1987;106:467–468.

132. Karram MM. Lower urinary tract infection. In: Ostergard DR, Bent AE, eds. *Urogynecology and urodynamics. Theory and practice,* 4th ed. Baltimore: Williams & Wilkins, 1996: 387–408.

133. Wathne B, Hovelius B, Mardh PA. Causes of frequency and dysuria in women. *Scand J Infect Dis* 1987;19:223–229.

134. Pfau A, Sacks T, Englenstain D. Recurrent urinary tract infection in postmenopausal women: prophylaxis based on understanding of the pathogenesis. *J Urol* 1983;129:1152–1160.

135. Stamey TA, Condy M, Mihara G. Prophylactic efficacy of nitrofurantoin macrocrystals and trimethoprim-sulfamethoxazonole in urinary infections: biologic effects on the vaginal and rectal flora. *N Engl J Med* 1977;296:780–788.

136. Martinez FC, Kindrachuk RW, Thomas E, et al. Effect of prophylactic low dose cephalexin on fecal and vaginal bacteria. *J Urol* 1985;133:994–998.

137. Aune A, Alraek T, LiHua H, et al. Acupuncture in the prophylaxis of recurrent lower urinary tract infection in adult women. *Scand J Prim Health Care* 1998;16:37–39.

138. Sobota AE. Inhibition of bacterial adherence by cranberry juice: potential use for the treatment of urinary tract infections. *J Urol* 1984;131:1013–1016.

139. Schmidt DR, Sobota AE. An examination of the anti-adherence activity of cranberry juice on urinary and nonurinary bacterial isolates. *Microbios* 1988;55:173–181.

140. Fleet JC. New support for a folk remedy: cranberry juice reduces bacteriuria and pyuria in elderly women. *Nutr Rev* 1994;52:168–170.

141. Frohne D. The urinary disinfectant effect of extract from leaves uva ursi. *Planta Med* 1970;18:1–25.

142. Gross AJ, Hummel G. Goethe almost died of urosepsis. *World J Urol* 1999;17:421–424.

143. Deshpande PJ, Sahu M, Kumar P. *Crataeva nurvala* Hook and Forest (Varuna)—the ayurvedic drugs of choice in urinary disorders. *Ind J Med Res* 1982;76:46–53.

144. *British herbal pharmacopoeia.* British Herbal Medicine Association, London, UK, 1983.

145. Bone K, Burgess N, McLeod D. Phytosynergistic prescribing. Portland, OR: Professional Complementary Health Formulas, 1994:69–70.

146. Curhan GC, Speizer FE, Hunter DJ, et al. Epidemiology of interstitial cystitis: a population based study. *J Urol* 1999;161:549–552.

147. Holm-Bentzen M, Lose G. Pathology and pathogenesis of interstitial cystitis. *Urology* 1987;29(suppl):8–13.

148. Hanno P. Interstitial cystitis and related diseases. In: Walsh P, et al., eds. *Cambell's urology.* Philadelphia: WB Saunders, 1998.

149. Pontari M, Hanno P, Wein A. Logical and systematic approach to the evaluation and management of patient suspected of having interstitial cystitis. *Urology* 1997;49(suppl 5A):114–120.

150. Nigro DA, Wein AJ. Interstitial cystitis: clinical and endoscopic feature. In: Sant GR, ed. *Interstitial cystitis.* Philadelphia: Lippincott-Raven, 1997.

151. Waxman JA, Sulak PJ, Kuehl TJ. Cystoscopic findings consistent with interstitial cystitis in normal women undergoing tubal ligation. *J Urol* 1998;160:1663–1667.

152. Hanno P, Levin RM, Monson FC, et al. Diagnosis of interstitial cystitis. *J Urol* 1990;143:278–281.

153. Parsons CL, Greenberg M, Gabal L, et al. The role of urinary potassium in the pathogenesis and diagnosis of interstitial cystitis. *J Urol* 1998;159:1862–1866.

154. Chambers GK, Fenster HN, Cripps S, et al. An assessment of the use of intravesicle potassium in the diagnosis of interstitial cystitis. *J Urol* 1999;162(part 1):699–701.

155. Gillenwater J, Wein A. Summary of the National Institute of Arthritis, Diabetes, Digestive, and Kidney Diseases workshop on interstitial cystitis. *J Urol* 1988;140:203–206.

156. Hanno PM, Landis JR, Matthews-Cook Y, et al. The diagnosis of interstitial cystitis revisited: lessons learned from the National Institutes of Health Interstitial Cystitis Database Study. *J Urol* 1999;161:553–557.

157. Koziol J, Clark D, Gittes R, et al. The natural history of interstitial cystitis: a survey of 374 patients. *J Urol* 1993;149:465–469.

158. Hwang P, Auclair B, Beechinor D, et al. Efficacy of pentosan polysulfate in the treatment of interstitial cystitis: a meta-analysis. *Urology* 1997;50:39–43.

159. Theoharides TC. Hydroxyzine therapy for interstitial cystitis. *Urol Clin North Am* 1994;21:113–119.

160. Sant G, La Rock D. Standard intravesicle therapies for interstitial cystitis. *Urol Clin North Am* 1994;21:73–83.

161. Stewart BH, Persky L, Kiser WS. The use of dimethylsulfoxide (DMSO) in treatment of interstitial cystitis. *J Urol* 1968;98:671–672.

162. Parsons CL. Interstitial cystitis. In: Ostergard DR, Bent AE, eds. *Urogynecology and urodynamics. Theory and practice,* 4th ed. Baltimore: Williams & Wilkins, 1996:409–425.

163. Lechevallier E. Interstitial cystitis. *Prog Urol* 1995;5:21–30.

164. Shanberg AM, Baghdassarian R, Tansey LA. Treatment of interstitial cystitis with the neodymium laser. *J Urol* 1985;134:885–888.

165. Bondavalli C, Schiavon L, Dall'oglio B, et al. Interstitial cystitis: surgical treatment. *Arch Ital Urol Androl* 1999;71:327–332.

166. Castello AJ, Crowe H, Agarwal D. Supratrigonal cystectomy and ileocystoplasty in management of interstitial cystitis. *Aust N Z J Surg* 2000;70:34–38.

167. Peeker R, Aldenborg F, Fall M. The treatment of interstitial cystitis with supratrigonal cystectomy and ileocystoplasty: difference in outcome between classic and nonulcer disease. *J Urol* 1998;159:1479–1482.

168. Geirsson G, Wang YH, Lindstrom S, et al. Traditional acupuncture and electrical stimulation of the posterior tibial nerve. A trial in chronic interstitial cystitis. *Scand J Urol Nephrol* 1993;27:67–70.

169. Fall M, Lindstrom S. Transcutaneous electrical nerve stimulation in classic and nonulcer interstitial cystitis. *Urol Clin North Am* 1994;21:131–139.

170. Chiken DC, Blaivas JG, Blaivas ST. Behavioral therapy for the treatment of refractory interstitial cystitis. *J Urol* 1993;149:1445–1448.

171. Scotti RJ, Ostergard DR. Urethral syndrome. In: *Urogynecology and urodynamics. Theory and practice,* 4th ed. Baltimore: Williams & Wilkins, 1996:339–359.

172. Zheng H, Wang S, Shang J, et al. Study on acupuncture and moxibustion therapy for female urethral syndrome. *J Trad Chin Med* 1998;18:122–127.

26

ANORECTAL DISORDERS IN GYNECOLOGIC PRACTICE

EDUCATIONAL OBJECTIVES

Medical Students	*Residents in Obstetrics/Gynecology*	*Practitioners*
APGO Objective No. 26	*CREOG Objective*	*ACOG Recommendation*
No specific recommendation	No specific recommendation	No specific recommendation

FUNCTIONAL ANATOMY

Anal Canal

The anal canal is the very distal part of the gastrointestinal tract and connects the rectum with the skin. The fusion between the anus and rectum is called the anorectal junction, and the part attached to the skin is called the anal verge. Laterally this structure merges with the puborectalis sling (discussed in Chapter 24). The length of the anal canal ranges from 2 to 6 cm (1), and its function is to prevent fecal material from leaking through its continence mechanism. The anal canal includes the anoderm, which is 2 to 3 cm above the dentate line, up to the level of the levator ani muscle (Fig. 26.1). Resting and squeezing forces create the closure pressure (the difference between maximum resting anal pressure and rectal pressure). These forces are an important factor in anal continence within the anal canal [a high-pressure zone in women ranges from 30 to 50 mm Hg, with an average of about 37 mm Hg (2)]. These forces decline with advancing age, particularly evident in the postmenopausal period (3).

Anal Sphincter Complex

The *internal anal sphincter* is the true sphincter of the gastrointestinal tract. It has a cylindrical configuration (4) and anteriorly creates the width of the anal sphincter in about 54% of the complex (5). The anterior and posterior wall thickness of the internal sphincter is equally distributed (6). The internal anal sphincter is an extension of the rectal, circular, smooth muscle layer and lies between the anal mucosa and the external anal sphincter (Fig. 26.2). The internal sphincter muscle migrates more that 1 cm (an aver-

age of 17 mm) above the proximal margin of the external sphincter muscle (7). The striated external anal sphincter muscle encapsulates the internal anal sphincter muscle, providing volunteer squeezing ability to the annual sphincter complex (6). Functionally, the internal sphincter muscle supplies about 85% of the maximal anal resting pressure responsible for anal continence (2).

The external anal sphincter muscle overlaps the internal sphincter and penetrates the internal sphincter to approximately 3.7 cm caudally (6). The posterior external anal sphincter is thicker (more pronounced in the proximal part) than the anterior aspect (4). Functionally, impulsive rectal distention stimulates the external anal sphincter, which supplies approximately 60% of the anal canal pressure and by doing so participates in continence; even so, it is not able to maintain continuous tone of the external sphincter muscle (8).

Morphologically, the external sphincter is divided into anatomic subdivisions in many modern texts (deep, superficial, and subcutaneous). However, a growing body of evidence shows that such division is difficult to substantiate anatomically and clinically (7).

Anorectal Symptomatology

The organ-specific anorectal interview for anorectal disorders usually oscillates among several common symptoms. When an organ-oriented symptom is present, it should be explored further with the focus on onset, frequency, duration, severity, location, aggravation, relief, and whether or not a symptom occurs only with bowel movement or exists independently. The leading symptom (if complex symptoms are present) should be established. To expedite a practitioner's mental diagnostic process, compartmentalization

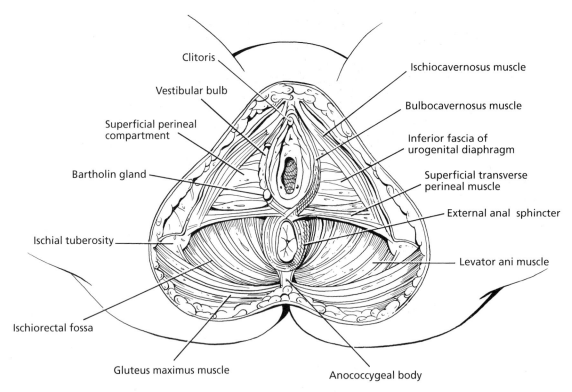

FIGURE 26.1. The anus and adjacent structures.

of a symptom with probable medical conditions is very helpful. One symptom may reflect several clinical scenarios; therefore, it is useful to group them under one umbrella to ease the initial step for evaluation. Nevertheless, it is clinical conviction that a well-obtained, organ-oriented, specific medical history helps establish a presumptive diagnosis in the majority of cases. The following symptoms may indicate associated conditions with a particular symptom.

Hematochezia or anorectal bleeding must be distinguished from melena (black, tarry stool). Melena usually reflects bleeding sources above the ligament of Treitz, where blood is exposed to hydrochloric acid (from the esophagus, stomach, or duodenum). When bleeding originates below the ligament of Treitz (in the jejunum, ileum, or colon), the stool color may be maroon or bright red).

Anorectal bleeding should be analyzed with a patient in reference to the following:

- Frequency
- Quantity
- Color (bright, maroon, and black) is noticed on underwear, toilet paper, in toilet bowl water
- Bleeding with or without clots

Anorectal bleeding can be associated with the following:

- Anal fissures
- Arteriovenous malformation
- Colorectal polyp or malignant neoplasia
- Hemorrhoids (internal or external)
- Inflammatory bowel disease

Pain and its characteristics, such as location, onset, frequency, radiation, duration, character, aggravation, and relief, should be explored. Pain and irritation in the anorectal area can be associated with the following clinical conditions:

- Abscess and fistula
- Anal fissure
- Hemorrhoids
- Levator syndrome
- Itching
- Sexually transmitted disease (STD)

Itching can be associated with the following conditions:

- Anal fissures
- Chronic discharge or diarrhea
- Dermatologic conditions of the anorectal area
- Excessive sweating
- Hemorrhoids
- Inappropriate hygiene
- Infection, particularly from a fungus or parasite

Discharge and its characteristics, such as frequency, quantity, location (anus or perineum), and consistency (liquid,

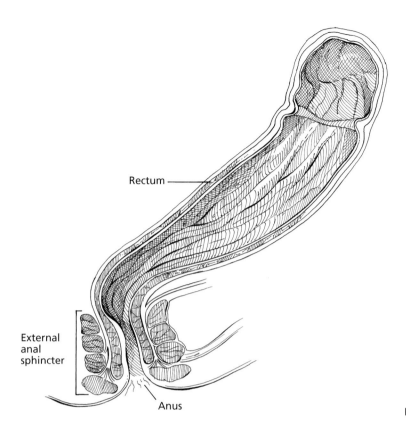

Rectum

External
anal
sphincter

Anus

FIGURE 26.2. The anus, rectum, and anal canal.

feces, blood-tinged, mucous, purulent), should be investigated. Discharge may be associated with physical activities or flatus, and may be a symptom of the following conditions:

- Anorectal abscess
- Anorectal fistula
- Fecal incontinence
- Recent surgery or trauma

Changes in stool habits may be attributed to the following:

- *Constipation* (related to diet, functional disorders, medication side effects, metabolic or endocrine disorders, hemorrhoids, polyps, or cancer)
- *Diarrhea* (related to infection, inflammatory bowel disease, irritable bowel syndrome, lactose intolerance, or medication side effects)
- *Incontinence*

Physical Evaluation

Examination of the anorectal area (proctologic examination) in a regular office setting (not furnished with a procto-table or Ritter table) is sufficient and effective. On a regular examining table a patient is placed in the left lateral decubitus position with the knee bent and drawn up to the chest. The buttocks will protrude a little over the table's edge (Sims position). Before a patient is placed in the left

lateral decubitus position, abdominal and inguinal inspection is usually performed.

Proctologic examination encompasses the following:

- Abdominal and inguinal inspection
- Buttocks and anoperineal inspection
- Anoscopy is designed to evaluate the anal canal and may assist in identifying internal hemorrhoids (often associated with corresponding external hemorrhoids) and anal fissures (tender and bleeds with ease).
- Digital rectal examination

Medical history combined with proctoscopic examination may provide the diagnosis of the following:

- *Anal or perianal abscess*— perineal area is red, swollen, and tender, with or without purulent drainage. On palpation an indurated or fluctuant mass can be established.
- Anal, perianal, or anal canal condylomata acuminata is a nontender lesion with the appearance of a wart. It may be present in a flat form that becomes visible after applying 3% to 5% vinegar, and white patches come to the surface.
- *Anal cancer* should be suspected when an ulcerative mass is present. By palpation the lesion is firm, fused with surroundings, fixed, and usually nontender. Biopsy with histologic confirmation establishes the definitive diagnosis.
- *Anal mucosal prolapse;* upon straining, anal mucosa comes out.

- *Fissure-in-ano* (a tear or split of the anoderm) usually indicates a chronic state when it imitates an ulcer. The affected area is tender and has an edematous tag. Increased guarding of sphincter muscle tone is often associated with an anal hypertrophic papilla.
- *External thrombosed hemorrhoids* present as a blue or purple swelling (grapelike appearance) at the anal verge. Internal hemorrhoids by palpation present as soft masses in this area.
- *Pilonidal cyst* located in the natal cleft is a cystic structure with hair present. When infected it may present as a *pilonidal abscess* (swelling, red, tender, with or without purulent drainage, and hair present).
- *Prolapsing hypertrophic papilla* is a mass that protrudes from the anal canal and is layered with the epidermis.
- *Pruritus ani* is usually present as symmetrically distributed itching around the anus. A red or white lichen like lesion of the skin with linear ulcerative appearance may have a leather like texture.
- *Hidradenitis suppurativa* is a chronic medical entity affecting the apocrine glands, subcutaneous tissue, and skin. The clinical picture includes induration of a single nodule or multiple discrete nodules of the skin with enlarged skin pores and tenderness. Medical history and physical examination including anoscopy and digital examination are usually sufficient to make the diagnosis. If any diagnostic question exists, a direct biopsy and histologic examination should rule out other conditions such as anal malignancy, Crohn disease, pilonidal disease, and cutaneous infection.
- *Treatment* with antibiotics reduces inflammation. Minocycline is effective in this condition. When hidradenitis suppurativa does not respond to conservative management, surgical management is recommended.
- *Foreign bodies* are associated either with using instruments for sexual stimulation or as results of assault. Anoscopic removal of foreign bodies is usually satisfactory treatment.

Laboratory

Simple tests for anal disorders can be performed in the office setting. Fecal occult blood testing usually is performed using a commercially available card (e.g., Hemoccult II), which turns dark blue in contact with hemoglobin (vitamin C when taken at a dose in excess of 250 mg/day, horseradish, and rare meat may produce false-negative results). Stool culture for microorganisms is indicated in association with persistent diarrhea.

Imaging Study

The following imaging study may be offered in anorectal disorders:

- Ultrasonography with a specially designed anorectal transducer
- Barium enema
- Defecography

Endoscopic Studies for Anorectal Disorders

- Anoscopy
- Flexible sigmoidoscopy
- Colposcopy can be used to identify the perianal area and lesions of the distal anal canal [particularly useful in a direct biopsy or identifying flat human papillomavirus (HPV) lesions]

Several anorectal disorders must be taken into account, such as Bowen disease, Paget disease, or inflammatory bowel disease, when considering the differential diagnosis. These conditions are beyond the scope of this presentation, and more information can be found in Chapters 13 and 14.

FECAL INCONTINENCE

A high prevalence of fecal incontinence in association with urinary incontinence and pelvic organ prolapse warrants an update in this field for clinicians providing primary care for women. A practitioner must become comfortable with inquiring about fecal incontinence among women patients. Because it is a socially embarrassing occurrence, fewer than 50% of women with fecal incontinence will volunteer to discuss this medical problem with their health-care providers (9). Conservative therapy and surgical reconstruction can improve symptoms in the majority of patients.

Definition

Fecal incontinence is the lack of feces evacuation control.

Incidence

The prevalence of fecal incontinence among women is estimated to be 0.4% to 17% and increases with advancing age (10). Approximately 35% to 50% of fecal incontinence coexists with urinary incontinence (11). In about 7%, pelvic viscera prolapse is associated with fecal incontinence (12).

Etiology

Several factors of coordination, such as colonic transit time, anorectal reflexes, rectal distensibility, sphincter complex function, stool volume, consistency, and mental function, are necessary to maintain fecal continence. Any abnormality or disorder among these factors may lead to fecal incontinence.

The following can disrupt the anal sphincter complex mechanism function:

- *Pudendal nerve* injury most commonly is encountered during parturition or chronic straining during defecation.
- *Anatomic structural injury* is usually associated with labor trauma, and approximately 35% of primiparous and 44% of multiparous women sustain injury to the anal sphincter complex during vaginal delivery (13). Midline episiotomy itself increases the risk for anal sphincter complex injury by 4- to 13-fold (14). Because approximately 50% of all vaginal deliveries are accomplished with midline episiotomy, the necessity of this obstetric procedure should be called into question (15). It is clinically recognized that anorectal surgery (e.g., therapeutic anal dilatation, hemorrhoidectomy, and rectovaginal fistula repair) may compromise anal sphincter complex integrity and function, leading to fecal incontinence.
- *Neuroanatomic causes* can be analyzed from two perspectives:
- Damage to the rectal reservoir by rectal distensibility (postradiation therapy, scleroderma, diabetes mellitus, and inflammatory bowel disease) or reduced rectal compliance (may manifest as fecal urgency).
- Dysfunctional anal sphincter complex secondary to anatomic structure injury or pudendal neuropathy.

Diagnosis

Pertinent medical history should include the following:

- Changes in usual bowel habit (frequency and consistency of stool)
- Duration of fecal leakage
- Need for perineal pad
- Leakage of gas, liquid or solid fecal materials
- Any conventional or alternative medication that may interfere or predispose to diarrhea or functional disorders of the anus and rectum
- Dietary habits
- Past pelvic surgery

Associated symptoms include the following:

- Fecal urgency
- Abdominal pain
- Social and life-style changes

Physical examination should include general examination and neurologic evaluation, with particular attention to the lower extremities and perineal and cutaneous-anal reflexes (when absence suggests pudendal neuropathy). More about neurologic examination is presented in Chapter 25.

Inspection of the sphincter complex and perineum may reveal the following:

- Visible keyhole-like distortion

- Trauma to the anus (most commonly caused by anal sexual intercourse and instruments used for sexual stimulation), which can produce low sphincter tone and low squeeze pressure
- Perineal descent or prolapse, observed with a Valsalva maneuver

Digital examination will disclose the following:

- A complete cloaca (absent or very thin perineum and rectovaginal septum)
- Low sphincter tone and low squeeze force (decreased, absence of contraction, or asymmetrical) with maximal squeezing effort of the anal sphincter complex (evaluation of the puborectalis muscle by palpation of the posterior wall of the rectum at the ano-rectal junction with voluntary contraction of the external sphincter muscle and the examining finger elevated anteriorly)
- Presence or absence of anorectal mass
- Presence or absence of stool impaction and stool consistency

Anoscopy should be performed in each case to rule out any abnormality associated with fecal incontinence, such as diverticula, hemorrhoids, fistulas, fissure, and polyps.

Anal manometry is recommended in all women with fecal incontinence. However, digital examination is an efficient tool in determining sphincter tone and actual contraction force.

Anal manometry is an office procedure in which a catheter is initially placed 5 to 6 cm into the anorectal canal then lowered in a step-down manner at 1-cm intervals while recording resting tone and squeeze pressure of the muscles. Normal volume is reflected at about 40 mm Hg resting pressure and 100 mm Hg squeeze pressure (16). Manometry provides information on anal continence mechanism by determining the following (16,17):

- *The threshold volume* of rectal distention that produces the first sensation of distension and a sustained feeling of urgency to defecate.
- *Rectal and anal canal compliance* is determined by dividing anal pressure by the volume. A fluid-filled balloon is connected to the manometry catheter and filled slowly with water. Pressure and volume measurements, at the first sensation of distention, the first urge to defecate, and the maximal tolerable volume, are determined and the pressure: volume ratio is established.
- *Amplitude and duration of voluntary contraction* of the external sphincter muscle is the ability to contract, the duration of contraction, and the force of contraction.
- *Anal canal resting tone and squeeze pressure* can be established.

Electromyography (EMG) provides information in reference to pudendal nerve integrity; although, it is rarely indicated in practice and should not be used alone (16,17).

Endoanal ultrasonography (endosonography) can determine the anal sphincter complex integrity or a defect associated with fecal incontinence in approximately 87% of cases. The initial results of sonography, of the anal sphincter complex, postulate that the majority of the anal sphincter complex is located at the level of the mid-anal canal. This examination can discriminate effectively between existing defects of the internal and external sphincter (18).

Anal endosonography has been performed immediately following vaginal delivery and has established that this technique can be used to diagnose clinically undetected anal sphincter tears that may be associated with subsequent fecal incontinence. Such early detection of anal sphincter injury during parturition presents an opportunity for instantaneous repair (19).

Defecography is a radiographic fluoroscopic examination to assess the rectum and pelvic floor during defecation and is performed on a barium-filled rectum. It is designed to provide clinical information on the following:

- Presence of structural abnormality
- Functional parameters (diameter of the anal canal and anorectal angle at rest and during straining)
- Puborectalis muscle indentation
- Rectal emptying
- Rectal prolapse

Defecography is particularly valuable for assessing obstructed defecation and for quantifying rectal emptying (17).

Differential Diagnosis

Functional fecal incontinence is defined as recurrent, uncontrolled passage of feces in the absence of anatomic or neurologic causes. The prevalence is estimated to be 2% to 7% (20). Retention of fecal material in the rectum may lead to fecal impaction in about 1.4%. The classification of functional fecal incontinence has been expanded to include incontinence associated with diarrhea and constipation. Therefore, irritable bowel syndrome with diarrhea-predominant symptoms is included in the category of functional fecal incontinence, because approximately 25% of these patients present with fecal incontinence. The diagnosis in the majority of patients can be made by a history of constipation or diarrhea and physical examination. Irritable bowel syndrome can usually be diagnosed when there is a large amount of fecal material in the rectum on digital examination or in the colon on abdominal palpation, and the presence of voluntary contraction of the external sphincter confirms appropriate efferent innervation. If necessary other studies, should be performed to rule out structural or neurologic abnormalities.

Conventional Therapy

For constipation-related fecal incontinence, habit training and laxatives (e.g., Lactuce 10 mg twice daily) with a weekly enema are recommended. Such management has been effective in over 90% of patients (21).

For diarrhea-related fecal incontinence, Loperamide Hydrochloride capsules (2 mg or oral suspension 1 mg/5 mL, not to exceed four doses per day), habit training and biofeedback are recommended.

Complementary Approach

For constipation, habit defecation training, acupuncture, biofeedback therapy, magnetic field therapy, craniosacral therapy, relaxology, sitz baths, hydrotherapy hypnosis, and meditation are suggested (22).

For diarrhea, acupuncture, habit defecation training, and biofeedback is recommended (22). No randomized controlled studies have reported on the effectiveness and safety of these complementary modalities.

Alternative Natural Therapy

Patient education, high-fiber diet, juice therapy, aromatherapy, homeopathic therapy, and life-style changes are offered for constipation or diarrhea.

For constipation, alternative remedies include aloe vera, *Asparagus officinalis,* castor oil plant, garlic (*Allium sativum*), and Chinese rhubarb (23). *For chronic diarrhea,* alternative remedies include American white pond lily, dogwood (*Cornus florida*), and tree of heaven (23)

RECTAL PROLAPSE

Rectal prolapse and its association with fecal incontinence is an uncommon entity. Internal or occult rectal prolapse and rectal intussusception do not project from the anal canal. In total (or full-thickness) rectal prolapse, the rectum slides down via the pelvic diaphragm and the anal canal (the distal rectum mucosa beyond the dentate line with straining).

Symptoms of rectal prolapse range from feeling that the rectum is falling out, changing bowel habit, feeling of incomplete evacuation, rectal bleeding, mucosal discharge, tenesmus, and fecal incontinence. Fecal incontinence and rectal prolapse coexist in 26% to 80% of cases. Rectal prolapse and uterine or vaginal prolapse occur concurrently in approximately 10% to 25% of cases, and rectal prolapse and urinary incontinence occur concurrently in an estimated 35% of cases. If these conditions are present and no symptoms of rectal prolapse are reported, the rectum should be examined for prolapse.

Diagnosis

Pertinent medical history and physical examination are sufficient to make a diagnosis of rectal prolapse. When regular proctologic examination does not identify rectal prolapse, a patient is asked to sit on the commode and strain. An examination is performed again, which may reveal rectal prolapse. If any doubt remains, proctosigmoidoscopy can be performed to confirm the diagnosis. Barium enema or colonoscopy should be performed to rule out colon abnormalities and defecography is indicated when concomitant pelvic viscera support or suspension dysfunction is present.

Therapy for total rectal prolapse consists of surgery (transanal, encirclement, or abdominal procedures). The abdominal approach yields the best results. Conservative pre- and post–operative management of constipation is essential.

Differential Diagnosis

Differential Diagnosis of rectal prolapse includes:

- Anal fissures—management includes fiber supplements, sitz baths, and topical anesthetic such as pramoxine (lidocaine jelly delays healing and may cause contact dermatitis). If this approach does not bring relief, surgery is recommended.
- Inflammation bowel disease should be treated accordingly.
- Mechanical obstruction of the anal canal requires surgery.

Conventional Therapy for Fecal Incontinence

A conventional therapy for fecal incontinence can be offered in three different categories:

Prophylaxis and early repair is a new concept that combines not only prevention of initial anal sphincter complex injury during parturition, but also uses endosonography to establish either external or internal (or both) anal sphincter tears. Clinically undetected postpartum anal sphincter complex tears can be established by endosonography with a documented sensitivity of 85% (19).

When obstetric laceration of the anal sphincter complex occurs immediately following vaginal delivery, overlapping sphincteroplasty yields positive results (24). If a randomized controlled study validates this initial approach, postpartum overlapping sphincteroplasty may significantly reduce the prevalence of fecal incontinence. In a view of recent data, there was no physical marker to reliably predict postpartum urinary or fecal incontinence (25). Postdelivery endosonography is the simple technique available (19).

Conservative therapy includes the following:

- Dietary modification
- Perineal resistant muscle exercise
- Biofeedback therapy

Surgical reconstruction techniques for the anal sphincter complex offer restoration of sphincter function of 15% to 80% depending on the type of operation. Currently, the following surgical techniques are used for sphincteroplasty:

- Overlapping sphincteroplasty yields an overall success rate of more than 70% when the anterior anal sphincter is reconstructed (26).
- End-to-end anastomosis yields a success rate of less than 60% (27)

Complementary Therapy

Patient Education

Fecal incontinence is a socially embarrassing and devastating condition. The practitioner must exercise discretion, sensitivity, and compassion when treating this condition. Meeting with a patient in a consultation room rather than in an examining room and providing a patient with necessary time to dress and use the bathroom after examination is usually helpful. Having a family member or friend present is comforting to some patients. Understanding the diagnostic process increases a patient's commitment and compliance. Once the diagnosis is reached, therapeutic options include conventional, complementary, and alternative approaches, and the pros and cons of therapy should be clearly presented. A patient's participation in the choice and execution of therapeutic measures is an essential aspect of not only their education to the condition, but also to their mindset in dealing with it. Printed or videotaped pertinent materials can ease the educational and decision-making processes for both patient and practitioner. Future communication should be established with reassurance of practitioner accessibility. Arranging contact between a newly diagnosed patient with fecal incontinence and an individual or support group of women with a similar health problem is very helpful.

Diet

Dietary modification is one of the management factors that each patient with fecal incontinence should be offered. Such a diet may include the following:

- Increase fiber intake.
- Avoid food consumption that may predispose or cause constipation (fewer than three bowel movements per week), diarrhea, or fecal urgency.

Acupuncture

Fecal incontinence improves with acupuncture therapy according to one clinical observation study (30). However, there are no additional data to confirm these findings.

Exercise

Perineal resistant muscle exercises or Kegel pelvic muscle exercises are described in more detail in Chapter 24. It has been suggested that approximately 63% of patients with fecal incontinence improve using this exercise (28).

Biofeedback

The biofeedback technique is presented in Chapter 25. Overall improvement of fecal incontinence can be achieved in more than 50% of cases (29).

Alternative Therapy

There is no specific reccommendation.

OTHER ANORECTAL CONDITIONS

In the gynecologic evaluation, a practitioner will encounter other anorectal conditions associated with fecal incontinence.

Hemorrhoids

Primary care physicians often see either external or internal hemorrhoids. The anorectal symptoms described earlier in this chapter can be present in association with hemorrhoids. Altered or difficult bowel movements are commonly reported. Constipation with infrequent defecation can be managed with conventional or alternative therapies as discussed previously. Anoreceptive sexual intercourse or manipulation for sexual stimulation can cause hemorrhoids to bleed. Visual inspection may show thrombosed external hemorrhoids, pruritus ani (erythema and excoriation of the skin), skin tags, and ulceration. The examination is performed with the patient in the jack-knife prone position (knee to chest), and anoscopy is used to evaluate internal hemorrhoids or fissures (it is helpful to separate the anal verge and inspect between the folds). Sigmoidoscopy is performed to identify other sources of a patient's symptoms, such as polyps, inflammatory bowel disease, or cancer. Prolapsing internal hemorrhoids should be distinguished from polyps, full-thickness rectal prolapse, and hypertrophied anal papillae.

Conventional internal hemorrhoid management consists of the *normalization of bowel habits* (from one to three times per day, to two to three times per week), by implementing a bowel management program (31):

- 25 to 30 g of fiber daily is recommended in the form of a fiber supplement or bulking agent (psyllium or a hydrophilic colloid such as Konsyl, Metamucil, Citrucil; 1 tablespoon of powder mixed in a glass of fluid or four to six tablets daily)
- Six to eight glasses of fluid per day
- Stool softener such as docusate sodium (Colace) or docusate calcium, one tablet once or twice daily
- Avoidance of deferring defecation or straining and appropriate perineal cleansing with soft toilet paper

Surgical therapy for internal hemorrhoids is indicated when internal hemorrhoids reach third or fourth degree prolapse, when the hemorrhoids are non-reducible or when they do not stay in place after repositioning. Hemorrhoidectomy is offered in such cases.

External hemorrhoids are defined as external hemorrhoidal vessels aggregated under the perianal skin just below the dentate line. As long as thrombosis does not occur within the vessels, external hemorrhoids will be asympto-

matic. Occasionally, swelling itself without thrombosis may produce symptoms. Thrombosed external hemorrhoids induce acute perianal pain and on examination present as a bluish grapelike lump tender to palpation. No bleeding is usually observed with external hemorrhoids as long as an ulcerative process is absent.

Treatment objectives for external thrombosed hemorrhoids are as follows:

- Pain relief with oral analgesic and warm tub baths.
- Local excision in the office setting is recommended when significant pain or ulceration is present. An anesthetic agent is used to infiltrate the area, thrombosed vessels are excised, and the skin is left open (incising the vessels with clot evacuation should be avoided due to the high rate of recurrence).

Alternative Therapy

Diet
Increasing consumption of raw vegetables, fruits, dried fruits, bran, and whole-grain breads will help to soften stools. Adequate fluid intake of six to eight 8-ounce glasses of liquid daily, including water, juices, and herbal tea, is advocated.

Other Steps
- Keeping legs elevated during defecation relaxes the anal muscles.
- Avoiding straining during evacuation prevents hemorrhoids from bleeding.
- Shortening the time of sitting on the toilet is advised.
- Using cold witch hazel compress helps shrink hemorrhoids.
- Walking 1 mile per day promotes digestion and defecation.

Anorectal Sexually Transmitted Diseases

Sexually transmitted diseases affecting the anorectal area are reaching epidemic proportions. It is estimated that approximately 10% of heterosexual women engage in anoreceptive intercourse. About 4% to 13% practice homosexual or bisexual sex (32). The following STD lesions can be identified on the perianal anal area or in the anal canal.

Condylomata Acuminata

Anal condylomata acuminata (anal warts) is caused by Human Papilloma Virus (HPV). There are over 70 identifiable subtypes of HPV, and the most commonly isolated forms from anal warts are subtypes 6 and 11 (associated with benign lesions); subtypes 16 and 18 are observed in dysplastic or malignant cells. Multiple subtypes may be present (32). The prerequisite for HPV penetration of the basal cell layers is the presence of microtrauma (sexual intercourse is the most common cause of microtrauma) to the epithelium. Upon entering the epithelium, HPV incubates for 3 weeks to 8 months (3 months average) and may remain in a subclinical state as a flat condylomata for many years. The epithelium and its surrounding stroma respond to virus invasion with hyperplasia. The risk of being infected by a carrier of HPV during a single sexual encounter is approximately 60% (33). To a lesser extent, HPV anal infection can be acquired through close contact alone, vertical transmission from a mother to her newborn, and autoinoculation. Risk factors that predispose a woman to HPV infection include multiple sexual partners, long-term oral contraceptive use, cigarette smoking, and immunosuppression [due to human immunodeficiency virus (HIV), drugs, or transplantation]. Malignant transformation occurs more often in patients with lesions located above the anal dentate line, in homosexuals, and in smokers (34).

Diagnosis

The diagnosis of anal condylomata acuminata is usually made by a typical gross appearance of lesions, which can be symptomatic (pain, pruritus, discharge, or bleeding). Flat warts are identified after 3% to 5% acetic acid is applied. HPV-affected epithelium presents as aceto-white patches detected by colposcopy magnification, magnifying glass, or the naked eye (35). Definitive diagnosis requires biopsy with histologic verification.

Differential Deagnosis

Differential diagnoses of anal warts include:

- *Skin tag*
- *Condylomata lata (secondary syphilis)*
- *Crohn disease*
- *Molluscum contagiosum*
- *Seborrheic keratosis*
- *Nevi*
- *Carcinoma*

Conventional Therapy

Human papillomavirus infection per se cannot be eradicated; although, treatment will remove the warts and ameliorate the patient's physical, emotional, and social trauma (33). It is a well-documented phenomenon that some warts will regress (36). There is no study to support the beneficial effect of any therapy if a patient presents with minor infection with little symptomatology and is in a stable monogamous relationship (33). Before commencing therapy, the entire anal canal should be inspected by proctoscopy with aceto-acid application through anoscopy with a colposcopy or other magnifying tool (37). It is a generally accepted practice to rule out other STDs (38).

There are several paradigms for HPV therapy.

Prevention is one of the most valuable tools for all STDs, including anal warts. A stable monogamous intimate relationship is the best therapeutic approach. A condom has

been suggested as a form of HPV prevention, but its effectiveness is compromised by the fact that it does not cover the scrotum (33).

Topical agents include the following:

- *Podophyllin*
- *Podofilox* or condylox 0.5% gel is an antimitotic drug that is either chemically synthesized or purified from the plant *Podophyllum peltatum.* It is prepared for external use only and is indicated for the treatment of a cutaneous part of the external genitalia and perianal areas. It is not recommended for mucosal application (i.e., on the anal canal or rectum). Hypersensitivity to the drug has been reported, and it should not be used during pregnancy or while breast-feeding. *Podofilox* is initially applied twice daily for 3 consecutive days, then is discontinued for 4 days. This cycle can be repeated until no visible warts are present or for a total of four cycles (39). *Condylox* is the only approved medication that can be self-administered by a patient at home.
- *Bichloracetic acid (BCA) and trichloroacetic acid (TCA)* are caustic medications that cause tissue sloughing. Both can be applied not only on the perineum and perineal areas but also on the anal canal mucosa. One of the medications is applied once per week, and sodium bicarbonate can be used to neutralize BCA or TCA to avoid skin irritation. Compared with podophyllin, BCA and TCA require fewer applications, and fewer treatment relapses are observed (40). These regimens are recommended when condylomata acuminata lesions smaller than 2 mm and limited disease are present (34)
- *5-Fluorouracil (5-FU)* has immunostimulative and antimetabolic properties. The 5% cream is applied on a daily basis and yields 50% to 75% condylomata acuminata eradication. Due to skin irritation, it is not widely used (34). As a preventive agent, 5-FU is used following ablative therapy on immunosuppressive patients. In such a clinical indication, 5-FU is commenced 4 weeks after an original ablative procedure and is administered twice weekly (40).

Immunotherapy in its clinical application applies antiviral properties. *Alpha-interferon* intralesional injections with a 30-gauge hypodermic needle yield an initial success rate of approximately 60% and a recurrence rate of 30%. Patients with either refractory or recurrent anal warts are good candidates for intralesional injections. Systemic administration has limited indications due to a high rate of undesirable side effects (40).

Ablative therapies for anal condyloma include cryotherapy, electrocautery therapy, and laser therapy. Such therapy is indicated when the condylomata are larger than 2 mm. A solution of 3% to 5% acetic acid should be used during all ablative procedures to identify flat condylomata acuminata.

Cryotherapy for anal warts is used weekly until after all lesions regress. Its effectiveness is compatible with TCA results (40). The recurrence rate is twice as high as with electrocautery therapy (41). A mixture of 1% lidocaine and epinephrine is injected with a 30-gauge hypodermic needle under each wart separately before cryotherapy application.

Electrocautery or CO₂ laser therapy is indicated for extensive disease and is executed under general or regional anesthesia. Both technologies can be applied to perform either condyloma ablation or excision. If anal warts are larger than 1 cm in diameter, excisional biopsy with a cold-knife is suggested to avoid a necrotic thermo-zone, which may obscure histologic examination. Electrocautery therapy has a lower recurrence rate than CO_2 laser, and there is no significant differences in postoperative pain, scaring, recuperation time, and healing time (42).

Alternative Therapy
Herbal Therapy

Mayapple (*Podophyllum peltatum*) or 25% podophyllin (*Podocon*) is an extract from the plant with cytotoxic properties (43). The extract is usually mixed with benzoin, which provides an adhesive component for better connection of the medication with warts. It is applied directly to the perianal wart and cannot be used in the anal canal because it is highly irritative to the skin. Protection of the skin surrounding the warts (e.g., with petroleum jelly) is required. Multiple applications of podophyllin at weekly intervals are needed. After 6 to 8 hours the applied area is washed off. As a single mode of therapy, the effectiveness of podophyllin is estimated to be 20% to 50%. Its use is contraindicated during pregnancy and while breast-feeding (40).

Other herbal remedies have been used in folk medicine for warts (23), including *garlic* (*Allium sativum*, applied externally to warts), *onion* (*Allium cepa*, also applied externally), and oats (*Aventa sativa*).

Herpetic Proctitis

Herpetic proctitis is cased by herpes simplex virus type 1 (HSV-1) in about 10% of cases and HSV-2 is responsible in over 85% of cases; occasionally varicella-zoster infects the perineal or anal canal area. HSV-2 is highly contagious, and recurrent outbreaks vary from less than one every 12 months to one per month. The incubation period lasts 4 to 21 days, and symptoms persist for 7 to 10 days. HSV-2 infection can extend to the anal canal or higher, to approximately 10 cm into the rectum (44). Infection manifests by small or large (or a mixture of both) vesicles with red areola, and ulcers occur when they rupture. HSV-2 usually causes itching, burning, rectal tenesmus (painful, long-standing, ineffective straining at stool), dyschezia (pain associated with rectal evacuation), local pain, and mucopurulent anal discharge. Such a clinical picture makes the working diagnosis of herpetic proctitis, and viral culture from vesicles is confirmatory. A microscopic examination of Giemsa-stained material obtained from ulcers by scrapings discloses multinucleated giant cells, or a direct biopsy, if indicated, can provide the diagnosis. Pain and its worsening during defecation can lead to psychogenic constipation that results in fecal impaction. Currently, no cure or vaccination is available.

Management of HSV infection, in an acute state, is treated with analgesic, stool softener, sitz baths, and an antiviral agent such as acyclovir (administered orally at a dose of either 400 mg three times daily or 200 mg five times daily for perianal infection; the dose must be doubled for infection of the anal canal, rectal involvement or primary herpetic proctitis).

The frequency of recurrence and the severity of symptoms can be reduced by continued suppressive administration of oral acyclovir 400 mg twice daily or 200 mg two to five times daily (34), or with famcyclovir or valacyclovir (36).

HIV and Acquired Immunodeficiency Syndrome

Over 1 million Americans are infected with HIV, and particularly affected are intravenous drug users and homosexuals. By practicing anoreceptive sexual intercourse, homosexuals are particularly prone to develop anorectal disorders such as fissures, ulcers, rectal abscesses, Kaposi sarcoma, anal neoplasia, sepsis related to STD infection, and death (44). It is estimated that approximately 34% of HIV-infected individuals will be diagnosed with an anorectal disorder (45).

Anorectal disorders associated with HIV can be analyzed from three different perspectives: general anorectal disorders, disorders with a distorted pathogenesis, and disorders unique to HIV.

General anorectal disorders include hemorrhoids and anal fissures. Conservative therapy is usually offered for these conditions.

A distorted pathogenesis is observed in such conditions as syphilis. More often, secondary forms of syphilis with condylomata lata are observed, and the tertiary syphilis regimen is suggested for any case of concomitant HIV infection and syphilis (46). Condylomata acuminata HPV types 16, 18, and 31 are the most commonly observed types in patients with HIV. These types of HPV often induce premalignant and malignant anal tissue transformation. Therapy does not differ from that used in the general population, but higher recurrence rates (10%–75%) are observed (34,47). HSV-2 is a predominant infection and is documented in about 94% of HIV cases, with 80% recurrence rates in HIV-positive patients (34). Treatment for HSV-2 in HIV-infected patients is recommended as follows (48): *primary* HSV, acyclovir 400 mg orally, three times daily for 10 days or until healed; *recurrent* HSV, acyclovir 400 mg orally, three times daily for 5 to 10 days or until healed; *suppressive therapy*, acyclovir 400 mg orally, two to three times daily for 10 days or indefinitely.

Anorectal disorders unique to HIV include *idiopathic anal ulcers* that must be diagnosed by direct biopsy [fissures, cancer, HSV, cytomegalovirus (CMV), mycobacterium avium complex (MAC), gonorrhea, chlamydia, syphilis, and fungus should be ruled out]. Therapy for idiopathic anal ulcers is surgical excision (47).

Recent clinical reports suggest the administration of oral or injectable steroids (49). *Depomondrol* (injectable steroid) intralesional injections are a promising new approach (50).

Anal intraepithelial neoplasia (AIN) ranges from AIN-I to AIN-III, or carcinoma *in situ*. In the general population, AIN is very infrequently diagnosed. Diagnostic annual screening with a Papanicolaou smear (which has a high false-negative rate, up to 70%) or an anoscopic direct biopsy is recommended. Observation with close follow-up every 6 to 12 months in low-grade AIN is recommended. In high-grade lesions, local excision, electrocautery, or laser (not advantageous over electrocautery or local excision) is used.

The prevalence of *non-Hodgkin lymphoma* in HIV-positive patients is estimated to be 3% to 10%. It is an aggressive condition in association with HIV. Management usually consists of chemotherapy, and excisional surgery is not recommended. In a case of obstruction by tumor, diverting colostomy is necessary (34).

Kaposi sarcoma is an epithelial malignancy that affects HIV-positive patients (particularly homosexuals and bisexuals) 20,000 times more frequently than is observed in the general population. Characteristic deep-purple red sessile nodules are identified on anoscopic examination. A direct biopsy with histologic verification provides a clue to the definitive diagnosis. Intralesional injection of chemotherapeutic agent or antiviral medication constitutes a management paradigm (34).

Cytomegalovirus prevalence is greater than 95% (affecting not only the anorectum but also the lungs, gastrointestinal tract, eyes, and central nervous system), and its clinical significance is manifested when CD4 counts are under 100 cells/mm^3 (diarrhea, abdominal pain, bleeding, lack of appetite, and weight loss). Physical findings include diffuse colitis and ulcers. Toxic megacolon and perforation can occur as sequelae of CMV. Intravenous administration of both *Ganciclovir* and *Foscarnet* comprises the treatment plan, and repeat therapy is often needed due to relapse (34).

Mycobacterium avium complex (MAC) is almost ever present in patients with CD4 counts under 100 cells/mm^3. A disseminated form clinically manifests with abdominal pain, watery diarrhea, dehydration, fever, excessive perspiration, bowel thickening, and weight loss. Clinical findings include hepatosplenomegaly and enlarged lymphatic nodes. The diagnosis is confirmed by direct biopsy, stool culture, and acid-fast staining stool sample. Sequelae of MAC infection in HIV-positive patients include anal bleeding, fistula formation, and colon obstruction. When untreated the survival time is under 6 months. Treatment extends survival to more than 1 year. The first line of therapy is *Clarithromycin* 500 mg orally twice daily or a combination of *Azithromycin* 500 mg with Ethambutol 15 mg/kg orally daily (34).

Syphilis

Anorectal manifestation of *syphilis* (infection with *Treponema pallidum*) includes primary ulcerative, nontender lesions known as *anal chancre*, which can present in single or multiple locations and occur 2 to 6 weeks or sometimes as long as 3 months after initial infection. Chancre is typically located at or near the anal verge. Clinical symptoms can be absent or present as mucoid discharge causing itching and offensive odor, tenesmus, and rectal pain. Untreated anal syphilis progresses to *secondary syphilis* (2–3 months after initial infection), with anal condylomata lata (a pale brown or large, pink, smooth verrucous perianal mass), which is very contiguous. Untreated *secondary syphilis* spontaneously resolves in about one third of cases, one third transform to *latent infection*, and one third progress to *tertiary syphilis* (1 year after initial infection, and can affect the central nervous system, cardiovascular system, hepatic system, renal system, any mucosal tissue, and the eyes). Any anal ulcer should be viewed as syphilis until proven otherwise. The diagnosis is reached by direct biopsy of the ulcer and by dark-field microscopic examination. Blood serologic testing (using the fluorescent treponemal antibody test) becomes positive early after infection. The Venereal Disease Research Laboratory test (VDRL) and the Rapid Plasma Reagin test (RPR) also should be given. The VDRL (can be false positive in autoimmune disorders) and RPR are good tests for evaluating treatment progress.

Therapy for all syphilis (if under 1 year's duration) is one intramuscular dose of 2.4 million U *Benzathine penicillin*. In penicillin-allergic patients, oral *Doxycycline* of 100 mg twice daily for 14 days is recommended. In tertiary/latent syphilis (lasting over 1 year), 2.4 million U is administered intramuscularly weekly for 3 consecutive weeks. In penicillin-allergic patients, oral *Doxycycline* 100 mg twice daily for 28 days is recommended. Neurosyphilis is treated with intramuscular injection of 2.4 million U *Benzathine* penicillin daily for 14 days plus oral probenecid 500 mg four times daily for 14 days. In penicillin-allergic patients, desensitization should be performed and penicillin therapy instituted afterward (36).

Gonorrhea

Anorectal gonorrhea is caused by *Neisseria gonorrhoeae* transmitted through anoreceptive intercourse or through autoinoculation from another location and causes cryptitis or proctitis (45,46). The incubation period ranges from 5 to 7 days and afterward becomes a symptomatic condition (bloody or thick mucopurulent anal discharge, itching, and tenesmus). Untreated gonorrhea can progress to *a disseminated form* causing endocarditis, meningitis, perihepatitis, and pancreatitis. Anoscopy without lubricant should be used (can contain an antimicrobial agent); if necessary, water on an anoscope will help to obtained a culture, or a blind culture can be performed. A sterile swab is inserted in the anal canal about 2 to 2.5 cm and rotated from side to side for a minimum of 30 seconds to collect material for a culture.

Any clinical suspicion of anal gonorrhea warrants empirical treatment with one dose *Ceftriaxone* 125 mg intramuscularly or oral administration of *Cefixime* 400 mg, *Ciprofloxacin* 500 mg, or *Oflaxacin* 400 mg. Due to the high coexistence of chlamydia with gonorrhea infection, the patient should be treated for chlamydia also.

Disseminated Gonorrhea is treated with intravenous medication or a combination of intravenous and oral medication for 7 to 10 days (36). Due to a 35% recurrence rate, follow-up anal culture is performed at 3-month intervals (46).

Chlamydia

Anal chlamydia infection is caused by *Chlamydia trachomatis* and can be transmitted via oral-anal or anal sexual intercourse, or by autoinoculation. The incubation period is 10 days, afterward becomes a symptomatic condition (fever, anal mucoid or bloody discharge, tenesmus, rectal pain) or an asymptomatic condition. Untreated anal chlamydia can result in perianal or anal abscesses, anal strictures, and fistulas. Chlamydia infection can mimic Crohn disease (46). Due to intracellular harboring, a swab culture is not as reliable as the microimmunofluorescent antibody titer (44). A rectal mucosa biopsy for a culture is a well recognized test, but it is invasive. A Ligase Chain Reaction urine test can confirm the diagnosis (36).

Therapy for chlamydia is accomplished either by a single oral dose of 1 g Azithromycin or oral Doxycycline 100 mg twice daily for 7 days (34). Combination treatment is recommended (36).

Complementary Therapy

No data are presently available for complementary therapies.

Alternative Therapy

There is no specific alternative therapy for anal STDs. However, alternative therapy can be used as a support treatment to add to conventional antibiotic management.

REFERENCES

1. Nivatvnges S, Stern HS, Fryd DS. The length of the anal canal. *Dis Colon Rectum* 1981;24:600–602.
2. Wunderlich M, Parks AG. Physiology and pathophysiology of the anal sphincter. *Int Surg* 1982;67:291–298.
3. Haadem K, Dahlstrom JA, Ling L. Anal sphincter competence in healthy women. Clinical implications of age and other factors. *Obstet Gynecol* 1991;78:823–827.
4. Aronson MP, Lee RA, Berquist TH. Anatomy of anal sphincter and related structures in continent women studied with magnetic resonance imaging. *Obstet Gynecol* 1990;76:846-851.
5. Fenne DE, Kriegshauser JS, Lee HH, ET AL. Anatomic and physiologic measurements of the internal and external anal sphincters in normal females. *Obstet Gynecol* 1998;91:369–374.
6. Strohbehn K. Normal pelvic floor anatomy. *Obstet Gynecol Clin North Am* 1998;25:683–705.
7. Delancey JO, Toglia MR, Perucchini D. Internal and external anal sphincter anatomy as it relates to midline obstetrical lacerations. *Obstet Gynecol* 1997;90:924–927.
8. Frenckner B. Ihre T. Influence of autonomic nerves on the internal anal sphincter in man. *Gut* 1976;17:306–312.
9. Leigh RJ, Tumberg LA. Fecal incontinence: the unvoiced symptom. *Lancet* 1982;1:134–151.
10. Thomas TM, Egan M, Walgrove A, et al. The prevalence of fecal and double incontinence. *Commun Med* 1984;6:216–220.
11. Caputo RM, Benson JT. Idiopathic fecal incontinence. *Curr Opin Obstet Gynecol* 1992;4:565–570.
12. Jackson SL, Weber AM, Hull TL, et al. Fecal incontinence in women with urinary incontinence and pelvic organ prolapse. *Obstet Gynecol* 1997;89:423–427.
13. Sultan AH, Kamm MA, Bartram CI. Anal sphincter disruption during vaginal delivery. *N Engl J Med* 1993;329:1905–1911.
14. Shiono P, Klebanoff MA, Carey JC. Midline episiotomies: more harm than good? *Obstet Gynecol* 1990;75:765–770.
15. Thacker SB, Banta HD. Benefits and risks of episiotomy: an interpretative review of the English language literature, 1860–1980. *Obstet Gynecol Surv* 1983;38:322-338.
16. Jackson SL, Hull TL. Fecal incontinence in women. *Obstet Gynecol Surv* 1998;53:741–747.
17. Whitehead WE, Wald A, Diamant NE, et al. Functional disorders of the anus and rectum. *Gut* 1999;45(suppl II):1155–1159.
18. Deen KI, Kumar D, Williams JG, et al. The prevalence of anal sphincter defects in fecal incontinence: a prospective endosonic study. *Gut* 1993;34:685–688.
19. Faltin DL, Boulvain M, Irion O, et al. Diagnosis of anal sphincter tears by postpartum endosonography to predict fecal incontinence. *Obstet Gynecol* 2000;95:643–647.
20. Nelson R, Norton N, Cautley E, et al. Community-based prevalence of anal incontinence. *JAMA* 1995:274:559–561.
21. Tobin GW, Brocklehurst JC. Fecal incontinence in residential homes for the elderly. Prevalence, aetiology and management. *Age Aging* 1986;15:41–46.
22. Chopra D, ed. *Alternative medicine. The definitive guide.* Tiburon, CA: Future Medicine Publishing, 1997.
23. *PDR for herbal medicines,* 2nd ed. Montvale, NJ: Medical Economics Company, 2000.
24. Sultan AH, Monga AK, Kumar D, et al. Primary repair of obstetric and anal sphincter rupture using the overlap technique. *Br J Obstet Gynecol* 1999;106:318–323.
25. Chliha C, Kalia V, Stanton SL, et al. Antenatal prediction of postpartum urinary and fecal incontinence. *Obstet Gynecol* 1999;94:689–694.
26. Wexner SD, Marchett F, Jagelman DG. The role of sphincteroplasty for fecal incontinence reevaluated: a prospective physiologic and functional review. *Dis Colon Rectum* 1991;34:22–30.
27. Blaisdell PC. Repair of the incontinent sphincter ani. *Surg Gynecol Obstet* 1940;70:692–697.
28. McIntosh LJ, Fraham JD, Mallett VT. Pelvic floor rehabilitation in the treatment of incontinence. *J Reprod Med* 1993;38:662–666.
29. Wald A. Biofeedback for fecal incontinence. *Ann Intern Med* 1981;95:146–149.
30. An XC, Zhao HS, Li XC, et al. Acupuncture treatment for disturbances in urination and defecation from sacral cryptorachischisis—a clinical observation of 254 cases. *J Trad Chin Med* 1986:95–98.
31. Orkin BA, Schwarrtz AM, Orkin M. Hemorrhoids: what the

dermatologist should know. *J Am Acad Dermatol* 1999;41: 449–456.

32. Frenczy A. Epidemiology and clinical pathophysiology of condylomata acuminata. *Am J Obstet Gynecol* 1995;172: 1331–1339.
33. Verdon ME. Issue in the management of human papillomavirus genital disease. *Am Fam Physician* 1997;55:1813–1816.
34. El-Attar SM, Evans DV. Anal warts, sexually transmitted diseases, and anorectal conditions associated with human immunodeficiency virus. *Primary Care* 1999;26:81–100.
35. Barrasso R. Latent and subclinical HPV external anogenital infection. *Clin Dermatol* 1997;15:349–353.
36. Drugs for sexually transmitted diseases. *Med Lett Drugs Ther* 1995;172:1331–1339.
37. Nagle D, Rolanddelli RH. Primary care office management of perianal and anal disease. *Prim Care* 1996;23:609–620.
38. Benson PM. What's new in sexually transmitted diseases. *Adv Dermatol* 1996;11:85–103.
39. von Krough G. Podophyllotoxin in serum: absorption subsequent to three day repeated applications of a 0.5% ethanolic preparation on condylomata acuminata. *Sex Trans Dis* 1982;9: 26–32.
40. Congilosi SM, Madoff RD. Current therapy for recurrent and extensive anal warts. *Dis Colon Rectum* 1995;38:1101–1107.
41. Billingham RP. Condyloma acuminata. In: Mazier WP, Levin DH, Luchtenfeld MA, et al., eds. Surgery of the colon, rectum and anus. Philadelphia: WB Saunders, 1995:313–321.
42. Billingham RP. Laser versus electrical cautery in the treatment of condyloma acuminata of the anus. *Surg Gynecol Obstet* 1982; 155:865–867.
43. Blumgarten AF. *Text book of materia medica, pharmacology and therapeutics,* 7th ed. New York: Macmilan, 1937:220, 223.
44. Wexner SD. Sexually transmitted diseases of the colon, rectum, and anus. The challenge of the 1990s. *Dis Colon Rectum* 1990; 33:1048–1062.
45. Wexner SD, Smith WB, Milsom JW, et al. The surgical management of anorectal diseases in AIDS and pre-AIDS patients. *Dis Colon Rectum* 1986:29:719–723.
46. Modesto VL, Gottesman L. Sexually transmitted diseases and anal manifestation of AIDS. *Surg Clin North Am* 1994;74:1433–1464.
47. Weiss EG. Wexner SD. Surgery for anal lesions in HPV-infected patients. *Ann Med* 1995;27:476–475.
48. Spach D, Hooton T. *The HIV manual.* New York: Oxford University Press, 1996.
49. Gopal DV, Hassaram S, Marcon NE. Idiopathic colonic inflammation in AIDS: an open trial of prednisone. *Am J Gastroenterol* 1997;92:2237–2240.
50. Viamonte M, Dailey TH, Gottesman L. Ulcerative disease of the anorectum in the HIV-positive patient. *Dis Colon Rectum* 1993;36:801–805.

27

BREAST DISORDERS

EDUCATIONAL OBJECTIVES

Medical Students (1)
APGO Objectives No. 44

Standards of surveillance of an
  adult women, including breast
  self-examination, physical
  examination, and mammography
Diagnostic approach to women with the
  chief complaint of breast mass, nipple
  discharge, or breast pain
History and physical findings that might
  suggest the following abnormalities:
    intraductal papilloma
    fibrocystic changes
    fibroadenoma
    carcinoma
    mastitis

Residents in Obstetrics/Gynecology(2)
CREOG Objectives

Benign conditions of the breast
Galactorrhea
Carcinoma of the breast:
  epidemiology
  invasive carcinoma

Practitioners (3)
ACOG Recommendations

Carcinoma of the breast
Epidemiology
Diagnosis
Biopsy
Occult lesions
Management
Prognostic factors
Estrogen use

Breast disorders affect females in pediatric, adolescent, reproductive, and postmenopausal groups. This chapter provides clinical information on the more commonly encountered benign, functional, and malignant disorders.

FEMALE BREAST EMBRYOLOGY

Milk lines (primitive mammary ridges) and epidermal cells start drifting into the mesenchymal tissue at 6 weeks of embryonic life. Primitive mammary ridges originally extend from the axilla to the inguinal area bilaterally, and by 10 weeks of embryonic age, upper and lower borders of milk lines go under involution, leaving only a thoracic uninvoluted area. The mammary glands and lactiferous ducts develop from mammary ridges. Each mammary gland produces primary and secondary buds. From secondary buds, solid cords originate (usually about 15–20 solid cords). The breast fibrous and the adipose tissue come from the proximate mesenchyme. At about 5 months of gestational age the breast areola develops. At birth, only the central duct is present, and shortly after delivery the nipple develops (the

nipple protrudes from the areola and embraces 10–15 terminal duct outlets). Apocrine glands within the areola are termed Montgomery glands. Between postpartum days 4 and 7, clear or cloudy breast discharge, termed colostrum (witch's milk), may be excreted, which usually resolves spontaneously. Maternal estrogen stimulation is responsible for this event.

Further female breast development remains suspended from the infant period until the pubertal thelarche stage is reached (4). Breast development during prepubertal and pubertal period is described in Chapter 2.

BREAST ANATOMY

The female breast is an anatomic structure that protrudes from the thorax and is customarily located between ribs 2 and 6 (Fig. 27.1). The mammary tissue covers the fascia of the pectoralis major muscle. The breast is a dome-shaped organ and the areola mammae, which is a circular area of pigmented skin 1.5 to 2.5 cm in diameter, is located centrally. Areolar tissues comprise bundles of smooth muscle whose function is to make the nipple erect. Montgomery gland secretion provides lubrication to the nipple.

The nipple (mammary papilla) is covered by wrinkled skin and is also pigmented. It is the gathering station for 15 to 20 lactiferous ducts, which create the ampulla (sinus lactiferi), partially within the nipple and partially under the nipple. From the ampulla the lactiferous ducts branch off and traverse radially to the chest wall, from which secondary tubules develop. These end in epithelial masses, creating the breast lobules (acinar structures). The terminal tubules and lobules reach full development only during pregnancy. The number of terminal tubules and lobules varies depending on the stage of life, with a peak during the reproductive period. The breast stoma is essentially composed of fatty and fibrous tissues, which together determine the size and consistency of the breast. The breast fascia and the pectoralis major muscle fascia separate the breast tissue from underlying muscle. The breast fascia divides the mammary gland into lobules and attaches to the skin, creating the Cooper suspensory ligaments in the upper part.

The blood supply is provided to the medial and central portion of the breast by the perforating branches of the internal mammary artery. The lateral thoracic, intercostal, subcapsular, and thoracodorsal arteries supply blood to the upper and upper-outer segment of the breast. Blood return is drained to the veins that traverse the arteries. Approximately 97% of the lymphatics drain to the axillary node, and the remaining 3% drain to the internal mammary lymphatic nodes.

Certain hormones influence breast anatomic development and function, while other hormones are necessary during the breast epithelial maturity stage. Multiple, synchronized hormonal biologic interactions are necessary for the mammary glands to reach anatomic and functional maturity. Three major hormones play an indispensable role in this process:

- *Estrogen* is responsible for ductal morphogenesis during the prepubertal period and epithelial growth thereafter. Hormone receptor–positive stromal cells mediate this process. Adipose tissue accumulation and storage also depend on estrogen activity. Specific estrogen breast receptors are scattered in the stroma (5).
- *Progesterone* is essential for lobuloalveolar development, and progesterone receptors are present in the breast ductal epithelium (6).
- *Prolactin* stimulates breast lobuloalveola to proliferate, functionally develop, and mature. These processes occur during pregnancy; although, they may take place as a result of a pathologic condition such as galactorrhea (7).

BREAST EVALUATION

The *medical history* for breast disorders is specifically oriented and should establish current symptomatology, reproductive performance and its association with symptoms, potential risk factors of breast cancer, and past and present medications that may influence past or present breast disorders.

Breast pain or *tenderness* and its fluctuation with the menstrual cycle or its persistent character should be established. A tender, thickening breast shortly before menses may indicate either an early pregnancy or fibrocystic disease.

Unilateral continuous pain in a postmenopausal woman and in a woman not on estrogen replacement therapy should raise suspicions of a malignant process. Bilateral pain also can be associated with cancer, but is less common.

Nipple discharge, either spontaneous or induced, may characterize a specific disorder:

- Milky nipple discharge is characteristic of galactorrhea. The clinician should obtain a history of past and present medications. Medications that cause galactorrhea are described in Chapters 3 and 11.
- Multicolored and gluey nipple discharge is present in ductal ectasia.
- Purulent nipple discharge is associated with mastitis.
- Watery nipple discharge is observed in papilloma or breast cancer.
- Serous or serosanguineous nipple discharge may be seen in breast cancer (unilateral, spontaneous, blood-tinged nipple discharge, particularly in postmenopausal women, is highly suspicious for malignancy), ductal ectasia, fibrocystic disease, or intraductal papilloma.

A history of a *self-discovered breast mass* should help establish how long the lump has been present, its behavior in terms of size and pain/tenderness during the menstrual cycle, and whether the pain fluctuates with menstrual cycles or is continuous. Skin discoloration, heat radiating from the

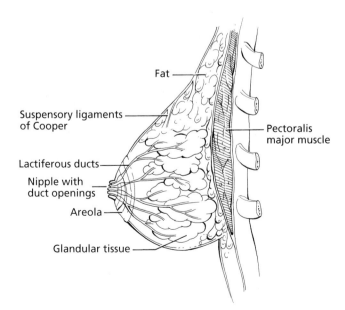

FIGURE 27.1. Internal breast structures.

tumor, vessel dilatation, and skin retraction (dimpling) may be reported.

Self-discovered skin dimpling on the breast is the result of shortening of the Cooper ligaments. This process is highly indicative of the presence of breast cancer.

Other symptoms may be related to recent or prior breast surgery (even abdominal or thoracic surgery may play a role in the development of galactorrhea), breast injury, and breast infection. Abnormal lactation indicates the need for appropriate clinical investigation.

Potential risk factors for breast cancer can be assessed by medical history. The most common risk factors for breast cancer development are previous breast cancer in the contralateral mammary gland and breast cancer in a first-degree relative, particularly when bilateral breast cancer occurred in the reproductive period.

Risk factors predisposing to breast cancer fall into the following categories:

- *Reproductive history*
  Menarche before age 12 or after age 17 years
  Chronic anovulatory menstrual cycles
  Menopause after the age 55 years or total menstrual years >40
  First term pregnancy after age 35 years
  Nulliparity
- *Benign breast neoplasia* (atypical lobular neoplasia)
- *Malignant neoplasia*
  Lobular carcinoma *in situ* (LCIS)
  Contralateral breast cancer
  Salivary gland cancer
  Uterine cancer
- *Family history of breast cancer*
  Premenopausal bilateral breast cancer in a first-degree relative (highest predisposition to develop breast cancer among all the risk factors)
  Postmenopausal bilateral breast cancer in a first-degree relative
  Premenopausal and postmenopausal breast cancer in a first-degree relative
- *Other Risk Factors*
  Advancing age
  Birthplace in North America or northern Europe
  White race
  High socioeconomic status
  Never being married
  Postmenopausal increased body mass index
  Increased breast density
  High breast asymmetry and larger breasts (predictor of, rather than an effect of, breast cancer)

CLINICAL BREAST EXAMINATION

The optimal time to perform breast examination is probably shortly after menses or before ovulation due to progressively increasing tenderness of the breast after ovulation.

The examination is customarily performed in different positions. The *standing position* is executed first with both arms at the sides resting on the hips, then with arms outstretched above the head (Fig. 27.2A–C). The following breast abnormalities should be detectable in this position:

- Breast general appearance, shape, size, symmetry, nipple position, and any deviation of the mammary gland from the midline
- Breast nipple inversion, skin discoloration, skin retraction, or dermatologic abnormalities (edema, nevi, eczematoid lesions, or ulcerations or cracks around the areola associated with Paget disease of the breast)
- Digital palpation beneath the lateral pectoralis major muscle, axilla, and supraclavicular area

The same abnormalities are assessed in the *supine position*, including looking for potential deep lesions (Fig. 27.2D):

- Visual inspection of the breast and chest wall
- Superficial palpation of the breast tissue, supraclavicular area, and axilla
- Deep palpation or the triple-touch technique against the chest wall and examination of the breast tissue, supraclavicular area, and axillary areas

The entire breast should be visually inspected and physically examined in an organized, systematic manner. The examination is customarily performed either clockwise or in a stripwise direction (rows). Each breast may be divided into four quadrants and a tail (Fig. 27.3). With the nipple at the center, an imaginary horizontal line connects the 3 and 9 o'clock positions, and a vertical line extends from the 12 to 6 o'clock positions. The four quadrants would then be the upper inner, upper outer, lower inner, and lower outer. A tail is created from the axillary area and attaches to the upper outer quadrant between the 9 and 11 o'clock positions (Fig. 27.3).

Division of the breast into quadrants assists not only in appropriate communication between specialists, but also provides valuable points of reference because 50% of breast cancer is diagnosed in the upper outer quadrant, approximately 18% beneath the nipple-areolar area, and about 15% in the lower inner quadrants.

Documentation of negative findings is as equally important to provide as positive findings. The specific risk factors, an appropriate schedule for a patient screening of breast cancer, and a follow-up plan should be in the record. A simple and abbreviated summary of breast evaluation should incorporate the following:

- Date of last menstrual period
- Date of last mammogram
- Current medication, particularly hormonal therapy and oral contraceptives
- Description of negative or positive findings
  Breast examination performed in the upright and supine position,
  Presence or absence of a dominant mass versus breast lumpiness

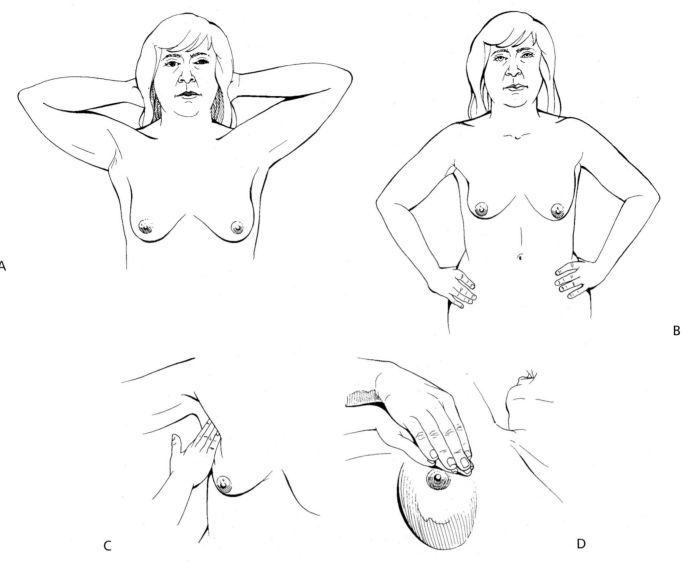

FIGURE 27.2. Breast examination. **A:** Skin changes or retraction, asymmetry, and prominent veins are best evaluated in this position. **B:** Pressure on the hips assists in the evaluation of skin retraction or skin dimpling. **C:** The upright position allows breast tail examination for enlargement of the axillary node. **D:** The supine position is most practical for superficial and deep palpation.

Presence or absence of nipple discharge
Presence or absence of lymphadenopathy

■ The schedule for the next breast evaluation and mammogram should be clearly stated. Mammography can detect appreciably smaller lesions (about 1.5 mm) than palpation (1.8 mm). Clinical breast examination is regarded as complementary to mammography (combined clinical breast examination and mammography yields positive findings of 9.2 in 1,000, and clinical breast examination alone yields positive findings in 8.8 in 1,000). Mammography alone can detect breast cancer in about 87% of cases). Mammographically detected cancer is smaller in size and the proportion of negative lymph nodes is greater.

The *breast self-examination (BSE)* technique should be explained to the patient, and the medical record should reflect it. BSE is executed similar to the way that clinical physical examination is performed (see description above). For several decades, BSE has been considered a factor that can decrease the mortality rate from breast cancer, although a large population study failed to substantiate this clinical conviction.

The American Cancer Society recommends conducting BSE on a monthly basis shortly after menses.

BREAST MASS EVALUATION

Following history and breast examination, a breast mass may be evaluated in several ways.

Imaging studies include: *ultrasonography, mammography, magnetic resonance mammography,* and *thermography.*

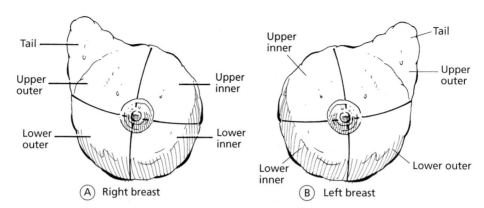

FIGURE 27.3. Quadrants of the breast and the tail for the right **(A)** and left **(B)** breasts.

The primary objectives of *ultrasonography* are to differentiate a breast cyst from a solid tumor and to establish the presence of breast complex mass (the presence of cystic and solid structures within the same mass). Ultrasonography is usually an adjunct to mammographic studies, but in selected cases may serve as the initial or sole imaging examination.

Mammography is currently considered the most valuable tool for early breast cancer detection and can reduce the mortality rate up to 30%. If the screening program is extended to women age 40 and older, it is estimated that the mortality rate could be reduced by 50%. Radiation exposure is low, approximately 0.5 rad. Mammography can identify a nonpalpable mass 1 to 2 mm in diameter and can definitively identify small calcifications, suggesting the presence of a malignant process. The overall accuracy of early breast cancer detection is estimated to be approximately 85%.

Magnetic resonance mammography may provide data regarding the nature of breast tumors. However, the phase of the menstrual cycle, during which this imaging study is performed may affect the specificity and be associated with an elevated false-positive rate of detection.

Thermography is performed in several countries, but this technology is not commonly performed in the United States.

Breast fine-needle aspiration cytology has been shown to distinguish benign from malignant breast lesions with great accuracy. It is a relatively simple procedure, particularly when a breast cyst has already been found. This modality is not only an effective diagnostic procedure, but is useful for determining appropriate therapy as well. A 22- to 25-gauge needle is used. Fine-needle aspiration should be preceded by mammography in women over 35 years of age. Fine-needle aspiration may also be used for cytologic diagnosis of solid tumors, but sensitivity (87%) and specificity (76%) are low. The projected false-negative rate of detection is 7.7%, and the false positive rate 1.2%. The technique for aspiration from a solid tumor differs from that for a cystic

tumor. Once the needle is inserted into the tumor, it is moved back and forth 8 to 10 times with suction applied constantly (two to three samples of the tumor are recovered). To obtain optimal cell collection (50%–87%), the syringe is placed in a container filled with cytofixative. It is customary practice to accept positive results as the definitive diagnosis and not to rely on negative results (open biopsy with tumor excision is a standard clinical approach in such situations).

Stereotactic core needle biopsy (CNB) is a new technology that allows tissue biopsy of suspicious findings to be obtained during mammography. This procedure minimizes the need for open biopsy, with a sensitivity of 71% to 100% and specificity of 85% to 100%. Modern radiographic equipment and an automated biopsy gun excises a core of tissue, and as many specimens can be removed as needed from suspicious areas. Core needle biopsy is cosmetically advantageous because it leaves only a minimal postoperative scar.

Breast open biopsy is a fundamental procedure in establishing a definitive diagnosis. In most instances, it can be executed under local anesthesia. In cases of small tumors or mammographically identified calcific areas, a radiographically guided J-wire placement (needle-localized biopsy) into a tumor or calcification may assist in removing a sample of the affected area. Frozen-section examination should be a part of needle-localized biopsy to determine the accuracy of the desired excision area.

The following scenarios are indications for breast open biopsy:

- Breast cyst will not completely regress following needle aspiration.
- Breast fluid is blood tinged on aspiration.
- Breast cyst recurs after aspiration.
- Serous or sanguineous nipple discharge, or ulceration or skin edema is present.
- Solid breast tumor (other than fibroadenoma) is diagnosed.

BENIGN BREAST DISORDERS

Congenital Breast Abnormality

Polythelia (supernumerary nipples) is defined as the presence of accessory breast nipple distribution along the primitive mammary ridges (milk ridges or milk lines) without breast ductal tissue. Such breast pathology can be associated with renal anomalies and neonates, and infants should be examined to exclude potential renal conditions (8). The surgical removal of supernumerary nipples is indicated only for cosmetic purpose (4).

Polymastia is the presence of breast tissue (ductal tissue) beneath the accessory nipples. This breast tissue may undergo a natural physiologic developmental and functional maturation process, leading to an increased lactation potential. Polymastia is also infrequently found beyond the customarily distribution of the milk ridges, such as in the middle part of the chest or over the scapula. The risk of benign or malignant neoplasia transformation can be expected in this abnormality. Surgical intervention is needed when a suspicious lesion is noted or for cosmetic concerns (4).

Athelia is the absence of the breast nipple. It is an exceedingly rare medical condition and is often linked to chest wall anomalies.

Amastia is the lack of breast tissue. It is an uncommon condition that frequently occurs with chest wall deformity.

The presence of athelia and amastia can be associated with *Poland syndrome*, which is characterized by the absence unilaterally or bilaterally of breast tissue. It involves varying degrees of deformity, aplasia of the pectoralis major muscle, and deformity of the chest wall, including the bony structures, rib deformities, webbed fingers, and radial nerve aplasia (9).

Asymmetry of the breast is commonly observed in early pubertal breast development (Tanner stages 2 and 4). During that period, reassurance is a sufficient tool in management, because a symmetric appearance eventually occurs in the majority of cases. Cosmetic concerns may be minimized by the use of padding of the smaller breast. A professionally custom-fitted padded bra can be obtained in commercial stores that specialize in accommodating postmastectomy patients. A padded bra is used transitionally while the smaller breast catches up to the larger one (9). When developmental asymmetry of the breast persists beyond age 18 (about 25% of cases) and contributes to psychological disturbances, plastic surgery reconstruction is recommended to avoid long-lasting emotional consequences. Either reduction mammaplasty of the larger breast or augmentation of smaller breast may provide satisfactory outcome. Bilateral reduction mammaplasty or unilateral reduction mammaplasty combined with contralateral mastopexy yields the best long-term results (10). Because breast implant surgery does not provide overall significant improvement when compared with plastic surgery itself, mammary gland implants should be avoided (11).

Breast hypoplasia is the presence of considerably smaller than average breast size (12). Adequate pubertal development with all secondary sex characteristics may nevertheless be present. In this clinical scenario, reassurance is the acceptable clinical course. Surgical breast augmentation is an option if the condition is contributing to psychological disturbances.

Abnormal pubertal developments, including ovarian failure, adrenal gland dysfunction, and hypothyroidism, may coexist with breast hypoplasia. Surgical augmentation mammaplasty is recommended in late adolescence or in adulthood.

More information on pubertal disorders is described in Chapter 2.

Tuberous breasts are characterized by an overdeveloped areola and nipple with underdeveloped vertical and horizontal diameters, with such a configuration resembling tuberous root plants (13). Surgical reconstructive surgery is recommended. The procedure chosen is dependent on the clinically identifiable deformity of the breast (14):

- Type I is defined as hypoplasia of the lower medial quadrant.
- Type II is defined as hypoplasia of the lower medial and lateral quadrants with sufficient skin.
- Type III is recognized when hypoplasia is similar to type II, but skin deficiency in the subareolar region is identified.
- Type IV is diagnosed when minimal breast base is present with severe breast constriction.

Macromastia (or breast hypertrophy or breast virginal hypertrophy) is a pathologic overgrowth of the breast before menarche and may occur unilaterally or bilaterally. Familial occurrence has been documented (4). The condition can be associated with the eating disorder bulimia nervosa, in which a patient attempts to compensate for body image (15). Oral contraceptives may accelerate the progress of hypertrophy and therefore should be avoided in this condition. Treatment for macromastia is surgical reduction mammaplasty (usually performed in late adolescence or early adulthood), which will significantly address not only the physical aspect of this disorder, but may also help to alleviate the psychological affects, including bulimia nervosa (16). A giant fibroadenoma or secondary lymphomas may produce similar symptoms and signs; therefore, excluding these conditions will aid in arriving at the definitive diagnosis of breast hypertrophy (17). Surgery itself does not prevent recurrence and including oral progesterone therapy is recommended following surgery. Progesterone alone can be administered, if conservative medical management is chosen (18).

Benign Breast Neoplasia

Proliferative breast disease is divided into two subtypes (19,20): proliferative breast disease without histologic atypia (1.5 to 2 times increase of breast cancer risk) and proliferative breast disease with atypical histological patterns of epithelial hyperplasia (risk of development breast cancer is 5%–10%). When a family history of breast cancer is present in this group, the risk of developing cancer within a period of 15 years increases to 20%.

Such changes in the breast should be identified and the diagnosis established, most commonly with the assistance of imaging studies (ultrasonography and mammography) and fine-needle biopsy. This nondominant proliferative breast disorder should be matched against benign dominant or malignant breast neoplasia.

Benign dominant breast neoplasia usually does not predispose to malignant transformation. Such tumors are described in the following sections.

Fibroadenomas

Fibroadenomas are predominantly benign breast neoplasms that affect young women (21,22); although, new fibroadenomas in women over 35 years have been reported as well (23). These tumors are common, accounting for 50% of all breast biopsy results. Fibroadenoma of the breast often spontaneously regresses (24). Malignant potential transformation of fibroadenoma is low, with the overall estimated risk of cancer 2.17 higher than in patients without the presence of this tumor. The risk increases when complex breast fibroadenoma is identified (fibroadenomas demonstrate mixed solid and cystic structure within the tumors or the presence of sclerosing adenosis, epithelial calcification, or papillary apocrine changes (21).

The diagnosis is essentially clinical and confirmed either by cytologic or histologic examination. The tumor is typically asymptomatic, located in the upper outer quadrant of the breast, unilateral [10% bilateral and multiple fibroadenoma in 10%–25% (25)] with an average size of 2 to 3 cm. However, the tumor may reach 10 to 15 cm (26), and even giant fibroadenomas have been reported (27). The skin over the tumor can be warm and dilated veins may be observed.

Physical examination is crucial in the detection of this tumor. Palpation may reveal a solid, firm, freely movable nontender mass, and no nipple discharge present.

Ultrasonography can assist in differentiating a pure solid tumor from a complex mass (24).

Magnetic resonance imaging has been gaining clinical attention, owing to its ability to distinguish benign from malignant growths (28).

Fine-needle aspiration cytology can differentiate malignant from benign breast tumors with great accuracy. In terms of cytologic accuracy for differentiating fibroadenomas from other benign processes, it has a sensitivity of 87% and specificity of 76% (29,30).

Core biopsy can provide documentation for the confident diagnosis of breast fibroadenoma (23).

The conservative medical approach is to provide reassurance because spontaneous regression of fibroadenomas often occurs and malignant degeneration is exceedingly low (23,24). Conservative surgical tumor excision by means of resection (open biopsy) also may be undertaken (23).

Fibrocystic Breast Disease

Fibrocystic disease is characterized by the presence of breast pain (mastalgia), breast tenderness, lumpiness, or cyst, as well as changes associated with the menstrual cycle. This condition predominantly affects women 25 to 50 years of age, with a prevalence of 50% during the reproductive years (31,32). The cause of this condition is unknown, but has been hypothesized as inadequate ovarian steroid production and secretion, because a typical histologic alteration in fibrocystic disease is observed in different menstrual phases, an in hyperprolactinemia (31,33). A tumor suppressor gene is postulated as a factor in fibrocystic disease, but such a gene has not yet been identified (34).

Food or beverages containing methylxanthines (chocolate, coffee, tea, and cola) have been postulated as substances that aggravate or even cause the disease, but clinicians disagree on this point (33,35).

The diagnosis is based on the symptom of mastalgia fluctuating during a menstrual cycle and getting progressively worse in the second phase of the cycle, with a peak shortly before menses. Pain eases with commencement of menstrual bleeding. The cyclicity of mastalgia is a significant parameter in clinical analysis.

Breast examination reveals defuse and frequently tender, multiple nodularities in both breasts. *Imaging studies* such as ultrasonography and mammography are often used not only to confirm clinical findings but also to differentiate benign from malignant lesions (36,37). Magnetic resonance imaging mammography has been used for some time, but fibrocystic changes associated with the menstrual cycle may lead to false-positive results (38).

Fine-needle aspiration cytology is often used in the diagnostic process of breast disorders (39).

Open breast biopsy is indicated if any suspicious lesion is present.

Conventional Therapy

Conventional therapy consists of conservative management:

- If symptoms are not severe, observation with reassurance may be a sufficient tool in the management of fibrocystic breast disease. It has been documented that spontaneous regression of benign cysts of the breast occurs in the majority of cases. Approximately 12% of cysts will not spontaneous regress within 5 years (40).
- Oral contraceptives pills can successfully decrease mastalgia in approximately 70% to 90% of cases (41).
- Oral medroxyprogesterone acetate, 20 mg daily in the second phase of a menstrual cycle, may provide relief (4,42).

However, a randomized controlled study did not document superiority of this mode of therapy over placebo (43).

- Oral danazol, 200-400 mg daily, significantly reduces symptomatology associated with fibrocystic disease (44,45).

Complementary Therapy

Patient Education

Patient education should be conveyed in reference to the nature and extent of the disease, available mode of diagnosis, and therapy available, including diet, nutritional supplements, and alternative remedies. The potential adverse reactions or interaction of conventional drugs and alternative remedies (including hormonal and non-hormonal therapeutic agents) should be presented. Physical and mental overwork without adequate rest may contribute to anovulation and continuous estrogen stimulation of the breast tissue. Combined spirit-mind-body stress reduction techniques may assist in the general well being of the patient. More details are presented in Chapters 3 and 5.

Diet

Diet in fibrocystic disease should address the following elements:

- Reduction of methylxanthine (caffeine, milk chocolate, bittersweet chocolate, chocolate cake, etc.) intake in foods (46)
- Reduction of methylxanthine (caffeine, coffee, tea, hot cocoa, cola, etc.) intake in beverages (46)
- Adoption of a low-fat (20% of calories) and high-carbohydrate diet is recommended. Such dietary modification not only can significantly reduce premenstrual breast pain, tenderness, and breast swelling within 6 months (47), but also reduces the area of mammographic density within 2 years (48).
- Increasing dietary fiber, such as whole grain, legumes, fruits, and vegetables, is advisable (49).
- Increasing consumption of seafood and seaweed is recommended (49).

Well-Fitting Bra

A well-fitting bra is a simple and frequently effective approach to assist a patient in coping with breast pain associated with fibrocystic disease (50).

Acupuncture

Acupuncture is recommended for benign breast disease, particularly when breast pain and swelling are present. Acupuncture itself yields 95% symptomatology reduction when compared with antiinflammatory drugs or multivitamin therapy (51). However, results of randomized controlled studies are needed to substantiate claims of safety and effectiveness.

Alternative Therapy

Vitamin A (150,000 IU per day orally for 3 months) is suggested for symptomatic benign breast disease (52). A randomized controlled study is needed to support the claims of safety and effectiveness of this therapeutic modality (4). The potential side effect of hepatotoxicity is a concern with high doses of beta-carotene.

Vitamin E (alpha-tocopherol, 600 IU per day orally) initially was reported to be a successful mode of therapy (49), but the results of subsequent randomized controlled studies have not supported this therapeutic claim (53,54).

Evening primrose oil (omega-6 fatty acid) is an effective and safe treatment for cyclic breast pain in approximately 45% of patients, which has been documented in a randomized controlled study at a total daily dose of 3,000 mg (either 1,000 mg three times daily or 1,500 mg twice daily) (55).

Natural Hormonal Therapy

Frequently, a vaginal micronized natural progesterone cream is suggested for cyclic breast pain associated with fibrocystic breast disease. A randomized double-blind placebo-controlled study showed no statistically significant effect of progesterone over placebo, and no major side effects were reported (56). Local application of micronized natural progesterone to the breast at a dose of one fourth to half a teaspoon in the second phase of the menstrual cycle also has been recommended (49), but lack of scientific data makes it difficult to promote such a clinical approach.

Herbal Remedy

The following herbal remedies have been suggested (49):

- *Yarrow leaf,* two to six 320- to 340-mg capsules daily or one-fourth to one teaspoon tincture, is recommended for breast fibrocystic disease. It is used in natural medicine practice, but no scientific data are available to support its use.
- *Phytolacca oil* is applied to the breast nightly for 2 weeks, then every other night. No data are available to support the efficacy and safety of this remedy.

Homeotherapy

Homeopathic treatment for breast fibrocystic disease includes the following (57):

- *Lapis albus,* in a dilution of 5 or 9 cH daily, is recommended when tender cystic structures are present.
- *Thuya,* in a dilution of 9 cH daily or 15 cH weekly, is suggested when cysts and indurated lumpiness are present.

No clinical scientific data are available to support these clinical approaches.

Breast Cysts

Breast cysts or mammary cysts are fluid collections within a lobular sac. The prevalence is estimated to be approximately

7% among adult women and predominantly affects women 40 to 50 years of age (58,59). Breast cysts arise as deviations of lobular natural involution associated with apocrine metaplasia of the breast epithelium (60). Cysts smaller than 3 mm have no pathologic significance and are considered microcysts. Cyst 3 mm or larger are macrocysts (59,61). Cysts can be solitary or multiple (most commonly associated with fibrocystic disease). Hormonal imbalance (hyperprolactinemia, luteal phase deficiency) may influence cyst formation, but hormonal aberration is neither a necessary, nor a sufficient factor to induce a breast cyst. It seems that psychogenic components may play a role in cystic formation (61).

The diagnosis is established by following the standard diagnostic protocol presented in this chapter, and the potential presence of breast cancer remains fundamental issue. Benign breast cyst transformation to malignancy is exceedingly low; the presence of macrocyst increases the breast cancer risk by three- to fourfold. Multiple recurrent cysts are associated with a small, but significant increase in breast cancer risk (59,61).

Conventional therapy consists of the following options (61):

■ Psychotherapy with or without tranquilizers.
■ Antiprostaglandin synthesis inhibitors.
■ Danazol, 200 to 400 mg daily.
■ Fine-needle aspiration.
■ Open biopsy with cyst extirpation (infrequently indicated).
■ Tamoxifen may promote breast cyst regression. Coincidentally, tamoxifen therapy for premenopausal breast cancer has induced regression of cysts in the contralateral mammary gland (62).

Cystosarcoma Phyllodes

Cystosarcoma phyllodes, or phyllodes tumor of the breast, is a fibroepithelial mass. It is an exceedingly rare tumor with a *prevalence* of 0.3% to 1% of all breast neoplasms (63). The nomenclature of this tumor may be misleading, because the term *sarcoma* usually has a malignant connotation. Clinically, cystosarcoma phyllodes is diagnosed in approximately 10% of all cases (64). The tumor may affect women of all ages, with approximately 5% of the women younger than 20 years (65) and about 26.9% postmenopausal women. White women are predominantly affected, 85.5% (66).

Etiology and natural behavior are not clearly understood, and no causation has been established between cystosarcoma phyllodes and oral contraceptives, nicotine use, diabetes mellitus, age of menarche, allergies, or family history of cancer. The tumors are classified according to international criteria as benign, borderline, and malignant (63).

The diagnosis is suggested on clinical observation of a large (3–5 cm in diameter) painless tumor with sudden growth acceleration and is well defined with firm and soft

areas. The mean age at diagnosis of this tumor is 46 years in adult women (63,66). The mean age at diagnosis of this tumor is 17.7 years among girls and women 10 to 24 (67). The standard diagnostic protocol for breast mass evaluation is applicable, but neither clinical nor imaging studies can distinguish benign from malignant processes.

The differential diagnosis includes fibroadenoma, fibrocystic disease, mastitis, abscess, medullary carcinoma, virginal hyperplasia, lipoma, and lymphoma (4,64).

Conventional therapy of benign cystosarcoma phyllodes is wide tumor resection with a 2 cm tumor-free zone. Benign tumor recurrences following resection have occurred and usually are detected an average of 18 months after initial operation (63). Recurrences most commonly accompany incomplete excision of the benign tumor and are observed in about 7.9% of cases. Rare or no recurrence is observed when the tumor is less than or equal to 2 cm. Further excision or mastectomy can prevent recurrence of the tumor (66,68,69).

Complementary-alternative therapy is not available.

Intraductal Papillomas

Benign intraductal papillomas arise from proliferation of cells in the terminal duct unit with projections into the ductal lumen (4,70). They most commonly affect women 20 to 40 years of age (71). However, among the adolescent population, they account for approximately 1.2% of all breast lesions (72). Intraductal papilloma is classified as a central or peripheral lesion. Peripheral papilloma may coexist in approximately 37.5%, with carcinoma in the terminal ductal-lobular units (73).

The diagnosis continues to be one of the most difficult diagnostic processes. The tumor may produce serosanguineous nipple or bloody discharge and is usually small and palpable in the areolar region, but it may reach giant proportions (up to 15 cm) (75). Evaluation is customarily conducted within the framework of standard diagnostic protocols for breast masses, described elsewhere in this chapter. Histology confirmation verifies the definitive diagnosis. *Conventional therapy* is surgical excision of the affected ductolobular unit.

Mammary Duct Ectasia

Mammary duct ectasia (duct ectasia syndrome, periductal mastitis, mammary dysplasia, mastopathy) is a benign entity characterized by dilatation of the subareolar duct and inflammatory changes with fibrosis reaction in collecting ducts. Mammary ductal ectasia is diagnosed preoperatively in approximately 4.2% of cases, and incidental postoperative findings are found in approximately 8.1% (76). This condition most commonly affects women 50 to 60 years of age (77) and is rarely observed among adolescents or young women (32).

The diagnosis may be presumed based on symptoms and clinical findings, yet the majority of cases do not produce any symptoms (78). The clinical course is characterized by a long history of tumor formation, nipple discharge, nipple retraction, and mastalgia. Nonpuerperal mammary abscess is frequently present (78).

Breast examination may reveal the presence of multicolored and sticky nipple discharge, nipple retraction, and tenderness to palpation, fistula formation, and subareolar mass/abscess formation.

Mammography may guide the diagnosis; ultrasonographic features show linear rosary-like dilatation, and pseudocystic ectasia may be present (77). The clinical and radiographic appearance of this entity may be indistinguishable from breast cancer (79).

The *differential diagnosis* includes other breast tumors associated with nipple discharge; excluding breast cancer is a fundamental objective.

Conventional therapy consists of excision of the central mammary tissue and larger ducts (76,79). When abscess is present, resection of the entire abscess yields better results than incision and drainage (80). Fistulas also require surgical removal with reconstruction of the nipple areolar area (76,78).

Complementary-alternative therapy is not presently available.

Mastitis

Mastitis breast infection during a nonpuerperal period (non-lactational) is unusual, and therefore of interest to gynecologic practice. Gram-positive and gram-negative microorganisms most commonly cause mastitis. Abscess formation is a sequela of breast infection. The infection can be transmitted locally from an infected skin area or can be associated with nipple piercing. Clinically, breast infection develops in the following phases:

- The cellulitis stage can be managed conservatively with antibiotics after fine-needle aspiration for cultures and sensitivity (81).
- Focal abscess is clinically diagnosed (painful mass, severe tenderness to palpation, and warm, edematous skin with or without fluctuant occurrence within the abscess) and documented by ultrasonography. Microbiologic culture can be obtained with percutaneous fine-needle cavity aspiration followed by treatment with antibiotics. If this approach is not successful, abscess drainage is necessary (81,82).
- Multiloculated abscess presents with similar symptoms and signs as focal abscess. An ultrasonographic study is helpful. Urgent surgical incision and drainage is required, but percutaneous aspiration of the abscess cavity for partial drainage can be used palliatively, followed by incision and complete drainage of the abscess (abscesses of >3 cm require definitive treatment by incision and drainage) (81,83).

Abscess formation may coexist with breast cancer. Clinical, mammographic, and sonographic examinations can be compromised to identify cancer in the presence of an abscess (81,84).

The growing popularity, particularly among adolescents and young women, of nipple piercing has increased the incidence of breast infection and breast abscess formation. The most common organisms associated with complications from nipple piercing are *Staphylococcus aureus, Pseudomonas aeruginosa,* and beta-hemolytic streptococci. Treatment is undertaken as described above (4,85).

BREAST CANCER

Definition

The presence of malignant neoplasia as a primary or secondary process within the breast tissue constitutes breast cancer.

Incidence

Breast cancer is the most common cancer among women, accounting for 32% of all newly diagnosed cancer (86)—175,000 new cases were diagnosed in 1999. The lifetime risk for developing breast cancer in the United States is one in nine (87). The incidence of invasive breast cancer has changed little since 1990. Early breast cancer detection has dramatically increased, and the mortality rate has been reduced by 11% for women under 50 years of age and by 6% in women over 50 years old. This improvement is due to the introduction of preventive programs, which commenced over a quarter century ago in the United States. Among African-American women, the incidence of breast cancer is higher in those under the age of 40 than in those over the age of 40 (88). Breast cancer is the second leading cause of overall cancer death in industrialized European countries and the United States (89). Nationwide, the breast cancer mortality rate, an essential parameter in cancer control, has decreased slightly since 1989. This decline is a reflection of early detection and improved management of the disease (90).

The prevalence of synchronous bilateral cancer is approximately 1% to 2%, and that of metachronous breast cancer is 5% to 6% (91).

Etiology

The cause of breast cancer has not yet been established. Epidemiologic data suggest that at least 50% of breast cancer may be interpreted by identifying potential risk factors (presented at the beginning of this chapter), and most breast cancers can be linked to environmentally induced mutations (90). Furthermore, inherited susceptibility to breast cancer development (5%–10% of all women with breast cancer) led to the discovery and identification of breast cancer susceptibility genes (germline mutation) BRCA 1 and BRCA 2, and commercial kits are now available for breast and ovarian cancer genetic testing. However, the risk identification associated with BRCA mutations may be less than previously estimated (92). For women with a positive family history of breast cancer or the presence of breast cancer bilaterally, BRCA 1 and BRCA 2 can play role as a predictor of breast cancer development in first-degree relatives (93). The presence of a germline mutation of BRCA 1 in patients under 50 years of age with breast cancer is predictive of developing breast cancer in the contralateral mammary gland in up to 40%, versus 12% in patients over 50. Therefore, the age at the time of primary cancer and BRCA 1 should be taken into account, when prophylactic mastectomy is considered (94).

Classification

Breast cancer classification is based on morphologic patterns and is divided into two types. Breast carcinoma of ductal epithelial origin is diagnosed as either ductal carcinoma *in situ* (DCIS) or invasive infiltrating ductal carcinoma (occurs in 72%). Breast carcinoma of lobular origin is diagnosed as LCIS or invasive infiltrating lobular carcinoma (10%–15%). The remaining 13% to 18% of breast cancer includes, Paget disease, inflammatory carcinoma, and sarcomas.

Diagnosis

The diagnostic process does not depart from the standard protocol for breast mass evaluation described earlier in this chapter.

Staging

Breast cancer clinical staging is based on the tumor-node-metastasis (TNM) system. The American Joint Committee on Cancer developed the breast cancer staging system, which categorized patients into similar groups for inter-center comparison. This staging is not adequate for segregating patients for selection of appropriate surgical treatment (95). The TNM staging system is summarized in Table 27.1 (2,3).

Clinical staging requires chest radiography, routine blood testing, and liver function studies. A bone scan is a part of pretreatment evaluation when an invasive breast tumor is present.

Some authorities also suggest performing lymphatic node mapping with lymphoscintigraphy due to the absence of significant drainage of outer quadrant breast tumors to the internal mammary nodal chain. Patients undergoing lymphatic mapping for management of breast cancer should have radiolabeled tracer and gamma probe sentinel node identification despite tumor location in the breast (96).

Breast cancer affects children in less than 1% of cases. However, the most common malignant breast neoplasia is secondary to diseases such as rhabdomyosarcoma, Hodgkin and non-Hodgkin lymphoma, and neuroblastoma, and is commonly reported as a metastatic disease. The foremost risk factor for breast cancer development in adolescents is an immediate positive family history of the disease. The most common symptom and sign is a breast mass. The evaluation protocol and therapeutic approach are similar to those for adult women and include genetic BRCA 1 and BRCA 2 testing (4).

Differential Diagnosis

- Breast benign neoplasia
- Benign causes of nipple discharge

Conventional Therapy

Surgery itself is not curative for breast cancer regardless of the extent of excision performed. This clinical realization has led to changes in clinical practice, and more conservative surgical approaches are being undertaken, eliminating classic radical mastectomy. Segmental resection or local excision combined with axillary dissection and followed by radiotherapy is frequently performed. *Lumpectomy, segmental mastectomy, or tylectomy* are surgical procedures that incorporate tumor resection and 2 to 3 cm of surrounding breast tissues. Axillary lymphadenectomy may or may not be indicated in association with lumpectomy and depends on clinical staging and histological type and grade of the tumor.

Quadrantectomy or partial mastectomy is designed to remove the breast quadrant in which the tumor is present and the lining of the chest muscle below the tumor.

Simple mastectomy is a procedure in which the entire mammary gland is removed with sampling of the axillary lymph nodes.

Modified radical mastectomy or total mastectomy removes the entire breast, axillary lymph nodes, and lining over the tumor chest muscles.

Radical mastectomy procedure incorporates extirpation of the entire breast, axillary lymph nodes, and underlying chest muscles (this procedure is infrequently performed in the United States and accounts for fewer that 5% of all surgeries performed for breast cancer).

A multidisciplinary approach (surgeon, radiation oncologist, and medical oncologist) has replaced a single specialty care in breast cancer management. Mammography plays a crucial role in conservative surgery, because multicentric disease may be present, occasionally requiring modified radical mastectomy with lymphadenectomy.

Breast cancer surgical staging has not been designed for clinical management and in many instances does not ade-

TABLE 27.1. TNM BREAST STAGING SYSTEM

	Primary Tumor (T)	Regional Nodes (N)		Pathologic Classification (pN)		Distant Metastasis (M)	
Stage	Definition	Stage	Definition	Stage	Definition	Stage	Definition
TX	Primary tumor cannot be assessed	NX	Regional node cannot be assessed	pNX	Regional node cannot be assessed	MX	Presence of distant metastasis cannot be assessed
T0	No evidence of primary tumor	N0	No regional node metastasis	pN0	No regional node metastasis	M0	No distant metastasis
TIS	Carcinoma in situ: intraductal carcinoma, lobular carcinoma Paget's disease of the nipple with no tumor	N1	Metastasis to movable ipsilateral axillary lymph nodes	pN1	Metastasis to movable ipsilateral axillary lymph nodes	M1	Distant metastasis includes ipsilateral suraclavicular lymph nodes
T1	Tumor ≤2 cm in greatest dimension	N2	Metastasis to ipsilateral axillary lymph nodes fixed to one another or to other structures	pN1a	Only micrometastases (none >0.2 cm)		
T1a	Tumor ≤0.5 cm in greatest dimension	N3	Metastasis to ipsilateral internal mammary lymph nodes	pN1b	Metastasis to lymph nodes(s) any >0.2 cm		
T1b	Tumor 0.5–1 cm in greatest dimension			pN1bi	Metastasis in 1–3 lymph nodes any >0.2 and <2 cm in greatest dimension		
T1c	Tumor 1–2 cm in greatest dimension			pN1bi i	Extension of tumor beyond the capsule of lymph node metastasis <2 cm in greatest dimension		
T2	Tumor 2–5 cm in greatest dimension			pN1bi v	Metastasis to lymph node ≥2 cm in greatest dimension		
T3	Tumor >5 cm in greatest dimension			PN2	Metastasis to ipsilateral axillary nodes that are fixed to one another or to other structures		
T4	Tumor of any size with direct extension to chest wall or skin			pN3	Metastasis to ipsilateral internal mammary lymph node(s)		
T4a	Extension to chest wall						
T4b	Edema or ulceration of the skin of the breast or satellite skin nodules confirmed to the same breast						
T4c	Both (T4a and T4b)						
T4d	Inflammatory carcinoma						

quately reflect clinical parameters. However, such staging is frequently used as a therapeutic guide. So, in order to meet educational objectives, this staging system is incorporated into this book presentation.

Carcinoma In Situ *Therapy*

Atypical epithelial hyperplasia, LCIS (lobular neoplasia), radial scar, and DCIS are considered high-risk lesions that predispose toward the future development of noninvasive or invasive breast carcinoma (97).

Ductal carcinoma in situ has a favorable prognosis (long-term survival rates approach 100% with appropriate management). In general, DCIS is viewed as a direct precursor to invasive breast carcinoma or an early, noninvasive ductal epithelial malignant neoplasia. Therefore, similar treatment rules are applicable as for an early invasive stage of breast carcinoma. According to the National Cancer DataBase, conservative surgery is applied to more than 50% of cases of DCIS with a low rate of radiotherapy utilization and a high rate of axillary lymphadenectomy (98). In many instances, such a trend may lead to either over or under treatment. Mastectomy achieves a nearly 100% curative rate but may represent overtreatment, mainly to those women who present with asymptomatic lesions with only mammographically documented disease. Axillary lymph node dissection of breast masses of less than or equal to 5 cm is not routinely recommended (lesions >5 cm have an increased risk for microinvasion and lymph node extension).

The rate of recurrence of DCIS with conservative surgery is approximately 20% (10% with invasive stage), with a potential long-term cure rate of at least 90%. When radiotherapy is added, the recurrence rate is reduced to 10% (5% with invasive stage), with a long-term cure rate of 95%.

A patient's selection of conservative breast surgery for DCIS should address not only the cosmetic and emotional aspects, but also factors that increase the rate for local recurrence:

■ Close microscopic observation of involved surgical specimen margins
■ Presence of necrosis
■ High-grade tumor differentiation (poorly differentiated tumor)

In view of the presence of these factors, radiation to the breast should be added as a part of breast-conserving therapy.

Patients with low-grade tumor without necrosis, tumor size up to 1.5 cm, and reliability and willingness to adhere to a close follow-up regimen can be considered for conservative surgery (97,99).

Lobular carcinoma in situ can be managed with nonoperative observation because it is considered an indicator

(marker) of potential increased risk for invasive breast carcinoma, but not as a precursor to it (100). Invasive lobular carcinoma may develop in approximately 20% to 25% of women with LCIS. LCIS is an asymptomatic lesion with no ability to grow as a mass, and mammography cannot identify LCIS. It is only documented by histology. When an invasive stage of lobular carcinoma occurs, it frequently is a multicentric and bilateral malignant process (101).

Management of LCIS takes many forms:

■ Nonoperative observation follow-up only has been suggested (102)
■ Chemoprevention with tamoxifen or some other agent has been recommended (101)
■ Bilateral modified mastectomy is offered, because bilateral invasive carcinoma *in situ* can occur. Such a radical approach is based on the Van Nuys Prognostic Index, which relates to histologic determination of tumor diameter and microscopic thickness of the margin-free zone specimen, and histologic grading of the tumor (103). If mastectomy is chosen, a unilateral procedure is inappropriate. Existing risk factors and patient anxiety (carcinophobia) of potential invasive breast carcinoma (up to 25%) warrants prophylactic bilateral mastectomy in selected patients.

Microinvasive Carcinoma Therapy

Microinvasion of breast carcinoma is defined as a malignant process migrating from the breast epithelium to the stroma and is less than or equal to 1 mm in diameter. DCIS may present with such invasive characteristics. LCIS is not likely to be accompanied by such stromal changes. In ductal microinvasive carcinoma, the therapy is individualized based on histologic criteria such as tumor diameter, microscopic thickness of the margin-free zone specimen, and histologic grading of the tumor (the Van Nuys Prognostic Index) (104,105).

Invasive Breast Carcinoma Therapy: Stage I and Stage II Management

Breast-conserving surgical therapy (commonly lumpectomy or segmental resection) with radiation is customarily extended to patients with disease in stages I and II. A meta-analysis of randomized studies on 10-year survival, comparing combined breast-conserving surgical therapy and radiation with total mastectomy, documented that survival rates for breast-conserving therapy are at least as high as those for total mastectomy. It also has been determined that lymph node status and tumor size does not significantly alter the relative survival rates. For node-positive patients, breast-conserving therapy may confer a relative survival advantage over total mastectomy. The effectiveness of total mastectomy without adjuvant radiation appears to be inferior to breast-conserving therapy for node-positive patients (106).

Radiation, as a part of breast-conserving therapy, is usually delivered to the whole breast at a dose of 4,500 to 5,000 cGy and a boost is directed to the tumor bed of 1,500 to 2,000 cGy. Patients with positive axillary lymph nodes receive radiation to the supraclavicular nodes. Irradiation customarily begins as soon as the incisional wound is healed (107).

In invasive stage I or II breast cancer with positive nodes, adjuvant chemotherapy with cyclophosphamide and doxorubicin (107) is usually recommended and is started concomitant with radiation therapy or in sequence (107,108). The initial results of preoperative chemotherapy for operable breast cancer seemed to yield favorable results, but the lack of a randomized controlled study makes it difficult to predict the role of such an approach (109).

Overall 5-year survival rates in the patient population treated with breast-conserving therapy and radiation is 85% to 89% as compared with 76% to 89% with total mastectomy (106,110,111).

In order to minimize the recurrence of breast cancer following breast-conserving therapy with radiation, the following elements should be considered:

- Surgeon's ability to completely resect the primary lesion with surgical margin-free tissues and without significant breast deformity.
- Single lesion versus multicentric lesions—solitary tumors foretell better results than multicenter primary lesions as documented by mammography. Scattered and widely separated lesions are better treated with modified radical mastectomy. Immediate cosmetic reconstruction is an appropriate approach (112). Consultation with a plastic surgeon should be scheduled before breast surgery, and support group information should be provided. Reconstructive breast surgery is a lengthy operation. Unexpected intraoperative findings may preclude immediate reconstructive breast surgery.
- Far-reaching intraductal cancer infiltration does not respond well to breast-conserving therapy.
- Women with large tumors (>5 cm in greatest dimension) in a small size breast are poor candidates for breast-conserving therapy.
- Women with central lesions infiltrating the nipple-areola complex are good candidates for breast-conserving therapy. However, cosmetic breast reconstruction is required after removing the breast mass. It is the surgeon's obligation to provide appropriate points of reference on the surgical specimen for the pathologist. Estrogen and progesterone receptor studies also should be requested. Appropriate microscopic tissue evaluation for a surgical margin state is essential in lumpectomy. If a microscopic margin-positive result (≤5 mm) is obtained, excision should extend beyond the surgical margin-free zone.

Drawbacks of breast-conserving therapy include exposure to extensive radiation, potential for tumor recurrence, and protracted postoperative treatment.

Follow-up for invasive breast cancer falls into two categories. Breast cancer screening for locoregional recurrence should be conducted twice yearly for 5 years, and every year thereafter if breast-conserving therapy has been implemented.

Surveillance for a second primary breast cancer on the contralateral breast is based on screening techniques (BSE, clinical breast evaluation, and mammography) when mastectomy has been chosen as a mode of treatment.

Advanced Breast Cancer Therapy

The following clinical criteria suggest the presence of local advanced breast cancer:

- Tumor size greater than 5 cm (T3)
- Fixed or matted N2 axillary lymphatic nodes
- Presence of inflammatory breast carcinoma

Therapy commences with chemotherapy (most commonly used drug combinations are cyclophosphamide, methotrexate, and 5-fluorouracil, or cyclophosphamide, doxorubicin, and 5-fluorouracil) for inoperable breast cancer. If a tumor responds to chemotherapy, surgery and radiotherapy may follow. In postmenopausal women, adjuvant tamoxifen is administered for 5 years. Patients with an intact uterus on tamoxifen should be closely monitored (with yearly gynecologic examination and possibly a yearly cytologic examination of endometrial aspirate) because tamoxifen is a remote potential risk for endometrial hyperplasia and endometrial cancer (approximately 0.5%).

Metastatic Breast Cancer

Metastatic breast disease is established by clinical evaluation and tests such as bone scan, computed tomography (CT), and liver function tests, and tumor markers are used. Metastatic breast cancer is a chronic illness. Because metastatic breast cancer is fatal, several forms of palliative therapies are available that are essentially designed to improve quality of life:

- Hormonal therapy should be offered based on breast receptor status. Estrogen receptor–positive patients may benefit from antiestrogen agents such as tamoxifen citrate (Nolvadex, 20 mg daily), with an expected response in approximately 60%. Estrogen receptor–positive patients have approximately an 8% to 10% better prognosis than estrogen-negative patients do at 5 years. When a progesterone receptor–positive status is present, patients will respond to hormonal therapy in about 80%.
- Oophorectomy is offered to premenopausal patients and is considered to be an endocrine-manipulative procedure, with response rates of 30% to 40%.

- Radiotherapy is used to control bone pain or prevent pathologic fractures.

Hormonal and combination chemotherapy is standard protocols for metastatic breast cancer, and radiotherapy is predominantly used for bone metastatic pain and central nervous system metastasis.

Complementary Therapy

Complementary and alternative therapies cannot replace conventional established therapies for breast cancer, but can be used as adjuncts. Complementary therapies may assist the patient in coordinating mind-spirit-body balance and by doing this can maximize quality of life. There is the mounting evidence that complementary and alternative remedies exhibit biologic activity, and they are readily available and widely used with and without physician consent. Data are available reporting initial successful outcomes of complementary and alternative therapies. However, scientific documentation is lacking in reference to the safety and efficacy of such approaches.

Patient Education

Patient education in a screening program for breast cancer is essential, because these programs are conceptually based on each individual's level of knowledge, allowing them to make the decision to participate in and to follow the recommendations of the early detection methods for breast cancer.

Breast Cancer Screening

Breast cancer screening is based on the following clinical criteria (112):

- Most common malignancy among women in the United States.
- Long preclinical phase of 1 to 2 years.
- Screening techniques (BSE, clinical breast examination, and screening mammography) are noninvasive and well tolerated, involve little radiation exposure, and are relatively inexpensive.
- Effective management with low morbidity is available for early stages of breast cancer.

Independent meta-analysis data support the notion that the relative risk of dying from breast cancer is reduced by 26% between ages of 50 and 74 years, when all screening techniques are implemented. Mammography is the most important screening tool. Yearly mammography among women 40 to 49 years of age decreases their breast cancer mortality rate by 20%. In younger women (25–39 years), BSE and clinical breast examination are recommended (4,112).

In summary, the American Cancer Society recommendation for breast screening is as follows:

- Monthly BSE
- Clinical breast examination every 1 to 3 years for women 20 to 39 years of age
- Yearly clinical breast examination from the age of 40 years on
- First mammographic examination at 40 years of age
- Follow-up mammographic examination every 1 to 2 years from ages 40 to 49 years
- Mammography annually after 50 years of age

Because breast cancer is predominantly environmentally induced (hereditary breast cancer accounts for 5%–10% of cases), patients should be made aware of the life-style factors predisposing to breast cancer and an appropriate plan should be established to eliminate such factors.

When to commence BSE education is debated. It seems logical to introduce such a program among adolescent girls, because breast cancer may affect this population (<1% of all breast tumors) (113). Initiation of BSE in this group is controversial and is only recommended for girls with a strong immediate family history of breast cancer and carriers of the BRCA 1 or BRCA 2 gene. BSE probably should begin at 18 years of age (4). Other screening techniques, such as clinical breast examination and mammography, should be a part of patient education. Patients should be made aware of the benefits of early breast cancer detection and its association with the high probability of cure and reduction of mortality rates by more than 26%. BSE and clinical breast examination are described earlier in this chapter.

The prevalence of breast cancer and the diagnostic process for evaluating a breast mass should be clearly described. Upon reaching the diagnosis of breast cancer, the nature and therapeutic options should be explained, including conventional, complementary, and alternative therapies. Breast cancer diagnosis is a devastating occurrence for the mind, body, and spirit. From the patient's perspective, the diagnosis of breast cancer, as with other types of cancer, is a hopeless/helpless situation. It is believed, but not scientifically documented, that a negative, emotional state may significantly inhibit a patient's natural instinct to cope with the disease. Psychotherapeutic intervention not only increases a patient's emotional ability to cope with cancer but also augments natural killer cell activity. The psychobiologic mechanism of cancer is a complex issue and should be considered in terms of psychoneuroimmunology (114). Despite this obvious psychological involvement and its sequelae among cancer patients, there is some scientific data on clinically appropriate psychological interventions (115).

It has been documented that women with breast cancer often turn to complementary or alternative medicine. About 72% of women in the United States attempt some form of alternative therapy at the time of initial diagnosis, and only 54% of these patients inform their physicians (116). The motivations for seeking such treatments include "maximizing quality of life," "seeking natural approaches to healing," and "looking to stay well when the disease is in remission" (117). An additional aspect of patient education is to assist in making informed choices in reference to unregulated "natural health" products. A knowledgeable physician should be the best source, not a retailer, to supply a remedy (118). It is imperative in the management of patients with breast cancer to accept and support their decision of using alternative therapies, because it provides the practitioner an opportunity to intervene when potential adverse effects or interactions may occur. Patients who turn to alternative remedies in addition to standard therapies are at greater psychological distress and need appropriate emotional support (119).

Family members, friends, and a support group should be extensively incorporated into an educational program.

Following breast surgery, some general advice as listed below, is an important aspect of a patient's preparation for this stage of the recovery process. Everyday activity may cause discomfort that can be minimized by providing the following simple information:

- Wearing loose-fitting clothes and gloves is advised.
- Avoiding sun overexposure is advised.
- Gentle exercise of the arm affected by axillary lymphadenectomy is advised.

Diet

Diet may play a significant role in environmental carcinogenesis of the breast and may account for approximately 35% of cases (120). Diets that induce rapid growth and lead to greater adult heights increase breast cancer risk. A dietary factor such as alcohol consumption (>29.9 g per day) increases the mortality rate from the disease (121). Dietary fat was previously implicated as a high risk factor in breast cancer development, but its role in breast cancer development is controversial (122).

A sedentary life-style and a high-calorie diet results in increased body mass and in the postmenopausal period is particularly associated with a higher risk of breast cancer (122,123).

Based on these clinical findings, diet modification and life-style changes are important considerations in breast cancer prevention and management.

A long-term weight reduction and maintenance program should include but not be limited to diet (see also Chapters 3 and 11). Lifestyle modification should increase physical exercise and limitation on alcohol consumption.

Because fruits and vegetables are rich in chemopreventive factors, they should be added to dietary programs. Based on data presented above, practical suggestions pertaining to dietary modification include increasing fruit (berries, apples, cherries, grapes, and plums) and vegetable consumption (especially onion and garlic), reducing fats, reducing cooked meat consumption, and avoiding alcohol to lower the risk of developing breast cancer (122,123).

Nutritional Supplements

Approximately 80.9% of patients with breast cancer in the United States are reported to use dietary supplements. The use of vitamin C, n-3 fatty acids, evening primrose oil, and herbal remedies increases as the patient's disease progresses. The use of miscellaneous supplements such as shark cartilage are directly associated with a more advanced stage of breast cancer at the time of diagnosis (124).

The following dietary supplements are suggested for patients with breast cancer or as a mode of prevention of breast cancer (125). However, scientific data to support the beneficial effects of nutritional supplements in breast cancer are insufficient to make a definitive recommendation.

Nutrients

The following nutrients are recommended to complement standard conventional treatment (125):

- Essential fatty acids, at the dose as directed on the label (promote proper cell reproduction)
- Coenzyme Q10, 100 mg daily (improves cellular oxygenation)
- Germanium, 200 mg daily (immunostimulant)
- Kyolic (garlic), two capsules three times daily (enhances immune system)
- Proteolytic enzymes, at the dose as directed on the label (free radical scavenger)
- Selenium, 200 to 400 μg daily (free radical scavenger)
- Shark cartilage (BeneFin), 0.5 mg per 1 pound of body weight (inhibits tumor growth and stimulates immune system)
- Brewer's yeast (a source of vitamin B)
- Choline, 100 mg three times daily (enhance estrogen synthesis)

Vitamins
- Vitamin A, 50,000 IU daily (enhances immune system)
- Vitamin B complex, 100 mg three times daily (promotes physiologic cell division and function and participates in hormone synthesis)
- Vitamin B_3 (niacin), 100 mg daily (promotes physiologic cell division and function and participates in hormone synthesis)
- Vitamin C, 5,000 to 20,000 mg daily in divided doses (anticancer agent)
- Vitamin E, 400 IU daily to begin, gradually increased to 1,000 IU daily (deficiency has been determined in breast cancer; participates in hormone synthesis and enhances immune system function)

Acupuncture

Acupuncture seems to benefit breast cancer patients significantly in relieving pain and improving arm movement following surgery and axillary lymphadenectomy (126). Despite improvements in antiemetic drug therapy, as many as 60% of patients treated with antineoplastic agents (chemotherapy) eventually experience nausea and vomiting (127). Based on scientific evidence, the National Institutes of Health Panel of Experts in Acupuncture released its consensus demonstrating the efficacy of acupuncture in the treatment of nausea and vomiting associated with chemotherapy (128).

Acupressure is recommended as therapy adjuvant to conventional antiemetic therapy for patients being treated with cytotoxic agents (chemotherapy). Application of an elastic wrist band with a stud over the acupuncture point P6 that is pressed regularly every 2 hours for 5 to 10 minutes will extend the effect of antiemetic drugs for 24 hours (129).

Finger acupressure seems to be beneficial in reducing nausea and vomiting associated with chemotherapy when applied bilaterally at P6 and ST36 acupressure points (130).

Electrical stimulation (10 Hz DC) at point P6 for 5 minutes before chemotherapy administration seems to be effective in preventing nausea and vomiting in 66% of patients (129). Both acupressure and electrical stimulation of acupuncture point P6 are awaiting clinical validation.

Pressure treatment for lymphedema also can improve outcome (131).

Group Support Therapy

Significant emotional distress occurs in approximately 80% of patients diagnosed with breast cancer. Mood disturbance, self-esteem, maladaptive coping responses, death-phobic feelings, anxiety, depression, fatigue, and emotional distress can all be significantly reduced with group psychotherapy (132,133). Group psychotherapy combined with hypnosis or self-hypnosis provides not only significant emotional support but also equips patients best in controlling pain sensation (134).

When breast cancer patients' own coping abilities are overstretched by the challenge of cancer, they rely on their "significant others" (partners, families, or friends). Providing a brief psychoeducational group program only for these significant others builds greater confidante support, greater marital satisfaction, and less mood disturbance (135).

Alternative Therapy

Alternative therapy is customarily used in conjunction with standard conventional therapy. Herbal remedies have been suggested for prophylactic use and for actual treatment of breast cancer.

Herbal Remedy

Camellia sinensis (green tea) has an active component of polyphenols that expresses inhibitory effects in carcinogenesis (136). Polyphenolic components also are present in fruits and vegetables and express antioxidants properties, which may reduce the risk for cancer (137). In a case con-

trol study, results indicated that increased consumption of green tea prior to clinical onset of breast cancer significantly improves stage I and II breast cancer outcome. The recommended daily dose of polyphenols is 300 to 400 mg. One cup of tea contains 80–106.6 mg of polyphenols (136).

Phragmites communis (reed herb) can be taken orally or by infusion and has been recommended for breast cancer. The recommended dose is 100 g of fresh foliage. Reed herb exhibits diuretic and diaphoretic effects (138). However, its proof of its effectiveness is lacking.

Homeopathy

Initial results from a randomized controlled study indicate that *belladonna* (7 cH dilution for 15–30 days following breast radiotherapy) provides statistically significant reduction of symptoms of radiodermatitis (skin discoloration, swelling, pain, and feeling of warmth). Neither chemotherapy nor hormonal therapy seems to interfere with belladonna's therapeutic effect (139).

REFERENCES

1. Association of Professors of Gynecology and Obstetrics (APGO). *Medical student educational objectives,* 7th ed. Washington, DC: 1997.
2. Council on Resident and Gynecology (CREOG). *Educational objectives core curriculum for residents in obstetrics and gynecology,* 5th ed. Washington, DC: CREOG, 1996.
3. American College of Obstetrician and Gynecologists (ACOG). Educational bulletin no. 158. Washington, DC: ACOG, 1991.
4. Templeman C, Hertweck SP. Breast disorders in the pediatric and adolescent patient. *Obstet Gynecol Clin North Am* 2000;27:19–34.
5. Cunha GR, Young P, Hom YK, et al. Elucidation of a role for stromal steroid hormone receptors in mammary gland growth and development using tissue recombinants. *J Mammary Gland Biol Neoplasia* 1997;2:393–402.
6. Hennighausen L. Molecular mechanisms of hormone controlled gene expression in the breast. *Mol Biol Rep* 1997;24:169–174.
7. Topper YJ, Freeman CS. Multiple hormone interactions in the developmental biology of the mammary gland. *Physiol Rev* 1980;60:1049–1106.
8. Kenney RD, Flipo JL, Black EB. Supernumerary nipples and renal anomalies. *Am J Dis Child* 1987;141:987–998.
9. Capraro VJ, Dewhurst CJ. Breast disorders in childhood and adolescence. *Clin Obstet Gynecol* 1975;18:25–50.
10. Kuzbari R, Deutinger M, Todoroff BP, et al. Surgical treatment of developmental asymmetry of the breast. Long term results. *Scand J Plast Reconstr Surg* 1993;27:203–207.
11. Sandsmark M, Amland PF, Samdal F, et al. Clinical results in 87 patients treated for asymmetrical breast. A follow-up study. *Scand J Plast Reconstr Surg* 1992;26:321–326.
12. Emans SJ, Laufer MR, Goldstein DP, eds. *Pediatric and adolescent gynecology,* 4th ed. Philadelphia: Lippincott-Raven, 1998.
13. Rees TD, Aston SJ. The tuberous breast. *Clin Plast Surg* 1976;3:339–347.
14. von Heimberg D, Exner K, Kruft S, et al. The tuberous breast

deformity: classification and treatment. *Br J Plast Surg* 1996;49: 339–345.

15. Kreipe RE, Lewand AG, Dukarm CP, et al. Outcome for patients with bulimia and breast hypertrophy after reduction mammaplasty. *Arch Pediatr Adolesc Med* 1997;151:176–180.

16. Greydanus DE, Parks DS, Farrell EG. Breast disorders in children and adolescents. *Pediatr Clin North Am* 1989;36:601–603.

17. Di Noto A, Pacheco BP, Vicala REA. Two cases of breast lymphoma mimicking juvenile hypertrophy. *J Pediatr Adolesc Gynecol* 1999;12:33–35.

18. Corriveau S, Jacobs SJ. Macromastia in adolescence. *Clin Plast Surg* 1990;17:151–160.

19. Page DL, Dupont WD. Indicators of increased breast cancer risk in human. *J Cell Biochem Suppl* 1992;16G:175–182.

20. London SJ, Connolly JL, Schnitt SJ, et al. A prospective study of benign breast disease and risk of breast cancer. *JAMA* 1992; 19;267:941–944.

21. Dupont WD, Page DL, Parl FF, et al. Long-term risk of breast cancer in women with fibroadenoma. *N Engl J Med* 1994;331: 10–15.

22. Tissier F, De Roquancourt A, Astier B, et al. Carcinoma arising within mammary fibroadenomas. A study of six patients. *Ann Pathol* 2000;20(2):110–114.

23. Foxcroft L, Evans E, Hirst C. Newly arising fibroadenomas in women aged 35 and over. *Aust N Z J Surg* 1998;68:419–422.

24. Greenberg R, Skornick Y, Kaplan O. Management of breast fibroadenomas. *J Gen Intern Med* 1998;13:540–645.

25. Diehl T, Kaplan DW. Breast masses in adolescent females. *J Adolesc Health Care* 1985;6:353–357.

26. Turbey WJ, Buntain WL, Dudgeon DL. The surgical management of pediatric breast masses. *Pediatrics* 1975;56:736–739.

27. Neinstein LS. Review of breast masses in adolescents. *Adolesc Pediatr Gynecol* 1994;7:119–129.

28. Kuhl CK. MRI of breast tumors. *Eur Radiol* 2000;10:46–58.

29. Dent DM, Cant PJ. Fibroadenoma. *World J Surg* 1989;13: 706–710.

30. Chhieng DC, Cangiarella JF, Waisman J, et al. Fine-needle aspiration cytology of spindle cell lesion of the breast. *Cancer* 1999; 25;87:359–371.

31. Kubista E. Diagnosis and therapy of fibrocystic breast disease. *Zentralbl Gynakol* 1990;112:1091–1096.

32. Harris JR, Henderson IC, Kellerman S, eds. *Breast disease.* Philadelphia: JB Lippincott, 1987.

33. Vorherr H. Fibrocystic breast disease: pathophysiology, pathomorphology, clinical picture and management. *Am J Obstet Gynecol* 1986;154:161–179.

34. Lunddin C, Mertens F. Cytogenetics of benign breast lesions. *Breast Cancer Res Treat* 1998;51:1–15.

35. Lubin F, Ron E, Wax Y. A case control study of caffeine-free diet on benign breast disease. *JAMA* 1985;253:2388–2392.

36. Drukker BH, deMendonca WC. Fibrocystic changes and fibrocystic disease of the breast. *Obstet Gynecol Clin North Am* 1987; 14:685–702.

37. Kossoff MB. Ultrasound of the breast. *World J Surg* 2000;24: 143–157.

38. Rieber A, Nussle K, Merkle E, et al. MR Mammography: influence of menstrual cycle on the dynamic contrast enhancement of fibrocystic disease. *Eur Radol* 1999;9:1107–1012.

39. Bedard YC, Pollett AF. Breast fine-needle aspiration. A comparison of ThinPrep and conventional smears. *Am J Clin Pathol* 1999:111:523–527.

40. Brenner RJ, Bein ME, Sarti DA, et al. Spontaneous regression of interval benign cyst of the breast. *Radiology* 1994;193: 365–368.

41. London RS, Sundarm GS, Goldstein PJ. Medical management of mammary dysplasia. *Obstet Gynecol* 1982;59:519–523.

42. Cox EB. Benign breast lesions and breast cancer. *Female Patient* 1986;11:52.

43. Maddox PR, Harrison BJ, Horobin JM, et al. A randomized controlled trial of medroxyprogesterone acetate in mastalgia. *Ann R Coll Surg Engl* 1990;72:71–76.

44. Dobrel A, Tobiassen T, Rasmussen T. Treatment of recurrent cyclical mastodynia in patients with fibrocystic breast disease. A double-blind placebo-controlled study—the Hjorring project. *Acta Obstet Gynecol Scand* 1984;123(suppl):177–184.

45. Gorins A, Perret F, Tournant B, et al. A French double-blind crossover study (danazol versus placebo) in the treatment of severe fibrocystic breast disease. *Eur J Gynaecol Oncol* 1984;5: 85–89.

46. Scott EB. Fibrocystic breast disease. *Am Fam Physician* 1987;36: 119–126.

47. Boyd NF, McGuire V, Shannon P, et al. Effect of a low-fat high-carbohydrate diet on symptoms of cyclic mastopathy. *Lancet* 19882:128–132.

48. Boyd NF, Greenberg C, Lockwood G, et al. Effects at two years of a lo-fat, high-carbohydrate diet on radiologic features of the breast: results from a randomized trial. Canadian Diet and Breast Cancer Prevention Study Group. *J Natl Cancer Inst* 1997; 89:488–496.

49. Hudson T. Women's encyclopedia of natural medicine. Lincolnwood, IL: Keats Publishing, 1999:89–96.

50. BeLieu RM. Mastodynia. *Obstet Gynecol Clin North Am* 1994; 21:461–477.

51. Ceffa GC, Chio C, Gandini G. Acupuncture in breast diseases. How, when and why. *Minerva Med* 1981;72:2239–2242.

52. Band PR, Deschamps M, Falardeau M, et al. Treatment of benign breast disease with vitamin A. *Prev Med* 1984;13: 549–554.

53. Ernster VL, Goodson WH 3rd, Hunt TK, et al. Vitamin E and benign breast "disease": a double-blind randomized clinical trial. *Surgery* 1985;97:490–494.

54. Meyer EC, Sommers DK, Reitz CJ, Mentis H. Vitamin E and benign breast disease. *Surgery* 1990;107:549–551.

55. Pye JSK, Mansel RE, Hughes LE. Clinical experience of drug treatment of mastalgia. *Lancet* 1985;2:373–377.

56. Nappi C, Affinito P, DiCarlo C, et al. Double-blind controlled trial of progesterone vaginal cream treatment for cyclical mastodynia in women with benign breast disease. *J Endocrinol Invest* 1992;15:801–806.

57. Holtzscherer A, Legros MS. *Pratique homeopathique en gynecologie.* Boiron, France: 1994.

58. Mechella M, DeCesare A, Lauretti MC. Cystic disease of the breast. Ten-year experience. *Minerva Chir* 1997;52:1327–1234.

59. Hughes LE, Bundred NJ. Breast macrocysts. *World J Surg* 1989; 13:711–714.

60. Haagensen DE Jr. Is cystic disease related to breast cancer? *Am J Surg Pathol* 1991;15:687–694.

61. Gorins A, Tournant B, Perret F, et al. Breast cysts. *Verh K Acad Geneeskd Bel* 1991;53:101–118.

62. Hurst JL, Mega JF, Hogg JP. Tamoxifen-induced regression of breast cyst. *Clin Imag* 1998;22:95–98.

63. Mallebre B, Ebert A, Perez-Canto A, et al. Cystosarcoma phyllodes of the breast. A retrospective analysis of 12 cases. *Geburtshilfe Frauenheilkd* 1996;56:35–40.

64. Vorherr H, Vorherr UF, Kutvirt DM, et al. Cystosarcoma phyllodes: epidemiology, pathohistology, pathology, diagnosis, therapy, and survival. *Arch Gynecol* 1985;236:173–181.

65. Amerson JR. Cystosarcoma phyllodes in adolescent females: a report of seven patients. *Ann Surg* 1970;171:849–853.

66. Holthouse DJ, Smith PA, Naunton-Morgan R, et al. Cystosarcoma phyllodes: the Western Australian experience. *Aust N Z J Surg* 1999;69:635–638.

67. Rajen PB, Croanor ML, Rosen PP. Cystosarcoma phyllodes in adolescent girls and young women: a study of 45 patients. *Am J Surg Pathol* 1998;22:64–69.

68. Moffat CJ, Pinder SE, Dixon AR, et al. Phyllodes tumors of the breast: a clinicopathological review of thirty-two cases. *Histopathology* 1995;27:205–218.

69. Zurrida S, Bartoli C, Galimberti V, et al. Which therapy for unexpected phyllodes tumor of the breast? *Eur J Cancer* 1992;28:654–657.

70. Obuchi N, Abe R, Kasai M, et al. Genesis and extension of intraductal papillomas of the breast–three dimensional morphological study. *Nippon Geka Gekkai Zasshi* 1983;84:500–507.

71. Oberman HA. Breast lesions in adolescent females. *Pathol Ann* 1979;1:175–201.

72. Neinstein LS, Atkinson J, Diament M. Prevalence and longitudinal study of breast mass in adolescents. *J Adolesc Health* 1993;14:277–281.

73. Kimijima I, Abe R, Ohuchi N, Akimoto M. Surgical treatment for intraductal proliferative lesions. *Nippon Geka Gekkai Zasshi* 1989;90:1406–1409.

74. Onnis GL, Chiarelli SM, DallaPalma P. Intraductal breast papilloma in an adolescent: case report. *Eur J Gynaecol Oncol* 1983;4:211–213.

75. Roy I, Meakins JL, Tremblay G. Giant intraductal papilloma of the breast: a case report. *J Surg Oncol* 1985;28:281–281.

76. Browning J, Bigrigg A, Taylor I. Symptomatic and incidental mammary duct ectasia. *J R Soc Med* 1986;79:715–716.

77. Naani MT, Bernabei P, Nocentini C, et al. Mammary duct ectasia: nosologic assessment. Features and echographic incidence. *Radiol Med (Torino)* 1993;85:748–752.

78. Petersen L, Graversen HP, Andersen JA, et al. The duct ectasia syndrome—an overlooked disease entity. *Ugeskr Laeger* 1993;155:1540–1545.

79. Miller SD, McCollough ML, DeNapoli T. Periductal mastitis. Masquerading as carcinoma. *Dermatol Surg* 1998;24:383–385.

80. Petersen L, Graversen HP, Andersen JA, et al. The duct ectasia syndrome. A prospective clinical study of patients with breast disease. *Ugeskr Laeger* 1993;155:1545–1549.

81. Ferrara JJ, Leveque J, Leveque J, et al. Nonsurgical management of breast infections in nonlactating women. A word of caution. *Am Surg* 1990;56:668–671.

82. O'Hara RJ, Dexter SP, Fox JN. Conservative management of infective mastitis and breast abscesses after ultrasonographic assessment. *Br J Surg* 1996;83:1413–1414.

83. Hook GW, Ikeda DM. Treatment of breast abscess with US-guided percutaneous needle drainage without indwelling catheter placement. *Radiology* 1999;213:579–582.

84. Crowe DJ, Helvie MA, Wilson TE. Breast infection. Mammographic and sonographic findings with clinical correlation. *Invest Radiol* 1995;30:582–587.

85. Tweeten SS, Rickman LS. Infectious complications of body piercing. *Clin Infect Dis* 1998;26:735–740.

86. Kesey JL, Bernstein L. Epidemiology and prevention of breast cancer. *Annu Rev Health* 1996;17:47–67.

87. Nohueria SM, Appling SE. Breast cancer: genetics, risks, and strategies. *Nurs Clin North Am* 2000;35:663–669.

88. Sondlik EJ. Breast cancer. Incidence, mortality, and survival. *Cancer* 1994;74(suppl):995–999.

89. Harper GR, Enlishbe BH. Prevention and screening for breast cancer. *Cancer Detect Prev* 1993;17:551–555.

90. Polednak AP. Epidemiology of breast cancer in Connecticut women. *Conn Med* 1999;63:7–16.

91. Donovan AJ. Bilateral breast cancer. *Surg Clin North Am* 1990;70:1141–1149.

92. Alberg AJ, Heltzlsouer KJ. Epidemiology, prevention, and early detection of breast cancer. *Curr Opin Oncol* 1997;9:505–511.

93. Gershoni-Baruch R, Dagan E, Fried G, et al. Significantly lower rates of BRCA 1/BRCA 2 founder mutation in Ashkenazi women with sporadic compared with familial early onset breast cancer. *Eur J Cancer* 2000;36:983–986.

94. Verhoog LC, Brekelmans CT, Seynaeve C, et al. Contralateral breast risk in influenced by the age at onset in BRCA 1–associated breast cancer. *Br J Cancer* 2000;83:384–386.

95. The American Joint Committee on Cancer. *The manual for staging of cancer*, 4th ed. Philadelphia: JB Lippincott, 1992.

96. Johnson N, Soot L, Nelson J, et al. Sentinel node biopsy and internal mammary lymphatic mapping in breast cancer. *Am J Surg* 2000;179:386–388.

97. Simmons RM, Osborne MP. The evaluation of high risk and pre-invasive breast lesions and the decision process for follow up and surgical intervention. *Surg Oncol* 1999;8:55–65.

98. Winchester DJ, Menck HR, Winchester DP. National treatments trends for ductal carcinoma *in situ*. *Arch Surg* 1997;132:660–665.

99. Delaney G, Ung O, Cahill S, et al. Ductal carcinoma *in situ*. Part 2: Treatment. *Aust N Z J Surg* 1997;67:157–165.

100. Gump FE, Kinne D, Schartz GF. Current treatment for lobular carcinoma *in situ*. *Ann Surg Oncol* 1998;5:33–36.

101. Gump FE. Lobular carcinoma *in situ* 9LCIS): pathology and treatment. *J Cell Biochem Suppl* 1993;17G:53–58.

102. Frykberg ER, Bland KI. *In situ* breast carcinoma. *Adv Surg* 1993;26:29–72.

103. Mosny DS. Surgical therapy strategies in carcinoma in of the breast. *Schwiez Rundsch Med Prax* 1998;87:516–519.

104. Frykberg ER, Bland KI. Management of *in situ* and minimally invasive breast carcinoma. *World J Surg* 1994;18(1):45–57.

105. Prasad ML, Osborne MP, Hoda SA. Observations on the histologic diagnosis of microinvasive carcinoma of the breast. *Anat Pathol* 1998;3:209–232.

106. Morris DA, Morris RD, Wilson JF, et al. Breast-conserving therapy vs mastectomy in early-stage barest cancer: a meta-analysis of 10-year survival. *Cancer J Sci Am* 1997;3:6–12.

107. Straus K, Lichter A, Lippman M, et al. Results of the National Cancer Institute early breast cancer trial. *J Natl Cancer Inst Monogr* 1992;11:27–32.

108. Fisher B, Bauer M, Margolese R, et al. Five-year results of a randomized clinical trial comparing total mastectomy and segmental mastectomy with or without radiation in the treatment of breast cancer. *N Engl J Med* 1985;312:665–673.

109. Mamounas EP, Fisher B. Preoperative chemotherapy for operable breast cancer. *Cancer Treat Res* 2000;103:137–155.

110. Fisher B, Redmond C, Poisson R, et al. Eight-year results of a randomized clinical trial comparing total mastectomy and lumpectomy with or without irradiation in the treatment of breast cancer. *N Engl J Med* 1989;320:822–828.

111. Lichter AS, Lippman ME, Danforth DN Jr, et al. Mastectomy versus breast-conserving therapy in the treatment of stage I and II carcinoma of the breast: a randomized trial at the National Cancer Institute. *J Clin Oncol* 1992;10:976–983.

112. Caffo O, Cazzolli D, Scalet A, et al. Current adjuvant chemotherapy and immediate breast reconstruction with skin expanders after mastectomy for breast cancer. *Breast Cancer Res Treat* 2000;60:267–275.

113. Ashikari R, Jun MY, Farrow JH. Breast carcinoma in children and adolescents. *Clin Bull* 1977;7:55–62.

114. Greer S. Mind-body research in psychooncology. *Adv Mind Body Med* 1999;15:236–244.

115. Kantor DE, Houldin A. Breast cancer in older women: treat-

ment, psychosocial effects, interventions, and outcomes. *J Gerontol Nurs* 1999;19–25:54–55.

116. Adler SR, Fosket JR. Disclosing complementary and alternative medicine use in the medical encounter: a qualitative study in women with breast cancer. *J Fam Pract* 1999;48:453–458.

117. Gray RE, Fitch M, Saunders PR, et al. Complementary health practitioners' attitudes, practices and knowledge related to women's cancers. *Cancer Prev Control* 1999;3:77–82.

118. Gotay CC, Dumitriu D. Health food store recommendations for breast cancer patients. *Arch Fam Med* 2000;9:629–698.

119. Burstein HJ, Gelber S, Guadgnoli E, et al. Use of alternative medicine by women with early-stage breast cancer. *N Engl J Med* 1999;340:1733–1739.

120. Eichholtzer M. Nutrition and cancer. *Ther Umsch* 2000;57:146–151.

121. Fuchs CS, Stampfer MJ, Colditz GA, et al. Alcohol consumption and mortality among women. *N Engl J Med* 1995;332:1245–1250.

122. Snyderwine EG. Diet and mammary gland carcinogenesis. *Rec Results Cancer Res* 1998;152:3–10.

123. Pujol P, Galtier-Dereure F, Bringer J. Obesity and breast cancer risk. *Hum Reprod* 1997;12(1):116–125.

124. Newman V, Rock CL, Faerber S, et al. Dietary supplement use by women at risk for breast cancer recurrence. The Women's Healthy Eating and Living Study Group. *J Am Diet Assoc* 1998;98:285–292.

125. Balch JF, Blach PA. *Prescription for nutritional healing,* 2nd ed. Garden City Park, NY: Avery, 1997:160–164.

126. He JP, Friedrich M, Ertan AK, et al. Pain-relief and movement by acupuncture after ablation and axillary lymphadenectomy in patients with mammary cancer. *Clin Exp Obstet Gynecol* 1999;26:81–84.

127. King CR. Nonpharmacologic management of chemotherapy-induced nausea and vomiting. *Oncol Nurs Forum* 1997;24(suppl):41–48.

128. NIH consensus conference. Acupuncture. *JAMA* 1998;4:280:1518–1524.

129. Dundee JW, Yang J. Prolongation of the antiemetic action of P6 acupuncture by acupuncture in patients having cancer chemotherapy. *J R Soc Med* 1990;83:360–362.

130. Dibble SL, Chapman J, Mack KA, Shih AS. Acupressure for nausea: results of a pilot study. *Oncol Nurs Forum* 2000;27:41–47.

131. Jacobson JS, Workman SB, Kronenberg F. Research on complementary/alternative medicine for patients with breast cancer: a review of biomedical literature. *J Clin Oncol* 2000;18:668–683.

132. Spiegl D, Bloom JR, Yalom I. Group support for patients with metastatic cancer. A randomized outcome study. *Arch Gen Psychiatry* 1981;38:527–533.

133. Spiegel D, Morrow GR, Classen C, et al. Group psychotherapy for recently diagnosed breast cancer patients: a multicenter feasibility study. *Psychooncology* 1999;8:482–493.

134. Spiegel D, Bloom JR. Group therapy and hypnosis reduce metastatic breast carcinoma pain. *Psychosom Med* 1983;45:333–339.

135. Bultz BD, Speca M, Brasher PM, et al. A randomized controlled trial of a brief psychoeducational support group for partners of early stage breast cancer patients. *Psychooncology* 2000;9:303–313.

136. Nakachi K, Suemasu K, Suga K, et al. Influence of drinking green tea on breast cancer malignancy among Japanese patients. *Jpn J Cancer Res* 1998;89:254–261.

137. Ahmad N, Mukhtar H. Green tea polyphenols and cancer: biologic mechanism and practical implications. *Nutr Rev* 1999;57:78–83.

138. *PDR for herbal medicine,* 2nd ed. Montvale, NJ: Medical Economics Company, 2000:639.

139. Balzarini A, Felisi E, Martini A, et al. Efficacy of homeopathic treatment of skin reactions during radiotherapy for breast cancer: a randomized, double-blind clinical trial. *Br Homeopath J* 2000;89:8–12.

28

APPROACH TO THE PATIENT'S APPROACH: CONTRACEPTIVES AND SEXUALITY

EDUCATIONAL OBJECTIVES

Medical Students (1) *APGO Objective No. 1–8*	*Residents in Obstetrics/Gynecology(2)* *CREOG Objectives*	*Practitioners (3)* *ACOG Recommendations*
Gynecologic history	Professional growth and development	Values, morals, and ethics
Examination	Ethics	Ethical principles:
Pap smear and culture	Communication skills	autonomy
Diagnosis and management plan	Information management	beneficence
Personal interaction and	Continuing medical education	justice
communication skills	Stress management	Ethical concepts:
Legal issues in gynecology	History	informed consent
Ethics in gynecology	Diagnostic studies and diagnosis	honesty
Preventive care and health	Patient education and consultation	confidentiality
maintenance	Screening	Decision-making
		Physician–patient
		Relationship with third
		parties
		Guidelines for decision
		making

PATIENT APPROACH

Communication Skill

Establishing a personal/professional relationship with a patient is essential in any medical practice; yet, gynecology requires developing an extraordinary skill in this area due to the intimacy of the specialty itself. Practitioners must earn a patients' trust. They must present themselves as knowledgeable, honest, sympathetic and they must be good listeners. Individualizing a patient's needs requires not only the ability to recognize different maturity levels (early, middle, and late adolescent, reproductive, menopausal, and postmenopausal periods), but also the ability to recognize the varying capacity of patients to understand and to reason. Physical maturity and cognitive maturation are not always concurrent; to some degree they may develop independent of one another. Nevertheless, the differences in the cognitive maturation process can be broadly categorized as follows (4).

The early adolescent period (11–14 years) is a puberty phase that is associated with rapid body image changes and the onset of menarche. At this particular stage, the cognitive ability of adolescent girls to predict the consequences of their actions has not yet developed. These patients may be self-absorbed and intensely preoccupied with their physical appearance, body image, and personal feelings and thoughts. They may be moody and opinionated, with the issue of sexuality dominating their thoughts.

Practitioners must develop the skill to cope with the specialized demands of this age group, especially regarding issues of sexuality, addressing pubertal abnormalities, and communicating with patients on the appropriate intellectual level. Most adolescents in this age group are troubled by physical developmental differences; therefore, reassurance is a necessary strategic treatment tool. Practitioners must develop the ability to discern an individual patient's ability to reason. They must also be able to communicate effectively with the patient's parents regarding the adolescent's associated emotional lability, indecisive behavior (alternately childish and adult), and the need for privacy, personal attention, and acceptance. Serious health problems should be clearly conveyed to the patient, and treatment options shared with parents or guardians only when the definitive diagnosis has been reached.

Self-abuse is a difficult subject, and adolescents often reject reasonable advice. For example, to assert that cigarette smoking is a health hazard may be a less effective deterrent than mentioning that smokers carry the smell on their hair, skin, and clothes.

The middle adolescent period (age 15-17 years) is characterized by the following attributes (4):

- Comfort level with changed body image is attained.
- Friends and friendship take precedence over self-involvement.
- Personal appearance, with particular attention to clothes and makeup, is emphasized.
- First sexual activity by most adolescent girls occurs in this period.
- Experimentation with alcohol, drugs, and smoking is frequently observed.

Taking these developmental aspects of adolescence into account is paramount for successful counseling of this group. A tactful approach to inquiry regarding the intimate aspects of the adolescent girl's life is essential. Practitioners must become skilled in counseling girls of this age regarding dangerous social interactions, including those of a sexual nature. It is crucial to acknowledge that girls in this group are still developing their abstract reasoning skills.

The late adolescent period (18–21 years) is characterized as follows (4):

- Abstract reasoning skills become more developed.
- Emotional intimacy of a more mature nature is expressed in relationships.
- Identity issues focus more on personal and vocational options.
- Feelings of ambiguous sexual orientation can occur in this period, with homosexual thoughts. Experiences may lead to emotional disorders such as anxiety, eating disorders, alcohol abuse, or practicing unsafe sex.

In this late adolescent period, young women may seek the support and guidance of a skilled practitioner more than they did in the preceding two stages, when family was the primary support mechanism.

To develop the appropriate skills to effectively manage disorders in this adolescent group, practitioners must understand the basic changes associated with age, maturity, and cognitive levels. They must have the fundamental clinical knowledge, as well as natural compassion, honesty and discretion. The practitioner must also have superior communication skills in order to cope not only with the physical and emotional aspects of the adolescent's life, but also with the more intimate aspects; including friendships, school performance, substance abuse, sexuality, and pregnancy. Practitioners must approach patients of this age in a nonjudgmental, non-patronizing, and non-moralizing way in order to be effective.

For any age group, the following skills are helpful to any clinician:

- Verbal expression should be appropriate for the patient's age, intellectual capacity, educational level, and social background.
- Patient education should be conveyed by a compassionate, cooperative, trustful practitioner with an implacable bedside manner. Effective communication and interpersonal skills are an integral part of treatment, and may be supported by clinical publications, illustrations, and audiovisual materials.

Ethics

Basic ethical concepts (autonomy, beneficence, justice, and futility) should be adapted to the practice of gynecology. These ethical principles should be applied with regard to informed consent, informative management within established practice norms, clinical research, and dispensing medical advice. The practitioner's attitude of availability and observation of confidentiality in patient interactions enhance a patient's emotional comfort and physical well being. An integral part of medical ethics for any medical practitioner is to develop a lifelong habit of self-education, self-assessment, and sharing with patients, their families, and other health-providers.

Gynecologic History

The patient's gynecologic history should be obtained using a structured approach that incorporates the following elements:

- Chief complaint or reason for seeing a practitioner.
- Menstrual history should include age of menarche, frequency (interval between the first day of menses and the first day of the next menstrual flow), duration, estimated amount, and last menstrual period. The presence of clots (smaller than dime is acceptable as normal), irregularity of menses and its potential relationship to coitus, and sexual habits should be established. A more detailed description of menstrual history is provided in Chapter 9.

- Current and past contraceptive method and reproductive plans.
- Number of pregnancies (G), abortions, preterm deliveries, term deliveries, and number of children alive (P), is expressed as; GoP0000.
- Infertility.
- Diethylstilbestrol exposure.
- Menopause symptoms and their management.
- Postmenopausal endometrial bleeding.
- Sexual life history and form of sexual practice (see also the later section on Sexual History Taking).
- Sexual abuse/assault.
- History of genital tract disorders, and its medical or surgical treatment.
- Sexually transmitted diseases and other pelvic inflammatory diseases.
- Breast disorders or mass including biopsy and family history of cancer
- Adjacent organs disorders such as urinary tract or lower intestinal tract
- Family medical history with particular attention to female members of immediate family.
- Current and past medication
- Allergy
- Review of central nervous system, gastrointestinal system, cardiovascular system, endocrine and metabolic systems, and urinary system.
- Social history (occupation, marital status, exercise, hobbies, alcohol, tobacco and or drug use).

The elements of the gynecologic medical history are rather straightforward, but because this is a sensitive topic for adolescent patients, excellent communication skills are needed. Such skills can be developed by observing the following (4,5):

- Initiate medical history from a non-treatment and general subject standpoint.
- Establish school performance (poor performance lowers self-esteem and may indicate high-risk health behaviors).
- Determine the patient's self-image (an injured self-image often coexists with adolescent depression and eating disorders such as anorexia and bulimia).
- Identify other symptoms of depression, such as decreased appetite, sleeping disorder, feelings of sadness with a tendency to cry easily, malaise, fatigue, headaches, and coexistent abdominopelvic disorders. At any given time, about 3%–5% of adolescent girls are affected by depression, and approximately 13%–18% of all adolescents will experience a severe depressive episode (6).
- Determine the presence or absence of suicidal feelings (suicidal intent constitutes immediate psychiatric referral).
- Potential substance use or abuse is best identified by indirect inquiry about her friends being involved in this activity followed by direct questioning of the patient. Type and amount of substance used and potential referral to a rehabilitation program should be discussed, if indicated.

- Discussing sexual activity is difficult, especially that involving high-risk behavior (unsafe sex practice). An adolescent patient can be passively involved in high-risk sexual activity through the high-risk behavior of a sexual partner.
- Determine contraceptive use.
- Suspected physical, sexual, or mental abuse must be reported, even though it involves (an acceptable) breach of confidentiality.

Physical Examination

Gynecology is a form of primary care for the female population and requires knowledge gained in both a general physical examination and a bimanual pelvic examination.

The *general physical examination* should include the following elements:

- *Weight and height* are taken, and body mass index (BMI) is calculated in kg/m^2.
- *General appearance* (facial expression and skin color; posture; warm, dry hands; good visual contact).
- *Vital signs* determine stable versus medically unstable status (pulse, blood pressure, body temperature, and respiratory rate).
- *Skin* evaluation.
- *Musculoskeletal system evaluation* should be performed, with particular attention to the presence of scoliosis (particularly in adolescents), fibromyalgia, fibrositis, tendonitis, and septic joints, which can be associated with gonorrhea.
- The *back* should be examined for mobility, bending limitations, and deformities, and for tenderness at the costovertebral angle.
- *Head, eyes, ears, nose, and throat* examination should be routine.
- *Neck* assessment should include visual inspection and palpation of the thyroid gland, lymph nodes, and carotid pulses.
- *Heart evaluation* includes percussion and auscultation to determine size, rhythm, and sound (murmurs).
- *Lung examination* is routinely performed by percussion and auscultation.
- *Breast and axilla examination* is described in great detail in Chapter 27.
- *Abdominal evaluation* is performed to establish general appearance (scaphoid, flat, obese, or distended) and any noticeable abnormality.
    Percussion can delineate size, organ boundaries, or the presence of a solid mass; ascites are identified by dullness on percussion. Increasing tympany may suggest intestinal obstruction.
    Auscultation may assist in detecting hypoactive or silent abdomen (ileus) or hyperactive intestinal peristaltic rushes. Bruits may indicate abdominal aneurysms.

Palpation is either superficial *or* deep in nature. It can identify hepato- or splenomegaly, an abdominal mass, ascites (valve sensation from intraabdominal fluid and shifting dullness on percussion), and tenderness or rebound tenderness.

Pelvic examination should include external genital examination, speculum examination, internal-external vaginal examination, and rectal bimanual examination. Drapes should cover both of the patient's legs and her abdominal areas, only the perineal-perianal area should be exposed. Elevating the patient's upper body to approximately 30 degrees will allow eye contact between the practitioner and patient. A patient's very first pelvic examination can be a traumatic experience. Therefore, the components of the examination should be explained in detail beforehand, and preparation may include supporting visual material such as illustrations and three-dimensional pelvic models.

The *external genital* examination should include visual inspection and palpation on all patients. The clinician can *visually inspect* the mons pubis (hair and skin), clitoral hood, labia majora, perineum, anal area, labia minora, urethral meatus and Skene glands, and Bartholin glands. The adolescent girl's developmental stage (Tanner stage) should be determined and any abnormalities noted (labial hypertrophy >5 cm from midline or microperforate or septate hymen may cause pathology; this topic is addressed in greater detail in Chapter 2). Pelvic-perineal muscle relaxation and contraction should be observed with the patient' squeezing and relaxing those muscles. The vaginal wall is inspected for descent or prolapse with the patient bearing down (imitating bowel movement). More anatomic details of the external genitalia and perianal area and their abnormalities are described in Chapters 13 and 26.

Palpation of the external genitalia should include physical palpation as well as cold or gentle needle touch to assess peripheral innervation integrity.

Speculum examination requires greater care and sensitivity when performed in adolescent patients. Several types of vaginal speculum are available, in various sizes, shapes, and designs, and are made of either plastic (disposable) or metal (undisposable).

Pediatric specula , such as a Graves speculum, are commonly used and recommended for examination of young girls.

A Pederson 2.5 × 9 cm *adolescent speculum* is well tolerated by sexually active adolescent patients, and a Huffman speculum is appropriate for virginal girls 10 years or older.

Adult specula are available in several sizes, and the majority of parous patients can be examined with a medium, Graves, or Pederson speculum. Postmenopausal women and those who exhibit atrophy also can be examined with adolescent specula.

Insertion of a speculum begins with warming and moistening or lubricating the speculum. Upon separation of the labia, the speculum is gently introduced and advanced with both blades closed until the cervix is visualized. Inspection of the cervix is initiated by observing the cervical lips, ectocervix, and external os of the cervical canal. Any abnormality should be noted and recorded. The vaginal fornices and walls also can be inspected by rotating and pulling back the speculum simultaneously. Cervicovaginal cytology samples, cervical cultures, and vaginal tissue can be obtained for microscopic examination with 0.9% sodium chloride (trichomonas or clue cells) or 10% potassium chloride (yeast infections). Cervicovaginal abnormalities and the Papanicolaou (Pap) smear technique are discussed in Chapters 15 and 17.

Bimanual pelvic examination is routinely performed with two fingers (the index and middle fingers inserted intravaginally). However, only one finger is used in patients with vaginal atrophy or stenosis, or in sexually inactive adolescent girls. The external hand (abdominal hand) is laid flat on the suprapubic area, and is used to bring the pelvic organs close to the internal examining hand. The following features are examined and recorded:

- Consistency of the *vaginal canal* and wall surface is determined. The internal hand (vaginal hand) examines the vaginal fornices for depth and consistency.
- Presence or absence of *the cervix* , its position in relation to the longitudinal axis of the vagina, and its alignment (in the posterior or anterior fornix) within the vaginal pool should be determined. The shape, consistency (soft or firm), mobility, and tenderness also should be established.
- *The uterus* is evaluated and the following parameters recorded:
  Size is reported as expected normal size or enlarged, and compared to gestational age accordingly.
  Shape can be normal (pear shaped), globular or irregular, symmetric or asymmetric.
  Consistency can be normal, soft, or firm.
  Position can be mid-position, antero- or retro–flexed, or antero- or retro–verted.
  Location can be midline or shifted to the right or left lower abdominal quadrant.
  Adnexa (ovarian and fallopian tube structure together) are situated on both sides of the uterus. Palpable ovaries or impalpable ovaries unilaterally or bilaterally should be noted (right side is more frequently palpable than left). Consistency, tenderness, and mobility also should be determined. Within 2 years of a postmenopausal period, the ovary should be unpalpable bilaterally.

Intervals of Gynecologic Screening Evaluation

The following clinical approach for gynecologic care is generally accepted:

- Pap smear should be obtained on an annual basis from the onset of sexual activity or the age of 18 years, for 3

TABLE 28.1. IMMUNIZATION PROGRAM

Immunization Type	Intervals
Tetanus-diphtheria booster vaccine	One dose between age 14 and 16 years
Influenza vaccine	Annually from age 65 years or if medically indicated otherwise
Pneumococcal vaccine	From age of 19 to 64 years with medical condition predisposing for pneumococcal infection
Measles, mumps, rubella	The absence of immunity evidence in all women of reproductive age
Hepatitis B vaccine	All women associated with professional exposure

consecutive years. If Pap smears are negative and patients are over 19 years of age, examination every 3 years is sufficient.

- Physical examination should be performed annually with or without the necessary blood test.
- Lipid profile every 5 years from age 19 to 64 years and every 3 to 4 years from age 65 years.
- Thyroid-stimulating hormone every 3 to 5 years after age 65 years.
- Mammography is recommended from age 40 years every other year, from age 50 years annually.
- Colon screening with colonoscopy every 3 to 5 years after age 50 years.

Immunization Recommendation

Immunization recommendation in gynecologic practice is presented in Table 28.1.

CONTRACEPTIVE METHODS AND STERILIZATION

Contraception is defined as voluntary pregnancy prevention, and the female partner is more likely to use contraception than the male partner. In the United States the pregnancy rate in 1996 was 104 pregnancies per 1,000 women 15 to 44 years of age, 9% lower than in 1990 (115.6/1,000). Since 1990 rates have decreased further:

- 8% for live birth
- 16% for induced abortion
- 4% for fetal losses

The teenage (15–19 years) pregnancy rate has declined considerably from 1990 and has been reported to be 98.7 per 1,000 women in 1996. Among factors contributing to this reduction are decreased sexual activity, increased condom use, and the adoption of injectable and implant contraceptives.

Barrier Methods

Barrier methods can be either of the *mechanical* or chemical type. Mechanical barriers can take the following forms:

Male condom use has increased in the past decade owing to its conferred protection from sexually transmitted diseases (STDs), including human immunodeficiency virus (HIV). Latex condoms are the most popular, and when used properly, failure rates are estimated to be approximately 1 to 5 per 100 women-years. About 2% of condoms can rupture, so it is advisable to use them in combination with vaginal spermicides.

Female condoms are latex or polyurethane vaginal pouches. They differ from male condoms by covering not only vaginal walls but also part of the vulvoperineal area. Female condoms provide the same pregnancy protection as male condoms, and provide additional vulvar STD protection. They also give women the contraceptive option ordinarily available only to men.

Diaphragm failure ranges from 2 to 15 instances per 100 woman-years. Diaphragms are differentiated from each other by different rim styles (arching spring, coil, and flat), and rim diameter range from 50 to 150 mm. The following points should be considered when fitting a patient for a diaphragm:

- It should cover the cervix.
- Posteriorly, the leading edge of the diaphragm should rest in the posterior vaginal fornix.
- Anteriorly, one or two fingers should fit between the proximal surface of the symphysis pubis and edge of the diaphragm.
- The patient must learn the proper position of the diaphragm.

The following principles should be applied for effective diaphragm use:

- Proper insertion and positioning.
- Intravaginal application of spermicides.
- Each consecutive act of coitus requires new application of spermicides without removing the diaphragm.
- The diaphragm should be left intravaginally for a minimum of 6 hours following intercourse.

The effectiveness of *cervical caps* is compatible with that of diaphragms. Because cervical caps are difficult to insert, they are not commonly used (the Femcap is relatively easier to fit and insert). They should be left in place for at least 6 hours following coitus. When inserted properly, a cervical cap can remain in place for several days. However, it must be removed during menses and can produce an offensive smell with time. Cervical caps are manufactured in four sizes, and spermicides do not have to be used with them.

The *vaginal sponge* is a dimpled polyurethane disk saturated with nonoxynol-9 spermicide. Its effectiveness is similar to that of chemical barriers. It is inserted into the vagina and left in the proximity of the cervix. It can be inserted up to 24 hours preceding coitus and can remain within the vagina for 24 hours after sexual intercourse.

Chemical barriers or spermicides are vaginal surface active and nontoxic, and are predominantly composed of nonoxynol-9 spermicide. The mechanism of action is to immobilize sperm. Over-the-counter products are offered in the form of creams, jellies, aerosol foams, foaming tablets, and vaginal suppositories. These agents exhibit not only spermicidal effects, but are also considered to be microbicidal agents, conferring some protection from STDs. No evidence is present that spermicides may cause congenital anomalies (8,9). Propranolol and 3β-sympathomimetic antagonists also demonstrate spermicidal properties, but clinical data are scarcely available.

Compliance and proper applications are essential. When sexual intercourse is repeated more than 1 hour after initial coitus, new application of a fresh agent is required regardless of other barrier methods used with spermicides. Approximately 4% of users of chemical contraceptives exhibit allergic reactions.

Medical Contraceptives

Medical contraceptives are a very effective form of birth control, if taken correctly and consistently.

The oral contraceptive (OC) pill or birth control pill is composed of synthetic estrogen (ethinyl estradiol or mestranol) and progestin (norethindrone, norethindrone acetate, ethynodiol diacetate, norethynodrel, norgestrel, levonorgestrel, desogestrel, or norgestimate). All progestins used in OC pills are 19-nortestosterone derivatives. Initially, monophasic (or fixed-dose or fixed-ratio) progestin/estrogen was developed. Today the progestin: estrogen ratio is often expressed as 1:20, 1:30, 1:35, or 1/50. The same proportion doses of estrogen and progestin components are taken for 21 consecutive days.

Phased pills are characterized by a varying progestin: estrogen ratio, which changes over the 21-day cycle. Biphasic combinations have two different progestin: estrogen ratios, and triphasic combinations have three different ratios that gradually decrease the total progestin dose (12%–20%) over the 21-day course. Multiphasic (biphasic or triphasic) OC pills are replacing monophasic pills. The fundamental concept in multiphasic composition of pills is to reduce the total dose of synthetic steroids being administered and to maintain contraceptive efficacy, decrease undesirable side effects, and control the cycle. Research theoretical data postulate that multiphasic formulations may be the safest among OC pills.

Dosing of the estrogen and progestin components in OC pills varies. *The 20-μg formulation* is a new low-dose product. The newest (Mircette) 21-day pill is a combination of 20 μg of ethinyl estradiol and 0.15 mg desogestrel followed by a 2-day pill-free interval, then 5 days of 10 μg of ethinyl estradiol. This OC formula failure rate is estimated to be 1.02 pregnancies per 100 woman-years (10).

The *30-, 35-, or 50-μg formulations* are composed of either ethinyl estradiol or mestranol (eventually metabolized to ethinyl estradiol); both express almost equal clinical potency. The progestin component varies from 0.15 to 1 μg. A 50-μg pill is the highest estrogen dose available in the United States.

The *mechanism of action* of oral contraceptive pills, regardless of formulation, is to suppress secretion with an inhibiting mid-cycle gonadotropin surge from the pituitary gland, caused by the inability of the pituitary to respond to the hypothalamic gonadotropin-releasing hormone. Consequently, the ovarian synthesis of estrogens and progesterone is transitionally eliminated (the suppressed ovarian steroid synthesis is restored spontaneously shortly after OC discontinuation). Endometrial atrophy and out-of-phase and endosalpinx function are induced. OC pills make the cervical mucus thick, viscid, dry, and impenetrable by sperm. However, OC pills do not induce a hypoestrogenic state. OC serum estrogen levels are similar to serum estrogen levels observed in the natural early follicular phase of the menstrual cycle (11). OC pills not only induce alterations in reproductive capacities, but also influence metabolic changes that directly relate to the estrogen or progestin component.

Synthetic estrogen may transitionally influence the following metabolic processes and symptoms (normalization occurs upon OC discontinuation):

■ Increasing the risk of thromboembolic disorders due to elevation of liver synthesis of a clotting factor such as fibrinogen, factor VII, or factor X
■ Increasing the risk of blood hypertension by increasing hepatic production of angiotensinogen
■ Increasing symptoms of nausea, depression, breast tenderness, and fluid retention

Synthetic progestins can be responsible for the following potential metabolic alterations or symptoms:

■ Influencing glucose metabolism may lead to hyperglycemia. This metabolic phenomenon is dose related.
■ Increasing weight (anabolic effect), acne, amenorrhea.

Both estrogen and progestin may affect the following:

■ *Lipid metabolism,* in which the estrogen component exhibits a beneficial effect by increasing high-density lipoprotein cholesterol (HDL-C) and by decreasing low-density lipoprotein cholesterol (LDL-C). On the other hand, the progestin component decreases HDL-C and increases LDL-C. Low-dose OC pills induce a negligible effect in this regard.
■ *Breakthrough bleeding* results from either a too-low dose of estrogen or a too-high dose of progestin.
■ *Amenorrhea* is induced by the same causes as presented in breakthrough bleeding, and OC pills with a higher estrogen formulation can treat both conditions.

- OC pills may induce *headaches*, but it is an uncommon event. Nonvascular, non-migraine-type headaches will not get worse while taking OC pills. If headache exacerbation occurs, OC pill discontinuation and headache evaluation is warranted. Symptoms of migraine-type headaches may get worse (50%), be unchanged (35%), or improve (15%). If an asymptomatic patient develops headaches associated with OC pills, OC pills should be discontinued, and clinical investigation of the headaches is indicated. Patients with migraines without auras and non-migraine headaches can probably safely use low-dose OC pills (e.g., 20-µg pills) (12).
- *Chloasma* (increased pigmentation of the face and other skin areas) is more accentuated with sunshine exposure and usually takes a long time to normalize upon discontinuation of OC pills.
- *Gallbladder disease* risk is significantly reduced by low-dose OC pills.
- *Cardiovascular disease* is relevant in cigarette-smoking women over 35 years of age (may predispose to myocardial infarction). Nonsmoking women may continue using of low-dose of OC pills until they have a menopausal period (13).
- Normotensive, nonsmoking women under 35 years of age taking low-dose OC pills are not at increased risk of either hemorrhagic or ischemic *stroke* (14).
- The rate of *thromboembolic disease* is estimated at 10 to 15 nonfatal venous thromboses per 100,000 OC pill users. The rate among OC nonusers is about 4 cases per 100,000. Thromboembolic disease among OC pill users is dose related; therefore, reducing the dose of both components may decrease the risk (15). Patients who take anticoagulants such as warfarin sodium can benefit from OC pills because this contraceptive method significantly reduces the risk of ovarian hemorrhage at the time of ovulation. Preventing pregnancy via OC pills in women on anticoagulant medication also confers protection against a teratogenic warfarin effect on a developing fetus as well as fetal intracranial bleeding.

The side effects of OC pills are listed as follows:

- *Breast cancer* risk (16):
  Duration of use demonstrates minimal influence.
  Current users have an increased relative risk of 1.24, and the risk reaches 1.0 10 years after OC pills have been discontinued.
  Users under 20 years of age have an increased relative risk of 1.59, but this risk vanishes 5 years after OC pills have been discontinued.
  Users who stop using the OC pill at 25 years of age have an increased risk of developing breast cancer at 35 years of age (1 per 10,000 users). By 45 years of age, the risk in these women declines to that of the general population. Users who stop using the OC pill at 40 years of age have an increased risk of

developing breast cancer at the age of 50 years (1 per 526), but that risk decreases by the age of 60 years (1 per 714).
- OC pill use does not increase the risk of developing *cervical cancer*, despite the controversy surrounding this subject (17).
- *Endometrial cancer* incidence is reduced by 50% when OC pills are used for at least 1 year. This protective effect lasts at least 10 years and is even greater among nulliparous than parous women (17).
- *Ovarian cancer* risk is reduced by OC pills, particularly epithelial type cancer. The protective effect of OC is directly related to the duration of use and extends for 10 years following 6 months of use (17).
- *Hepatocellular adenoma* is a benign condition and can be induced by OC pills. The incidence is estimated to be 1 in 30,000 to 250,000 users, and the incidence increases with the duration of use. Hepatocellular adenoma usually regresses spontaneously after discontinuation of OC pills (17).

Contraindications to OC pills include the following:

- Age over 30 years and cigarette smoking
- Active liver disease (e.g., hepatitis)
- Coronary artery disease or history of congestive heart failure
- Cerebrovascular disease
- Current use of rifampin
- Diabetes mellitus with vascular complications
- Estrogen-dependent malignancy (breast and endometrium) or undiagnosed but suspected malignancy
- History of coagulopathy, deep vein thrombosis, or pulmonary embolism
- Hypertensive disease, either uncontrolled or untreated [some authorities suggest that a low-dose pill (20 µg) can be offered, but caution should be exercised]
- Intestinal malabsorption syndrome
- Pituitary prolactinoma
- Suspected or known pregnancy
- Undiagnosed abnormal genital bleeding
- Systemic lupus erythematosus

There is no significant increased risk of congenital anomalies if OC pills are taken during an initial stage of pregnancy. Fertility after discontinuation of oral contraceptive is delayed and varies from patient to patient, reaching expected fecundability of the general population within 1 year. OC pills do not increase the abortion rate, chromosomal aberrations or congenital anomalies.

"Mini-pills" oral contraceptives are a contraceptive method of hormonal suppression of ovulation [incomplete blocking of positive-feedback mechanisms leading to inadequate luteinizing hormone (LH) pituitary surges], altering endometrial and cervical mucus with progestin administration alone. The dose of progestin is constant and depends

on progestin's hormonal potency. Norethindrone at a dose of 0.35 mg (*Micronor* or *Nor-QD*) and DL-norgestrel (*Ovrette*) are commonly used. These progestin microdoses are administered in a continuous, nonstop mode. Due to common abnormal endometrial bleeding (endometrial irregular shedding or asynchronized out-of-phase endometrium), mini-pills are not frequently prescribed. Nevertheless, in women who present with contraindications to estrogen (e.g., cardiovascular disease, uncontrolled hypertension, age >35 years, cigarette smokers, and lactating women). The failure rate of mini-pills is estimated to be 2 to 7 pregnancies per 100 women-years, and the rate of ectopic pregnancy is increased (decreased fallopian tube function).

The *injectable hormonal contraceptive method* is equally effective as OC pills or surgical sterilization. The mechanism of this contraceptive method is based on the same principles as those of mini-pills. Intramuscular injection of Depo-Provera (depo-medroxyprogesterone acetate in microcrystalline suspension) at the dose of 150 mg every 3 months is recommended. Unpredictable endometrial bleeding, spotting, and weight gain (average of 2.27 kg or 5 pounds in the first year and less in subsequent years) are the most commonly reported complications. There are no significant changes in carbohydrate, lipid, and protein metabolism, and there is no increased risk for breast cancer, cervical cancer, ovarian cancer, or liver cancer. No teratogenic risk effect has been documented if pregnancy occurs, and long-term fertility is not affected (16). The infrequent mode of administration (four times per year) and high efficacy with good safety makes this form of contraceptive very attractive to women (and adolescents) who have a problem with complying with the schedule of OC pills.

Subdermal implants (Norplant) provide sustained release of progestin from implants. The contraceptive mechanisms are the same as those described for mini-pills. Shortly after removing Silastic implants, reproductive capacity returns. Levonorgestrel subdermal silicone rubber rods (each containing 36 mg of dry crystals) slowly release progestin at the rate of 80 µg per day within the first year and 30 µg thereafter for a total contraceptive effect lasting 5 years. The six rods (each is 34 mm long and 2.4 mm in diameter) are surgically inserted in the subdermal area of the upper inner arm under local anesthesia. The contraceptive effect is comparable with that of surgical sterilization, with annual cumulative pregnancy rate <1.0/100 (18). Side effects include abnormal endometrial bleeding (two thirds of cases), weight gain, acne, and headaches. There are few contraindications to this contraceptive method. Surgical removal under local anesthesia is recommended every 5 years.

Intrauterine Devices

The contraceptive mechanism of intrauterine devices (IUDs) is based on hostility to the sperm, ovum, and fertil-

ized ovum (19). Whether or not an IUD causes abortion remains controversial. A properly inserted IUD will prevent intrauterine pregnancy at a rate of 96% to 99%, but has not demonstrated a capacity to prevent extrauterine pregnancy. A higher rate of ectopic pregnancy (although the IUD itself does not increase the risk of ectopic pregnancy) than intrauterine pregnancy has been observed when conception occurs with the IUD in place (20). It is an appropriate method of contraception for women with low-risk of STD exposure (stable, monogamous sexual life), for women who have completed their families, and for women who do not wish to undergo sterilization. Two IUDs have been approved and are available for use in the United States. The *copper-bearing IUD*, *ParaGard* (TCu 380 A), is effective for up to 10 years. The *progestin-release IUD* (*Progestasert*, which releases 65 µg of progestin per day) is effective for 1 year and should be replaced annually.

From a practical point, IUD insertion is best performed during menses, but it can be inserted on any day of the menstrual cycle provided that the patient is not already pregnant. Postpartum insertion is usually executed 4 to 8 weeks after delivery.

The most frequently reported complications associated with IUDs are excessive abnormal endometrial bleeding and secondary dysmenorrhea. These symptoms are responsible for almost 50% of copper-type IUD removal.

Absolute *contraindications* for IUD use include the following:

- Abnormal endometrial bleeding (undiagnosed)
- Pelvic infection (suspected or known)
- Pelvic malignancy (suspected or known)
- Pregnancy (suspected or known)

Relative contraindications include:

- Nulliparity
- High-risk sexual behavior
- Abnormal Pap smear
- Abnormal shape of the uterine cavity
- Corticosteroid therapy, immune suppression, chemotherapy, vulvar heart disease

Mitral valve prolapse will require one prophylactic dose of antibiotic when the IUD is inserted. If pregnancy occurs with the IUD visible and the protruding IUD string from the external os of the cervical canal is present, the IUD should be removed to avoid abortion or premature delivery (risk of spontaneous abortion or premature delivery increases two- to four–fold with the IUD in place). When the IUD string is missing, the device can be removed at delivery.

Female Surgical Sterilization

Female surgical sterilization is defined as voluntary, permanent occlusion or removal of either the fallopian tubes or uterus. There are several methods of interruption or obliteration of the fallopian tubes.

Mechanical occlusion can be performed through laparoscopy, laparotomy (mini-laparotomy), or colpotomy. The incidence of pregnancy with the following mechanical occlusion techniques is 20 pregnancies per 1,000 tubal sterilizations:

- *The Pomeroy technique* or partial resection of the fallopian tubes bilaterally (the midsections of the tubes are ligated with absorbable suture and the tubal segment is excised over the ligation suture).
- *The Parkland modification* of the Pomeroy technique also involves segmental resection of the fallopian tubes, but two separate ligation sutures are used, and the segment of the tube between the sutures is removed.
- *The Irving technique* consists of tubal double ligation with sutures, division between sutures, and burial of the proximal ligated end into the myometrial tunnel.
- *The Uchida technique* is based on ligation and segmental resection of the fallopian tubes, submersion of the proximal stump under the mesosalpinx, and approximation of the mesosalpinx edges with purse-string sutures.
- *The Kronner technique or fimbriectomy* is a simple ligation of the tube before the fimbriated end of the Fallopian tube followed by excision of the fimbriae.

Tubal occlusion with unipolar electrocoagulation (the 10-year cumulative probability of pregnancy is 7.5 per 1,000 tubal sterilizations) or *bipolar electrocoagulation* (10-year cumulative probability of 25 pregnancies per 1,000 tubal sterilizations) is customarily performed via laparoscopy (21).

Tubal occlusion with *clip sterilization* is usually performed laparoscopically, and the spring clip method yields a 10-year cumulative probability of pregnancy of 36.5 per 1,000 tubal sterilizations (21).

Tubal occlusion with a *Silastic ring* applied via laparoscopic approach has a 10-year cumulative probability of pregnancy of 18 per 1,000 tubal sterilizations (21).

Hysterectomy is an exceedingly rare method of sterilization in the United States.

The complications of female tubal sterilization include the following:

- Complications associated with surgery
- Complications associated with general anesthesia
- Ectopic pregnancy (one third of all pregnancies)
- Postsurgical chronic pelvic pain

Tubal ligation reversal is possible in selected cases but involves major reconstructive surgery under general anesthesia, and success rates vary.

Natural Contraceptive Methods

Several methods of natural contraception are commonly used.

The rhythm method is considered an ineffective method of pregnancy prevention. The technique is dependent on the natural infertile period during the menstrual cycle. Calendar calculation, cervical mucus quality, and basal body temperature are used to establish the fertile period of each cycle. Upon reaching the predicted potential phase of conception, sexual abstinence should be observed to avoid pregnancy. The following factors limit the effectiveness of this technique:

- Individual variation of intervals of the menstrual cycle
- Inability to comply with the method
- Duration of sperm survival

Coitus interruptus is dependent on the male partner's awareness of impending ejaculation and the ability to withdraw the penis from the vagina beforehand. The technique is ineffective for several reasons:

- The deposition of sperm before orgasm can be reached
- Frequent ejaculation near the vaginal orifice
- Failure to exercise the self-control to withdraw

Postcoital douche presumably flushes out the ejaculate with water, vinegar solution, or other products. This method is also ineffective.

Emergency Contraceptive

An emergency method of postcoital contraception, or "morning after pill," is used after unprotected coitus or a contraceptive accident to prevent pregnancy. The mechanisms of this form of contraceptive are based on two principles: either to delay or to suppress ovulation or to inhibit the implantation process of the fertilized ovum (22).

Estrogen alone may be used as follows:

- Ethinyl estradiol, 5 mg daily for 5 days orally
- Conjugated estrogens, 30 mg daily for 5 days orally
- Injectable conjugated estrogens, 50 mg daily for 2 days injected intramuscularly

Progestin alone may be used in the form of D-norgestrel 0.4 mg in one oral dose within 3 hours after intercourse.

An estrogen/progestin combination (*Ovral*) is composed of ethinyl estradiol 50 μg/DL-norgestrel 0.5 mg. The first dose (two tablets) should be taken within 72 hours of unprotected coitus, and two more tablets are taken 12 hours later. Prior to the first dose, antiemetic medication can be administered to reduce the nausea and vomiting associated with this method. This emergency contraceptive method is the one most commonly used in the United States and is approximately 75% effective.

Other emergency contraceptive regimens include *Mifepristone* (RU486), 50 to 100 mg daily for 4 days in the mid-luteal phase of the menstrual cycle; danazol, 400 mg oral initial dose followed by 400 mg 12 hours later; or insertion of a copper-T IUD within 5 days of coitus.

Complementary Contraceptives

Patient Education

Contraception and sexual education are very personal subjects. Traditionally, and in many instances culturally, these educational aspects are considered a family responsibility. This stance has been tested in the face of teenage pregnancy, abortion, and pregnancy complications. Many elementary and high schools include sexuality and contraceptive curricula. Information and education about contraception has become more accessible, and recent statistics indicate a trend of declining teenage pregnancy. Patient education should incorporate the physiology of puberty, menstrual cycle, sexuality, personal hygiene, sexual intercourse, and high-risk sexual behavior (those that lead to pregnancy, STDs, and HIV infection). A girl's preparation for appropriate contraception according to her health condition, reproductive period, and stage of family completion should be an integral part of education. Potential side effects, complications, and failure rates of contraceptive methods should be presented, and available alternative methods should be described. Safe sex practice, pregnancy prevention, STDs, and potential for hepatitis B transmission by the sexual route should be incorporated into any educational curriculum. Methods of male contraception also should be included in patient education.

Nutritional Supplements

Nutritional supplements are offered for women on OC pills to compensate for the metabolic alterations induced by the pills. Several formulations are offered, and one such regimen is listed as follows (23):

- Folic acid, 800 μg to 2.5 mg
- Vitamin B_{12}, 100 to 1,000 μg
- Vitamin B_6 (pyridoxine), 50 to 100 mg
- Vitamin B_2 (riboflavin), 5 to 10 mg
- Vitamin C, 500 to 3,000 mg
- Zinc, 15 to 45 mg

This formulation is recommended daily for the duration of OC pill administration.

Alternative Contraceptives

Historically, many herbs, including Rue, Tansy, and Queen Anne's lace, were used as a form of contraceptive. These herbs are now known to induce abortion rather than to prevent pregnancy (24).

Postcoital vaginal douching with diet cola is one folk medicine recommendation, reported anecdotally in clinical data. A laboratory *in vitro* study documented the spermicidal properties of Coca-Cola (25).

The following *herbal contraceptive methods* have been recommended in folk medicine, but their effectiveness and safety have not been documented (26):

- *Burning bush* (*Dictamnus albus*), one cup three times daily of infusion prepared with 20 g of dried herb in 1 L of water.
- *Caster oil plant* (*Ricinus communis*) is prepared for internal use as a contraceptive method.
- *Cat's claw* (*Uncaria tomentosa*), specially prepared, is taken in the form of liquid, one cup at a time during menses, to prevent pregnancy for 3 to 4 years (27).
- *Jack-in-the-pulpit* (*Arisaema atrorubens*) is used for contraceptive purposes by the Hopi Indians.
- *Rue* (*Ruta graveolens*) is used in folk medicine as a contraceptive and an abortive agent.

SEXUALITY

Sexual Development

Development of human sexuality begins at the time of conception, when the Y chromosome is or is not transferred and genetic determination is accomplished. Sexual orientation and behavior are affected not only by the hormonal milieu, but also by one's own personality, environmental factors (immediate family, peers, and friends), emotional state, and socioeconomic condition. Such complex and multifactorial processes contribute to an individual's sexual identity and preferences, such as heterosexual, homosexual (homosexual experience and homosexual identity are two distinct entities), bisexual, or asexual. Patients looking for their sexual identity may adopt other unusual sexual behaviors, such as exhibitionism, transvestism, voyeurism, pedophilia, necrophilia, and zoophilia. There is not enough scientific data to determine the causes of these sexual aberrations.

The determination of *sexual identity* is a complex process that involves the following components (28):

- *Biologic and physical differences* between men and women (chromosomes, hormones, external genitalia, gonads, and secondary sex characteristics).
- *Gender identity* includes a set of feelings, attitudes, beliefs, thoughts, and expectations.
- *The social role of sexual identity* is greatly influenced by family, social, cultural, and daily life experiences.
- *Sexual orientation* is defined as a consistent pattern of sexual excitement toward the opposite gender or the same gender.
- *Sexual identity* results from internal and external experiences and eventually leads to one's sexual life-style.

Sexual Physiology

Human sexual physiology (sexual responses or sexual function, or human response cycle) is essential for the clinical comprehension of sexual dysfunction. The sexual response cycle can be initiated by audiovisual or other sensual stimulation or by physical caressing, foreplay, masturbation, and sexual intercourse. Sexual response is a cascade process that is considered to be a cycle, and its complexity is analyzed within the following neurophysiologic phases (29).

The libido, desire, or appetitive phase is controlled by the dopamine-sensitive excitatory and inhibitory center located in the central nervous system. Positive or negative sexual impulses travel from the brain via the spinal cord to the spinal sexual reflex centers, which are responsible for excitement and orgasm phases. This phase is characterized by psychological sexual interest and can last from minutes to hours.

The arousal or excitement phase is considered to be a reflex in response to stimulation (endings of the sensory nerve endings). It is governed by the parasympathetic nervous system and provides genital sexual transformation and extragenital changes. Efferent stimuli are conducted from the external genitalia through the pelvic nerve to the uterovaginal nerve plexus. Afferent impulses run through the dorsal clitoral nerve to the pudendal nerve and to the sacral centers. The excitement phase may last from minutes to hours.

Genital sexual transformation is associated with vascular engorgement that leads to the following:

- Clitoral length and diameter enlargement.
- Vaginal vascular transudate increases vaginal lubrication in normoestrogenic or hyperestrogenic women (hypoestrogenism compromises this mechanism).
- Tenting and expansion of the upper part of the vagina.

Extragenital changes include the following:

- Breast nipple erection.
- Increased breast size.
- Engorgement of the areola.
- Occurrence of the sex flush (transient erythematous changes on the face, neck, and chest) is present in approximately 75% of women during this sexual function phase.
- Increased blood pressure.
- Increased heart rate.
- Enhanced body muscle tension.

The *orgasm phase* is also a reflex response to appropriate stimulation, which must be sufficient in duration and intensity. This phase is managed by the sympathetic nervous system, which produces the levator sling and a series of reflex clonic contractions in the genital musculature. The extragenital orgasmic phase manifests as follows:

- Sex flushes at maximal intensification
- Heart rate and respiratory rate at maximal intensification
- Elevation of blood pressure

The orgasmic phase or climax is the shortest among all sexual function phases and usually lasts 5 to 15 seconds.

The *refractory or resolution phase* induces a sensation of well being and usually lasts from a few minutes to hours.

Sexual Behaviors

Masturbation can provide a learning tool about sexual responsiveness and its acceptance varies within different cultures. *Self-masturbation* begins as a learning process of self-discovery and commences before age 13 in both girls and boys (boys report self-masturbation more frequently than girls do). *Partner masturbation*—either heterosexual or among girls themselves—is a common form of sexual experimentation.

Noncoital behaviors are most commonly reported as feeling the breast directly or indirectly (through clothing), or feeling of sex organs (the penis or female external genitalia) directly or indirectly. This is a common sexual practice to avoid vaginal penetration.

Oral sex with cunnilingus (oral stimulation of the female external genitalia) and fellatio (oral stimulation of the penis) is often practiced among virginal and non-virginal girls and young women. It is a frequent sexual practice and is gaining popularity among adolescents. This experience is prevalent among heterosexuals, homosexuals, and bisexuals.

Anal sex is also a frequent sexual practice and is experienced among all sexual orientation groups.

Sexual intercourse (vaginal penetration with the penis) has become a more frequent practice among adolescents in the past 25 years (47.7% of all girls experience sexual intercourse—65.6% of black girls, 45.7% of Hispanic girls, and 44% of white girls). However, there is no scientifically established normative sexual timetable for initiating coitus. Biopsychological factors such as pubertal maturity, family characteristics, relationships, and psychosocial context influence the initiation of sexual intercourse. Adolescents engaging in sexual intercourse have been categorized as follows:

- *Delayer* —has never had sexual intercourse
- *Anticipator* —has not experienced coitus, but has a 50% chance of initiation within 1 year
- *One-timer* —experienced one episode of sexual intercourse
- *Steady* —encountered multiple episodes of sexual intercourse only with one partner
- *Multiple* —had several episodes of sexual intercourse with more than one partner

Knowing which of these categories describes the patient helps the clinician to address any sexual dysfunction and to establish an appropriate individual health-care plan.

Same-gender experiences during the adolescent period do not predict homosexual orientation. *Homosexual identity* (lesbianism) is a development process that includes the following events (28):

- *Sensitization* is a generalized feeling of being different from other girls.
- *Identity confusion* (14–16 years) involves expression of interest in the same sex interest, along with internal confusion, conflict, and anxiety due to feelings of being sexually different from peers.

- *Identity assumption* (21–23 years) is a formal self-identification as homosexual. In this stage an individual establishes contact with positive homosexual role models, experiences homosexual experimentation, and explores the homosexual community.
- *Commitment* (before age 28 years) is integration of homosexual identity (open homosexual relationship, disclosure of homosexual identity to family and non-homosexual friends or acquaintances, and adoption of homosexual life-style).

Bisexual orientation may begin during adolescence and persist throughout life, or may convert either to heterosexual or homosexual identification.

SEXUAL DYSFUNCTION

Definition of Sexual Dysfunction

Sexual dysfunction is the decreased, disturbed, or absence of sexual interest or sexual responses to adequate stimulation.

Incidence

There are insufficient data in the literature to determine the incidence or prevalence of sexual dysfunction according to age group. In general, it can be presented for the age range of 18 to 73 years in the following groups (30–32):

- Lack of sexual desire is estimated at 33% to 38%.
- Lack of excitement (lubrication) ranges from 14% to 18%.
- Lack of orgasm (anorgasmia) is estimated to occur in 15% to 24%.
- Lack of pleasure occurs in 16% to 21%.

Etiology

The causes of sexual dysfunction are unknown but are considered to be multifactorial, probably influenced by health (physical and emotional), life-style, sociocultural characteristics, and sexual experiences. However, some risk predictors for sexual dysfunction in women have been identified (32):

- Decrease in household income
- Emotional problems or stress
- Ever sexually forced by a man
- Ever sexually touched as a child
- History of STDs
- Urinary tract symptoms
- Poor to fair health
- Previous abortion

Classification

Sexual dysfunction can be classified as follows:

- Primary sexual dysfunction—realistic sexual expectation has never materialized.

- Secondary sexual dysfunction—prior sexual function within realistically expected norm.
- Situational sexual dysfunction—the functions of sexual responses are present in some situations but not in others.

Diagnosis

Because sexual dysfunction can affect any component of the sexual cycle, appropriate and phase-specific symptoms should be established. Determining the pertinent medical history and symptoms is essential in sexual dysfunction clinical practice.

Sexual History Taking

The following categories of female sexual dysfunction must be explored by taking an appropriate sexually oriented history.

Sexual desire (libido) disorders are considered to be a partially testosterone- and androstenedione-dependent phenomenon (33). Traumatic head injury, temporal lobe epilepsy, acromegaly, depression, and back injury decrease libido (34). Sexual desire can be compartmentalized in several categories.

Hypoactive sexual desire is characterized by a persistent or recurrent insufficiency or absence of sexual fantasies or desire for sexual activity. This phase of sexual response cycle can be affected by a woman's general physical and psychological health (particularly depression), hormonal abnormalities, medication (tricyclic antidepressants, monoamine oxidase inhibitors, selective serotonin reuptake inhibitors, Lithium, and other antipsychotic medications), and recreational drugs (35). Sudden influential negative events may include the following:

- Death in family or close friend
- Aging or child leaving home
- Ongoing stressful relationship
- Job loss

Sexual aversion is a recurrent or persistent avoidance of or aversion to coitus. This form of sexual desire dysfunction can be associated with the following:

- History of physical or sexual abuse
- Vaginismus
- Dyspareunia (either superficial or deep dyspareunia)
- Extensive negative and unexpressed feelings about relationship
- Aversion to semen is a phobic form of the disorder and is very difficult to treat

The level of sexual desire can be determined by direct or indirect questioning (36):

- Feelings of sexual desire—almost never or never, a few times, sometimes, most times, almost always, or always
- Patient's self-rating of desire—none or very low, low, moderate, high, or very high

- Sexual relationship—very dissatisfied, moderately dissatisfied, equally satisfied/dissatisfied
- Presence or absence of aversion to semen or other aspects of sexual life

Sexual arousal disorder is defined as the absence or partial lack of physical signs of arousal during the excitement phase of the sexual response cycle, with other phases being intact. Among clinical signs, lubrication is the most prominent. Lack or insufficient lubrication may lead to different degrees of discomfort during coitus and in extreme cases makes sexual intercourse impossible to tolerate. Estrogen deficiency compromises blood flow within the vaginal mucosa and results in decreased lubrication

Taking a sexual history in reference to arousal dysfunction can help establish the cause (36). The severity of *vaginal dryness during sexual intercourse* can be established by how often coitus is attempted despite the existence of vaginal dryness (did not attempt, almost always or always attempted, more than half the time, about half the time, much less than half the time, almost never, or never). It is often associated with hypoestrogenism.

The severity of *discomfort during sexual intercourse* can be established based on frequency of attempted coitus regardless of experiencing coital pain (the same expected answers as stipulated above) and how many times sexual intercourse is attempted per month (0, 1–2, 3–4, 5–6, 7–10, or >11).

Vaginal ballooning (tenting) following total hysterectomy can be compromised and cause deep dyspareunia due to the following:

- Intravaginal scaring
- Shortening of the vagina
- Decreasing vasocongestion
- Loss of uterine contraction associated with sexual stimulation

Whether or not supracervical uterine amputation (supracervical hysterectomy) affects the stability of sexual function has not been definitively established (37).

In addition to history of prior abdominal or pelvic surgery (perineal surgery, pelvic lymphadenectomy, pelvic exonerations, vascular surgery on the iliac or aorta vessels, and other pelvic surgery), a history of pelvic inflammatory disease and STDs should be obtained.

Vaginal stenosis, adhesion, and scarring may follow radiotherapy for genital tract malignancies. Complications associated with radiation therapy may reduce vaginal lubrication and may cause dyspareunia.

Orgasmic disorder is defined as the persistent or chronic recurrent inability to reach orgasm (anorgasmia). This condition can be classified as follows:

- Lifelong anorgasmia or primary anorgasmia (the woman never reaches orgasm during sexual intercourse) is estimated to affect about 10% of women.

- Intermittent anorgasmia (situational anorgasmia) is reported in approximately 50% of women.

The causes of female anorgasmia can be categorized as follows:

- Traumatic or unpleasant sexual experiences (sexual molestation or rape).
- Psychotropic medications (*Thioridazine*, *Fluphenazine*) or major tranquilizers (e.g., *Diazepam*) may produce anorgasmia. Antidepressants also may be responsible for orgasmic disorders (35).
- Alcohol consumption and recreational drugs can interfere with reaching orgasm.
- Environmental contact with pesticides, lead, vinyl chloride, and mercury may produce anorgasmia.
- Anorgasmia of physical origin can follow pelvic surgery or spinal cord injury or surgical intervention.
- Emotional disorders or interpersonal unsatisfactory relationship.

Orgasmic experiences can be further established by inquiring about frequency of orgasm during sexual intercourse or sexual stimulation (never, almost never, a few times, sometimes, most times, almost always, or always). A patient may also self-rate the degree of clitoral sensation during sexual intercourse or sexual stimulation: not at all, very low, low, moderate, high, or very high (34).

Sexual satisfaction disorder is multifactorial and is influenced by psychosocial, interpersonal (particularly with her partner), environmental, cultural, general health, current and past medication, religious denomination, and family characteristics. These parameters should be explored during sexual history taking.

Discomfort or pain during the sexual experience is a common occurrence among women with a sexual dysfunction. *Dyspareunia* is chronic recurrent genital pain generated before, during, or after sexual intercourse. It is a heterogeneous disorder with latent overlapping causes, leading to depression, anxiety, and sexual dysfunction. It may be caused by anatomic anomalies or anatomically acquired abnormalities such as postdelivery or postsurgical scarring, vaginal stenosis, pelvic inflammatory disease, or endometriosis. Dyspareunia is sub-classified as follows:

- *Superficial dyspareunia* is pain during pineal insertion and is usually caused by vulvovestibular or vaginal disorders, or the dysfunctional ballooning of the upper half of the vagina.
- *Deep dyspareunia* occurs upon deep pineal penetration and is frequently experienced after surgery, pelvic inflammatory disease, and pelvic endometriosis. Pelvic relaxation, urinary tract, and anorectal disorders also may be responsible for deep dyspareunia.
- *Diffuse dyspareunia* is the presence of superficial and deep penetration pain. Long-lasting diffuse dyspareunia is highly refractory to treatments.

Vaginismus is recurrent chronic involuntary contraction of the distal third of the vagina and makes pineal penetration of the vagina difficult. This condition may be triggered by an abusive sex experience (unpleasant sexual experience, rape, incest), psychological factors such as unexpressed negative feelings toward a sex partner, fear of pain, and stress regarding or desire for pregnancy.

In summary, the history for evaluation of female sexual dysfunction should include the following elements:

- Marital status
- Menstrual patterns
- Parity and form of delivery
- Sexual identification and form of sexual practice
- Sexual abuse
- Medical disorders
- Gynecologic or abdominal surgery
- Current and past medications
- Substance abuse
- Emotional or psychiatric disorders

Physical Examination

The physical examination and pelvic examination should be undertaken as described in the section on Patient Approach at the beginning of this chapter. Particular attention should be directed to the following elements:

- *The vulvovestibular condition* should be assessed. Vulvovestibulitis, vulvar edema, erythema, or excessive discharge should be excluded. Fourchette irritation or increased muscle tone may suggest vaginismus. The Bartholin glands and Skene glands should be palpated to rule out tenderness. Postepisiotomy induration or tenderness should be excluded.
- The *vaginal* evaluation should focus on the presence or absence of vaginal stenosis, adhesions, strictures, constricting bands, and vaginal congenital abnormalities, as well as posthysterectomy vaginal depth. Vaginal vault induration or tenderness to palpation or motion should be ruled out. Vaginal suspension and support disorders, such as descent, prolapse, or vaginal wall anatomic abnormalities (entero-, recto-, or cystoceles) should be ruled out. Postradiotherapy fibrosis or stricture should be noted. Vaginal mucosa atrophy in hypoestrogenic women (postmenopausal or postoophorectomized women) and hyperandrogenic women should be noted.
- *Cervical* tenderness to palpation and to motion should be either established or ruled out.
- *Uterine* fixed retroflexion may produce deep dyspareunia, uterine posterior wall tumors (predominantly leiomyomata), or adenomyosis (globular and tender uterus). Chronic endometritis can lead to sexual dysfunction.
- *Posterior cul-de-sac* examination may show the presence of tenderness or nodularity, which can suggest endometriotic implants.
- *Levator ani* tenderness may suggest the presence of myalgia.
- *An adnexal mass* also may contribute to sexual dysfunction.
- *Anorectal* and urinary tract evaluation should be included.
- Imaging technology should be used as indicated.

Laboratory Testing

Initial laboratory testing is usually performed based on history and physical findings as follows:

- Complete blood count and erythrocyte sedimentation rate, and hemoglobin A1C or other appropriate laboratory tests, when chronic medical condition are present
- Fasting blood chemistry (SMA-20) and hepatitis panel
- Urinalysis or urine culture (if indicated)
- Hormonal evaluation as indicated, which often includes serum thyroid profile, testosterone levels, luteinizing hormone, and follicle-stimulating hormone (long-lasting low libido constitutes indication for endocrinologic evaluation)
- HIV testing
- Serum levels for toxins such as lead, mercury, pesticides, and vinyl chloride, among others
- Pap smear
- Vaginal wet mount evaluation or cervical culture (if the cervix is absent, cultures culture can be obtained from the urethra)

Differential Diagnosis

The differential diagnosis of sexual dysfunction should include the following:

- Endocrine disorders
- Chronic illness
- Long-term medication use
- Psychiatric or emotional disorders
- Substance abuse

Conventional Therapy

Conventional therapy is aimed toward the specific affected phase of sexual cycle responses.

Sexual desire disorder therapies depend on the underlying cause. Therapy for *hypoactive sexual desire disorders* is described as follows.

Testosterone therapy frequently provides gratifying results, despite side effects such as acne, alopecia, facial skin oiliness, hirsutism, virilization, and fluid retention (38). Because menopausal status may be related to lower sexual desire, therapeutic effort is directed to this particular group of women (39). In the United States a combination of 0.625 mg esterified estrogen and 1.25 mg methyltestosterone, or 1.25 mg esterified estrogen and 2.5 mg methyl-testosterone is given. This combination may produce undesirable androgenic effects and may adversely influence the serum lipoprotein profile (40).

Oral testosterone administration creates undesirable supraphysiologic serum peak testosterone levels at a dose as low as 20 mg testosterone undeconate. The paucity of relevant data in the literature makes the use of oral testosterone questionable (41).

Recent advances with a transdermal *Testosterone* matrix patch, which releases 150 μg per day (applied twice weekly), is a promising treatment for low-libido patients (41).

Initial data indicate that subcutaneous testosterone implants at a dose of 50 mg may be effective in enhancing libido without inducing virilizing side effects (42). In general, testosterone replacement is not recommended while a postmenopausal woman is on estrogen therapy. Women who demonstrate hyperandrogenic signs also are not good candidates for treatment with testosterone or other androgenic agents. Absolute contraindications for testosterone treatment are pregnancy, lactation, and suspected androgen-dependent benign or malignant neoplasia.

Antidepressants may assist in the treatment of low sexual desire associated with clinical depression; however, at the beginning of therapy this form of therapy may decrease libido.

Individual or couples therapy is indicated when no causative medical disorder is present (43).

Sexual aversion disorder therapy incorporates individual counseling (desensitization and cognitive-behavioral therapy is recommended on an individual basis). Aversion to semen is a phobic condition, and treatment may be difficult. In libido-related sexual aversion disorders, couples psychotherapy may be indicated, especially when emotional differences, conflict, or issues of dominance are present.

Sexual arousal therapy is focused on improving lubrication. Estrogen replacement therapy increases vaginal mucosa function and is recommended in hypoestrogenic women, because estrogen deficiency is related to lubrication and dyspareunia. An estrogenic vaginal cream also can be applied (39). Estrogen replacement therapy should be considered first in the treatment of insufficient lubrication in postmenopausal or castrated women. Estrogen replacement therapy is discussed in further detail in Chapter 12.

Topical nonhormonal vaginal lubricants are recommended in normoestrogenic women to ease vaginal discomfort associated with insufficient lubrication and pineal traction.

Orgasmic disorder therapy includes the following:

- Psychotherapy to enforce positive body image, relaxation techniques, acceptance of sexual feelings, and sensual touching
- Self- or partner masturbation
- Traditional sex therapy, either individual, couples, or group

Such therapeutic approaches may aid the patient in achieving orgasm via masturbation in approximately 90% and via sexual intercourse in about 75% (44).

Therapy for dyspareunia targets the underlying condition associated with this form of sexual disorder. Such treatment may include conservative medical therapy such as hormone replacement or conservative surgical or surgical execrative intervention. When the cause of dyspareunia cannot be identified, individual, couples, or group therapy should be offered. Simply changing the sexual position may eliminate pain, particularly when uterine retroflexion is present.

Therapy for vaginismus is recommended with two simultaneous approaches: relaxation technique and dilators to increase the vaginal diameter (gradually increasing self or partner's finger insertion), ultimately with gradual pineal introduction into the vagina. Women who present with sexual phobias require psychotherapy with application of systemic desensitization techniques.

Complementary Therapy

Practitioner Education

Adequate knowledge of fundamental human sexuality, the ability to evaluate and manage sexual dysfunction, and sufficient time in practice to cope with sexual problems are essential in assisting a female patient in this very intimate aspect of life. It is difficult for physicians to dissociate from their own cultural views on sexuality and to explore comfortably a female patient's or both partners' sexual issues from a scientific perspective without appropriate preparation. To impose on a patient a practitioner's own unscientific convictions and experiences regarding sexuality is not only improper but also harmful. Identification of patients with sexual dysfunction and recognition of the practitioner's own limitation's in clinical evaluation and management skills are paramount to successful therapy. A practical knowledge of the sexual response cycle and its potential disturbance is crucial to helping patients. Distinguishing simple from multiple disorders, establishing the duration of the disorder, and identifying primary, secondary, and situational characteristics of sexual dysfunction will promote appropriate care. The following points should be established:

- Single sexual dysfunction (one phase of sexual response cycle is affected)
- A stable versus unstable sexual and interpersonal relationship
- Sexual dysfunction is present no longer than 1 year

Clinical recognition of simple cases of sexual dysfunction will help the practitioner initiate therapy with a better chance for a successful outcome. In contrast to simple sexual dysfunction, a complex or multiple sexual dysfunction (two or more dysfunctions of the sexual response cycle are present) requires the expertise of an adequately trained and an experienced sex therapist. Even with primary disorders that have existed for longer than 1 year (especially if the relationship with the partner is unstable), patients will benefit from the expert treatment of a sex therapist, as will those who have disorders of the desire or excitement phase. Providing health care that addresses sexual aspects requires that the clinician be familiar with the physiology of sexuality, its dysfunction, tactful and careful sexual history taking, and therapeutic diversities. A practitioner who embraces sexual treatments should incorporate the generally accepted model of PLISSIT. P stands for permission (open and understandable permission to cope with sexuality by incorporating natural instinctive sexual behavior within acceptable norms); LI stands for limited information (providing a patient with pertinent limited amounts of information); SS stands for specific suggestion (providing a patient with a specific suggestion pertinent to her sexual issue); IT stands for intensive therapy (usually provided by a sex therapist).

It is also worthwhile to mention that well-designed weight reduction and maintenance program may be the only treatment that patient needs, because obesity can cause sexual function disturbances (48).

Patient Education

Because sexual expectations in modern society are high, sexual function and positive pleasurable effect and a planned child are deserved rewards. However, sexual intercourse carries negative aspects such as unwanted pregnancy and STDs, as well as the potentially deadly HIV infection or chronic and debilitating hepatitis B infection. To secure a rewarding sexual life, patient education should include all aspects of contraception and prevention, not only from pregnancy but from infection. Such education should be delivered as a continuous process, not just as part of a sporadic school curriculum. Patient education is best initiated in childhood, when a child poses her first question about her genitalia or natural physiologic occurrences in sexuality (45–47). It should be considered an ongoing process, into which should gradually be introduced the importance of physical hygiene and body-mind-spirit techniques for mental well being throughout life. Education should incorporate topics of sexual orientation, understanding the physiology of puberty, menses, reproduction, mental and spiritual development, and culture and norms governing life, including sexuality. A healthy sexual initiation and the value of a satisfactory monogamous sexual relationship are essential. The physiology of the sexual response cycle should be explicitly and implicitly presented to women with early symptoms of sexual response cycle dysfunction. Making women aware of the importance of early diagnosis and the availability of treatments for sexual dysfunctions is the best care a physician can provide for prevention and treatment. Psychosocial, cultural, mental and physical health, age, the use of drugs or smoking, and family characteristics have a great impact on women's sexual function.

Therefore, educating patients about these aspects may improve sexual expression and experience significantly. A prior traumatic or emotionally and physically unpleasant sexual experience, as well as an underlying chronic illness, may compromise a woman's intimate life dramatically. A healthy un-stressful life-style, the ability to implement relaxation techniques (including mind-body connection through meditation), a low-fat, high-fiber diet, enhanced with fresh fruits and vegetables, and physical and mental hygiene will positively influence sexual performance. Exercise and weight reduction is also an important aspect, because obesity itself may predispose to disturbances of sexual function (48).

Hypnotherapy

Hypnosis can be an effective form of therapy for sexual dysfunction; although, due to the paucity of supporting scientific data, this promising treatment is only occasionally used for dysfunction management (49).

Biofeedback Therapy

Visual feedback and audio feedback can improve arousal in sexual response phase dysfunction. The treatment is applied in two sessions, each consisting of six visual or audio feedback 3-minute exercises. Visual feedback therapy yields superior results over audio feedback for overall control of sexual arousal dysfunction (50). Biofeedback halved probe insertion (in contrast with other solid dilators, such as Sims dilators) as an adjunct treatment to psychotherapy for vaginismus can yield satisfactory results (51). However, this technique should be recommended with caution due to the lack of well-documented clinical scientific results.

Alternative Therapy

Herbal Remedies

Herbal remedies are often used in the general treatment of underlying medical conditions. *Hypericum perfortum* (St. John's wort) can be effectively used and is well tolerate for mild to moderate depression, as is *Valeriana officinalis* for insomnia (52). At present, the absence of scientific evidential data in the clinical literature limits any recommendations for herbal medical treatment of specific phase dysfunctions of the sexual response cycle. However, anecdotal reports have mentioned the following unproved herbal remedies (26):

- *Damiana* (*Turnera diffusa*), in 380-, 384-, 395-, and 450-mg daily capsules, is offered as a treatment for sexual disorders.
- *Muira-puama* (*Ptychopetalum olacoides*), 0.5 g daily in a single dose or 0.5 to 2 mL three times daily, is recommended for sexual disorders.

REFERENCES

1. Association of Professors of Gynecology and Obstetrics (APGO). *Medical student educational objectives,* 7th ed. Washington, DC: APGO, 1997.
2. Council on Resident and Gynecology (CREOG). *Educational objectives core curriculum for residents in obstetrics and gynecology,* 5th ed. Washington, DC: CREOG, 1996.
3. American College of Obstetrician and Gynecologists (ACOG). *Educational bulletin no. 136.* Washington, DC: ACOG, 1989.
4. Hampton HL. Examination of the adolescent patient. *Obstet Gynecol Clin North Am* 2000;27:1–18.
5. Beach R, ed. Contemporary adolescent gynecology. *Med Economics* 1995;1:6–12.
6. American Medical Association (AMA). *AMA guidelines for adolescent preventive service (GAPS).* Chicago, IL: AMA, 1994.
7. Ventura SJ, Mosher WD, Curtin SC, et al. Trends in pregnancies and pregnancy rates by outcome: estimates for the United States, 1976–1996. *Vital Health Stat 21* 2000;56:1-47
8. Harlap S, Shiono PH, Ramcharan S. Congenital abnormalities in the offspring of women who used oral and other contraceptives around the time of conception. *Int J Fertil* 1985;30:39–47.
9. Warburton D, Neugut RH, Lustenberger A, et al. Lack of association between spermicide use and trisomy. *N Engl J Med* 1987; 317:478–482.
10. Mircette Study Group. An open-label, multicenter, noncomparative safety and efficacy study of Mircette, a low-dose estrogen-progestin oral contraceptive. *Am J Obstet Gynecol* 1998;179(suppl):2.
11. Dericks-Tan JSE, Kock P, Taubert HD. Synthesis and release of gonadotropin: effect of an oral contraceptive. *Obstet Gynecol* 1983;62:687–690.
12. Chang CL, Donaghy M, Poutler N. Migraine and stroke in young women: case-control study. The World Health Organization Collaborative Study of Cardiovascular Disease and Steroid Hormone Contraception. *BMJ* 1999;318:13–18.
13. The World Health Organization Collaborative Study of Cardiovascular Disease and Steroid Hormone Contraception. Acute myocardial infarction and combine oral contraceptives: results of an international multicenter case-control study. *Lancet* 1997; 349:1202–1209.
14. The World Health Organization Collaborative Study of Cardiovascular Disease and Steroid Hormone Contraception. Acute myocardial infarction and combine oral contraceptives: ischaemic stroke and combined oral contraceptives of an international multicenter case-control study. *Lancet* 1997;348:489–510.
15. Spitzer WO, Lewis MA, Heinemann LAJ, et al. Third-generation oral contraceptives and risk of venous thromboembolic disorders: an international case control study. *BMJ* 1996;312:83–90.
16. Collaborative Group on Hormonal Factors in Breast Cancer. Breast cancer and hormonal contraceptives: collaborative reanalysis of individual data on 53,297 women with breast cancer and 1,000,239 women without breast cancer from 54 epidemiological studies. *Lancet* 1996;347:1713–1727.
17. Nelson AL. Counseling issues and management of side effects for women using depot medroxyprogesterone acetate contraception. *J Reprod Med* 1996;41:391–400.
18. Sivin I, Mishell DR Jr, Diaz S, et al. Prolonged effectiveness of Norplant capsule implants: a 7-year study. *Contraception* 2000; 61:187–194.
19. World Health Organization (WHO). Mechanism of action, safety, and efficacy of intrauterine devices. *WHO Tech Rep Ser* 1987;753:791.
20. Diaz S, Croxatto HB, Pavez M, et al. Ectopic pregnancies associated with low dose progestagen-releasing IUDs. *Contraception* 1980;22:259–269.
21. Peterson HB, Xia Z, Huges JM, et al. The risk of pregnancy after tubal sterilization: findings from the US Collaborative Review of sterilization. *Am J Obstet Gynecol* 1996;174:1161–1170.
22. Wellbery C. Emergency contraceptive. *Arch Fam Med* 2000;9: 624–646.
23. Hudson T. *Women's encyclopedia of natural medicine.* Lincolnwood, IL: Keats Publishing, 1999:74.
24. Fissell ME. Natural contraceptives. *Womens Health Primary Care* 1999;2:670.
25. Umpierre SA, Hill JA, Anderson DJ. Effect of "cola" on sperm motility. *N Engl J Med* 1985;131:1351.
26. *PDR for herbal medicine,* 2nd ed. Montvale, NJ: Medical Economics Company, 2000.
27. Cabieses F. *The saga of the cat's claw.* Lima, Peru: Via Lactera Editores, 1994.
28. Blythe MJ, Rosenthal SL. Female adolescent sexuality. *Obstet Gynecol Clin North Am* 2000;27:125–141
29. Leif HI. Inhibited sexual desire. *Med Aspect Hum Sexuality* 1977;7:94–95.
30. Rosen RC, Taylor FJ, Leiblum SR, et al. Prevalence of sexual dysfunction in women: results of a survey study of 329 women in an outpatient gynecological clinic. *J Sex Marital Ther* 1993;19: 171–188.
31. Laumann EO, Gagnon JH, Michael RT. *The social organization of sexuality: sexual practice in the United States.* Chicago, IL: University of Chicago Press, 1994.
32. Laumann EO, Paik A, Rosen RC. Sexual dysfunction in the United States. Prevalence and predictors. *JAMA* 1999;281:537–544.
33. Matteo S, Rissman EF. Increased sexual activity during the midcycle portion of the human menstrual cycle. *Horm Behav* 1984; 18:249–255.
34. Blumer D, Walker AE. The neural basis of sexual behavior. In: Benson DF, Blumer D, eds. *Psychiatric aspect of neurologic disease.* New York: Grune & Stratton, 1975.
35. Meston CM, Gorzalka BB. Psychoactive drugs and human sexuality. The role of serotinergic activity. *J Psychoactive Drugs* 1992; 24:1–40.
36. Kaplan SA, Reis RB, Kohen IJ, et al. Safety and effectiveness of slidenafil in postmenopausal women with dysfunction. *Urology* 1999;53:481–486.
37. Kikku P. Supravaginal uterine amputation vs. hysterectomy: effects on coital frequency and dyspareunia. *Acta Obstet Gynecol Scand* 1983;62:141–145.
38. Redmond GP. Hormones and sexual function. *Int J Fertil Womens Med* 1999;44:193–197.
39. Avis NE, Stellato R, Crawford S, et al. Is there an association between menopause status and sexual functioning. *Menopause* 2000;7:297–309.
40. Hickok LR, Toomey C, Speroff L. A comparison of esterified estrogens with and without methyltestosterone: effect on endometrial histology and serum lipoproteins in postmenopausal women. *Obstet Gynecol* 1993;82:919–924.
41. Buckler HM, Robertson WR, Wu FCW. Which androgen replacement therapy for women? *J Clin Endocrinol Metab* 1998; 83:3920–3924.
42. Davis SR, McCloud PI, Strauss BJG, et al. Testosterone enhances estradiol's effect on postmenopausal bone density and sexuality. *Maturitas* 1995;21:227–236.
43. Leiblum SR, Rosen RC, eds. *Sexual desire disorders.* New York: Guilford, 1988.
44. Heiman J, LoPiccolo J. *Becoming orgasmic: a sexual and personal growth program from women,* 2nd ed. New York: Simon & Schuster, 1988.
45. Ostrzenski A. Level of sexual education and sexual experiences among female university students in Wroclaw. *Pol Tyg Lek* 1972; 2:75–77.

46. Ostrzenski A. Level of sexual education among women from rural areas. *Pol Tyg Lek* 1972;30:1180–1181.
47. Ostrzenski A. Level of sexual education among female blue collar worker. *Pol Tyg Lek* 1972;52:2080–2082.
48. Sasaki Y, Arai T. Obesity and disturbance of sexual function. *Nippon Rinsho* 1997;55:3007–3011.
49. Gilmore LG. Hypnotic metaphor and sexual dysfunction. *J Sex Marital Ther* 1987;13:45–57.
50. Hoon EF. Biofeedback-assisted sexual arousal in females: a comparison of visual and auditory modalities. *Biofeedback Self Regul* 1980;5:175–191.
51. Barnes J, Bowman EP, Cullen J. Biofeedback as an adjunct to psychotherapy in the treatment of vaginismus. *Biofeedback Self Regul* 1984;9:281–289.
52. Ernst E. Herbal medications for common ailments in the elderly. *Drug Aging* 1999;15:423–428.

29

MEDICAL/LEGAL ASPECTS OF GYNECOLOGY

EDUCATIONAL OBJECTIVES

Medical Students (1)
APGO Objective Nos. 63 and 64

Sexual assault:
  child sexual assault victim
  adult sexual assault victim
  acquaintance rape
Domestic violence:
  prevalence and incidence
   of violence against women
  elder abuse
  child abuse
  assessment of the involvement
   of any patient in domestic violence
   situations counseling patients for
   short-term safety
  counseling patients regarding local
   support agencies for long-term
   management and resources
Counseling patients requiring resources
  for batterers and perpetrators of
  domestic violence

Residents in Obstetrics/Gynecology(2)
CREOG Objectives

Crisis intervention:
  History
  Physical examination
  Diagnostic studies
  Diagnosis
  Management
  Follow-up

Practitioners (3)
ACOG Recommendations

Sexual assault:
  Incidence
  Psychological impact
  Assault assessment kits
  Medical evaluation
  Legal concerns
  Counseling
  Follow-up
  Special circumstance

SEXUAL ASSAULT

Definition

The definition of sexual assault varies from state to state and in general can be expressed as an unconsented natural or unnatural sexual act by force or by deception. The term *sexual abuse* is used interchangeably with *sexual molestation, sexual abuse, rape, incest,* and *sexual victimization.*

Incidence

In the United States, the incidence of adult sexual assault is estimated to be 200 cases per 100,000 people (4); the incidence of child sexual abuse is 45 cases per 100,000 children (5).

Classification

- Occasional rape
- Marital rape
- Date (acquaintance) rape

Diagnosis

Before a formal evaluation of the alleged sexual assault victim is initiated; written, informed consent (in the presence of a witness) for medical evaluation, treatment, collection of specimens, photographs, and the release of information to legal authorities is required. The history part of sexual assault should also be obtained in the presence of a witness and carefully recorded using a patient's own statements, phrases, and words (time; place; circumstances; type of forceful intercourse, such as vaginal, oral, anal, or combination; and degree of penetration). Also, last menses, contraceptive use, and knowledge of pregnancy should be recorded.

Sexual assault symptoms are not specific, and clinical information should include a general gynecologic history (see Chapter 28) and target history

Emotional symptoms should be recorded on a sexual assault form, which usually comes with the assault assessment kits provided by a state agency, and may include the following:

- Anxiety, low self-esteem, depression, withdrawal
- Interpersonal relationship difficulty, social dysfunction, or work or school problems
- Sleep disorder
- Sexual disorders
- Out of ordinary sexual behavior following the assault

The victim's activities following the alleged sexual victimization should be recorded:

- Changing clothing
- Having bath
- Douching
- Taking any medication

Physical signs and their evidential preservation include the following:

- Photography of clothing and victim's body, with particular attention to bruises and wounds.
- Clothing collection should be handled directly as little as possible, properly labeled, and single items placed in separate paper bags.

Physical examination should include the following:

- Removal of seminal samples from the skin
- Fingernail scraping
- Trimming pubic hairs matted with semen
- Combing pubic hair
- Cutting head hair and securing it for forensic evidence

Oral cavity examination should include the following:

- Swabs for semen are obtained if the alleged assault occurred within 6 hours.
- Microbiologic culture for *Gonococcus* and other sexually transmitted diseases.
- Saliva specimen should be obtained with clean gauze or filter paper and preserved for future reference.

Perineal and perianal evaluation should include assessment of the external genitalia for injuries and abrasions (colposcopic examination should be incorporated for this part of the evaluation).

A vaginal speculum evaluation (a water-lubricated and warmed speculum is inserted) consists of the following:

- Vaginal contents are assessed; if present, aspiration is performed and specimen is placed in a test tube, sealed, and labeled.
- A specimen is obtained from the posterior vaginal fornix using a saline-saturated, cotton-tipped swab. The specimen is smeared on a glass microscopic slide, air-dried, labeled, and placed in a test tube.
- The vaginal pool is washed with 4 mL saline, and the contents are aspirated, placed in a test tube, sealed, and labeled. Microscopic examination may document the presence of motile sperm if evaluation is conducted not later than 6 hours following the assault.
- Vaginal and cervical lacerations and abnormalities are recorded and colposcopic examination is undertaken.
- Papanicolaou smear is taken.
- Cervical microbiologic cultures or DNA probe for sexually transmitted diseases are performed.

Anal evaluation includes the following:

- Lacerations and foreign material, if present, should be recorded and secured.
- Rectal swabs should be obtained.
- Microbiologic culture for *Gonococcus* and other sexually transmitted diseases should be taken.
- Dry-mount slides should be prepared and secured.

Pelvic examination is performed and any abnormality recorded (see the section on Pelvic Examination in Chapter 28).

The following *laboratory tests* should be ordered:

- Pregnancy test
- Blood type
- Rapid Plasma Reagin (RPR)
- Substance abuse toxicology levels
- Urine analysis
- Microbiologic cultures from each orifice (oral, anal, vaginal) involved in the event

Conventional Therapy

For *pregnancy prophylaxis*, see the section on Emergency Contraceptives in Chapter 28. Prophylaxis for sexually transmitted diseases (gonococcal, chlamydial, trichomonal, and bacterial vaginosis infections) includes all of the following modalities:

- Ceftriaxone, 125 mg single dose intramuscularly
- Metronidazole, 2 g single dose orally
- Doxycycline, 100 mg twice daily for 7 days

If the patient has a contraindication to the above prophylaxes, second-line prophylaxis may be offered according to recommendations from the Centers for Disease Control and Prevention (see Chapter 17). Hepatitis B prophylaxis with virus vaccination also should be given.

A *follow-up* visit should be scheduled 2 weeks after initial evaluation that includes the following:

- Wet-mount evaluation from vaginal secretions.
- Microbiological cultures for *Neisseria gonorrhoeae* and *Chlamydia trachomatis* if prophylactic treatment has not been instituted.
- Blood samples for serologic evaluation should be obtained.
- Pregnancy test—if pregnancy is established to be a result of sexual assault, a patient should receive counseling on the options available to her (accepting the pregnancy and child, putting the baby up for adoption, or undergoing a medically induced abortion). On September 28, 2000, the U.S. Food and Drug Administration approved *Mifepristone* (RU-486) as an early pregnancy abortion pill, and it is available under the brand name *Mifeprex*.

Subsequent follow-up visit is usually offered 12 weeks following the initial evaluation and incorporates tests for microorganism infections and the following serologic tests:

- Syphilis
- Human immunodeficiency virus (HIV; the test should be repeated at 6 months)
- Hepatitis B is ordered if hepatitis B virus vaccination was not administered at the initial evaluation

Counseling is an essential part of treatment and should be integrated into the management plan. The long-term cumulative physical and emotional effects of sexual violence are overwhelming, and are similar to or worse than those associated with a major chronic illness. Therefore, immediate, follow-up, multilevel counseling is necessary that includes support from family, friends and other specialized organizations.

The physician's role in the legal proceedings of the sexual assault victim is well defined:

- Forensic evaluation of a victim with documentation of physical and emotional status consistent with the use of force or deception to have a natural or unnatural sexual act
- Forensic specimen collection and preservation
- Notification of the state or local child protective service agency about suspicions of sexual abuse, if the victim is a minor
- Testimony in legal proceedings

Complementary Therapy

Hypnosis

Hypnosis in the treatment of victims of sexual abuse can help to reconstruct their memories of the experience, both by reviewing them with greater control over their physical sense of comfort and safety and by harmonizing painful memories with a sense of control. Hypnotherapy is particularly useful in coping with post-traumatic stress disorder following sexual victimization (7).

DOMESTIC VIOLENCE

Definition

Physical, sexual, psychological, and economic coercive or assault behavior occurring between a spouse or partner, a child, or elderly person that results in physical injury or emotional disturbance is considered domestic or family violence.

The physical aspect of domestic violence includes: pushing, slapping, kicking, hitting, beating, threatening with a weapon, throwing an object, or throwing an object at the victim.

Sexual violence incorporates forced natural or unnatural sexual acts.

Psychological abuse includes intimidation, verbal abuse or verbal threat, and social isolation.

Economic abuse integrates deprivation of food, clothing, money, transportation, or health care.

The battered wife (woman) syndrome is a complex of symptoms occurring as a result of deliberate, severe, and repeated (more than three times) acts of violence against a woman by her partner that may lead to minimal injury or bruises (8). The battering cycle usually occurs in three phases (9):

- The tension-building phase includes name-calling, verbal intimidation, hostility, or non-explosive dissatisfaction, and mild physical pushing.
- Uncontrollable tension discharge phase incorporates verbal and physical attacks cause emotional dysfunction and physical injuries; in self-defense, women may injure or murder the attacker.
- Apologetic phase is an attacker apologizes, asks for forgiveness in remorse, promises to control his or her anger, and presents victim with gifts.

The prevalence of domestic violence in the United States is unknown. Violence by men against women is estimated to occur in the range of 9.7% to 29.7% in nonpregnant women and approximately 0.9% to 21% during pregnancy (10). Women who are battered prior to a pregnancy, experience more violence during pregnancy (40%–60%) than to women who were not battered before becoming pregnant (11). Domestic violence is the most common origin of nonfatal injury inflicted on inner-city women in the United States (12) and increases the risk of fatal violence (homicide) (13).

Before medical evaluation, *informed consent* for collecting forensic evidence of physical abuse (photos) and examination should be conducted as described earlier for sexual assault.

Risk factors for domestic (family) violence behavior include the following (14,15):

- Consumption or abuse of alcohol
- Use or abuse of illicit drugs
- Family history of domestic violence during childhood
- Raised by a single parent
- Married as a teenager
- Pregnancy before marriage

A *variety of symptoms* can lead a practitioner to explore the presence of domestic violence (3):

- Headaches
- Insomnia
- Choking sensation
- Hyperventilation
- Gastrointestinal symptoms
- Chest, pelvic, and back pain
- Emotional symptoms of anxiety, embarrassment, frequent crying, evasiveness, or passiveness

Physical examination may provide evidence of prior (scars or burns, particularly cigarette burns) or recent domestic violence (wearing sunglasses to hide an eye injury, bruises on the breast or abdomen, or cuts and open wounds).

It is essential that a practitioner address the abuse by treating injuries and providing emotional support. If suicidal tendency is present, appropriate referrals should be made. The availability of support services such as shelters and emotional, financial, and legal support should be presented. If a victim decides to return home, she should be given the phone numbers of resource agencies and instructed to prepare and execute an exit plan should she decide to leave (16):

- Packed change of clothes for herself and children
- Cash, checkbook, and documentation for other accounts
- Identification papers, driver's license, and professional license
- Children's books and toys
- A precise plan for where to go at any time if the situation calls for it

A physician's legal responsibility varies from state to state in domestic violence. In a case of battered women, only a few states obligate a physician to report suspicion or proven cases of domestic or family violence with partner abuse (3). In 1994, the federal Violent Crime Control and Law Enforcement Act provided legal protection for those women who are victims of domestic violence.

INFORMED CONSENT

Informed consent is not only legal but is an ethical obligation to provide a patient with necessary up-to-date, knowledgeable and well-versed data concerning her particular clinical matter or procedures. Based on such educated infor-

mation, a patient (not a physician) makes a decision about medical conservative or invasive medical care.

Well-structured informed consent should incorporate the following elements:

- Nature and extent of illness.
- Nature, extent, and complexity of the treatment, including surgical interventions, with disclosure of the proposed type of surgical intervention (recognized, experimental, especially hazardous, or solely cosmetic).
- Benefits of such therapeutic approach.
- Expected results of the specific treatment (not guaranteed results) and what such offered treatment will not accomplish.
- Success rate under similar clinical conditions.
- Potential complications of the treatment and the known risks associated with conservative therapy or surgical intervention. The risk factors should incorporate potential fatal outcome, if such risk is documented.
- Alternative conservative and/or surgical therapies available for a patient's specific illness and their likelihood of success, imperfect success, or failure.
- Intraoperative discovery of unexpected pathology and formal patient's instruction on how it should be approached.
- A practitioner's own experience in managing such a medical entity and its inherent potential complications associated with the mode of therapy.

It is important to make sure that a patient fully understands a proposed mode of therapy. Informed consent can not be structured on patient's questions and answers only, because it will require medical knowledge and practical experience to cover specific areas of therapeutic modalities. Therefore, it is solely the physician's responsibility to fulfill this obligation and delegating this task to other medical personnel is not advisable. Informed consent should be well documented in a patient's medical record, signed, and witnessed.

Minors and Informed Consent

Minors (adolescents) who request reproductive health services can obtain them on their own consent; however, the majority of adolescents get the services with the consent of their parents or guardians. Some states challenge this right and try to modify state minor consent statutes, particularly in a view of obtaining contraceptives or inducing abortion (17).

Clinical Research and Informed Consent

Clinical, scientific research with informed consent (including experimental surgery), in which a human is a scientific subject, requires balancing the following major aspects (18):

- To meet the highest clinical research standard with the highest standard of ethics

- To prepare and to present informed consent that will incorporate all standard parameters (see above), particularly with regard to assessing the risks and benefits of research protocol
- To establish the relationship between the risks of a protocol and the informed consent of research subjects
- To disclose the research design, including a randomized, blinded, and placebo-controlled study (a patient should know that there is a 50:50 chance of not receiving the real treatment)
- To disclose the accompanying anesthesia (its informed consent should be incorporated), if it is planned
- To disclose all possible risks and complications of medication used in the research protocol

The tendency in clinical research is to emphasize the more beneficial aspects of the protocol than the potential risk factors (19,20). Therefore, the potential risks and potential benefits should be presented equally in informed research protocols in order to allow a patient to make her decision.

REFERENCES

1. Association of Professors of Gynecology and Obstetrics (APGO). *Medical student educational objectives,* 7th ed. Washington, DC: APGO, 1997.
2. Council on Resident Education in Obstetrics and Gynecology (CREOG). *Educational objectives core curriculum for residents in obstetrics and gynecology,* 5th ed. Washington, DC: CREOG, 1996.
3. American College of Obstetrician and Gynecologists (ACOG). *Educational bulletin no. 242.* Washington, DC: ACOG, 1997.
4. U.S. Department of Justice. *Criminal victimization 1994. Bureau of Justice statistics bulletin. National crime victimization survey.* Washington, DC: U.S. Government Printing Office, 1996.
5. Sedlak AJ, Brooadhurst DB. *Third national study of child abuse and neglect.* Washington, DC: U.S. Government Printing Office, 1996.
6. Sadler AG, Booth BM, Nielson D, et al. Health-related consequences of physical and sexual violence: women in the military. *Obstet Gynecol* 2000;96:473–480.
7. Spiegl D. Hypnosis in the treatment of victims of sexual abuse. *Psychiatr Clin North Am* 1989;12:295–305.
8. Parker B, Schumacher SN. The battered wife syndrome and violence in the nuclear family of origin: a controlled pilot study. *Am J Public Health* 1977;67:760–761.
9. Walker LE. *The battered women syndrome.* New York: Springer, 1984.
10. Ballard TJ, Salzman LE, Gazmararian JA, et al. Violence during pregnancy: measurement issue. *Am J Public Health* 1998;88:274–276.
11. Parker B, McFarlane J. Nursing assessment of battered women. *Matern Child Nurs J* 1991;16:161–164.
12. Grisso JA, Wishner AR, Schwarrz DF, et al. A population-based study of injuries in inner-city women. *Am J Epidemiol* 1991;134:59–68.
13. Kellermann AL, Mercy JA. Men, women and murder: gender-specific differences in rates of fatal violence and victimization. *J Trauma* 1992;33:1–5.
14. Vinken RM. Family violence. Aids to recognition. *Postgrad Med* 1982;71:115–122.
15. Thompson J, Canterino JC, Feld SM, et al. Risk factors for domestic violence in pregnant women. *Prim Care Update Obstet Gynecol* 2000;7:138–141.
16. Helton A. Battering during pregnancy. *Am J Nurs* 1986;86:910–913.
17. English A. Reproductive health service for adolescents. *Obstet Gynecol Clin North Am* 2000;27:195–211.
18. Maclin R. The ethical problem with sham surgery in clinical research. *N Engl J Med* 1999;341:992–996.
19. Advisory Committee on Human Radiation Experimentation. New York: Oxford University Press, 1996.
20. National Bioethics Advisory Commission (NBAC). Research involving persons with mental disorders that may affect decision-making capacity. Rockville, MD: NBAC, 1998.

30

CONVENTIONAL DRUG AND ALTERNATIVE THERAPY INTERACTION

EDUCATIONAL OBJECTIVES

Medical Students (1) *APGO Objective*	*Residents in Obstetrics/Gynecology (2)* *CREOG Objective*	*Practitioners (3)* *ACOG Recommendation*
No specific recommendation	No specific recommendation	No specific recommendation

The use of herbs in medical practice flourished until the seventeenth century, when scientifically formulated pharmacologic agents began to progressively dominate the medical field (4). Currently, a renaissance in the use of herbal remedies in mainstream medicine is being observed. In the United States, the acceptance of herbal remedies by the general population is growing. In 1997, the rate of use increased by 380% when compared with 1990 (5). This is a public-driven phenomenon without the medical community's full acceptance. Therefore, many patients are hesitant to share their self-healing approaches with their physicians for the following reasons:

■ Patients accept herbal remedies as natural products or food, which they interpret as meaning "safe" by the majority of users, as opposed to medicine.
■ Inadequate information in reference to safety and efficacy of herbs.
■ Fear of disapproval by a physician.
■ Perception of the patient of the physician's lack of knowledge.
■ Physician's lack of understanding of a patient's motivation to use herbs.
■ Patient's ability to control her health problem(s).

A physician's personal conviction that herbs are nothing more than placebos may lead to dismissal of herbs as a therapeutic trend in medicine. That patients use herbs is an undeniable fact, and unsupervised administration may cause health hazards or interact with conventional drugs. Therefore, it is necessary for physicians to adopt an attitude of acceptance regarding herbal treatment, and to learn about such alternative therapies and their potential interference with conventional treatment. The field of gynecology is not immune from this trend and in fact is even more affected than some other specialties. The process of incorporating questions about alternative therapy into history taking does not require new skills. However, patients' responses will require knowledge for their interpretation. Therefore, physician history taking should embrace the following:

■ Type, dose, and form of preparation of herbal remedies
■ Side effect and severity produced by herbal remedies
■ Type and dose of dietary supplements taken concomitantly with or independently from herbal remedies
■ Type and dose of other over-the-counter or prescription medication taken concomitantly with herbal remedies
■ Who provides advice for herbal remedies or supplemental nutrients, or over-the-counter drugs (an herbalist, pharmacist, naturopathic practitioner, acupuncturist, or natural healer)

Adverse reactions to herbs or dietary nutrient supplements can be attributed to inherent toxicity, dose, idiosyncratic reactions to herbs with allergic reactions, anaphylaxis, and herb-drug potential interactions. Additional potential problems exist within manufacturing and quality control regarding the amount of active ingredient and contamination. Herbs also may be inappropriately or incompletely labeled. Herbs, as natural products, are not subject to the same vigorous scrutiny as standard pharmaceuticals. Therefore, theoretical (potential) and actual herb-drug interactions and adverse reactions to herbs are difficult to appropriately judge.

There are several reasons for patients turning to herbal remedies (6–8):

■ Sense of taking action and control of their health problem.
■ Medical professional care is not immediately available, too costly, or too time consuming.

- Cultural and religious factors.
- Public conviction that natural herbal products are healthier than conventional agents.
- Limited public knowledge about the actual and potential toxicity of herbs.

It is the general conviction of allopathic practitioners that complementary and alternative therapeutic remedies are not appropriately tested in well designed, adequately powered, and randomized controlled clinical trials. Therefore, these remedies are labeled as unscientific, where as the Conventional remedies are of course labeled scientific. Since the 1960s, the U.S. Food and Drug Administration has set the standard for approving any new medication, but many therapies introduced before that time do not meet these criteria and are still commonly used (e.g., warfarin, heparin, or aspirin). The American College of Chest Physicians (ACCP) Consensus Conference on Antithrombotic Therapy documented that only 24% of the 1986 recommendations were evidence based, and 55% of recommendations were based on uncontrolled clinical observational studies. In 1998, the same group established that 44% of recommendation met the grade A standard for evidence-based recommendations (9,10).

The type of study and its design determines the level of medical evidence and is classified as follows (11):

- *Grade A* consists of a clinical study
  Level I: Large randomized trials with clear-cut results and low risk of error

- *Grade B* consists of a clinical study
  Level II: Small randomized trials with uncertain results and moderate to high risk of error (B1)
  Level III: Nonrandomized, contemporaneous controls (B2)
- *Grade C*
  Level IV: Nonrandomized, historical controls (C1)
  Level V: No controls, case series only (C2)

Complementary/alternative therapies (unconventional therapies) are grade C at best and predominantly are based on case reports. They therefore represent the weakest grade of recommendation. As previously stated, many conventional therapeutic modalities are based on grade C recommendations, and because they come from the mainstream of modern Western medicine they are generally accepted. Based on the same grade of study, unconventional therapies are not incorporated into conventional practice because most well trained physicians have not been introduced to the therapeutic armamentarium of complementary/alternative medicine. Most conventional doctors are not adequately exposed to unconventional therapies and feel uncomfortable making management decisions in this field. This scenario presents a challenge for integrating conventional and complementary/alternative therapies in the field of gynecology.

Table 30.1 lists the most frequently used herbal remedies and commonly administered prescription medication in gynecology and summarizes the potential and actual herbal-drug interactions. It is designed to guide students, residents, and practitioners in the possible adverse reactions and potential interactions associated with use in gynecologic practice.

TABLE 30.1. POTENTIAL HERB–DRUG INTERACTIONS

Herb	Indication/Dose	Side Effects	Contraindications	Drug Interactions Potential	Drug Interactions Actual	Type of Evidence for Use
Allspice (12)	Dysmenorrhea Bruises Common cold Intestinal gas	GI symptoms Skin rash Seizures with excessive use	Chronic GI illness History of cancer Increased risk for cancer	Iron Other mineral supplements	Not determined	Anecdotal (12)
Aloe (12–18)	Oligomenorrhea Herpes Acne Skin irritation Common cold Constipation Depression Diabetes Capsules, 75 mg, 100 mg, 200 mg Juice 99.6% Gel, 98%, 99.6%	Abortion Premature delivery Diarrhea Dehydration Intestinal spasms Skin irritation Allergy Hypokalemia Increased adverse effect of corticosteroids	Menorrhagia Intermenstrual bleeding Menses Pregnancy Lactation	Cardiac glycosides (digoxin, lanoxin) Diuretics (lasix, edecrin, demadex, bumex) Cardiac antiarrhythmics Corticosteroids	Oral antidiabetic agents (16)	Grade B₁ (16) Inconclusive clinical evidence (14,15) No beneficial clinical effect (14,18)
American cransebill (12)	Birth control Abnormal endometrial bleeding Vaginal discharge Bladder inflammation Tincture, 2–4 cc 3 times daily	Liver damage	Pregnancy Lactation	Not determined	Not determined	No beneficial clinical effect (12)
Angelica (12,15,19)	Menopausal symptoms Osteoporosis Dysmenorrhea Tincture, 1.5 g daily dose	Dizziness Faint feeling Photodermatosis May pose a cancer risk	Pregnancy Lactation Peptic ulcer Diabetes	Cumadin (unusual bleeding or bruises Aspirin Laxative Antacids	Not determined	No beneficial clinical effect (12) Unproven use in folk medicine (19)

(continued)

TABLE 30.1. (CONTINUED)

Herb	Indication/Dose	Side Effects	Contraindications	Drug Interactions		Type of Evidence for Use
				Potential	Actual	
Belladonna (15,19)	Colic-like uterine cramps Liver and gallbladder disorder Muscular pain GI colic pain Asthma Dray extract, 0.3 g daily dose	No adverse reaction is reported with appropriate dose Toxicity is dose related and fatal dose related to the atropine content of 5–50 g (corresponds to 100 mg of atropine content)	Not reported	Tricyclic antidepressants (increases the anticholinergic effect) Antiarrhythmic agents (decreased therapeutic effects) GI motility drugs (decreased activity)	Not determined	Use in folk medicine for colic-like pain (19)
Black catechu (12)	Birth control Chronic gonorrhea Cracked nipples Diarrhea Dried extract, 0.3–2 g daily	Constipation Dizziness Hypotension	Pregnancy Lactation	Immune-suppressant drugs Antihypertensive agents (synergistic action) Narcotics for pain (worsen constipation)	Not determined	Unproven use in folk medicine (19)
Black cohosh (12,15,19–22)	Vasomotor symptoms due to menopause or oopherectomy Premenstrual syndrome (PMS) 80 mg daily for 6 months; also is available with St. John's Wort	Nausea Vomiting Hypotension Dizziness Miscarriages in large doses	Pregnancy (increased spontaneous abortion) Lactation	Antihypertensive agents (synergistic action)	Not determined	Grade C$_2$ for vasomotor symptoms (21) in large doses Anecdotal for PMS
Black haw (12,19)	Dysmenorrhea Miscarriage prevention Extract in a form of tea	Stomach upset	Allergy Pregnancy Lactation	Cumadin (increases bleeding potential)	Not determined	Anecdotal

424

Herb (references)	Uses and dosage	Adverse effects	Contraindications	Drug interactions		Evidence
Blue cohosh (12,19,23,24)	Amenorrhea, Dysmenorrhea, Threatened abortion; Capsules, 500 mg; Liquid extract 1:1 in 70% ethanol, 0.5–1 mL 3 times daily	Chest pain, Diarrhea, Stomach cramps, Hypertension with headaches, blurred vision, or seizures	Pregnancy, Lactation, Heart condition	Antihypertensive agents; Medication for angina pectoris (Nitroglycerine Sorbitrate, Vascor, Inderal, Cardizem Calan, Adalat); Nicotine replacement agents (Nicorrette, Nicoderm)	Not determined	Grade C2 and anecdotal
Boldo (12,25,26)	Dysmenorrhea, Gonorrhea, Syphilis; Dried extract, 2.5 g daily	Decreased coordination, Hyporeflexes, Seizures	Pregnancy, Lactation, Central nervous system disorder, Respiratory tract disorders	Not determined	Not determined	Anecdotal
Buchu (12,27)	Genital tract infection, Urinary tract infection; Tincture, 1–2 cc, orally 3–4 times daily	Increases menstrual flow, Increases abortion rate, GI symptoms, Liver damage, Renal dysfunction	Pregnancy, Lactation, Preexisting renal dysfunction or infection, or liver disorder	Cumadin (increases bleeding potential)	Not determined	Anecdotal
Burning bush (19)	Amenorrhea, Birth control; Infusion, 1–2 g dried herb to 1 cup of water, 2–3 times daily after meals	Not recorded	Not determined	Not determined	Not determined	Anecdotal
Butterbur (12,23)	Genital tract spasm, Urinary tract spasm	Abdominal pain or pressure, Difficulty urinating, Constipation, Difficulty breathing, Difficulty swallowing, Skin, eye, or stool discoloration, GI symptoms, Predisposes to liver damage and cancer	Pregnancy, Lactation, Asthma, Liver disorder	Atropine	Not determined	Anecdotal

(continued)

TABLE 30.1. (CONTINUED)

Herb	Indication/Dose	Side Effects	Contraindications	Drug Interactions			Type of Evidence for Use
				Potential	Actual		
Cacao tree (12)	Prevention of pregnancy stretch marks External use in a form of butter or syrup	Allergic reaction	Not determined	Not determined	Not determined		Use in folk medicine
Caraway (12,19)	Dysmenorrhea Dyspeptic complaints Essential oil, 1–3 drops in a single dose	Diarrhea Mucus membrane irritation	Allergy	Not determined	Not determined		Use in folk medicine
Castor oil plant (19,23,26–28)	Birth control	Acute intestinal pain (appendicitis-like) Allergy Nausea Vomiting Dehydration Electrolyte imbalance	Pregnancy Lactation Abdominal pain obstruction	Not determined	Not determined		Anecdotal
Catnip (12)	Dysmenorrhea Laxative Capsule, 380 mg Tincture, 2–4 mL orally 3 times daily	Headaches Nausea Vomiting	Pregnancy Lactation	Cardiac glycosides	Not determined		Use in folk medicine
Cat's claw (12,15,19,29,30)	Birth control (inhibition of ovarian steroid) synthesis Antiviral Antiinflammatory Capsule 250–500 mg, daily dose 250–1,000 mg	Acute renal failure	Pregnancy Lactation	Antihypertensive agents (synergistic action) Cumadin (increases bleeding potential) Iron (decreased therapeutic effect of iron)	Not determined		Grade C_2 and anecdotal

	Indications/Dosage	Adverse effects	Contraindications	Drug interactions		Use in folk medicine
Celandione (12,19,23,27)	Genitalia warts Fluid extract 1:1 in 25% ethanol for 2 weeks at a time (local toxicity)	Nausea Fatigue Insomnia Hypotension Drowsiness Liver damage Frequent urination	Pregnancy Lactation Liver disorder GI disorder	Cardiac glycosides Narcotics Oral antidiabetic agents Sulfa drugs	Not determined	
Chamomile (12,19,31–39)	Dysmenorrhea Antispasmodic, tea (1 tablespoon of flower heads in a cup of hot water for 10–15 min, four times daily) (31) Antiinflammatory 3–10% ointment or cream (32,33) Sedative, tea or capsules 125 mg, 354 mg, and 360 mg, 3–4 times daily mg, or 100% oil	Allergy Hay fever Asthma Anaphylactic reaction Conjunctivitis Nausea Vomiting (34–36) Influences on coordination (influences driving or operating machinery with large dose) Adverse reaction is rare (39)	Pregnancy (may trigger miscarriages; potentially teratogenic) Lactation Allergy Hay fever Asthma Prior anaphylactic reaction	Anticoagulants (37) (warfarin) Sedatives (excessive sedation, syncretic action)	Not determined	Antispasmodic [effective and safe, grade A evidence (31)] Antiinflammatory [topical application—no statistically significant differences, grade A evidence (32)] Sedative effect [Grade C_1 evidence (38)]
Chaste tree (12,19,40–43)	Endometrial bleeding Infertility Inadequate lactation Hyperprolactenemia (40) Premenstrual syndrome (41) Dray berries 20–40 mg daily (42) or capsules, 3.5–4.3 mg daily, or 50–70%, 40 drops of extract (19,42)	GI symptoms Abdominal–pelvic cramps Acne formation Transient headaches (41) Allergic reaction (41) Increases menstrual flow (12) Side effects seem to be rare (<2%) (42)	Pregnancy Lactation Hormonal replacement therapy (42,43)	Dopamine-receptor antagonists (haloperidol) may weaken or block the effects of Chaste tree (19) Oral contraceptive pills (may decrease the efficacy) (45)	Not determined	Inadequate luteal phase defect due to hyperprolactenemia [grade A evidence (40)] Premenstrual syndrome [grade C_1 evidence (41,44)]

(continued)

TABLE 30.1. (CONTINUED)

Herb	Indication/Dose	Side Effects	Contraindications	Drug Interactions Potential	Actual	Type of Evidence for Use
Clary (12,46)	Dysmenorrhea Warm compress with four drops of essential oil Premenstrual syndrome Decreased libido Inhalation with 2 drops of essential oil	Increased menstrual flow Headaches Drowsiness Euphoria	Pregnancy Lactation Estrogen-dependent or -sensitive cancer Hypermenorrhea	Alcohol (increases effect)	Not determined	Anecdotal
Couchgrass (12,47)	Premenstrual syndrome Urinary tract infection Capsule, 380 mg, once daily Tablet, 60 mg, 2–3 tablets, 1–2 per day	Electrolyte imbalance Skin irritation	Not determined	Not determined	Not determined	Anecdotal
Cranberry (48–53)	Urinary tract infection (UTI) prevention for sexually active women Concentrated juice extract (commercial is only 10–20% pure) 300 mL (10 oz) (48) Capsule extracts, 300–400 mg, 1 capsule daily (49,50)	No adverse reaction at these doses	Not determined	Not determined	Not determined	Grade B$_1$ (48,49), Grade C$_2$ (50) [no clinical definitive data to support for prevention (52)] No evidence to support therapeutic effect in UTI (53)
Damiana (19,54)	Sexual dysfunction Capsule 380–450 mg daily	No side effects at recommended doses	Not determined	Not determined	Not determined	Anecdotal

428

Herb (refs)	Use / Dosage	Adverse effects	Contraindications	Interaction	Drug interaction	Efficacy
Devil's claw (12,37,55)	Dysmenorrhea; Menopause symptoms; Capsule 200–750 mg (4.5 g daily); Tinctures; Tea	No side effects at recommended doses	Gastric or duodenal ulcer; Pregnancy (may cause uterine contraction and miscarriage); Breast-feeding	Cardiac antiarrhythmic medication	Warfarin [increased risk for bleeding (37)]	Anecdotal
DHEA (12,56–60) (natural steroid found in the yam plants with no receptors identified in the human body)	Enhancing libido (56); Slowing down aging (56); Menopause symptoms (56); Capsules 5 mg, 25 mg, 50 mg (25–50 mg is average dose); Time-released tablet 15 mg daily	Hirsutism; Insomnia; Mood lability; Behavioral changes; Irritability with increased aggressiveness; Decreased HDL cholesterol (57); Increased risk of breast cancer (58)	Pregnancy; Lactation with breast-feeding; Hormonally dependent malignancy	Tobacco smoking and alcohol consumption may increase DHEA activity (59)	Reduces serum bioactive testosterone and androstenedione (60) but increases serum total testosterone levels (58); Increases serum endogenous estradiol levels (58)	Anecdotal
Dong quai (12,37,61–63)	Dysmenorrhea; Irregular menstrual cycle; PMS (61); Menopause symptoms; Tablets 0.5 mg or raw root (4.5–30 g boiled or soaked in wine)	Bleeding; Skin sensitivity to sunlight; Diarrhea; Fever; Adverse reaction is rare with good safety profiles (61)	Bleeding disorders; Suring menses; Following miscarriage; Hypomenorrhea; Pregnancy; Diabetes (increase blood glucose level)	Not determined	Warfarin (increased risk for bleeding (37,62,63)	Anecdotal and grade C_2; Menopause symptoms [no significant effect, grade B_1 (64)]
Echinacea (14,15,39,65–69)	Lower urinary tract infection (65); Common cold (14); Capsule 300–400 mg three times daily (tid) (14) or tablet 335 mg tid; Tincture 30–50 drops tid (39)	Anaphylaxis (67); Skin rash; Pruritis; Dizziness; Undetermined long-term (>6 weeks) effect on the immune system (potential immunosuppressive) (14,39); Hepatotoxicity (69)	Multiple sclerosis; Collagenosis; HIV infection; Tuberculosis infection (65,68)	Corticosteroids and cyclosporine [immunostimulating effect of echinacea may offset immunosuppressive effect of corticosteroids and cyclosporine (66)]	Not determined	Inconclusive evidence (14)

(continued)

TABLE 30.1. (CONTINUED)

Herb	Indication/Dose	Side Effects	Contraindications	Drug Interactions Potential	Drug Interactions Actual	Type of Evidence for Use
Evening primrose oil (15,19,70,71)	Mastalgia (70) PMS (71) Menopausal hot flashes (19) Capsule 500 mg or 1,300 mg (3–4 g daily in divided doses) (19)	Seizure (lowers the inconclusive seizures threshold	Seizure disorder	Anticonvulsant agents	Not determined	Anecdotal (19) and inconclusive [grade B₁ evidence (15,71)]
False unicorn root (12,19)	Menstrual dysfunctions Dysmenorrhea Menopause symptoms Tincture 5–10 drops daily	Occasionally gastric cramps	Pregnancy Lactation with breast-feeding	Not determined	Not determined	Anecdotal
Fennel (12,19)	Menstrual dysfunction Oil 0.1–0.6 mL for 2 weeks	Allergy	Pregnancy Lactation with breast-feeding	Not determined	Not determined	Anecdotal
Garlic (14,15, 19,66,77–80)	Dysmenorrhea Bloating Common colds High pressure (19) Hyperlipidemia (14) Fresh bulb (2–5 g),, oil, extract, (dried powder 0.4–1.2 g)0 Capsule 300–900 mg daily	Contact dermatitis Stomach upset Reflux Headaches Offensive breath odor Antiplatelets (14,77)	Elective surgery (7–10 days prior to surgery) Pregnancy Lactation with breast-feeding	Increased drug absorption by intestinal vasodilatation (15) Inhibition of iodine uptake (78) Antidiabetic oral agents (may potentiate hypoglycemia) (39)	Warfarin and antiplatelet agents (14,15,62,66)	Lowering total cholesterol, triglyceride, and blood pressure [grade B₁ evidence (79,80)] Gynecology (anecdotal)

Herb (refs)	Uses and dosage	Side effects	Contraindications	Drug interactions		Evidence
Ginger (19,39,66,81–84)	Preventing postanesthesia nausea and vomiting following laparoscopic gynecology surgery (powdered root, 1 g) (81) Preventing nausea/vomiting due to chemotherapy (capsule 250–1,000 mg 3–4 times daily or tea: steep powder or fresh root) (39) Motion sickness (stick consumed during travel) (82,83)	No serious side effects GI upset (mild) (39) Contact dermatitis (rare) (84)	Pregnancy Lactation with breast-feeding (39) Gallstone (19)	Warfarin (may increase anticoagulant effect of Warfarin) (66)	Not determined	Grade B₁ evidence (81–83)
Ginkgo biloba (39,62,65, 69,85–91)	Premenstrual symptoms (85) Sexual disorder antidepressant-induced (mainly orgasmic and less libido or arousal phase) (86,87) Memory enhancement (88) Capsule 60–120 mg 3 times daily	GI upset (mild) Allergy Headaches Skin reaction Heart palpitation (89,65)	Pregnancy Lactation with breast-feeding Elective surgery (7–10 days prior to surgery)	Not determined	Warfarin and NSAIDs (increased bleeding) (62,63,69,89) Thiazide diuretic (causing hypertension) (90) Monoamine oxidase (MAO) inhibitor (may compete for MAO inhibitor) (91)	PMS [grade B₁ evidence (85)] Sexual disorder [grade B₁ evidence (86)] Memory enhancement [grade B₁ evidence (88)]

(continued)

TABLE 30.1. *(Continued)*

Herb	Indication/Dose	Side Effects	Contraindications	Drug Interactions			Type of Evidence for Use
				Potential	**Actual**		
Goldenseal (12,19)	Dysmenorrhea Irregular menstruation Capsule or tablet 250–540 mg (average 750 mg in divided dose) Dried root 0.5–1 g three times daily	GI symptoms Mouth sores Sleepiness Respiratory depression Slow pulse, asystole Numbness or prickling in the arms and legs Skin inflammation Leucopoenia	Heart disease Vascular disease Pregnancy Lactation with breast-feeding Operating machines or driving a car	Warfarin Beta blockers Calcium channel blockers Cardiac glycosides Alcohol	Not determined		Anecdotal
Gotu kola (12,23)	Birth control Capsule 250–450 mg (average 450 mg) daily	Burning Itching Drowsiness Sedation	Diabetes Pregnancy Lactation Hypertension	Antidiabetic Drugs reducing cholesterol	Not determined		Anecdotal
Great burnet (19)	Menorrhagia Menopause symptoms Extract, juice, or tea	Not determined	Not determined	Not determined	Not determined		Folk medicine
Green tea (12,19,101–106)	Improved prognosis in stage I and II breast cancer (≥5 cups/day prior malignancy occurrence) (101) Lowering cholesterol (8-week therapy reduces serum cholesterol up to 4%) (102,103) Potentially preventive effect against cancer in humans (104–106) Capsule 100 mg 3–4 times daily (3 cups of green tea contains 240–320 mg) (19)	Not determined at the recommended doses (19)	<5 cups during pregnancy	Chemotherapy with adriamycin (12) Alkaline medication (green tea decreases resorption) (19) Drinking milk may reduce the tea's antioxidant effect (12)	Not determined		Grade C₁ evidence

432

Common name (References)	Medicinal uses and dosage	Adverse effects/toxicity	Contraindications	Drug interactions	Efficacy
Hops (12,23,45)	Menopause symptoms; Extract 2–4 mg daily (provides a sedative effect)	Sedation; Allergy; Mental slowness; Blisters	Estrogen-dependent cancer; Pregnancy; Lactation (23,45)	Alcohol; Anticholinergic; Antidepressant; Antihistamines; Antipsychotic	Anecdotal
Jequirity (19)	Contraceptive (abortifacient)	Toxicity	Toxicity	Not determined	Folk medicine
Kava (12–14, 19,107–111)	Menopausal symptoms; Anxiety (induces relaxation, promotes sleep, improves interpersonal interaction) (107); Capsule root extract 100–500 mg (150–300 mg daily with daily dose of Kava 50–240 mg); Tincture 30 drops tid; Infusion ½ cups (twice daily); The drug should be administered with food or liquid (19)	No health hazard with proper dose; Hallucinogenic (13); Reducing motor reflexes (reduces coordination) and may cause dyskinesia (driving and operating machinery can be affected) (109); Hepatotoxicity (110); Skin reactions (111)	Pregnancy; Lactation with breast-feeding (45); Parkinson's disease (19)	Not determined; Sedative agents and augments and prolongs sedation and hypnotics (15); Alprazolem (can result in coma) (66,69); Anesthetics (prolongs sedation time) (15); Alcohol (concomitant use causes hypnotic action) (19); L-dopa (antagonizing the effect of dopamine) (12,19)	Anxiety [grade B$_1$ evidence (108)]; Menopause (anecdotal)
Kelpware (12)	Menstrual irregularities; Inflammatory bladder disease; Soft extract 200–600 mg daily	Excessive urination; Excessive thirst; Elevation of plasma glucose; Liver damage	Pregnancy; Lactation with breast-feeding; Diabetes; Malignancy; Kidney disorder; Liver disease; Heart conditions	Thyroid hormone (increase therapeutic effect); Anticoagulants	Anecdotal

(continued)

TABLE 30.1. (CONTINUED)

Herb	Indication/Dose	Side Effects	Contraindications	Drug Interactions		Type of Evidence for Use
				Potential	Actual	
Khella (12,23,112)	Dysmenorrhea Capsule, tablet, tea, and injectable (average daily dose of 20 mg of khellin) (12)	Allergy Sleeplessness Sunlight sensitivity (mild) Liver enzyme elevation GI symptoms (prolong use) Vertigo (prolong use) Hypotension (mild) (12)	Pregnancy Lactation with breast-feeding (23) Liver disease Angina symptoms	Cardiac glycoside (112)	Warfarin (augments bleeding) Calcium channel blockers (enhances lowering pressure) (12)	Anecdotal
Lady's Mantle (12,19)	Dysmenorrhea Menstrual irregularities Menopausal symptoms (12,19) The average is 5–10 mg of herb (19)	No side effects with designated dose Liver damage (potential risk)	Pregnancy Lactation with breast-feeding	Not determined	Not determined	Folk medicine
Licorice or liquorice (19,15, 26,27,45,66,69, 113–118)	Antiinflammatory (19)	Hypokalemia (113) Hypertension (114) Cardiac arrest (115) Ventricular tachycardia (116) Chronic fatigue (117) Mineralocorticoid excess syndrome (sodium and water retention, loss of potassium, limit renine-angiotensin-aldosterone system) (118)	Kidney insufficiency (45) Hypertension (26) Prolonged use (>4–6 weeks) (45) Pregnancy (26,27) Liver disorder (26) Diabetes (45)	Estrogen (augments estrogen effect) (15) Monoamine oxidase inhibitors (increased side effects) (15,66) Oral contraceptive (OC) pills increase sensitivity to licorice (113)	Anti-hypertension diuretics (26,69) (non–potassium-sparing and can offset the effect of spironolactone Cardiac glycoside (increases arrhythmia) (27,69) Corticosteroids (increased plasma levels) (15)	Anecdotal
Lovage (12,19)	Menstrual irregularity Urinary tract infections Tea 1 cup several times a day between meals (4–8 g of herb daily)	Low potential of skin sensitivity to UV	Pregnancy Lactation with breast-feeding	Anticoagulant agents	Not determined	Folk medicine

Herb	Indication/Dosage	Side Effects	Contraindications	Drug Interactions		Evidence
Lungwort (12)	Hypermenorrhea; Tincture 1–4 mL tid	GI symptoms (mild); Skin inflammation	Pregnancy; Lactation with breast-feeding	Anticoagulant agents	Not determined	Folk medicine
Madder (12)	Oligomenorrhea; Amenorrhea; Tincture (liquid extract 20 drops tid for 2 months)	Galactorrhea (red-tinged); Perspiration, saliva, tears, or urine can be red-tinged (contact lenses can be stained)	Pregnancy; Lactation with breast-feeding	Not determined	Not determined	Folk medicine
Marjoram (12)	Oligomenorrhea; Amenorrhea; Dysmenorrhea; Tincture ½–1 teaspoon tid; Tea (1–2 teaspoons of dried leaves/flowers no more than 3 cups daily)	No side effects with recommended dose	Pregnancy	Not determined	Not determined	Not determined
Motherwort (12,19)	Amenorrhea; Dysmenorrhea; Tincture 2–6 mL daily; Liquid extract (1:1) 2–4 mL tid	No health hazards with proper dose; Skin sensitivity to light; Prolong bleeding	Pregnancy; Sunlight exposure; Thrombocytopenia	Warfarin (augments bleeding); Beta blockers	Not determined	Folk medicine
Mugwort (12,19)	Hypermenorrhea; Tincture 2.5 mL tid (dried herb 15 g in 500 mL of water); Menopausal symptoms; Tincture 5 mL 30 min before bedtime	Allergy; Skin reactions	Pregnancy; Lactation with breast-feeding; Hematological disorders	Warfarin (augments bleeding)	Not determined	Folk medicine
Nettle (12)	Abnormal endometrial bleeding; Tincture ¼–1 teaspoon twice daily (bid)	GI symptoms; Hives	Pregnancy; Lactation with breast-feeding	Diuretics (hypokalemia)	Not determined	Folk medicine

(continued)

TABLE 30.1. (*CONTINUED*)

Herb	Indication/Dose	Side Effects	Contraindications	Drug Interactions		Type of Evidence for Use
				Potential	**Actual**	
Oak (12,19)	Abnormal endometrial bleeding: 2 capsules tid Tea 1 cup tid (3 g of herb) Vaginal discharge: douche (boiling for 15 min 20 g of oak/1 L of water)	No health hazard with proper dose GI symptoms Abdominal pain Kidney disorder Liver damage Death may occur from tannic acid enemas or extended use on skin	Pregnancy Lactation with breast-feeding Skin damage	Atropine Caffeine Cardiac glycosides Morphine Nicotine Quinine Heavy metal salts such as iron or gold	Not determined	Folk medicine
Oregano (12,19)	Dysmenorrhea Capsule 450 mg, 2 capsules orally bid Oil: few drops to juice Tea: 1 cup several times daily	No adverse reaction in designated dose	Iron-deficiency anemia	Iron (decreases absorption)	Not determined	Folk medicine
Parsley (12,19,45)	Menstrual irregularities Capsule 430–455 mg (average daily dose 1 g) Tea: 2–3 cups daily (1–2 g of the leaf or root) Liquid extract 2–4 mL tid	No side effects determined	Allergy to the herb Pregnancy Lactation with breast-feeding Heart condition Hypotension Liver disease Kidney insufficiency Peptic ulcer	Antihypertension agents Antidepressants Narcotic pain medications	Not determined	Folk medicine
Pennyroyal (12,19,23,27,45)	Amenorrhea Uterine leiomyomata Premenstrual syndrome Tea: 2 cups daily of 1–2 teaspoons of dried herb for 1 cup of boiling water); overdose (>5 g) can be fatal	Hepatotoxicity (particularly oil) Abdominal cramps GI symptoms Lethargy Dizziness Confusion Hallucination Malaise	Pregnancy Lactation with breast-feeding Liver disorder Kidney disorder Seizure	Biaxin Diflucan Nizoral Tagamet Zithromax	Not determined	Anecdotal

Herb	Uses/Dose	Side Effects	Contraindications	Drug Interactions		Evidence
Poke (pokeweed) (12,19)	Breast inflammation or abscess Dysmenorrhea Usual dose is 60–100 mg daily	All parts of the herb are poisonous (cooking reduces toxicity) Central nervous symptoms, including coma Tachycardia Hypotension Respiratory dysfunction Headaches GI symptoms Blood disorders	Pregnancy Lactation with breast-feeding Allergy Driving or operating machinery	Antabus (poke contains alcohol) Alcohol Sedatives Tranquilizers Narcotic medications Muscle relaxant Antiseizure drugs Oral contraceptive Fertility drugs	Not determined	Anecdotal
Queen Anne's lace (12,23,27,45)	Menstrual irregularity Tea: no dose established	Increased skin sensitivity to sunlight Increased frequency of urination Occasionally may cause bradycardia, hypotension Decrease mental alertness	Pregnancy Lactation with breast-feeding	Antihypertensive agents Cardiac glycosides Antianxiety drugs Sedatives Muscle relaxant Pain medication	Not determined	Anecdotal
Ragwort (12,19)	Dysmenorrhea Menstrual irregularities External use only	Carcinogenic GI symptoms Jaundice Abdominal pain Fever Fatigue Coughing	Pregnancy Lactation with breast-feeding	Not determined	Not determined	Folk medicine
Red clover (12,13,78, 119,120)	Menopause symptoms (phytoestrogens used for natural estrogen replacement therapy) Tablet 100 mg Capsule 200–430 mg Tincture 2–6 mL tid Tea Raw sprouts	Breast enlargement and tenderness Nausea Bloting Menstrual irregularity Weight gain No significant influence on the lipoprotein profiles (119) It is considered unopposed to estrogen therapy, and the impact on the endometrium should be recognized	Pregnancy or planning pregnancy Lactation with breast-feeding Estrogen-dependent cancer Coagulation disorders	Tamoxifen (Nolvadex) or raloxifene (Evista) effectiveness can be reduced by red clover	Warfarin (augments bleeding) (120) Aspirin Oral contraceptive pills	Anecdotal

437

(continued)

TABLE 30.1. (CONTINUED)

Herb	Indication/Dose	Side Effects	Contraindications	Drug Interactions Potential	Drug Interactions Actual	Type of Evidence for Use
Rosemary (12,19,26,45)	Oligomenorrhea Amenorrhea Dysmenorrhea Induction of abortion (2,19) Tincture: single dose of 20–40 drops daily Rosemary wine (20 g of herb added in 1 l of wine, standing for 5 days)	No health hazards with suggested dose (19) Increased skin sensitivity to sunlight GI symptoms Skin irritation	Pregnancy or planning pregnancy (12,26,45) Allergy (12)	Antabuse (contains alcohol)	Not determined	Folk medicine
Rue (12,19,23,45)	Dysmenorrhea Oligomenorrhea Birth control (12,19) Capsule (daily dose of the herb is 0.5–1 g) tid Tea: 2 cups daily (12,19)	No health hazards with suggested dose (19) Increased skin sensitivity to sunlight (photosensitization) Increased risk of miscarriage (12)	Pregnancy or planning pregnancy (23,45) Excessive exposure to ultraviolet light (45) Renal insufficiency (45)	Cardiac glycosides Antihypertensive agents (12) Fertility drugs (decreased effectiveness) (12)	Not determined	Folk medicine
Safflower oil (12,19,23,45)	Menstrual irregularities (12,19) To induce abortion (19) Capsule 390 mg (the average daily dose is 3 g with a single dose of 1 g)	Not determined	Pregnancy or planning pregnancy (23,45) Lactation with breast-feeding (12) Peptic ulcer (45) Hemorrhagic disorders (45)	Immune system suppressants: Imuran, Prograf, Sandimmune (12)	—	Folk medicine
Sassafras (12,19)	Venereal disease To enhance performance Extract (1:1 in 25% alcohol) 2–4 mL orally tid Tincture 5 g daily	Carcinogenic	Due to carcinogenic effect, the herb should not be used (19)	Not determined	Not determined	Anecdotal
Shepherd's purse (12,19)	Hypermenorrhea Premenstrual syndrome Extract 10–15 g/day	No health hazards with suggested dose (19)	Pregnancy Lactation with breast-feeding (12)	Not determined	Not determined	Folk medicine

Herb	Uses/Dose	Toxicity/Side effects	Pregnancy/Lactation	Antabuse (contains alcohol)	Not determined	Anecdotal
Skullcap (12)	To enhance chemotherapy for cancer Capsule 425–429 mg tid Tea: dried herb 1–2 g tid Tincture: 1:5 in 45% alcohol, 1–2 mL orally tid	In large dose can be toxic and cause irregular heart beats, contusion, stupor Twitching Liver damage	Pregnancy Lactation with breast-feeding	Antabuse (contains alcohol)		
Soybean (19,121–127)	Menopause symptoms (121,122) Osteoporosis (prevention and therapy) (123,124) The average preventive dose is 16–20 g (32–40 mg of isoflavones) daily (125) and therapeutic dose is 24–30 g (48–60 mg isoflavones) (125)	No health hazards with suggested dose (19) GI symptoms (mild) (19) Allergy (124)	Pregnancy or planning pregnancy (in animal study, physiologic markers and/or morphologic changes of sexual differentiation were altered) (126) Lactation with breast-feeding	Not determined	Estrogens (synergic actions) (127) Antibiotics change isoflavone metabolism (124) Warfarin (augments bleeding) (124)	Menopause (anecdotal evidence) Osteoporosis (inconclusive evidence) (123,126) Lipoprotein profiles (no effect on HDL cholesterol; decreases total and LDH cholesterol, and triglyceride) (125)
St. John's wort (12,14,20,68, 129–134)	Menopause symptoms (76.4% psychosomatic symptoms improvement) (128) Premenstrual syndrome (50% improvement in symptom severity) (129) Depression (mild-moderate form improvement up to 55%) (14,20,130) Tablet 300 mg tid (standardized to 0.3% hypericin) (14,128–130)	Dry mouth Headaches Sweating asthenia Nausea Dizziness Withdrawals (131) Photosensitivity (14)	Allergy Pregnancy Lactation with breast-feeding (12)	Tyramine (food or beverages such as Chianti wine, beer, aged cheese, chicken liver, chocolate, bananas or meat tenderizers) (12)	Oral contraceptive pills Warfarin Cyclosporin Amphetamines (132) Cardiac glycoside (133) Antidepressants: (a) Monoamine oxidase inhibitors (potentiate effectiveness; (b) Selective serotonin reuptake inhibitors (potentiate effectiveness) (68) Photosensitizer drugs (e.g., tetracycline or piroxicam) (134)	Menopause [grade C_2 evidence (128)] Premenstrual syndrome [grade C_2 (129)] Mild-to-moderate depression [grade B_1 evidence(130)] Moderate-to-severe depression (the putative evidence available)

(continued)

TABLE 30.1. (CONTINUED)

| Herb | Indication/Dose | Side Effects | Contraindications | Drug Interactions | | Type of Evidence for Use |
				Potential	Actual	
Stavia (19)	Birth control Cut herb for oral administration	No health hazards with suggested dose	Not determined	Not determined	Not determined	Folk medicine
Tea tree oil (12,19)	Vaginal infections (12) Disinfect (19) Oil 0.4–100% used internally and externally	No health hazards with suggested dose (9) GI symptoms Decreased coordination	Allergy Pregnancy Lactation with breast-feeding (12)	Not determined	Not determined	Folk medicine
Thyme (12,19)	Dysmenorrhea (12) Cough Bronchitis (13) Extract (12–14%), 1–2 g is taken 1–3 times daily Tea: 1.5–2 g dried herb tid Cough syrup, 1 teaspoon orally every 2 hours as needed	No health hazards with suggested dose (19) GI symptoms Cracked lips Dizziness Headaches Muscle weakness Bradycardia Decreased respiratory rate Tongue irritation from toothpaste (12)	No health hazards with suggested dose (19) Pregnancy Lactation with breast-feeding Allergy Heart condition GI disorder (12)	Not determined	Not determined	Dysmenorrhea (anecdotal evidence) (12) Cough and bronchitis [grade C_1 evidence (19)]
True unicorn root (12)	Menstrual irregularities Tea or liquid extract	In large dose, GI symptoms may occur	Pregnancy Lactation with breast-feeding GI disorder	Sedatives Antihistamines Seizure agents Narcotics for pain Tranquilizers	Not determined	Anecdotal
Turmeric (12,19)	Amenorrhea Bruising Cystitis Tincture: 10–15 drops bid or tid Tea: 2–3 cups between meals Powder (1.5–3 g/day bid or tid after meal)	No health hazards with suggested dose (19)	Pregnancy Lactation with breast-feeding Bleeding disorder (12) Gallstones Biliary duct obstruction (19)	Warfarian Immune system suppressant Nonsteroidal antiinflammatory drugs (12)	Not determined	Anecdotal

Herb	Uses/Dosage	Adverse effects	Contraindications/Cautions	Drug interactions	Efficacy
Valerian (12,14,15,19, 39,135,136)	Anxiety Insomnia 400 mg at night (14,39) Tea: 2–3 g/1 tsp, tid (39)	No health hazards with suggested dose (19) Fatigue Tremor Headaches Paradoxical insomnia (14,39) Morning sedation (135) Hepatotoxicity (136)	Pregnancy Lactation with breast-feeding (12) Driving or operating machinery for several hours following valerian administration	Sedatives Hypnotic agents Alcohol Antihypertensive Anesthetics (prolongation of sedation time) (15,137)	Not determined Inconclusive evidence (14)
Wild yam (12,19)	Dysmenorrhea Menopause symptoms Wild yam is used as an active component of semisynthetic agent (DHEA) (19) Capsule 200 mg, 400 mg, 505 mg, or 535 mg Liquid extract (1:1 or 1:2); 250 mg/mL (19)	No health hazards with suggested dose (19) Masculinizing effect (acne, oily skin, hirsutism, menstrual irregularities may occur at the dose of 25 mg of DHEA) Headaches (12)	Pregnancy Lactation with breast-feeding Hormone-dependent malignancy (12)	Estrogen (synergistic effect) Antiinflammatory effect of indomethacine is decreased (19)	Not determined Anecdotal
Yarrow (12,19,23, 26,27,45)	Breast fibrocystic disease Menstrual irregularities	No health hazards with suggested dose (19) Allergy Photosensitivity Bleeding (12)	Pregnancy (23,27,45) Lactation with breast-feeding (12) Allergy (19,26)	Warfarin Antihypertensive Sedatives Tranquilizers Narcotic pain drugs Antiseizure agents Muscle relaxants (12)	Not determined Folk medicine

GI, gastrointestinal.

441

REFERENCES

1. Association of Professors of Gynecology and Obstetrics (APGO). *Medical student educational objectives,* 7th ed. Washington, DC: APGO, 1997.
2. Council on Resident and Gynecology (CREOG). *Educational objectives core curriculum for residents in obstetrics and gynecology,* 5th ed. Washington, DC: CREOG, 1996.
3. American College of Obstetrician and Gynecologists (ACOG). *Educational bulletins.* Washington, DC: ACOG, 2000.
4. Trevelyan J. Herbal medicine. *Nurse Times* 1993:89:36–38.
5. Eisenberg DM, Davis RB, Ettner SL, et al. Trends in alternative medicine use in the United States, 1990–1997: results of a follow-up national survey. *JAMA* 1998;280:1569–1575.
6. Brown JS, Marcy SA. The use of botanicals for health purposes by members of a prepaid health plan. *Res Nurs Health* 1991;14:339–350.
7. Gill GV, Redmond S, Garratt F, Paisey R. Diabetes and alternative medicine: cause for concern. *Diabetes Med* 1994;11:210–213.
8. Gesler WM. Therapeutic landscapes: medicinal issues in light of the new cultural geography. *Soc Sci Med* 1992;34:735–746.
9. First ACCP Conference on Antithrombotic Therapy. *Chest* 1986 (conference supplement).
10. Fifth ACCP Conference on Antithrombotic Therapy. *Chest* 1999 (conference supplement).
11. Sackett DL. Rules of evidence and clinical recommendations on the use antithrombotic agents. *Chest* 1986;89(suppl):2–3.
12. Fetrow CW, Avila JR. The complete guide to herbal medicines. Springhouse, PA, 1999.
13. Winslow LC, Kroll DJ. Herbs as medicines. *Arch Intern Med* 1998;158:2192–2199.
14. Mar C, Bent S. An evidence-based review of 10 most commonly used herbs. *Best Practice* 1999;171:168–171.
15. Hardy ML. Herb-drug interactions: an evidence-based table. *Alternative Med Alert* 2000;6:64–69.
16. Bunyapraphatsara N, Yongchaiyudha S, Rungpitarangsi V, et al. Antidiabetic activity of aloe vera L. juice II. Clinical trial in diabetes mellitus patients in combination with glibenclamide. *Phytomedicine* 1996;3:245–248.
17. Reynolds T, Dweck AC. Aloe vera leaf gel : a review update. *J Ethnopharmacol* 1999;68:3–37.
18. Vogler BK, Ernst E. Aloe vera: a systemic review of its clinical effectiveness. *Br J Gen Pract* 1999;49:823–828.
19. *PDR for herbal medicines.* Montvale, NJ: Medical Economics Company, 2000.
20. Rotblatt MD. Herbal medicine: a practical guide to safety and quality assurance. *Best Practice* 1999;171:172–175.
21. Vorberg G. Treatment of menopausal symptoms. *ZFA* 1984;60:626–629.
22. Shaw CR. The perimenopausal hot flashes: epidemiology, physiology, and treatment. *Nurse Pract* 1997;22:55–56, 61–66.
23. Farnsworth NR, Bingel AS, Cordell GA, et al. Potential value of plants as sources of new antifertility agents I. *J Pharm Sci* 1975;64:535–598.
24. Scott CC, Cohen KK. The pharmacologic action of N-methylcytisine. *Therapeutics* 1943;79:334–341.
25. Speisky H, Cassels BK. Boldo and Boldine: an emerging case of natural drug development. *Pharm Res* 1994;29:1–12.
26. Wichti M, ed. *Herbal drugs and phytopharmaceuticals.* Boca Raton, FL: CRC Press, 1994.
27. Brinker F. *The toxicology of botanical medicines,* 2nd ed. Sandy, OR: Eclectic Medical, 1996.
28. Scarpa A, Guerci A. Various uses of the castor oil plant (*Ricinus communis* L.), a review. *J Ethnopharmacol* 1982;5(2):117–122.
29. Rodriguez H, Massey PJ, Rodriguez K. Inhibition of steroid hormone production by a nutrition supplement "una de Gato" or "cat's claw." *Biol Reprod* 1998;58:208–214.
30. Hilepo JN, Bellucci AG, Mossey RT. Acute renal failure caused by "cat's claw" herbal remedy an a patient with systemic lupus erythematosus. *Nephron* 1997;77:361–369.
31. Weizman Z, Alkrinawi S, Goldfarb D, et al. Efficacy of herbal tea preparation in infantile colic. *J Pediatr* 1993;122:650–652.
32. Maiche AG, Grohn P, Maki-Hokkonen H. Effect of chamomile cream and almond ointment on acute radiation skin reaction. *Acta Oncol* 1991;30:395–396.
33. Fidler P, Loprinzi CL, O'Fallon JR, et al. Prospective evaluation of a chamomile mouthwash for prevention of 5-FU-induced oral mucositis *Cancer* 1996;77:522–525.
34. Benner MH, Lee HJ. Anaphylactic reaction to chamomile yea. *J Allergy Clin Immunol* 1973;52:307–308.
35. Subiza J, Subiza JL, Hinojosa M, et al. Anaphylactic reaction after the ingestion of chamomile tea: a study of cross-reactivity with other composite pollens. *J Allergy Clin Immunol* 1989;84:353–358.
36. Subiza J, Subiza JL, Alonso M, et al. Allergic conjunctivitis to chamomile tea. *Ann Allergy* 1990;65:127–132.
37. Heck AM, DeWitt BA, Lukes AL. Potential interactions between alternative therapies and warfarin. *Am J Health Syst Pharm* 2000;57:1221–1227.
38. Paladini AC, Marder M, Viola H, et al. Flavonoids and the central nervous system: from forgotten factors to potent anxiolytic compounds. *J Pharm Pharmacol* 199;51:519–526.
39. O'Hara MA, Kiefer D, Farrel K, et al. A review of 12 commonly used medical herbs. *Arch Fam Med* 1998;7:523–536.
40. Milewicz A, Gejdel E, Sworen H, et al. *Vitex agnus* extract in the treatment of luteal phase defects due to latent hyperprolactinemia. Results of randomized placebo-controlled double-blind study. *Arzneimittelforschung* 1993;43:752–756.
41. Reichert R. Comparing vitex and vitamin B_6 for PMS. *Q Rev Nat Med* 1998;9:19–20.
42. Foster S. Herbs for your health. Loveland, CO: Interweave, 1996.
43. Chaste tree. In: *The review of natural products. Facts and comparisons.* St. Louis: MO, 1998.
44. Leigh E. Vitex more effective than pyridoxine in PMS. *Herbal Gram* 1998;42:16–19.
45. McGuffin M, Hobbs C, Upton R, et al., eds. *Botanical safety handbook.* Boca Raton, FL: CRC Press, 1997.
46. Ulubelen A, Topcu G, Eris C, et al. Terpenoids from salvina sclarea. *Phytochemistry* 1994;36:971–974.
47. Reynolds J, ed. *Martindale: the extra pharmacopoeia,* 21st ed. London: Royal Pharmaceutical Society of Great Britain, 1996.
48. Avron J, Monane M, Gurwitz JH, et al. Reduction of bacteriuria and pyuria after ingestion of cranberry juice. *JAMA* 1994;271:751–754.
49. Walker EB, Barney DP, Mickelsen JN, et al. Cranberry concentrate: UTI prophylaxis. *J Fam Pract* 1997;45:167–168.
50. Faxman B, Geiger AM, Palin K, et al. First-time urinary tract infection and sexual behavior. *Epidemiology* 1995;6:162–168.
51. Brown D. *Herbal prescription for better health.* Rocklin, CA: Prima Publishing, 1996.
52. Jepson RG, Mihaljevic L, Craig J. Cranberries for preventing urinary tract infections. *Cochrane Database Syst Rev* 2000;2:CD001321.
53. Jepson RG, Mihaljevic L, Craig J. Cranberries for treating urinary tract infections. *Cochrane Database Syst Rev* 2000;2:CD001322.
54. Wagner H, Wiesenauer M. *Phytotherapie. Phytopharmaka und pfanzliche homoopathika.* New York: Fischer-Verlag, 1995.

55. Brooks S, ed. Botanical toxicology. *Protocol J Botan Med* 1995; 1:147–158.

56. Scolnick AA. Scientific verdict still out on DHEA. *JAMA* 1996; 276:1365–1367.

57. Morales AJ, Haubrich RH, Hwang JY, et al. The effect of six months treatment with 100 mg daily dose of dehydroepiandrosterone (DHEA) on circulating sex steroids, body composition and muscle strength in age-advanced men and women. *Clin Endocrinol (Oxf)* 1998;49:421–432.

58. Dorgan JF, Longcope C, Stanczyk FZ, et al. Plasma sex steroid hormone levels and risk of breast cancer in postmenopausal women. *J Natl Cancer Inst* 1999;91:380–381.

59. Katz S, Morales AJ. Dehydroepiandrosterone (DHEA) and DHEA-sulfate (DS) as therapeutic options in menopause. *Semin Reprod Endocrinol* 1998;16:161–170.

60. Roberts E. The importance of being dehydroepiandrosterone sulfate (in the blood of primates): a longer and healthier life? *Biochem Pharmacol* 1999;57:329–346.

61. Hardy ML. Herbs of special interest to women. *J Am Pharm Assoc (Wash)* 2000;40:234–242.

62. Fugh-Berman A. Herb-drug interaction. *Lancet* 2000;355: 134–138.

63. Smolinske SC. Dietary supplement-drug interactions. *J Am Med Womens Assoc* 1999;54:191–192, 195.

64. Hirta JD, Swiersz LM, Zell B, et al. Does dong quai have estrogenic effects in postmenopausal women? A double-blind, placebo-controlled trial. *Fertil Steril* 1997;68:981–986.

65. Ko R. Adverse reactions to watch for in patients using herbal remedies. *Best Pract* 1999;171:181–186.

66. Miller LG. Herbal medicinals. *Arch Intern Med* 1998;158: 2200–2211.

67. Mullins RJ. Echinacea-associated anaphylaxis. *Med J Aust* 1998; 168:170–171.

68. *The review of natural products: St. Louis Missouri.* Philadelphia: JB Lippincott, 1998.

69. Miller LG. Herbal medicinals: selected clinical consideration focusing on known or potential drug-herb interactions. *Arch Intern Med* 1998;158:2200–2211.

70. McFayden IJ, Forrest AP, Chetty U. Cyclic breast pain—some observations and the difficulties in treatment. *Br J Clin Pharmacol* 1992;46:161–164.

71. Budeiri D, Li Wan POA, Dorman JC. Is evening primrose oil of value in the treatment of premenstrual syndrome? *Control Clin Trials* 1996;17:60–68.

72. Johnson ES, Kadam NP, Hylands DM, et al. Efficacy of feverfew as prophylactic treatment of migraine. *BMJ* 1985;291: 569–573.

73. Murphy JJ, Heptinstall S, Mitchell JR. Randomized double-blind placebo-controlled trial of feverfew in migraine prevention. *Lancet* 1988;2:189–192.

74. Vogler BK, Pittler MH, Ernst E. Feverfew as a preventive treatment for migraine: a systemic review. *Cephalgia* 1998;18: 704–708.

75. Hausen BM. A six-year experience with composite mix. *Am J Contact Dermat* 1996;7:94–99.

76. Makheja AN, Bailery JM. A platelet phospholipase inhibitor from the medicinal herb feverfew (*Tanacetum parthenium*). *Prostaglandins Leukot Med* 1982;8:653–660.

77. Jappe U, Bonnekoh B, Hausen BM, et al. Garlic-related dermatoses: case report and review of the literature *Am J Contact Dermat* 1999;10(1):37–39.

78. Kasseler WJ, Blanc P, Greenblatt R. The use of medicinal herbs by human immunodeficiency virus-infected patients. *Arch Intern Med* 1991;151:2281–2288.

79. Vordberg G, Schneider B. Therapy with garlic: results of a placebo-controlled, double-blind study. *Br J Clin Pract* 1990; 69(suppl):7–11.

80. Stevinson C, Pittler MH, Ernst E. Garlic for treating hypercholesterolemia. A meta-analysis of randomized clinical trials. *Ann Intern Med* 2000;133:420–429.

81. Phillips S, Ruggier R, Hutchinson SE. *Zingiber officinale* (ginger)—an antiemetic for day case surgery. *Anesthesia* 1993;48: 715–717.

82. Langer E, Greifenberg S, Gruenwald J. Ginger: history and use. *Adv Ther* 1998;15:25–44.

83. Schid R, Schick T, Steffen R, et al. Comparison of seven commonly used agents for prophylaxis of seasickness. *J Travel Med* 1994;1:203–206.

84. Kanerva L, Estlander T, Jolanki R. Occupational allergic contact dermatitis from spices. *Contact Dermatitis* 1996;35: 157–162.

85. Tamborini A, Taurelle R. Value of standardized *Ginkgo biloba* extract (Egb 761) in the management of congestive symptoms of premenstrual syndrome. *Rev Fr Gynecol Obstet* 1993;88: 447–457.

86. Cohen AJ, Bartlik B. *Ginkgo biloba* for antidepressant-induced sexual dysfunction. *J Sex Marital Ther* 1998;24:139–143.

87. Rosen RC, Lane RM, Menza M. Effects of SSRIs on sexual function: a critical review. *J Clin Psychopharmacol* 1999;19: 67–85.

88. LeBars PL, Katz MM, Berman N, et al. A placebo-controlled, randomized trial of an extract of *Ginkgo biloba* for dementia. North American EGb Study Group. *JAMA* 1997;278: 1327–1332.

89. Rosenblatt M, Mindel J. Spontaneous hyphema associated with ingestion of *Ginkgo biloba* extract. *N Engl J Med* 1997;336: 1108.

90. Shaw D. Kolov LCS, Murray V. Traditional remedies and food supplements: a 5-year toxicological study (1991–1995). *Drug Safety* 1997;17:342–356.

91. White HL, Scates PW, Cooper BR. Extracts of *Ginkgo biloba* leaves inhibit monoamine oxidase. *Life Sci* 1996;58: 1315–1321.

92. Palmer BV, Montgomery ACV, Monteiro JC, Ginseng and mastalgia. *BMJ* 1978;1:1284.

93. Greenspan EM. Ginseng and vaginal bleeding. *JAMA* 1983; 249:2018.

94. Koren G, Randor S, Martin S, et al. Maternal ginseng use associated with neonatal androgenization. *JAMA* 1990;264:2866–2869.

95. Awang DV. Maternal use of ginseng and neonatal androgenization. *JAMA* 1991;266:363.

96. Cupp MJ. Herbal remedies: adverse effects and drug interactions. *Am Fam Physician* 1999;59:1239–1245.

97. Jones BD, Runikis AM. Interaction of ginseng with phenelzine. *J Clin Psychopharmacol* 1987;7:201–202.

98. Becker BN, Greene J, Evanson J, et al. Ginseng-induced diuretic resistance. *JAMA* 1996;276:606–607.

99. Wiklund IK, Mattsson LA, Lindgren R, et al. Effect of standardized ginseng extract on quality of life and psychological parameters in symptomatic postmenopausal women: a double-blind, placebo-controlled trial. Swedish Alternative Medicine Group. *Int J Clin Pharmacol Res* 1999;19:89–99.

100. Vogler BK, Pittler MH, Ernst E. The efficacy of ginseng. A systemic review of randomized clinical trials. *Eur J Clin Pharmacol* 1999;55:567–575.

101. Nakachi K, Suemasu K, Takeo T, et al. Influence of drinking green tea on breast cancer malignancy among Japanese patients. *Jpn J Cancer Res* 1998;89:254–256.

102. Yang TT, Koo MW. Hypocholesterolemic effect of Chinese tea. *Pharmacol Res* 1997;35:505–512.

103. Yang TT, Koo MW. Chinese green tea lowers cholesterol level through an increase in fecal lipid extraction. *Life Sci* 200;66: 411–423.

104. Imai K, Suga K, Nakachi K. Cancer-preventive effects of drinking green tea among a Japanese population. *Prev Med* 1997;26: 769–775.

105. Mukhtar H, Ahmad N. Green tea in chemoprevention of cancer. *Toxicol Sci* 1999;52:11–117.

106. Bushman JL. Green tea and cancer in humans: a review of the literature. *Nutr Cancer* 1998;31:151–159.

107. Uebelhack R, Franke L, Schewe HJ. Inhibition of platelet MAO-B kava pyrone-enriched extract from Piper ethysicum Forster (kava-kava). *Pharmacopsychiatry* 1998;31:187–192.

108. Pittler MH, Ernst E. Efficacy of kava extract for treating anxiety: systemic review and meta-analysis. *J Clin Psychopharmacol* 2000;20:84–89.

109. Singh YN. Kava: an overview. *J Ethnopharm* 1992;37:13–45.

110. Strahl S, Ehret V, Dahm HH, et al. Necrotizing hepatitis after taking herbal remedies. *Dtsch Med Wochenschr* 1998;123: 1410–1414.

111. Jappe U, Franke I, Reinhold D, et al. *J Am Acad Dermatol* 1998; 38:104–106.

112. Varonos DD, Voukydes PC, Nikitopoulou GC. Digitoxin antagonism by visnadin. *J Pharm Sci* 1962;51:1013–1014.

113. De Klerk GJ, Nieuwenhuis MG, Beutle JJ. Hypokalemia and hypertension associated with use of liquorice flavored chewing gum. *BMJ* 1997;314:731–732.

114. Russo S, Mastropasqua M, Mesetti MA, et al. Low doses of liquorice can induce hypertension encephalopathy. *Am J Nephrol* 2000;20:145–148.

115. Montoliu J. Liquorice-induced cardiac arrest. *BMJ* 1977;2: 1352–1353.

116. Eriksson JW, Carlberg B, Hillorn V. Life-threatening ventricular tachycardia due to liquorice-induced hypokalaemia. *J Intern Med* 1999;245:307–310.

117. Baschetti R. Liquorice and chronic fatigue syndrome. *N Z Med J* 1995;108:259.

118. Olukoga A, Donaldson D. Liquorice and its health implications. *J R Soc Health* 2000;120:83–89.

119. Howes, JB, Sullivan D, Lai N, et al. The effect of dietary supplementation with isoflavones from red clover on the lipoprotein profiles of post menopausal women with mild to moderate hypercholesterolaemia. *Atherosclerosis* 2000;152:143–147.

120. Argento A, Tiraferri E, Marzaloni M. Oral anticoagulants and medical plants. An emerging interaction. *Ann Ital Med Int* 2000;15:139–143.

121. Albertazzi P, Pansini F, Bonaccorsi G, et al. The effect of dietary soy supplementation on hot flushes. *Obstet Gynecol* 1998;91:6–11.

122. Albertazzi P, Pansini F, Bottazzi M, et al. The effect of dietary soy supplementation on hot flushes. *Obstet Gynecol* 1999;94:229–231.

123. Potter SM, Bauman JA, Teng H, et al. Soy protein and isoflavones: their effects on blood lipids and bone density in postmenopausal women. *Am J Clin Nutr* 1998;68(suppl):1375–1379.

124. Knight DC, Eden JA. A review of the clinical effects of phytoestrogens. *Obstet Gynecol* 1996;87(part 2):897–904.

125. Anderson JW, Johnstone BM, Cook-Newell ME. Meta-analysis of the effects of soy protein intake on serum lipids. *N Engl J Med* 995;333:276–282.

126. Levy JR, Faber KA, Ayyash L, et al. The effect of prenatal exposure to the phytoestrogen genistein on sexual differentiation in rats. *Proc Soc Exp Biol Med* 1995;208:60–66.

127. Gambacciani M, Ciaponi M, Cappagli B, et al. Effects of combined low dose of the isoflavone derivative ipriflavone and estrogen replacement on bone mineral density and metabolism in postmenopausal women. *Maturitas* 1997;28:75–81.

128. Grube B, Walper A, Wheatley D. St. John's wort extract: efficacy for menopausal symptoms of psychological origin. *Adv Ther* 1999;16:177–186.

129. Stevinson C, Ernst E. A pilot study of *Hypericum perforatum* for the treatment of premenstrual syndrome. *Br J Obstet Gynaecol* 2000;107:870–876.

130. Gaster B, Holroyd J. St. John's wort for depression: a systematic review. *Arch Intern Med* 2000;24:160:152–156.

131. Woelk H for the Remotiv/Imipramine Study Group. *BMJ* 2000;321:536–539.

132. Johne A, Brockmoller J, Bauer S, et al. Pharmacokinetic interaction of digoxin with an herbal extract from St. John's wort (*Hypericum perforatum*). *Clin Pharmacol Ther* 1999;66:338–345.

133. Beade-van Dijk PA, van Galen E, Lekkerkerker JF. Drug interactions of *Hypericum perforatum* (St. John's wort) are potentially hazardous. *Ned Tijdschr Geneeskd* 2000;144:811–812.

134. Miller LG. Herbal medicinals: selected clinical consideration focusing on known or potential drug-herb interaction. *Arch Intern Med* 1998;158:2200–2211.

135. Reichert R. Valerian clinical monograph. *Q Rev Nat Med* 1998; 207–215.

136. Can TY, Tang CH, Critchley JA. Poisoning due to an over-the counter hypnotic, Sleep-Qik (hyoscine, cyprohepta dine, valeriam). *Postgrad Med J* 1995;71:227–229.

SUBJECT INDEX